Protein Purification and Analysis III

Methods and Applications

Protein Purification and Analysis III – Methods and Applications

Publisher: iConcept Press Ltd.
Cover design: Pineapple Design Ltd.
Interior design: iConcept Press Ltd.
Typesetting and copy editing: iConcept Press Ltd. and Pineapple Design Ltd.

ISBN: 978-1-922227-66-9

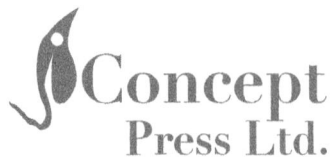

ꝓConcept
Press Ltd.

www.iconceptpress.com

Contents

Preface

Proteins are biochemical compounds consisting of one or more polypeptides typically folded into a globular or fibrous form, facilitating a biological function. A polypeptide is a single linear polymer chain of amino acids bonded together by peptide bonds between the carboxyl and amino groups of adjacent amino acid residues. The sequence of amino acids in a protein is defined by the sequence of a gene, which is encoded in the genetic code. The complexity and sheer number of proteins in a cell are impediments to identifying proteins of interest or purifying proteins for function and structure analysis. Thus, reducing the complexity of a protein sample or in some cases purifying a protein to homogeneity is necessary. *Protein Purification and Analysis* discusses varies aspect related to protein analysis. There are totally three volumes. This book is the last volume.

There are totally 12 chapters in this book. Chapter 1 describes *in vivo* and *ex vivo* approaches for determining the role of an olfactory receptor protein in the detection of its cognate agonist and various analogs. Surprising responses of the olfactory receptor to unrelated compounds is also discussed. Chapter 2 reviews the recent studies on the features of PTEN in the signalling pathways involved in several diseases as emerging evidences suggest that PTEN enzymatic activity will not cover the entire mechanism of the ability. Chapter 3 proposes site-directed mutagenesis approach for determining the structure-function relationships of neurotransmitter transporters. Both the benefits and limitations are discussed. In addition, basic methods and related experimental protocols for the site-directed mutagenesis study are reviewed. Chapter 4 proposes a new approach for the structural-functional analysis of G protein-coupled receptors and heterotrimeric G proteins, which is based on the use of synthetic peptides corresponding to functionally important regions of the proteins, and for the development of selective regulators of hormonal signalling systems on the basis of these peptides.

Chapter 5 discusses the use of solid-phase supports, mainly reversed-phase silica-gel, as a media on which to immobilize and react peptides in order to facilitate various protein chemistry analyses. The main focus is on phosphorylation analysis, yet a wide range of chemical reactions can be performed on these supports sequentially, which improves reaction rates, recoveries and sample purities. Chapter 6 summarizes the current evidence which supports the involvement of molecular mechanisms observed in the course of chondrocyte progression through the growth plate in cartilage matrix destruction in osteoarthritis. This can provide new approaches for the treatment of the disease by targeting signalling pathways responsible for chondrocyte phenotypic modifications. Chapter 7 describes the role of flotillins and c-Cbl-associated protein (CAP) in the nuclear trafficking and membrane localization of FRS2. Flotillins, CAP and fibroblast growth factor receptor substrate 2 (FRS2) are regulators signal transduction, which interact with each other. Chapter 8 suggested that using 2D/3D LC-MS/MS and carbonate extraction plus Triton X-114 extraction of isolated microsomes should significantly improve the coverage of microsomal membrane proteome. Moreover, the presented methods in the chapter should easily translate to the development of a quantitative proteomics to analyze liver disease-related microsome proteins for biomarker discovery and mechanism clarification of a liver disease.

Chapter 9 provides comprehensive methods for the identification of aberrant hyper/hypo-methylated genes using the MeDIP-chip and MassARRAY. miRNAs, as small noncoding RNAs, not only regulate the expression of hyper/hypo- methylation genes directly but also regulate methylation levels and gene expression indirectly through histone and DNA methylation modification. Chapter 10 discusses the effect of water molar tate on the properties and delivery profiles of dopamine from nanostructured sol-gel silica. Chapter 11 attempts to solve the waste water recycle problem by using biorefinery approaches, as this approach could utilize wastewater without treatment or with only slight treatment prior to use. Chapter 12 discusses how the combination of system analysis and information theory can be a reliable strategy for the determination of the Shannon entropy, bitrate and capacity of signaling pathways and genetic networks.

Editing and publishing a book is never an easy task. Each chapter in this book has gone through a peer review, a selection and an editing process so as to guarantee its quality. Without the supports and contributions of the authors and reviewers, this book can never be able to complete. We would like to thank all of the authors in this book and all of the reviewers who participated in the reviewing process: Hiroyoshi Ariga, Wayne L. Backes, Catherine Baugé, I Bókkon, Sharmila Chattopadhyay, Pedro Rodriguez Cutillas, Jeroen den Hertog, Michael J. Duryee, Antonio Ferrante, Christophe Flahaut, Nicholas J Gibson, Vipul Gohel, Ramon Hurtado-Guerrero, Anti Kalda, Rajashri D. Kamble, Galina Karpova, Kyoko Kofuji, Satoshi Kubota, Ramesh Chander Kuhad, Yun Jong Lee, Yung-Feng Lin, Shabaz Mohammed, SundaraBaalaji Narayanan, Verena Niggli, Keith K. Parker, R. Daniel Peluffo, Richard I Samuels, Matthias Schmitz, Rosalia C.M. Simmen, Ingebrigt Sylte, Shin-Ichiro Takahashi, Masaharu Takigawa, Jose A. Viscarra, Magali Waelbroeck, Robert Yung-Liang Wang, M G Waugh, Peter J Woolf, Silvio Zaina and Lei Zhou. We hope that you, the reader, will find this book interesting and useful. Any advices please feel free and are always welcome to tell us.

iConcept Press Ltd
May 2014

Analysis of Odorant Receptor Protein Function in the Yellow Fever Mosquito, *Aedes aegypti*

Joseph C. Dickens
Invasive Insect Biocontrol and Behavior Laboratory
Henry A. Wallace Beltsville Agricultural Research Center, Plant Sciences Institute
United States Department of Agriculture, Agricultural Research Service, USA

Jonathan D. Bohbot
Invasive Insect Biocontrol and Behavior Laboratory
Henry A. Wallace Beltsville Agricultural Research Center, Plant Sciences Institute
United States Department of Agriculture, Agricultural Research Service, USA

Alan J. Grant
Invasive Insect Biocontrol and Behavior Laboratory
Henry A. Wallace Beltsville Agricultural Research Center, Plant Sciences Institute
United States Department of Agriculture, Agricultural Research Service, USA

1   Introduction

Insect odorant receptors (ORs) are ligand-gated ion channels formed by a pair of proteins: a canonical receptor protein that gives the protein complex its specificity and an obligatory co-receptor named Orco (Nakagawa *et al.*, 2005; Sato *et al.*, 2008; Wicher *et al.*, 2008). These ORs and accessory proteins including odorant binding proteins (OBPs) (Vogt *et al.*, 1999), odorant degrading enzymes (ODEs) (Vogt *et al.*, 1985) and sensory neuron membrane protein (SNMP) (Vogt *et al.*, 2009) are expressed by the molecular machinery of olfactory sensory neurons (OSNs) associated with individual sensilla. The ORs are embedded in the cell membrane of dendrites housed within the sensillum. Odorants may be solubilized in the sensillum lymph by OBPs or deactivated by ODEs. Odorants interact either alone, or in combination with a transporting OBP (Xu *et al.*, 2005), with the OR complex leading to the opening of an ion channel resulting in depolarization of the cell and subsequent action potentials. While it is possible to record action potentials from individual sensory cells located within single sensilla, the contribution of each molecular component (OR, OBP, ODE or SNMP) to the olfactory process is difficult to ascertain. Thus, a comparative approach in which components of the system are isolated for examination and compared to their function in the animal may be necessary in order to better understand their roles.

The study of OR function was made possible by their initial discovery and characterization in the fruit fly *Drosophila melanogaster* (Clyne *et al.*, 1999b; Gao & Chess, 1999; Vosshall *et al.*, 1999). Subsequently, ORs have been characterized from insects within several orders including moths, beetles, ants, bees and mosquitoes (Krieger *et al.*, 2003; Robertson & Wanner, 2006; Wanner *et al.*, 2007; Hallem *et al.*, 2006). For the yellow fever mosquito, *Aedes aegypti* (L.), the expression patterns of ORs have been localized to specific olfactory organs such as the antennae, maxillary palps and proboscis (Bohbot *et al.*, 2007) (Figure 1A). Of special interest is the fact that only three ORs (OR7, OR8 and OR49) are expressed in the maxillary palps of *Ae. aegypti* males and females, and one of these ORs, Orco (formerly known as OR7), is the obligate co-receptor.

The maxillary palps of *Ae. aegypti* (Figure 1A) possess a single type of basiconic sensillum (Figure 1B) which number approximately 21 in males and 35 in females (McIver, 1982). Each of these sensilla contains the dendritic processes of three OSNs (Grant & O'Connell, 1996). The "A" neuron producing the largest amplitude spike or action potential responds to CO_2; an adequate stimulus for the "B" neuron with the intermediate spike amplitude is unknown; the "C" neuron with the smallest amplitude spike responds specifically to the host attractant 1-octen-3-ol (Figure 1C). Since detection of CO_2 was shown to involve gustatory receptors (Jones *et al.*, 2007) and individual OSNs express only one OR, the "B" and "C" neuron must express either OR49 or OR8 (Figure 1D). Heterologous expression of ORs in *Xenopus laevis* oocytes coupled with two-microelectrode voltage clamp (TEVC) recordings showed OR8-Orco to be responsive to 1-octen-3-ol (Bohbot & Dickens, 2009), supporting the hypothesis that the "C" neuron in these basiconic sensilla on the maxillary palps express OR8-Orco.

Here we describe *in vivo* and *ex vivo* approaches for determining the role of the protein OR8 in the detection of its cognate agonist 1-octen-3-ol and various analogs. We also discuss surprising responses of the receptor to unrelated compounds. Detailed accounts of the methods and procedures described herein have been published elsewhere and are open access (Bohbot & Dickens, 2009; Grant & Dickens, 2011).

2   Methods

2.1   *In vivo* characterization of OR function: Single cell recordings

Single cell recording (SCR) from neurons housed within the basiconic sensilla on the maxillary palps reveals the sensitivity and specificity of responses of the neurons to odorants. This technique was first used by Boeckh (1962) to record responses of single OSNs in a beetle, but since that time has been applied to many orders of insects. SCR reveals the action potential code sent to the brain for processing and integration with inputs from other sensory modalities. This multimodal message is sent to effectors directly resulting in overt behavior or adjustment of behavioral thresholds.

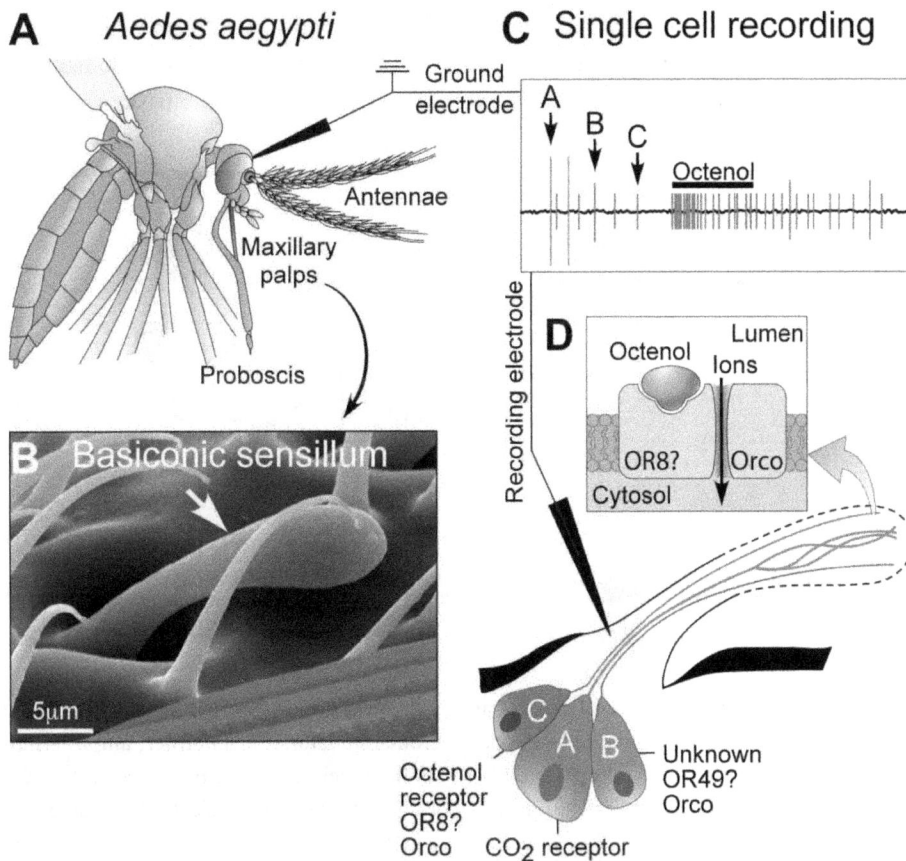

Figure 1: A. Female *Ae. aegypti* mosquitoes have three main olfactory appendages: the antennae, the maxillary palps and the proboscis. **B.** Scanning electron microscope image of a basiconic sensillum located on the surface of the maxillary palps. **C.** Schematic representation of a single cell recording. A basiconic sensillum typically houses three neurons that are categorized based on the size of their action potentials (APs). The "A" cell (green) generates the largest APs when stimulated with CO_2. What activates the medium-sized "B" cell (blue) is unknown. The "C" cell (red) generates the smallest APs when exposed to octenol. **D.** *In vivo* and *ex vivo* studies strongly suggest that the OR8-Orco complex confers octenol sensitivity to the "C" cell.

2.1.1   Mosquito sources

Eggs of *Ae. aegypti* were obtained from various sources (the Walter Reed Army Institute of Research in Silver Springs, MD, USA or The Center for Medical and Veterinary Entomology, USDA, ARS in Gainesville, FL, USA). Eggs are placed in plastic compartments filled with water and hatch within three days. Larvae are fed with fish food (Tetramin®) and adult mosquitoes are provided with a 10% sucrose solution. It takes 5 to 7 days for mosquitoes to develop from eggs to adults when reared at 27^0C (12h:12h L:D) and 70% relative humidity. The age of adult mosquitoes was continuously monitored and recorded.

2.1.2   Mosquito preparation

Mosquitoes are cold-anesthetized for approximately 45 seconds at 10^0F. Insect olfactory sensilla offer an ideal platform for recording responses of single OSNs to odorants. Individual sensilla generally house two or three receptor neurons (Figure 1D), which are electrically isolated from neurons located within other sensilla. An individual *Ae. aegypti* adult is fastened to a glass microscope slide using double stick tape and the maxillary palps are positioned in a manner to provide access to the basiconic sensilla.

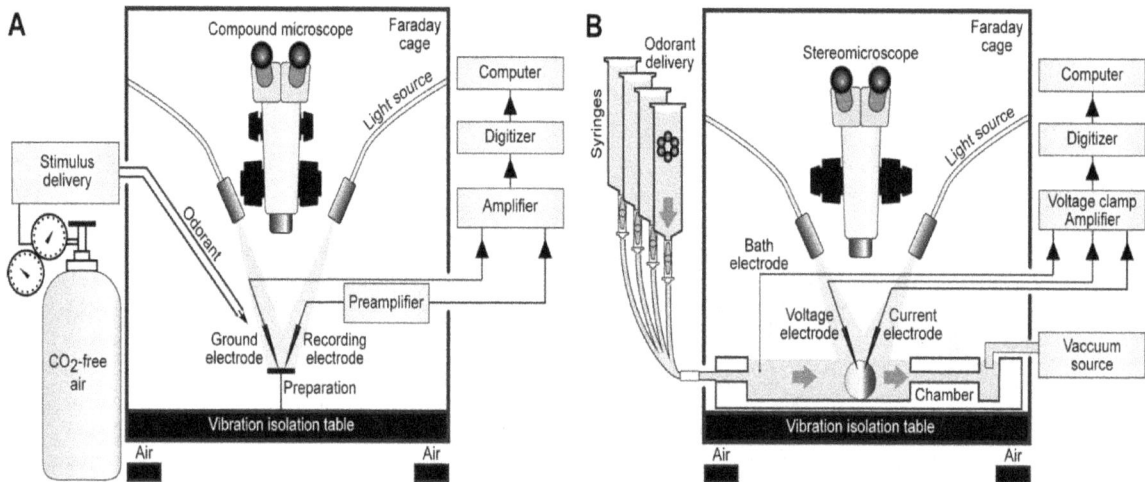

Figure 2: A. Set-up used for single cell electrophysiological recordings from olfactory sensory neurons utilizes a high power compound microscope, micromanipulators, preamplifier, amplifier, digitizer and computer. Odorants are administered by a stimulus delivery system connected to a CO_2-free air source to keep the "A" cell silent during recordings. **B.** Two-microelectrode voltage clamp set-up for the study of *Xenopus* oocytes expressing *Ors* includes a stereomicroscope, coarse manipulators, amplifier, digitizer and computer. Solutions of odorants kept in syringes deliver their load to the oocyte chamber. The bath level is kept constant using a vacuum source. Both set-ups are protected from electrical noise and mechanical vibrations using a Faraday cage and a vibration table, respectively.

2.1.3   Single cell recording

Under optical control usually 600-800x, high power micromanipulators (e.g., Leitz or Eppendorf) are used to insert a sharpened tungsten electrode in or near the base of a single sensillum (Figure 1D). The recording electrode is constructed from tungsten wire 0.125-0.25mm diameter and electrolytically sharpened (using a saturated potassium nitrite solution) to a tip of less than 1 μm. An indifferent or ground electrode also constructed from sharpened tungsten wire is placed elsewhere in the body of the mosquito and connected to ground (Figure 1A). Electrical signals recorded by the recording electrode are amplified and conditioned prior to visualization on a computer monitor and an optional oscilloscope (Figure 2A). The AutoSpike software used here for the collection and analysis of electrophysiological recordings from insect sensilla using a microcomputer is available from Syntech in Kirchzarten, Germany (Appendix).

In order to determine functional characteristics of the octenol receptor neuron purportedly expressing OR8 (Figure 1D), the preparation was exposed to the optical isomers of 1-octen-3-ol and closely related compounds (Grant and Dickens, 2011). Here, measured aliquots of serial dilutions of the experimental odorants are applied to strips of filter paper which are then placed into glass odor cartridges. In order to avoid unwanted stimulation of the "A" neuron (the CO_2 receptor) thus masking the response of the smaller "C" neuron, synthetic air with minimal amounts of CO_2 is used to carry molecules of the experimental odorant evaporating from the filter paper over the preparation (Figure 2A). Stimulus duration is 1 sec.

2.1.4   Enantioselectivity of the octenol receptor cell

Experimental odorants were selected in order to evaluate the relative importance of various structural features of the cognate agonist, 1-octen-3-ol (Figure 3). For example, 1-octen-3-ol has a chiral carbon at the 3-position, thus the existence of two enantiomers: (R)-(-)-1-octen-3-ol and (S)-(+)-1-octen-3-ol. In the related compound 1-octen-4-ol, the chiral center is displaced to the 4-position. The role of carbon chain length was examined by testing compounds one carbon longer (1-nonen-3-ol) and one carbon shorter (1-hepten-3-ol). The saturated analog, 3-octanol, was tested to determine the importance of the double bond at the 1-position. The effect of 1-octen-3-one was evaluated to show the importance of the hydroxy group.

A high degree of specificity was observed in responses of the "C" neuron assumed to express OR8. Sensitivity of the neuron to (R)-(-)-1-octen-3-ol was 100 - 1000x greater than for its enantiomer, (S)-(+)-1-octen-3-ol. The same was true for the rest of the odorants tested indicating strict structural requirements of a ligand for interaction with the odorant receptor. However, other proteins present in the receptor lymph such as OBPs and ODEs might be involved in the specificity. Thus the need to heterologously express OR8 to better understand its contribution.

2.2   *Ex vivo* characterization of OR function: Heterologous expression in *Xenopus laevis* oocytes

The discovery of hundreds of ORs in mosquitoes and other organisms has increased the demand for pharmacological means to study their physiological properties. While *in vivo* techniques provide a physiological context for the presumed OR of interest, the specific functional contribution of a receptor protein may be best achieved in a heterologous expression system. In the following example, we have used the oocytes of the African clawed frog *Xenopus laevis* as an *ex vivo* system to study the pharmacological properties of the mosquito octenol receptor OR8-Orco.

The experimental benefits with working with *Xenopus laevis* include:

- Inexpensive and low maintenance laboratory animal.

- Ease to harvest and impale due to the oocyte abundance and size (Figure 4).

- Frogs can be reused for future oocyte collection.

- Low expression levels of endogenous channels.

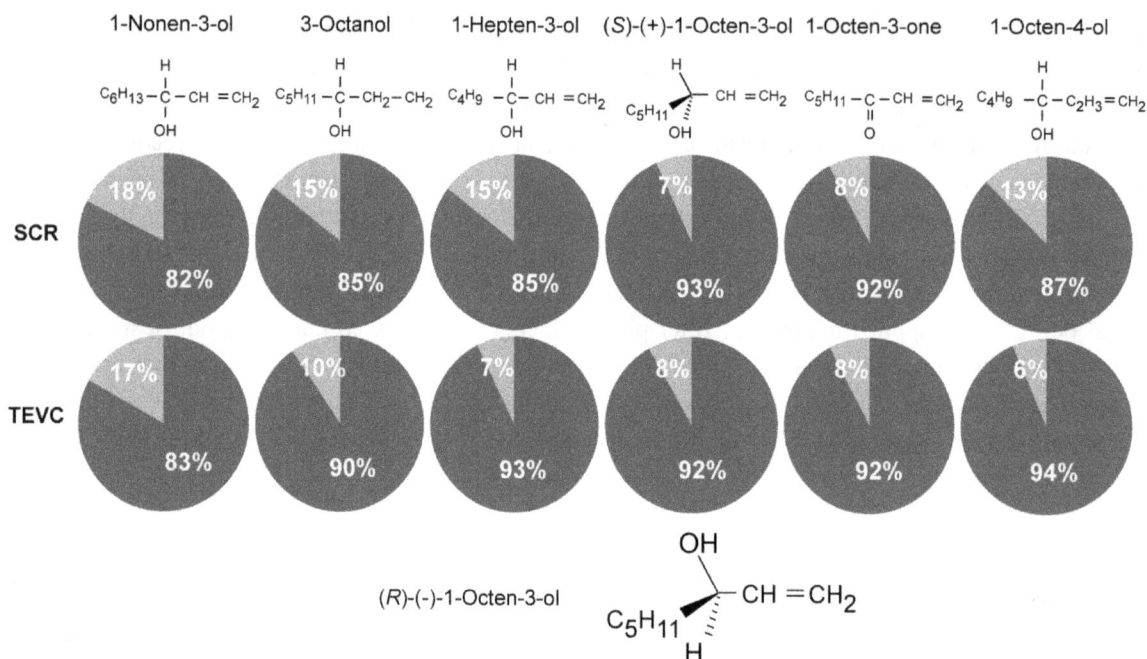

Figure 3: Experimental odorants used to determine the structural features required for OSN and OR8-Orco activation. Responses to octenol analogs (yellow) relative to the most active compound, (*R*)-(-)-1-octen-3-ol (blue), are shown as pie charts. Results from single cell (SCR) and two-microelectrode voltage clamp (TEVC) recordings are shown in the top and bottom row, respectively.

- High yield protein expression from multiple species of exogenous mRNA (e.g., *Or8* and *Orco*).

The high expression levels of membrane proteins by oocytes permit the recordings of large current responses in resulting from the effects of potential ligands or drugs. The equipment used for a typical TEVC set-up can be found in the appendix.

2.2.1   Oocyte procurement

Preparation of oocytes for injection begins with the surgical removal of the ovaries from a cold-anesthetized animal. The animal is placed in a container filled with ice water for at least 15 min until postural righting reflex is lost. The frog is then sacrificed by severing and destroying the spinal cord. An abdominal incision provides easy access to the ovaries, which are harvested and transferred to a container filled with Ca^{2+}-free Ringer's. Alternatively, only part of the ovary may be harvested. In this case, the incision site is sutured, allowing for re-use of the animal following recovery.

2.2.2   Oocyte isolation and preparation

Stage V and VI oocytes, which are characterized by a clear separation between the animal and vegetal poles (Figure 4), are manually isolated from the ovarian tissue in Ca^{2+}-free Ringer's under a stereomicroscope. Collected oocytes are then washed several times with Ca^{2+}-free Ringer's (to minimize the damaging effect resulting from protease activation) until most traces of blood and small particles are removed.

The oocytes are then treated with a room temperature collagenase solution (Appendix) for 30 min to 2 hrs under constant and gentle rocking. This important step assures the removal of the the follicular layer surrounding the oocyte. It is not necessary to remove the vitelline membrane to record whole-cell currents (Figure 4). If the digestion is allowed to proceed longer than necessary, the viability of the oocyte will be compromised. Oocytes are then serially washed with Ca^{2+}-free Ringer's, Ca^{2+}-free Ringer's supplemented with gentamycine (50µg/mL) and equilibrated in incubation medium (Appendix). Under a dissecting stereomicroscope, healthy oocytes are hand-selected and left in the incubation medium at 18^0C until injection.

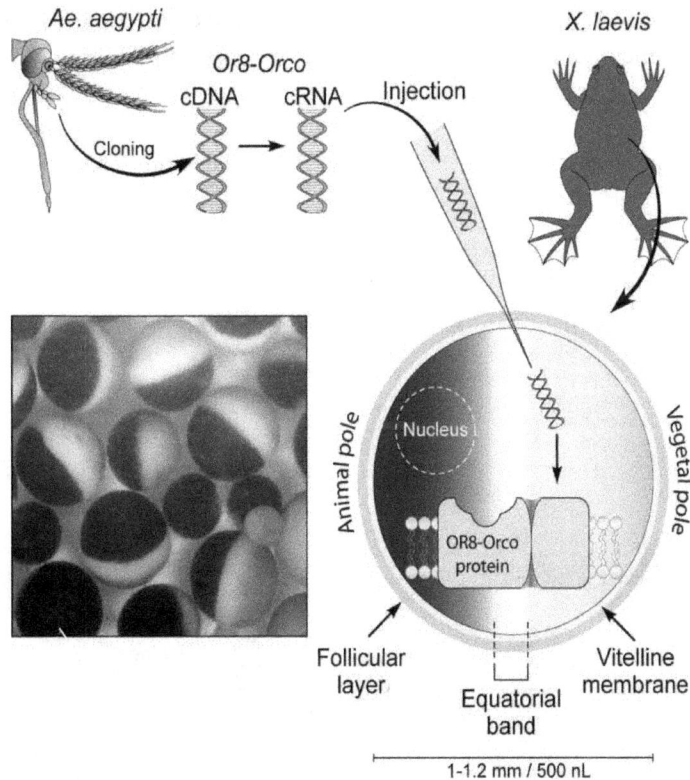

Figure 4: Heterologous expression of *OR8-Orco* in *Xenopus laevis* oocytes. The *Or8* and *Orco* genes are cloned from cDNA extracted form the mosquito maxillary palp tissue and cRNA-transcribed *in vitro*. Ovaries (~10,000 oocytes) are surgically removed from a female *Xenopus laevis* frog. Oocytes are then mechanically isolated, defollicled by collagenase treatment and individually sorted for injection.

2.2.3   cRNA preparation and synthesis

Both *Or8* and *Orco* genes are PCR amplified from maxillary palp cDNA and subsequently cloned into the pENTR vector and subcloned into the pSP64DV expression vector (Lu, Qiu et al. 2007). *In vitro* transcription of complementary RNA (cRNA) is carried out using linearized pSP64DV vector with either the T7 or SP6-RNA polymerase (Bohbot, Jones et al. 2010). cRNA reactions are scaled up in order to generate several micrograms of products stored at −80°C as 1 µL aliquots (final concentration of 3,000µg/µL for each gene).

2.2.4   Cytoplasmic injection of cRNA into oocytes

Equal molar quantities of cRNA are prepared prior to injection and kept on ice. One microliter of *Or8*, *Orco* and nuclease-free water are mixed together to produce a final concentration of 1,000 µg/µL (for each cRNA species) injection solution. Glass capillaries are pulled using a vertical one-stage pipette puller (see appendix), mounted on the mounting rod of the injector and back-filled with mineral oil and cRNA (Figure 4). Care must be taken in order to avoid air bubbles in the pipette. Oocytes are then transferred into an oocyte injection plate and aligned so that the injector punctures the membrane around the equatorial band, away from the animal pole where the nucleus is located (Figure 4). The injector is set to inject 27.6 nL or ~9 ng of *Or8* and *Orco* cRNA, which should allow for the injection of ~100 oocytes. Injected oocytes are stored at 18^0C in incubation medium for three days to allow for expression of the OR complex in the outer cell membrane of the eggs (Figure 5). Incubation periods may vary depending on the cRNA species.

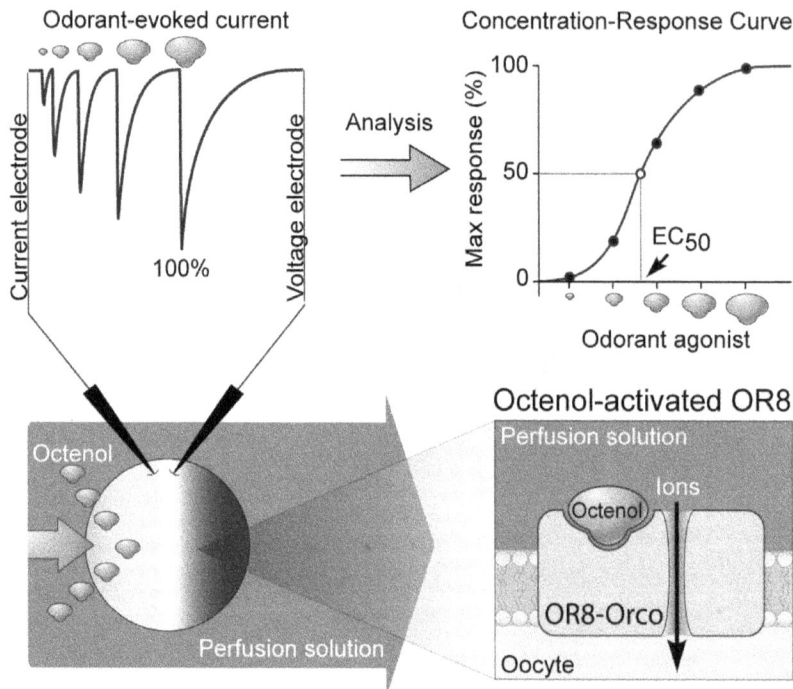

Figure 5:   Following injection, oocytes express large quantities of the receptor complex. OR-expressing oocytes are placed in a perfusion chamber and two microelectrodes are inserted into the oocytes.   Oocytes are then exposed to increasing concentrations of odorants (orange) and the resulting odorant-evoked currents are recorded.   Data is analyzed using a minicomputer equipped with the appropriate neuroscience software.

2.2.5   Two-microelectrode voltage clamp of oocytes

TEVC of oocytes is a standard electrophysiological technique whereby the oocyte membrane is artificially maintained at a desired holding potential or voltage clamp. Any deviation from this command in response to agonist activation of expressed ORs is measured by the voltage electrode and is corrected by a second electrode that passes more or less current to the oocyte in order to restore the preset voltage-clamp. Therefore, whole-cell currents flowing through the collective activation of ORs are constantly monitored by the current electrode (Figure 5).

The oocyte is placed into the perfusion chamber, which is connected to a gravity-driven perfusion system upstream and to a vacuum source downstream (Figure 2B). Experimental oocytes are continuously bathed in Ringer's solution. The same odorants tested for the *in vivo* studies are used for stimulation of the oocytes. Serial dilutions are prepared from molar concentrations of the odorants in Ringer's solution and placed in 50 mL syringes (Figure 2B). Since most odorants have little water solubility, dimethyl sulfoxide (DMSO) is used as a carrier to ensure delivery of the odorant to the preparation. Exposure of the oocyte to odorants lasts 8 sec. The oocyte is impaled with two microelectrodes pulled using the pipette puller mentioned above. These pipettes are filled with a 3 M KCl solution; chlorided silver wires inserted into the capillaries serve as electrodes. The voltage and current microelectrodes are mounted on coarse manual manipulators and positioned above the oocyte under a stereomicroscope. Once in the perfusion solution (Ringer's solution), the offset between the voltage electrode and the bath electrodes is adjusted to zero. Gentle pressure is then applied to the surface of the oocyte membrane until penetration occurs and the amplifier detects the resting potential ($\sim$-40 mV). The amplifier is then set on fast voltage-clamp (-80 mV) mode. The analog electrical signal from the amplifier is converted into a digital signal by the digitizer connected to a computer. A vibration table and a Faraday cage are used to protect the preparation from movement and electrical interference (Figure 2B). Responses to odorants are determined by exposure of the preparation to experimental odorants diluted in the Ringer solution.

Whole-cell odorant evoked currents are processed by the data acquisition and analysis software pCLAMP10 and displayed, as current traces, on the computer screen. The collected data can then be analyzed to generate concentration-response curves and extrapolated EC_{50} values (Figure 5).

2.2.6   Enantioselectivity of OR8-Orco in oocytes

Similar to results obtained from *in vivo* recordings from the "C" neuron in the basiconic sensilla on the maxillary palps, responses of the oocytes expressing OR8-Orco were highly specific for (R)-(-)-1-octen-3-ol. Based on EC_{50} values calculated from dose-response curves for each experimental odorant, the decrease in potency of related compounds relative to (R)-(-)-1-octen-3-ol ranged from nearly 6,000x for 3-octanol, the most effective analog, to 39,000 for 1-octen-4-ol, the least effective compound tested (Bohbot *et al.*, 2009). Surprisingly, the insect repellents, 2-undecanone and callicarpenal, also activated oocytes expressing the OR8-Orco complex (Bohbot *et al.*, 2011). In an attempt to compare results from SSR and TEVC studies, the response of each analog was compared to the (R)-(-)-1-octen-3-ol response at 0.05 µg and 10^{-6} M, respectively (Figure 3). These values were chosen because they were the lowest quantities evoking responses across all tested compounds.

3   Conclusions

Functional characterization of proteins is complex. A principal problem is the isolation of the protein of interest in a system that allows for controlled studies, minimizing contributions from other factors. Thus, ideally a comparison of measures of protein specificity and function should be made both *in vivo* and *ex vivo* while considering variables present in each system.

The octenol receptor cell and the OR8-Orco complex are specifically tuned toward (*R*)-(-)-1-octen-3-ol, bearing little flexibility to accommodate the most minute change to its chemical structure. Moreover, these results validate using these complementary approaches to study the function of insect receptors.

In the paradigm presented here, both OBPs and ODEs present *in vivo,* as well as potentially other proteins, could have played roles in the sensitivity and specificity of OR8-Orco for (*R*)-(-)-1-octen-3-ol and related compounds. Heterologous expression of the receptor complex allowed not only for verification of the role of OR8 in octenol detection, but also clarified the importance of OR8-Orco in the specificity of the octenol receptor neuron *in vivo.*

Appendix

Additional information on the methodologies and results on the topic addressed in this chapter can be found in the following open access research articles: Bohbot, J. D. & Dickens, J. C. (2009). Characterization of an enantioselective odorant receptor in the yellow fever mosquito *Aedes aegypti. PLoS ONE* 4(9): e7032. doi:10.1371/journal.pone.0007032. Grant, A. J. & Dickens, J. C. (2011). Functional characterization of the octenol receptor neuron on the maxillary palps of the Yellow Fever mosquito, Aedes aegypti. *PLoS ONE* 6(6): e21785. doi:10.1371/journal.pone.0021785

List of equipments and reagents used for two-electrode voltage clamp recordings

Solutions and reagents
Ringer's solution (pH 7.6, 96 mM NaCl, 2 mM KCl, 5 mM MgCl2, 5 mM HEPES and 0.8 mM CaCl2)
Enzyme solution (Ca^{2+}-free Ringer's supplemented with 2mg/mL collagenase from *Clostridium hystoliticum*)
Oocyte incubation medium (Ringer's solution supplemented with heat-inactivated horse serum (5%), tetracycline (50 mg/mL), streptomycin (100 mg/mL) and sodium pyruvate (550 mg/mL)
Equipment
Recording oocyte chamber (RC-3Z, Warner Instruments)
Incubator (Model 2005, VWR)
Digitizer Digidata 1440A and Electrophysiology Data Acquisition and Analysis Software pCLAMP10 (Molecular Devices)
Oocyte clamp (OC-725C, Warner Instruments)
Microprocessor-controlled injector (Nanoliter 2000, World Precision Instruments)
Glass capillaries for injection (177.8 x 1.14 x 0.053 mm, L x OD x ID, Warner Instruments)
Glass capillaries for recording (75 x 1.2 x 0.053 mm, L x OD x ID, Warner Instruments)
Needle/Pipette puller (Model 730, Kopf)
Two stereomicroscopes (injection and recording)

List of the equipments used for single cell recordings

Stimulus controller (CS-55, Syntech)
Data-acquisition amplifier/controller (IDAC 4, Synthec) and Autospike software (Syntech)
Pre-amplifier (Grass)
Audio monitor (AM10, Grass)
Vibration table (ISO Tab-L tabletop, Fabreeka)

Faraday cage (manually constructed or commercially available at Fabreeka)

References

Boeckh, J. (1962). Elektrophysiologische Untersuchungen an einzelnen Geruchsrezeptoren auf der Antenne des Totengräbers (Necrophorus, Coleoptera). Zeitschrift für Vergleichende Physiologie, 46, 349-353.

Bohbot, J. D. & Dickens, J. C. (2009). Characterization of an enantioselective odorant receptor in the yellow fever mosquito Aedes aegypti. PLoS ONE 4(9): e7032. doi:10.1371/journal.pone.0007032.

Bohbot, J., Pitts, R. J., Kwon, H. W., Rutzler, M., Robertson, H. M., & Zwiebel, L. J. (2007). Molecular characterization of the Aedes aegypti odorant receptor gene family. Insect Molecular Biology, 16, 525-537.

Bohbot, J. D., Fu, L., Le, T.C., Chauhan, K. R., Cantrell, C. L., & Dickens, J. C. (2011). Multiple activities of insect repellents on odorant receptors in mosquitoes. Medical and Veterinary Entomology, 25, 436-444.

Bohbot, J. D., Jones, P. L., Wang, G., Pitts, R. J., Pask, G. M., & Zwiebel, L. J. (2011). Conservation of indole responsive odorant receptors in mosquitoes reveals an ancient olfactory trait. Chemical Senses, 36, 149-160.

Clyne, P. J., Warr, C. G., Freeman, M. R., Lessing, D., Kim, J. & Carlson, J. R. (1999). A novel family of divergent seven transmembrane proteins: candidate odorant receptors in Drosophila. Neuron, 22, 327-338.

Gao, Q. & Chess, A. (1999). Identification of candidate Drosophila olfactory receptors from genomic DNA sequence. Genomics, 60, 31-39.

Grant, A. J. & Dickens, J. C. (2011). Functional characterization of the octenol receptor neuron on the maxillary palps of the Yellow Fever mosquito, Aedes aegypti. PLoS ONE 6(6): e21785. doi:10.1371/journal.pone.0021785.

Grant, A. J. & O'Connell, R. J. (1996). Electrophysiological responses from receptor neurons in mosquito maxillary palp sensilla. In Block, G. R. & Cardew, G. Olfaction in mosquito-host interactions. Chichester, UK: Wiley. (pp. 233-253).

Hallem, E., Ho, M. G., & Carlson, J. R. (2004). The molecular basis of odor coding in the Drosophila antenna. Cell, 117, 965-979.

Jones, W. D., Cayirlioglu, P., Kadow, I. G., & Vosshall, L. B. (2007). Two chemosensory receptors together mediate carbon dioxide detection in Drosophila. Nature, 445, 86-90.

Krieger, J., Grosse-Wilde, E., Gohl, T., Dewer, Y. M., Raming K, & Breer, H. (2004). Genes encoding candidate pheromone receptors in a moth (Heliothis virescens). Proceedings of the National Academy of Sciences (USA), 101, 11845-11850.

Lu, T., Qiu, Y. T., Wang, G., Kwon, J. Y., Rutzler, M., Kwon, HW., Pitts, R. J., van Loon, J. J. A., Takken, W., Carlson, J. R., & Zwiebel, L. J. (2007). Odor coding in the maxillary palp of the malaria vector mosquito Anopheles gambiae. Curr Biol 17, 1533-1544.

McIver, S. B. (1982). Sensilla of mosquitoes (Diptera: Culicidae). Journal of Medical Entomology, 19, 489-535.

Nakagawa, T., Sakurai, T., Nishioka, T., & Touhara, K. (2005). Insect sex-pheromone signals mediated by specific combinations of olfactory receptors. Science, 307, 1638-1642.

Robertson, H.M. & Wanner, K. W. (2006). The chemoreceptor superfamily in the honey bee, Apis mellifera: expansion of the odorant, but not gustatory, receptor family. Genome Research, 16, 1395-1403.

Sato, K., Pellegrino, M., Nakagawa, T., Nakagawa, T., Vosshall, L. B., & Touhara, K. (2008). Insect olfactory receptors are heteromeric ligand-gated ion channels. Nature, 452, 1002-1006.

Vogt, R. G., Riddiford, L. M., & Prestwich, G. D. (1985). Kinetic properties of a sex pheromone-degrading enzyme: The sensillar esterase of Antheraea polyphemus. Proceedings of the National Academy of Sciences (USA), 82, 8827-8831.

Vogt, R. G., Callahan, F. E., Rogers, M. E., & Dickens, J. C. (1999). Odorant binding protein diversity and distribution among insect orders, as indicated by LAP, an OBP-related protein of the true bug, Lygus lineolaris (Hemiptera: Heteroptera). Chemical Senses, 24, 481-495.

Vogt, R.G., Miller, N.E., Litvack, R., Fandino, R.A., Sparks, J., Staples, J., Friedman, R., & Dickens, J.C. (2009). The insect SNMP gene family. Insect Biochemistry and Molecular Biology, 39, 448-456.

Vosshall, L.B., Amrein, H., Morozov, P. S., Rzhetsky, A., & Axel, R. (1999). A spatial map of olfactory receptor expression in the Drosophila antenna. Cell, 96, 725-736.

Wicher, D., Schafer, R., Bauernfeind, R., Stensmyr, M.C., Heller,R., Heinemann,S.H., & Hansson, B. S. (2008). Drosophila odorant receptors are both ligand-gated and cyclic-nucleotide-activated cation channels. Nature, 452, 1007-1011.

Xu, P., Atkinson, R., Jones, D. N. M., & Smith, D. P. (2005). Drosophila OBP LUSH is required for activity of pheromone-sensitive neurons. Neuron, 45, 193-200.

Functions for the Tumor Suppressor PTEN in Cell Biology and Diseases

Yasuko Kitagishi
Department of Environmental Health Science
Nara Women's University, Japan

Mayumi Kobayashi
Department of Environmental Health Science
Nara Women's University, Japan

Satoru Matsuda
Department of Environmental Health Science
Nara Women's University, Japan

1   Introduction

PTEN (phosphatase and tensin homolog deleted on chromosome 10) is a tumor suppressor gene that is frequently deleted or mutated in a variety of human cancers such as gliomas, prostate, melanomas and endometrial cancers (Jiang & Liu, 2009; Carracedo *et al.*, 2011). The gene product PTEN is a dual-specificity phosphatase which has both protein phosphatase activity and lipid phosphatase activity that antagonizes PI3K activity. Cells that lack *PTEN* have constitutively higher levels of PIP3 and activated downstream targets (Torres *et al.*, 2001) (Figure 1). PTEN functions as a lipid phosphatase of PIP3, which is the product of a potent protooncogenic PI3K. However, a lot of known *PTEN* mutations in tumors are located corresponding outside of the catalytic site, and the mutant proteins exhibit normal phosphatase activity (Song *et al.*, 2012). This may suggest that tumor suppressive functions are distinct from those mediated by the catalytic activity, as the mutants still possess the phosphatase activity. Because wildtype has no enzymatic activity other than phosphatase activity, the phosphatase independent function is likely to result from changes in protein-protein interactions. The inactivation of tumor suppression by somatic mutation of PTEN may be caused by the lack of key PTEN interaction partners.

It is evident that PTEN contact the plasma membrane to regulate PIP3 level, yet it appears mainly cytosolic (Downes *et al.*, 2004). Therefore, identifying interacting partners of a PTEN mutant retaining phosphatase activity may uncover novel PTEN regulatory functions involved in a phosphatase independent manner. Protein-protein interactions are likely to be an important mechanism to regulate protein function. For the purpose, affinity purification coupled with mass spectrometry is a powerful tool for deciphering protein interaction networks (Shi *et al.*, 2012). Proteins from an affinity-purified sample are separated by one-dimensional SDS-PAGE, and after tryptic in-gel digestion, the resulting peptides are then analyzed by mass spectrometry. The protein interactors of a target protein can be identified by direct comparison of the peptide ratios between affinity-purified proteins. However, finding universal methods for removal of nonspecific interactions to retain specific interaction is difficult. The yeast two-hybrid screening system is also useful, which is the widely used genetic assay to identify and characterize novel protein interactions. The system has been adapted to cover an increasingly wide range of applications. For example, the interaction between PTEN function and adipocyte specific fatty acid binding protein FABP4 is of particular interest (Gorbenko *et al.*, 2010). In addition, recent studies have revealed a functional ubiquitin pathway for PTEN protein degradation (Maezawa *et al.*, 2008). In this review, we summarize the current research of how PTEN binds to the interaction partners as well as lipid bilayer to transduce signals downstream and what are the implications for diseases-associated biology.

2   Expression, Structure and Characteristics of PTEN

The human genomic *PTEN* locus consists of nine exons on chromosome 10q23.3, encoding a 5.5 kb mRNA that specifies a 403 amino-acid open reading frame. The translation product is a 53 kDa protein with homology to tensin and protein tyrosine phosphatases (PTPs). *PTEN* is ubiquitously expressed throughout early embryogenesis in mammals (Knobbe *et al.*, 2008). In addition, early growth regulated transcription factor 1 (EGR1), peroxisome proliferator activated receptor γ (PPARγ), p53, and activating transcription factor 2 (ATF2) can transcriptionally upregulate *PTEN* (Shen *et al.*, 2006; Pan *et al.*, 2007; Lee *et al.*, 2007), while transforming growth factor (TGF)-β, nuclear factor kappaB (NF-κB), and JUN negatively regulate *PTEN* expression (Yang *et al.*, 2009; Han *et al.*, 2008; Vasudevan *et al.*, 2007).

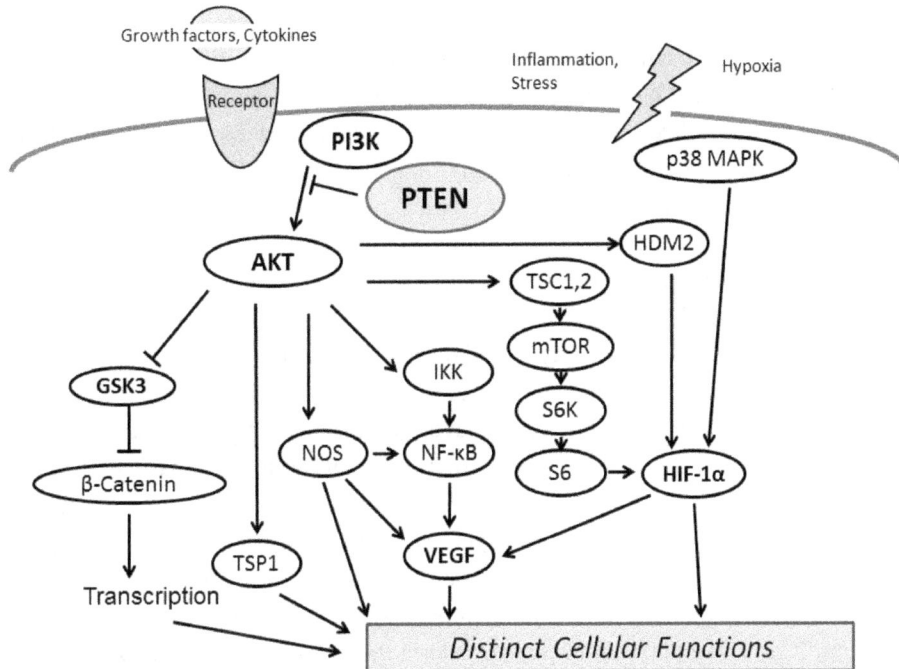

Figure 1: Schematic representation and overview of PTEN/PI3K/AKT signaling. Examples of molecules known to act on the regulatory pathways are shown. Note that some critical pathways have been omitted for clarity.

Interestingly, rosemary extract represses *PTEN* expression in K562 leukemic culture cells (Yoshida *et al.*, 2011). Methylation of the *PTEN* promoter can result in transcriptional silencing of the *PTEN* gene at the mRNA level (Mueller *et al.*, 2012). Some microRNAs such as miR-21, miR-19a, and miR-214 inhibit *PTEN* through targeting the 3'-untranslated region of *PTEN*, leading to inhibition of *PTEN* translation (Schwarzenbach *et al.*, 2012). PTEN activity can also be regulated by the posttranslational regulation including phosphorylation, acetylation, and oxidation (Singh & Chan, 2011).

Schematic structure of the PTEN protein is shown in Figure 2. PTEN protein consists of N-terminal phosphatase, and C-terminal C2, and PDZ (PSD-95, DLG1, and ZO-1) binding domains. The PTEN CX5R(S/T) motif resides within an active site that surrounds the catalytic signature with three basic residues, which are critical for PTEN lipid phosphatase activity. The structure endows PTEN with its preference for acidic phospholipid substrates such as PIP3. PTEN lipid phosphatase activity regulates AKT kinase pathway through modulation of PIP3 levels, regulating cell cycle progression, apoptosis, migration, and cell proliferation (Tsugawa *et al.*, 2002). The C2 domain in the C-terminal region of PTEN can also regulate cell migration (Raftopoulou *et al.*, 2004), which supports target the protein to move to the membrane through its affinity and regulate the phosphatase activity. Truncation or mutation of the C2 domain makes the protein unstable and accelerates protein degradation (Wang *et al.*, 2008). In addition, the C-terminus of PTEN contains two PEST (proline, glutamic acid, serine and threonine) sequences involved in protein degradation (Georgescu *et al.*, 2000). A PTEN mutation within a binding site of PICT1, which controls stability of PTEN, affects the protein level of PTEN and thereby reduces its enzymatic activity in the cells (Sasaki *et al.*, 2011). Overexpression of MAGI-2 has been shown to restore

PTEN stability (Subauste *et al.*, 2005). Akt activation leads to HIF-1a stabilization, whereas PTEN attenuates hypoxia-mediated HIF-1a stabilization (Li *et al.*, 2005). The instability of mutant PTEN and the reduction of HIF1a degradation have been shown to involve protein interactions. Casein kinase II-mediated phosphorylation stabilizes the PTEN protein by preventing its proteasomal degradation and caspase-proteolysis (Torres *et al.*, 2003). Accordingly, inhibition of the Casein kinase II-mediated PTEN phosphorylation results in increased PTEN activity and a reduction of AKT activity. The PDZ-binding sites allow interactions with PDZ containing proteins and the formation of PTEN associated complexes. Mutations in the PDZ domain for the regulatory proteins of PTEN may affect its ability through the PTEN activity (Ikenoue *et al.*, 2008).

PTEN negatively regulates the activity of PI3K/ AKT signaling through converting PIP3 to PIP2. The PIP3 is the principal second messenger of the PI3K pathway that mediates receptor tyrosine kinase signaling to the survival kinase AKT. Increased levels of PIP3 at the membrane cause PH domain-containing proteins such as AKT and PDK-1 to co-localize, resulting in the kinases-mediated phosphorylation and activation (Howes *et al.*, 2003). The activated AKT phosphorylates target proteins involved in cell survival, cell cycling and metabolism. Cell cycle mediators affected by AKT and PTEN levels include the forkhead transcription factors and glycogen synthase kinase (Nakamura *et al.*, 2000; Mulholland *et al.*, 2006). PTEN acts as regulator of maintaining basal levels of PIP3 below a threshold for those signaling activation. PTEN also plays an important role in the induction of apoptotic cell death signals in cells when cells lose contact with the extracellular matrix (Fournier *et al.*, 2009).

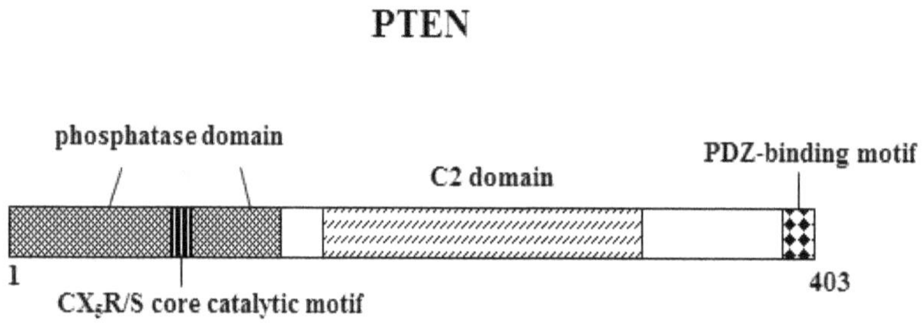

PTEN

Figure 2: Schematic structures of human PTEN protein. The predicted consensual domain structures for each protein are depicted. Note that the sizes of protein are modified for clarity. C2 domain: a structural domain involved in targeting proteins to cell membranes; PDZ: a common structural domain in signaling proteins (PSD95, Dlg, ZO-1, etc)

3   PTEN involved in Cancer

Because PTEN protein has been shown to play an important role in regulating proliferation and invasion of many cancer cells, PTEN is considered as an authentic tumor suppressor. The relevance of the PI3K pathway in cancer is focused by the numbers of components within the cascade whose activity is found altered. Actually, *PTEN* is one of the most mutated and deleted tumor suppressors in human cancer. Loss of heterozygosity studies have also suggested that *PTEN* may play an important role in advanced cancers (Tysnes & Mahesparan, 2001). In addition, alterations of *PTEN* in tumors are associated with a poor prognosis (Ohgaki & Kleihues, 2007). Germ line mutations of *PTEN* are the cause of *PTEN* hamartoma tumor syndromes (Cowden syndrome, Bannayan-Riley-Ruvalcaba syndrome, *PTEN*-related Proteus syndrome, Proteus-like syndrome) with increased risk for the development of cancers (Hobert & Eng, 2009). Cowden syndrome is autosomal dominant familial syndrome characterised by hamartomas, acral keratosis and multiple papillomas (Farooq *et al.*, 2010). Bannayan–Riley–Ruvalcaba syndrome is perceptible by macrocephaly, lipomatosis and hemangiomatosis (Litzendorf *et al.*, 2011). Cowden syndrome is thus caused by germline mutations of *PTEN*. In mouse models, however, complete inactivation of both copies of the *PTEN* gene results in embryonic death. *PTEN*-null embryos exhibit poorly organized ectodermal and mesodermal layers (Di Cristofano *et al.* 1998; Suzuki *et al.*, 1998). On the other hand, the *PTEN* heterozygous knockout mice are able to complete embryogenesis, which develop multiple organ neoplasms (Podsypanina *et al.*, 1999). So, several features observed in the *PTEN* heterozygous knockout mice are similar to those seen in Cowden syndrome. In contrast, overexpression of *PTEN* induces growth suppression by promoting G1 arrest (Weng *et al.*, 2001). This cell cycle arrest requires lipid phosphatase activity of PTEN and can be rescued with the introduction of constitutively active forms of PI3K or AKT. However, it is reported that *PTEN* constructs with point mutations in the loop regions of the C2 domain show reduced migration suppressing activity but retained catalytic activity (Raftopoulou *et al.*, 2004). Overexpression of *PTEN* also correlates with decreased total levels of cyclin D1, a key molecule regulated by AKT for cell cycle control (Vartanian *et al.*, 2011). Furthermore, PTEN regulates AKT activity so that the cell cycle inhibitor protein p27kip1 is increased (Dellas *et al.*, 2009; Yang *et al.*, 2002).

Increased proliferation, survival and motility are main cellular effects associated with the increased PIP3 level that contribute to its tumorigenic effects. Actually, dysregulation of the PI3K/PTEN/AKT pathway has been found in many malignant cancers. PTEN exerts its tumor-suppressive effect by dephosphorylating PIP3, thereby negatively regulating AKT activation and the survival pathway. Inactivating mutations in the *PTEN* gene are also common in tumors, indicating that elevated levels of PIP3 confer an advantage to cancer cells. PTEN deficiency leads to increased cell motility. Reintroducing the wild-type PTEN, but not the catalytically inactive PTEN, reduces the enhanced cell motility of PTEN deficient cells (Liliental *et al.*, 2000), suggesting that PTEN negatively controls cell motility through its phosphatase activity. Conversely, an absence of PTEN function may allow unregulated cell spreading and invasion, which might contribute to metastasis. Despite the main role of PTEN as a negative regulator of the PI3K pathway, studies report a number of tumor suppressive activities for PTEN that are used within the nucleus, where catalysis of PIP3 may not seem to represent a major function (Planchon *et al.*, 2008). The nuclear PTEN activities may include the regulation of genomic stability (Shen *et al.*, 2007), cell cycle progression, and gene expression.

4   Other diseases-associated functions of PTEN

4.1   Parkinson's Disease

As analyses have revealed many PTEN-binding proteins to different signaling cascades, PTEN may perform other functions besides the tumor suppressing activity (Figure 3). Actually, tissue-specific deletion of PTEN can result in autoimmunity, glucose dysregulation or neurological deficits, in addition to carcinogenesis. One of them, PTEN may be involved in a disease state such as Parkinson's disease (PD) (Rochet *et al.*, 2012). The PD is a neurodegenerative disorder characterized by degeneration of dopaminergic neurons in substantia-nigra of midbrain. Several evidences imply that genes associated with familial PD regulate cell death and/or the cell cycle related to AKT/PTEN pathway. For example,

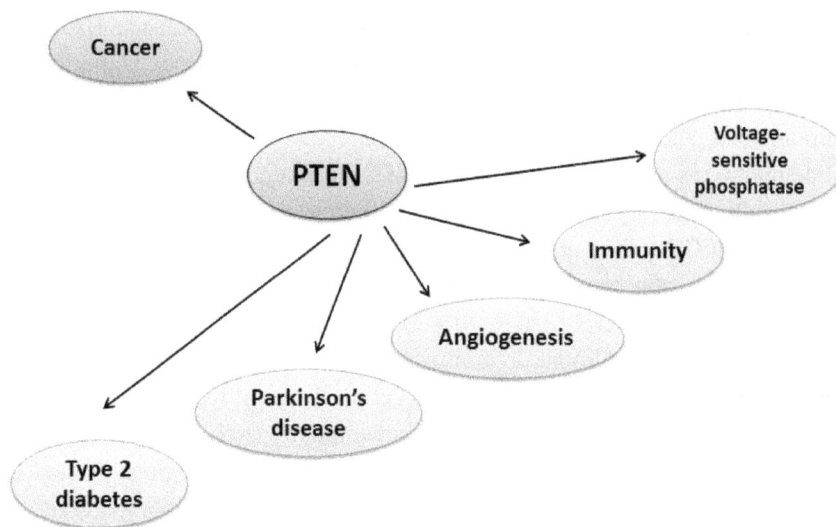

Figure 3: Implication of PTEN in various diseases. PTEN may be involved in other diseases including Diabetes and Parkinson's disease besides cancer.

deletions of Parkin, a PD related gene, in Drosophila result in AKT activation (Yang *et al.*, 2005). Furthermore, PTEN-induced putative kinase 1 (PINK1), which encodes a kinase downregulated in the absence of PTEN, has been identified as the sixth locus (PARK6) associated with familial PD (Plun-Favreau *et al.*, 2007). PINK1 is transcriptionally transactivated by the PTEN gene. The biochemistry of the neurodegeneration in PD points to mitochondrial oxidative stress as the mechanism driving neuronal cell death. The PINK1 is a mitochondrially targeted serine/threonine kinase, which is linked to autosomal recessive early onset PD (Poole *et al*, 2008; Poole *et al*, 2010). The PINK1 may exert a protective effect on the cell that is abrogated by the mutations, resulting in increased susceptibility to cellular stress. These findings provide a molecular link between mitochondria and the pathogenesis of PD.

4.2   Type 2 Diabetes

Type 2 diabetes is characterized by diminished pancreatic β-cell function. Insulin signaling within the β-cells has been shown to play an important role in maintaining the function of the β-cells. Under basal conditions, enhanced insulin-PI3K signaling via deletion of PTEN leads to increased β-cell mass (Stiles *et al.*, 2006). Mice with PTEN deletion in pancreatic cells show increase the β-cell mass because of both increased proliferation and reduced apoptosis. In particular, the relationship between PTEN function and adipocyte-specific fatty-acid-binding protein FABP4 is of interest inβ-cell signaling (Gorbenko *et al.*, 2010). The interaction of PTEN to FABP4 suggests a role for this phosphatase in the regulation of lipid metabolism and cell differentiation (Tsuda *et al.*, 2009). Tissue targeted deletion of PTEN lead to improved insulin sensitivity in the insulin-responsive tissues and protects from diabetes. PTEN has been shown to be upregulated in insulin resistance model of insulin/ insulin-like growth factor-1 signaling ablation in β-cells (Vellai *et al.*, 2006). Furthermore, PTEN is a key negative regulator of insulin-stimulated glucose uptake in vitro and in vivo (Wong *et al.*, 2007). The partial reduction of PTEN is enough to elicit enhanced insulin sensitivity and glucose tolerance. PTEN expression in pancreatic islets is also upregulated in models of type 2 diabetes (Wang *et al.*, 2010). So, PTEN exerts a critical negative effect upon β-cell function. In this way, PTEN in type 2 diabetes could be a therapeutic target to prevent the degeneration of β-cells.

4.3   Angiogenesis

PTEN also modulates angiogenesis via down-regulating PI3K/AKT pathway in types of cells (Okumura *et al.*, 2012). Although the effects of PTEN on invasion of hematopoietic cells and its clinical significance remains to be further elucidated, PTEN would be a candidate target to be addressed for inhibiting angiogenesis along with the treatment of leukemia. Recent study has demonstrated that in addition to suppress AKT activation, PTEN also controls the activity of Jun N-terminal kinase (JNK), which contributes to the increased expression of angiogenic cell growth and survival factor by stabilizing the endothelial-like growth factor (VEGF) that stimulates blood vessel formation. Studies have suggested that PTEN mutations can influence the activity of the VEGF (Jiang *et al.*, 2009; Kanwar *et al.*, 2011). Mutation of PTEN can also destabilize hypoxia inducible transcription factor 1a (HIF-1a), a molecule that drives VEGF transcription (Jiang *et al.*, 2008). PTEN knockout endothelial cells cause embryonic lethality due to endothelial cell hyper-proliferation and impaired vascular remodeling, whereas conditional PTEN knockout endothelial cells enhance neovascularization and tumor angiogenesis to increase tumor growth (Hamada *et al.*, 2005).

4.4   T/B cell Immunity

PTEN opposes PI3K activity and influences the selection of developing thymocytes (Wong *et al.*, 2012). PTEN conditional deficiency then causes autoimmune disease, T-cell hyper proliferation, and lymphoma. PTEN deletion in T cells has revealed the importance of PIP3 regulation for T-cell development through positive and negative selection of the T-cells (Johnson *et al.*, 2008). PTEN-deficient peripheral T cells are highly responsive to TCR stimulation, resulting in autoimmune pathology (Liu *et al.*, 2010). Activated T cells secrete increased amounts of cytokines and show a bias towards Th2 lineage. Consequently, PIP3 down-regulation by PTEN is required for properly limiting T-cell responses and maintaining the self-tolerance. The PI3K pathway has also come to the front position as a critical signaling circuit in B cell differentiation and function (Baracho *et al.*, 2011). PI3K signaling is attenuated via elevated PTEN expression and reduced CD19 signaling in newly formed B cells, conferring increased susceptibility to apoptosis. In the absence of PTEN, sustained activation of the PI3K pathway results in a break of tolerance and the generation of autoantibody-producing cells (Browne *et al.*, 2009). Correspondingly, loss of PTEN promotes B cell formation, which contributors to antibody responses to multivalent antigens.

4.5   Voltage sensitive phosphatase

The voltage-sensitive phosphatases (VSPs) hydrolyze phosphoinositides on depolarization of plasma membrane potential, representing a principle for the electrical activity into the transduction of biochemical signals. VSPs dephosphorylate the 5' position of the inositol ring of PIP3 and PIP2 upon voltage depolarization. The VSPs consist of a transmembrane voltage-sensor domain and a cytoplasmic phosphatase domain with sequence similarity to PTEN (Liu *et al.*, 2012). The cytoplasmic region of VSP, however, lacks the region corresponding to the COOH-terminal region and the PDZ-binding motif of PTEN. A unique feature of this protein is that depolarization-induced motions of the voltage sensor activate the PIP3 and PIP2 phosphatase activities. VSP is expressed in testis, sperm, blood cells, nervous system, and epitheliums. Patterns of membrane-potential changes may lead to alteration of cell morphology in these VSP-expressing cells. A chimeric protein made by fusing the PTEN to the voltage sensor of the prototypic VSP shows voltage-sensitive and PTEN-like enzymatic activity in a depolarization dependent manner, suggesting that PTEN may also function as a VSP in vivo (Lacroix *et al.*, 2011). Future studies are necessary to gain insights into physiological roles of activities of VSP and PTEN.

5   Perspective

PTEN may be regulated at multiple levels including transcription, protein stability, phosphorylation, and so forth. As PTEN is regulated by phosphorylation and degradation via ubiquitin/proteasome system, this targeting may offer a potential therapeutic modality for the treatment of those PTEN-related diseases. Furthermore, oxidative stress can inactivate PTEN. Understanding these regulations is crucial for therapeutic intervention and the effective design of novel therapeutics. Further mechanistic studies are needed in order to understand the precise molecular mechanisms of diseases with PTEN alteration.

Acknowledgments

This work was supported by grants-in-aid from the Ministry of Education, Culture, Sports, Science and Technology in Japan. In addition, this work was supported in part by the grant from SHIN-EI Pharmaceutical Co., Ltd.
Competing interests statement: The authors declare that they have no competing financial interests.

Abbreviations

PTEN: phosphatase and tensin homologue deleted on chromosome 10
PIP3: phosphatidylinositol 3,4,5-triphosphate
PIP2: phosphatidylinositol 4,5- bisphosphate
PI3K: phosphoinositide-3 kinase
PTP: protein tyrosine phosphatase
PPAR: peroxisome proliferator-activated receptor
VSP: voltage-sensitive phosphatase
LOH: Loss of heterozygosity

References

Baracho, G. V., Miletic, A. V., Omori, S. A., Cato, M. H., & Rickert, R. C. (2011). Emergence of the PI3-kinase pathway as a central modulator of normal and aberrant B cell differentiation. Curr Opin Immunol, 23, 178-183.

Browne, C. D., Del, Nagro, C. J., Cato, M. H., Dengler, H. S., & Rickert, R. C. (2009). Suppression of Phosphatidylinositol 3,4,5-Trisphosphate Production Is a Key Determinant of B Cell Anergy. Immunity, 31, 749–760.

Carracedo, A., Alimonti, A., & Pandolfi, P. P. (2011). PTEN level in tumor suppression: how much is too little? Cancer Res, 71, 629-633.

Dellas, A., Jundt, G., Sartorius, G., Schneider, M., & Moch, H. (2009). Combined PTEN and p27kip1 protein expression patterns are associated with obesity and prognosis in endometrial carcinomas. Clin Cancer Res, 15, 2456-2462.

Di Cristofano A., Pesce B., Cordon-Cardo C., Pandolfi P. P. (1998). Pten is essential for embryonic development and tumour suppression. Nat Genet, 19, 348-355.

Downes, C. P., Walker, S., McConnachie, G., Lindsay, Y., Batty, I. H., & Leslie, N. R. (2004). Acute regulation of the tumour suppressor phosphatase, PTEN, by anionic lipids and reactive oxygen species. Biochem Soc Trans, 32, 338-342.

Farooq, A., Walker, L. J., Bowling, J., & Audisio, R. A. (2010). Cowden syndrome. Cancer Treat Rev, 36, 577-583.

Fournier, M. V., Fata, J. E., Martin, K. J., Yaswen, P., & Bissell, M. J. (2009). Interaction of E-cadherin and PTEN regulates morphogenesis and growth arrest in human mammary epithelial cells. Cancer Res, 69, 4545-4552.

Georgescu, M. M., Kirsch, K. H., Kaloudis, P., Yang, H., Pavletich, N. P., & Hanafusa, H. (2000). Stabilization and productive positioning roles of the C2 domain of PTEN tumor suppressor. Cancer Res, 60, 7033-7038.

Gorbenko, O., Panayotou, G., Zhyvoloup, A., Volkova, D., Gout, I., & Filonenko, V. (2010). Identification of novel PTEN-binding partners: PTEN interaction with fatty acid binding protein FABP4. Mol Cell Biochem, 337, 299-305.

Hamada, K., Sasaki, T., Koni, P. A., Natsui, M., Kishimoto, H., Sasaki, J., Yajima, N., Horie, Y., Hasegawa, G., Naito, M., Miyazaki, J., Suda, T., Itoh, H., Nakao, K., Mak, T. W., Nakano, T., & Suzuki, A. (2005). The PTEN/PI3K pathway governs normal vascular development and tumor angiogenesis. Genes Dev, 19, 2054-2065.

Han, S., Ritzenthaler, J. D., Zheng, Y., & Roman, J. (2008). PPARbeta/delta agonist stimulates human lung carcinoma cell growth through inhibition of PTEN expression: the involvement of PI3K and NF-kappaB signals. Am J Physiol Lung Cell Mol Physiol, 294, L1238-L1249.

Hobert, J. A. & Eng, C. (2009). PTEN hamartoma tumor syndrome: an overview. Genet Med, 11, 687-694.

Howes, A. L., Arthur, J. F., Zhang, T., Miyamoto, S., Adams, J. W., Dorn, G. W. 2nd, Woodcock, E. A., & Brown, J. H. (2003). Akt-mediated cardiomyocyte survival pathways are compromised by G alpha q-induced phosphoinositide 4,5-bisphosphate depletion. J Biol Chem, 278, 40343-40351.

Ikenoue, T., Inoki, K., Zhao, B., & Guan, K. L. (2008). PTEN acetylation modulates its interaction with PDZ domain. Cancer Res, 68, 6908-6912.

Jiang, B. H. & Liu, L. Z. (2008). AKT signaling in regulating angiogenesis. Curr Cancer Drug Targets, 8, 19-26.

Jiang, B. H. & Liu, L. Z. (2009). PI3K/PTEN signaling in angiogenesis and tumorigenesis. Adv Cancer Res, 102, 19-65.

Johnson, T. A., Tsutsui, S., & Jirik, F. R. (2008). Antigen-induced Pten gene deletion in T cells exacerbates neuropathology in experimental autoimmune encephalomyelitis. Am J Pathol, 172, 980-992.

Kanwar, J. R., Kamalapuram, S. K., & Kanwar, R. K. (2011). Targeting survivin in cancer: the cell-signalling perspective. Drug Discov Today. 16, 485-494.

Knobbe, C. B., Lapin, V., Suzuki, A., & Mak, T. W. (2008). The roles of PTEN in development, physiology and tumorigenesis in mouse models: a tissue-by-tissue survey. Oncogene, 27, 5398-5415.

Lacroix, J., Halaszovich, C. R., Schreiber, D. N., Leitner, M. G., Bezanilla, F., Oliver, D., & Villalba-Galea, C. A. (2011). Controlling the activity of a phosphatase and tensin homolog (PTEN) by membrane potential. J Biol Chem, 286, 17945-17953.

Lee, Y. R., Yu, H. N., Noh, E. M., Kim, J. S., Song, E. K., Han, M. K., Kim, B. S., Lee, S. H., & Park, J. (2007). Peroxisome proliferator-activated receptor gamma and retinoic acid receptor synergistically up-regulate the tumor suppressor PTEN in human promyeloid leukemia cells. Int J Hematol, 85, 231-237.

Li, Y. M., Zhou, B. P., Deng, J., Pan, Y., Hay, N., & Hung, M. C. (2005). A hypoxia-independent hypoxia-inducible factor-1 activation pathway induced by phosphatidylinositol-3 kinase/Akt in HER2 overexpressing cells. Cancer Res, 65, 3257-3263.

Liliental, J., Moon, S. Y., Lesche, R., Mamillapalli, R., Li, D., Zheng, Y., Sun, H., & Wu, H. (2000). Genetic deletion of the Pten tumor suppressor gene promotes cell motility by activation of Rac1 and Cdc42 GTPases. Curr Biol, 10, 401-404.

Litzendorf, M., Hoang, K., & Vaccaro, P. (2011). Recurrent and extensive vascular malformations in a patient with Bannayan--Riley--Ruvalcaba syndrome. Ann Vasc Surg, 25, e15-e19.

Liu, L., Kohout, S. C., Xu, Q., Müller, S., Kimberlin, C. R., Isacoff, E. Y., & Minor, D. L. Jr. (2012). A glutamate switch controls voltage-sensitive phosphatase function. Nat Struct Mol Biol, 19, 633-641.

Liu, X., Karnell, J. L., Yin, B., Zhang, R., Zhang, J., Li, P., Choi, Y., Maltzman, J. S., Pear, W. S., Bassing, C. H., & Turka, L. A. (2010). Distinct roles for PTEN in prevention of T cell lymphoma and autoimmunity in mice. J Clin Invest, 120, 2497-2507.

Maezawa, S., Hayano, T., Koiwai, K., Fukushima, R., Kouda, K., Kubota, T., & Koiwai, O. (2008). Bood POZ containing gene type 2 is a human counterpart of yeast Btb3p and promotes the degradation of terminal deoxynucleotidyltransferase. Genes Cells, 13, 439-457.

Mueller, S., Phillips, J., Onar-Thomas, A., Romero, E., Zheng, S., Wiencke, J. K., McBride, S. M., Cowdrey, C., Prados, M. D., Weiss, W. A., Berger, M. S., Gupta, N., & Haas-Kogan, D. A. (2012). PTEN promoter methylation and activation of the PI3K/Akt/mTOR pathway in pediatric gliomas and influence on clinical outcome. Neuro Oncol, 14, 1146-1152.

Mulholland, D. J., Dedhar, S., Wu, H., & Nelson, C. C. (2006). PTEN and GSK3beta: key regulators of progression to androgen-independent prostate cancer. Oncogene, 25, 329-337.

Nakamura, N., Ramaswamy, S., Vazquez, F., Signoretti, S., Loda, M., & Sellers, W. R. (2000). Forkhead transcription factors are critical effectors of cell death and cell cycle arrest downstream of PTEN. Mol Cell Biol, 20, 8969-8982.

Ohgaki, H. & Kleihues, P. (2007). Genetic pathways to primary and secondary glioblastoma. Am J Pathol, 170, 1445-1453.

Okumura, N., Yoshida, H., Kitagishi, Y., Murakami, M., Nishimura, Y., & Matsuda, S. (2012). PI3K/AKT/PTEN Signaling as a Molecular Target in Leukemia Angiogenesis. Adv Hematol, 2012, 843085.

Pan, L., Lu, J., Wang, X., Han, L., Zhang, Y., Han, S., & Huang, B. (2007). Histone deacetylase inhibitor trichostatin a potentiates doxorubicin-induced apoptosis by up-regulating PTEN expression. Cancer, 109, 1676-1688.

Planchon, S. M., Waite, K. A., & Eng, C. (2008). The nuclear affairs of PTEN. J Cell Sci, 121, 249-253.

Plun-Favreau, H., Klupsch, K., Moisoi, N., Gandhi, S., Kjaer, S., Frith, D., Harvey, K., Deas, E., Harvey, R. J., McDonald, N., Wood, N. W., Martins, L. M., & Downward, J. (2007). The mitochondrial protease HtrA2 is regulated by Parkinson's disease-associated kinase PINK1. Nat Cell Biol, 9, 1243-1252.

Podsypanina K., Ellenson L. H., Nemes A. et al. (1999). Mutation of Pten/Mmac1 in mice causes neoplasia in multiple organ systems. Proc Natl Acad Sci USA, 96, 1563-1568.

Poole, A. C., Thomas, R. E., Andrews, L. A., McBride, H. M., Whitworth, A. J., & Pallanck, L. J. (2008). The PINK1/Parkin pathway regulates mitochondrial morphology. Proc Natl Acad Sci U S A, 105, 1638-1643.

Poole, A. C., Thomas, R. E., Yu, S., Vincow, E. S., & Pallanck, L. (2010). The mitochondrial fusion-promoting factor mitofusin is a substrate of the PINK1/parkin pathway. PLoS One, 5, e10054.

Raftopoulou, M., Etienne-Manneville, S., Self, A., Nicholls, S., & Hall, A. (2004). Regulation of cell migration by the C2 domain of the tumor suppressor PTEN. Science, 303, 1179-1181.

Rochet, J. C., Hay, B. A., & Guo, M. (2012). Molecular insights into Parkinson's disease. Prog Mol Biol Transl Sci, 107, 125-188.

Sasaki, M., Kawahara, K., Nishio, M., Mimori, K., Kogo, R., Hamada, K., Itoh, B., Wang, J., Komatsu, Y., Yang, Y. R., Hikasa, H., Horie, Y., Yamashita, T., Kamijo, T., Zhang, Y., Zhu, Y., Prives, C., Nakano, T., Mak, T. W., Sasaki, T., Maehama, T., Mori, M., & Suzuki, A. (2011). Regulation of the MDM2-P53 pathway and tumor growth by PICT1 via nucleolar RPL11. Nat Med, 17, 944-951.

Schwarzenbach, H., Milde-Langosch, K., Steinbach, B., Müller, V., & Pantel, K. (2012). Diagnostic potential of PTEN-targeting miR-214 in the blood of breast cancer patients. Breast Cancer Res Treat, 134, 933-941.

Shen, W. H., Balajee, A. S., Wang, J., Wu, H., Eng, C., Pandolfi, P. P., & Yin, Y. (2007). Essential role for nuclear PTEN in maintaining chromosomal integrity. Cell, 128, 157-170.

Shen, Y. H., Zhang, L., Gan, Y., Wang, X., Wang, J., LeMaire, S. A., Coselli, J. S., & Wang, X. L. (2006). Up-regulation of PTEN (phosphatase and tensin homolog deleted on chromosome ten) mediates p38 MAPK stress signal-induced inhibition of insulin signaling. A cross-talk between stress signaling and insulin signaling in resistin-treated human endothelial cells. J Biol Chem, 281, 7727-7736.

Shi, T., Zhou, J. Y., Gritsenko, M. A., Hossain, M., Camp, D. G. 2nd, Smith, R. D., & Qian, W.J. (2012). IgY14 and Super-Mix immunoaffinity separations coupled with liquid chromatography-mass spectrometry for human plasma proteomics biomarker discovery. Methods, 56, 246-253.

Singh, G. & Chan, A. M. (2011). Post-translational modifications of PTEN and their potential therapeutic implications. Curr Cancer Drug Targets, 11, 536-547.

Song, M. S., Salmena, L., & Pandolfi, P. P. (2012). The functions and regulation of the PTEN tumour suppressor. Nat Rev Mol Cell Biol, 13, 283-296.

Stiles, B. L., Kuralwalla-Martinez, C., Guo, W., Gregorian, C., Wang, Y., Tian, J., Magnuson, M. A., & Wu, H. (2006). Selective deletion of Pten in pancreatic beta cells leads to increased islet mass and resistance to STZ-induced diabetes. Mol Cell Biol, 26, 2772-2781.

Subauste, M. C., Nalbant, P., Adamson, E. D., & Hahn, K. M. (2005). Vinculin controls PTEN protein level by maintaining the interaction of the adherens junction protein beta-catenin with the scaffolding protein MAGI-2. J Biol Chem. 2005, 280, 5676-5681.

Suzuki A., de la Pompa J. L., Stambolic V. et al. (1998). High cancer susceptibility and embryonic lethality associated with mutation of the PTEN tumor suppressor gene in mice. Curr Biol, 8, 1169-1178.

Torres, J., Navarro, S., Roglá, I., Ripoll, F., Lluch, A., García-Conde, J., Llombart-Bosch, A., Cervera, J., & Pulido, R. (2001). Heterogeneous lack of expression of the tumour suppressor PTEN protein in human neoplastic tissues. Eur J Cancer, 37, 114-121.

Torres, J., Rodriguez, J., Myers, M. P., Valiente, M., Graves, J. D., Tonks, N. K., & Pulido, R. (2003). Phosphorylation-regulated cleavage of the tumor suppressor PTEN by caspase-3: implications for the control of protein stability and PTEN-protein interactions. J Biol Chem, 278, 30652-30660.

Tsuda, M., Inoue-Narita, T., Suzuki, A., Itami, S., Blumenberg, M., & Manabe, M. (2009). Induction of gene encoding FABP4 in Pten-null keratinocytes. FEBS Lett, 583, 1319-1322.

Tsugawa, K., Jones, M. K., Sugimachi, K., Sarfeh, I. J., & Tarnawski, A. S. (2002). Biological role of phosphatase PTEN in cancer and tissue injury healing. Front Biosci, 7, e245-e251.

Tysnes, B. B. & Mahesparan, R. (2001). Biological mechanisms of glioma invasion and potential therapeutic targets. J Neurooncol, 53, 129-147.

Vartanian, R., Masri, J., Martin, J., Cloninger, C., Holmes, B., Artinian, N., Funk, A., Ruegg, T., & Gera, J. (2011). AP-1 regulates cyclin D1 and c-MYC transcription in an AKT-dependent manner in response to mTOR inhibition: role of AIP4/Itch-mediated JUNB degradation. Mol Cancer Res, 9, 115-130.

Vasudevan, K. M., Burikhanov, R., Goswami, A., & Rangnekar, V. M. (2007). Suppression of PTEN expression is essential for antiapoptosis and cellular transformation by oncogenic Ras. Cancer Res, 67, 10343-10350.

Vellai, T., McCulloch, D., Gems, D., & Kovács, A. L. (2006). Effects of sex and insulin/insulin-like growth factor-1 signaling on performance in an associative learning paradigm in Caenorhabditis elegans. Genetics, 174, 309-316.

Wang, L., Liu, Y., Yan, Lu, S., Nguyen, K. T., Schroer, S. A., Suzuki, A., Mak, T. W., Gaisano, H., & Woo, M. (2010). Deletion of Pten in pancreatic β-cells protects against deficient β-cell mass and function in mouse models of type 2 diabetes. Diabetes, 59, 3117-3126.

Wang, X., Shi, Y., Wang, J., Huang, G., & Jiang, X. (2008). Crucial role of the C-terminus of PTEN in antagonizing NEDD4-1-mediated PTEN ubiquitination and degradation. Biochem J, 414, 221-229.

Weng, L. P., Gimm, O., Kum, J. B., Smith, W. M., Zhou, X. P., Wynford-Thomas, D., Leone, G., & Eng, C. (2001). Transient ectopic expression of PTEN in thyroid cancer cell lines induces cell cycle arrest and cell type-dependent cell death. *Hum Mol Genet, 10, 251-258.*

Wong, G. W., Knowles, G. C., Mak, T. W., Ferrando, A. A., & Zúñiga-Pflücker, J. C. (2012). HES1 opposes a PTEN-dependent check on survival, differentiation, and proliferation of TCRβ-selected mouse thymocytes. *Blood, 120, 1439-1448.*

Wong, J. T., Kim, P. T., Peacock, J. W., Yau, T. Y., Mui, A. L., Chung, S. W., Sossi, V., Doudet, D., Green, D., Ruth, T. J., Parsons, R., Verchere, C. B., & Ong, C. J. (2007). Pten (phosphatase and tensin homologue gene) haploinsufficiency promotes insulin hypersensitivity. *Diabetologia, 50, 395-403.*

Yang, G., Ayala, G., De, Marzo, A., Tian, W., Frolov, A., Wheeler, T. M., Thompson, T. C., & Harper, J. W. (2002). Elevated Skp2 protein expression in human prostate cancer: association with loss of the cyclin-dependent kinase inhibitor p27 and PTEN and with reduced recurrence-free survival. *Clin Cancer Res, 8, 3419-3426.*

Yang, Y., Gehrke, S., Haque, M. E., Imai, Y., Kosek, J., Yang, L., Beal, M. F., Nishimura, I., Wakamatsu, K., Ito, S., Takahashi, R., & Lu, B. (2005). Inactivation of Drosophila DJ-1 leads to impairments of oxidative stress response and phosphatidylinositol 3-kinase/Akt signaling. *Proc Natl Acad Sci U S A, 102, 13670-13675.*

Yang, Y., Zhou, F., Fang, Z., Wang, L., Li, Z., Sun, L., Wang, C., Yao, W., Cai, X., Jin, J., & Zha, X. (2009). Post-transcriptional and post-translational regulation of PTEN by transforming growth factor-beta1. *Cell Biochem, 106, 1102-1112.*

Yoshida, H., Okumura, N., Kitagishi, Y., Nishimura, Y., & Matsuda, S. (2011). Ethanol extract of Rosemary repressed PTEN expression in K562 culture cells. *Int J appl Biol pharm Technol, 2, 316-322.*

Site-directed Mutagenesis for the Identification of Ligand-binding Sites on Na$^+$/Cl$^-$-dependent Neurotransmitter Transporters

Chiharu Sogawa
Department of Dental Pharmacology
Okayama University, Japan

Norio Sogawa
Department of Dental Pharmacology
Okayama University, Japan

Shigeo Kitayama
Department of Dental Pharmacology
Okayama University, Japan

1   Introduction

Neurotransmitter transporters at the plasma membrane terminate synaptic neurotransmission by recycling the released neurotransmitter into neuronal and/or glial cells. There are two major subclasses of plasma membrane transporter: high-affinity glutamate transporters and Na^+ and Cl^- (Na^+/Cl^-)-dependent neurotransmitter transporters (neurotransmitter sodium symporters: NSSs) (Iversen, 1971). These subsets of transporters from the human genome also form the solute carrier (SLC)1 gene family and SLC6 gene family, respectively. The latter subclass is the largest and includes monoamine (dopamine (DA), noradrenaline (NA), and serotonin (5-HT)), amino acid (γ-aminobutyric acid (GABA), glycine, and proline), and osmolyte (betaine, creatine, and taurine) transporters (Yamauchi *et al.*, 1992; Amara & Kuhar, 1993; Borden *et al.*, 1995). There are also three subclasses of intracellular transporter: vesicular amine transporters (the SLC18 gene family), vesicular inhibitory amino acid transporters (the SLC32 gene family), and vesicular glutamate transporters (SLC17 gene family) (Gether, *et al.*, 2006).

The transporters for monoamines, such as the DA transporter (DAT), NA transporter (NET), and 5-HT transporter (SERT), are of particular interest since the 1950s when they were found to be targets of drugs of abuse and/or antidepressants and involved in various neuronal disorders including drug dependence, depression, and movement disorders such as Parkinson disease (PD) (Gether *et al.*, 2006). Therefore, elucidating the function and physiological role of these transporters should be the first step to clarifying their importance in pathophysiology and the development of treatments for these diseases.

Cloning the cDNA of these transporters has facilitated subsequent researches and resulted in further understanding of their roles in neurotransmission. In 1990, GABA transporter cDNA was the first to be cloned (Guastella *et al.*, 1990), followed by the cloning of NET (Pacholczyk *et al.*, 1991), DAT (Giros *et al.*, 1996), SERT (Blakely *et al.*, 1991), and other members of this gene family (Bröer & Gether, 2012). Information of their nucleotide sequences and deduced amino acid sequences was important for determining the structure-function relationship of the transporters. The cellular and molecular aspects of these transporters need to be elucidated to clarify their physiological and pathological relevance, because alterations to the structure, function, and expression of these transporters may produce anatomical and functional divergences, resulting in the involvement of a number of neurological and psychiatric disorders.

An essential property of NSSs is the ability to co-transport Na^+ ions with the substrate. Large differences in terms of transport stoichiometry have been reported between the substrate and Na^+ ion. Different ionic stoichiometries have also been observed among individual members of the monoamine transporter subclasses. DAT involves the co-transport of two Na^+ ions and one Cl^- ion (Gu *et al.*, 1994), whereas NET and SERT translocate the substrate with one Na^+ ion and one Cl^- ion (Gu *et al.*, 1996; Rudnick *et al.*, 2006). These differences may result in changes in the membrane potential and also substrate transport. Previous mutagenesis studies identified some critical residues that appeared to be involved in ion dependence and selectivity (Keshet *et al.* 1995).

The X-ray crystal structure of the bacterial homologue of the mammalian NSSs, *Aquifex aeolicus* leucine transporter (LeuT), confirmed the original structural topology predicted based on protein primary sequence and further extended understanding at atomic level (Yamashita *et al.*, 2005). Subsequent studies with LeuT revealed the ligand-binding domain for tricyclic antidepressants (TCAs) (Singh *et al.*, 2007; Zhou *et al.*, 2007). Given the difficulties in crystallizing mammalian transporters, site-directed mutagenesis, in conjunction with the crystal structure of LeuT, has been a helpful method for understanding the structure-function relationships of NSS. Addressing the differences in pharmacological profiles between LeuT and mammalian NSS, in combination with site-directed mutagenesis, has been a rational strategy to localize domains and residues critical for ligand interactions. Combination of site-directed mutagenesis with functional characterization of the mutant transporters has the capability to provide structural information and identify the functional role of specific protein sequences. Transporters for monoamines are particularly relevant to drug dependence, mood abnormalities, and other neurological disorders. Therefore, understanding the structure-function relationships of these transporters could provide clues to clarify their pathophysiological significance and thereby develop new strategies to treat the neuronal disorders mentioned above.

In this review, we addressed the site-directed mutagenesis approach for determining the structure-function relationships of membrane protein including NSS. Different methodologies for mutagenesis have been developed to introduce mutations at predetermined sites or regions in NSS. However, mutations can cause misfolding of the protein or improper insertion of the protein into the membrane, which can lead to loss of function. If loss of function is due to a lack of expression at the plasma membrane, it is difficult to conclude about the functional role of amino acid residues in the transporter protein. Therefore, the reason for loss of function should be accurately ascertained. We discuss both the benefits and limitations associated with site-directed mutagenesis. In addition, we gave a review over basic methods and related experimental protocols for the site-directed mutagenesis study of NSS.

2   Cellular and Molecular Aspects of NSSs

2.1   First Stage: Biochemical Approaches

Chemical transmission at synapses was established in the 1930s by Henry Dale and Otto Loevi in contrast to the electrical transmission theory proposed by physiologists. The process of these conflicting events was called "the war of soups and sparks" (Valenstein, 2005). Although Dale and Loewi used eserin to identify the action of acetylcholine (ACh), and considered that the termination of cholinergic transmission was achieved by the enzymatic degradation of ACh, they did not confirm the termination of neurotransmission for other neurotransmitters such as noradrenaline (NA).

Unlike ACh, the synaptic transmission of other classical neurotransmitters is terminated by uptake rather than enzymatic degradation. In the 1960s, Axelrod developed the basis of the uptake system and its physiological and pharmacological significance in neurotransmission (Axelrod et al., 1961). He established not only the physiological relevance of the uptake system, but also its pharmacological importance by demonstrating the inhibitory action of imipramine, an antidepressant, on NA uptake by sympathetic nerve endings.

This opened avenues for the development of antidepressant drugs and drugs for related neural disorders, and provided the basis for the uptake system as a drug target. Many researchers worked in this field because this recognition was important. One such achievement was the dopamine (DA) uptake system as a cocaine receptor, based on the DA hypothesis of the action of cocaine as a psychostimulant (Giros et al., 1996).

One approach to identify the structure-function relationship of DA uptake such as the DA transporter (DAT)/cocaine receptor was the development of binding agents according to receptor binding techniques (Kilty et al., 1991).

Another approach was protein purification and reconstitution. The protein that governs the uptake system for γ-aminobutyric acid (GABA) was first purified by Kanner's group, who succeeded in reconstituting it in liposomes, which resulted in demonstrating the Na^+/Cl^- -dependent uptake of GABA (Kanner, 1994). This led to the identification of GABA transporter (GAT) cDNA, as mentioned below.

SLC number / Common name	Endogenous substrate	Protein variation	Reference
SLC6A1/GAT1	GABA		Guastella *et al.* (1990)
SLC6A2/NET	NA/DA	C-t var1	Pacholczyk *et al.* (1991)
		C-t var2	
SLC6A3/DAT	DA/NA		Kilty *et al.* (1991)
SLC6A4/SERT	5-HT		Blakely *et al.* (1991)
SLC6A5/GlyT2	Glycine	GlyT2a,	Smith *et al.* (1992)
		GlyT2b	
SLC6A6/TauT	Taurine		Liu *et al.* (1992a)
SLC6A7/PROT	Proline		Fremeau *et al.* (1992)
SLC6A8/CT1	Creatine		Mayser *et al.* (1992)
SLC6A9/GlyT1	Glycine	GlyT1a	Guastella *et al.* (1992),
		GlyT1b	Liu *et al.* (1992b)
		GlyT1c	
		GlyT1d	
		GlyT1e	
SLC6A11/GAT3	GABA, β-alanine		Borden *et al.* (1992)
SLC6A12/BGT1	GABA, betaine		Yamauchi et a. (1992)
SLC6A13/GAT2	GABA, β-alanine		Borden *et al.* (1992)

Table 1: Nomenclature and overview of the SLC6 gene family neurotransmitter transporters.

2.2 Second Stage: cDNA Cloning through Different Strategies

Kanner and his colleagues purified a rat brain GAT protein (Radian *et al.*, 1986). They partially digested this protein, and obtained peptides to read amino acid sequences. They screened the cDNA library with oligo-probes made by information obtained from amino acid sequences of the peptides from the GAT protein, and succeeded in obtaining GAT-1 cDNA in 1990 (Guastella *et al.*, 1990).

Amara's group used other techniques, such as "expression cloning", to identify the NA transporter (NET) (Amara & Kuhar, 1993). Comparing these findings, it was hypothesized that GAT1 and NET consisted of a new gene family. Based on the homology of their nucleotide and deduced amino acid sequences, other transporters for classical neurotransmitters including DA (DAT), 5-HT (SERT), GABA (GAT2 and GAT3), and glycine (GLYT1 and GLYT2) have been identified. Furthermore, cDNA cloning of transporters for amino acids (proline) and osmolites (betaine, creatine, and taurine) confirmed that these transporters belonged to the gene family of the NSS, such as SLC6 (Table 1). Some transporters have splice variants that result in different peptide sequences. Bröer & Gether reviewed a synopsis of the biochemical and pharmacological properties of SLC6 family transporters (Bröer & Gether, 2012).

2.3   Third stage: X-ray crystallography of LeuT with different ligands

An analysis of the crystal structure of the bacterial homologue, LeuT from *Aquifex aeolicus* (Yamashita *et al.*, 2005) to the mammalian NSS revealed molecular insights into the SLC6 family. The amino acid sequences between the LeuT and human transporter homologues were aligned using Psi-BLAST. Clusters of high sequence conservation, including functionally important residues, were shown to be distributed throughout the primary structure, although the overall sequence identity between the eukaryotic and prokaryotic counterparts was only 20-25% (Yamashita *et al.*, 2005). There was an unexpected structural repeat in the first ten transmembrane domains (TMDs) that related TMD1-5 with TMD6-10 around the pseudo-twofold axis of symmetry located in the membrane (Figure 1). The pseudo-repeats were oriented antiparallel to one another with the two central TMDs, 1 and 6, which were unwound near the substrate and Na^+ binding sites, located halfway across the lipid bilayer. Helix 1 and 6 are therefore subdivided in to helix 1a/1b and helix 6a/6b. This unwinding structure was important for understanding the structure-function relationship because it exposed helix dipoles for the maintenance carbonyl oxygen and amide nitrogen in substrate binding and Na^+ coordination. Beuming *et al.* (2006) presented a comprehensive sequence alignment of all known prokaryotic and eukaryotic NSS using bioinformatics tools, and the resulting alignments were validated by comparisons with experimental data. The alignment of a number of regions, including TMDs 4, 5, and 9, as well as extracellular loops (ELs) 2, 3, and 4, differed from the one proposed LeuT protein. They showed that important similarities and differences among the sequences of the NSS were related to determine the selectivity of substrate binding and regulate the function of transport.

NSSs are membrane-spanning proteins that couple the thermodynamic movement of molecules (substrates) and ions across lipid bilayer membranes. These transporters assume at least three conformational states: outward-open, occluded, and inward-open. Access to either side of the membrane bilayer is controlled by extracellular and intracellular gates (Jardetzky 1966). An examination of the structure of the crystallized LeuT protein revealed this structure to be an "occluded form" with the substrates leucine, along with two Na^+ ions (Yamashita *et al.*, 2005). Subsequent studies added further structural models by indicating an occluded form with tricyclic antidepressant (TCA) (Singh *et al.*, 2007; Zhou *et al.*, 2007) and an outward-facing form with the competitive inhibitor tryptophan (Singh *et al.*, 2008). The structure of the TCA-LeuT complex revealed a TCA binding pocket, called the "extracellular vestibule", composed of 7 amino acid residues located approximately 11 Angstroms above the substrate leucine binding site, and accommodated with extracellular loop 4. Previous reports on the crystal structures of LeuT elucidating the architecture of neurotransmitter transporters demonstrated the existence of a substrate-and ion-bound occluded conformation. However, understanding of the mechanisms and structure-function relationships in neurotransmitter transporters was incomplete due to the absence of LeuT structures in the outward-open and inward-open states. Recently, Krishnamurthy and Gouaux (2012) reported the crystal structures of LeuT mutants in complexes with conformation-specific antibody fragments in the substrate-free outward-open and apo inward-open states. The transporter was shown to have an outward-open conformation in the absence of a substrate, but in the presence of sodium. The inward-open conformation involved large-scale conformational changes, including TMDs 1,2,5,6, and 7, a marked significant moves; while the remaining helices formed a scaffold. Helix 1a, in particular, was shown to bend around the center, which opened cytosolic access. These changes closed the extracellular gate, opened an intracellular vestibule, and largely disrupted the two Na^+ sites, thereby providing a mechanism by which ions and substrates were released to the cytoplasm.

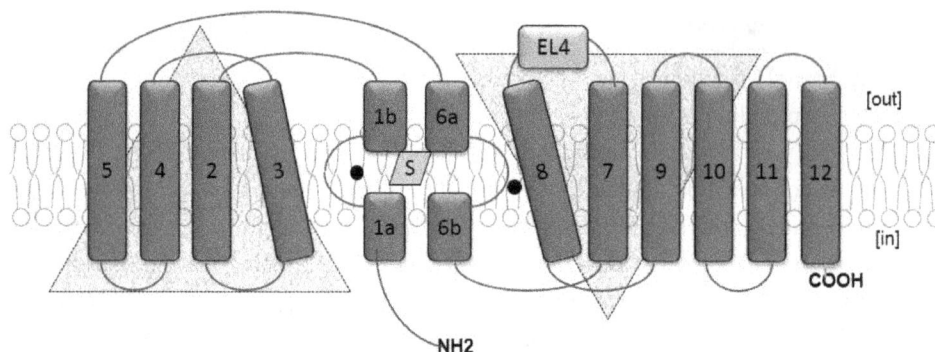

Figure 1: Schematic presentation of the topological model of the neurotransmitter transporter. A model of LeuT in the plasma membrane based on its crystal structure. S: the substrate leucine, closed circle: Na^+.

3   Approaches to Identify the Transporter-ligand Interaction by Site-directed Mutagenesis: Methodological Considerations

Site-directed mutagenesis changes the genetic code for a protein sequence and generates a mutant protein with a slightly different structure. Several different methodologies for mutagenesis have been developed to introduce mutations at predetermined sites or regions of NSSs. We summarize the major types of mutagenesis approaches.

3.1   Site-directed Mutagenesis

A previous study demonstrated that many mutant transporters could be generated with the site-directed mutagenesis method, which recently used a double-stranded DNA vector containing the insert to be mutated and two synthetic complementary oligonucleotides with the desired mutation. After the denaturation of double-strand DNA, oligonucleotides were allowed to anneal to the insert DNA, and high-fidelity DNA polymerase from heat-resistant bacteria was used to synthesize complementary strands to generate the mutated plasmid with staggered nicks. The parental plasmid was digested with DpnI endonuclease, which only digests methylated DNA leaving the *in vitro* synthesized mutant plasmid intact. The plasmid was then transformed into a strain of competent bacterial cells appropriate for the vector.

Kitayama *et al.* (1992) described the possible functional significance of polar amino acids lysing within three hydrophobic regions of DAT by expressing DAT cDNAs mutated in these polar residues. A single-stranded template for mutagenesis was derived from pcDNA/DAT1, and mutated by annealing oligonucleotides corresponding to the mutant sequences, *in vitro* synthesis and ligation of the mutant strand, nicking of the nonmutant strand, digestion of the nonmutant strand, and repolymerization and ligation of the gapped DNA. The replacement of aspartate at position 79 with alanine, glycine, or glutamate markedly reduced the uptake of [^{3}H] dopamine and reduced the mutants' affinity for the tritium-labeled cocaine analog. These results demonstrated that the aspartate residue lying within the TMD1 is crucial for DAT function and cocaine binding. Some other reports showed the important amino acids on DAT, SERT, and NET for cocaine binding by site-directed mutagenesis studies: Val152 (TMD3) (Lee *et al.*, 2000), and Tyr175 (Tyr176 in SERT) (TMD3) (Chen *et al.*, 1997). Cherubino *et al.* (2009) investigated the mutated GABA transporter as an interesting model for the study of the functional interaction between TCAs and selective serotonin reuptake inhibitors (SSRIs) with NSSs. The GABA transporter rGAT1 has been characterized in detail, and has already been reported to be affected by TCAs. The aspartate in position 401 of LeuT corresponds to lysine 448 in rGAT1. This amino acid, located at the beginning of TMD10, forms a pocket where TCAs bind to inhibit transport. They decided to investigate the antidepressant effects of the lysine 448 mutant of rGAT1 replaced with alanine, aspartate, and glutamate. The different effects elicited by the application of desipramine to the rGAT wild type and mutants confirmed the key role of this residue located in TMD10 in interactions with drugs (Cherubino et al., 2009).

3.2   Functional Chimeras between the Two Closely Related Monoamine Transporters

The construction of chimeric transporters can be useful to identify the functional domains of transporters and reveal interesting aspects of their structure-function relationships. Chimeric proteins were constructed by an *in vivo* method that generates chimeras within bacteria transformed with linear plasmid DNA containing a single copy of each parental cDNA in a tail-to-head configuration. The other simple way is to use restriction enzyme sites. If there is no available site, the introduction of restriction sites is carried out by site-directed mutagenesis without changing the coding amino acid residues (Mitrovic et al., 1998).

Overlap extension PCR, also known as fusion PCR, may be useful in carrying out the directed joining of cloned DNA sequences. This method uses PCR-based genetic recombination to generate linear DNA fragments composed of two or more distinct cDNAs with specific junction sites in order to create plasmids that express chimeric protein. Chimeric oligonucleotides are used to amplify the individual fragments of each gene of interest. An insertion fragment and two flanking fragments are prepared. The insertion fragment has an overlap region at both ends, and each of the two flanking fragments contains an overlap region at its 5'end. When the insertion and flanking fragments are combined into a secondary PCR (fusion-PCR), the overlapping sequences anneal to each other and are able to serve as priming sites that allow the 3' extension by DNA polymerase, resulting in a hybrid template. The hybrid template is then further amplified with the outermost primer pair.

To identify the regions important for the function and expression of the transporters, chimera has been made between different transporters, e.g., DAT and NET (Giros et al., 1994; Buck & Amara, 1995; Barker et al., 1995). Chimeras were useful because DAT and NET are similar, but still have distinct pharmacological differences. Chimeras between NET and SERT were constructed in which the predicted external loops of SERT were replaced one at a time with a corresponding sequence from NET (Smicun et al., 1999). Sensitivity to antidepressants was known to be different between species. A chimera study between human and rat SERT identified the region responsible for drug sensitivity (Barker et al., 1995).

3.3   Cysteine-scanning Mutagenesis (SCAM) for the Determinants of Transporter Function

Application of the substituted-cysteine accessibility method (SCAM) can be utilized for indirectly probing the structure and conformational dynamics of protein function in various membrane proteins. SCAM provides an approach to systematically map the residues on the water-accessible surface of a protein. Consecutive residues in putative membrane-scanning segments are mutated to cysteine and the mutant proteins are expressed in heterologous cells. Conformational changes in a protein may result in changes in the accessibility of substituted cysteines as assessed by their rates of reaction with polar sulfhydryl-specific reagents.

Cysteine substitution combinations with chemical modifications of the introduced cysteine residues to probe the accessibility of various regions to aqueous environments have been used to determine the functional properties of the NSSs (Javitch, 1998; Seal & Amara, 1998). Javitch used the SCAM method to determine the residues that line the transport pathway, as well as those that form the surface of the binding sites for substrates and inhibitors in DAT. To investigate the structural determinants underlying transport by the glutamate transporter EAAT1, Seal & Amara mutated each of 24 highly conserved residues (P392 to Q415) to cysteine. They proposed that this domain formed a reentrant membrane loop at the cell surface and may comprise part of the translocation pore for substrates and cotransported ions.

3.4   Computer-assisted Modeling of the Transporters

In a recent study, known high-resolution protein structures with LeuT were analyzed by the structural superposition of core TMDs (Jeschke, 2013). Structure superposition, computation of elastic network models and covariance matrices, and fitting were performed with software. Structural transitions between different conformations were analyzed in relative TMD arrangements using LeuT together with several other proteins. The relative arrangement of the TMDs was controlled by the functional state rather than by the properties of the individual proteins. A major conformational change was observed between the outward-open and inward-open states of the protein.

The crystal structure of LeuT was used as a template for the molecular modeling of monoamine transporters, such as DAT, SERT, and NET (Ravna et al., 2009). Various kinds of software were used for sequence alignment, visualization, and homology modeling. ICMPocketFinder was used to explore possible drug binding pockets. Two putative drug binding sites (pockets 1 and 2) were identified in each transporter, and, in DAT, cocaine, and clomipramine, were docked into binding pocket 1 and pocket 2, respectively. Pocket 1 is the leucine binding site in LeuT, which involved TMDs 1, 3, 6, and 8. Pocket 2, corresponding to the clomipramine binding site in the crystal structure of the LeuT-clomipramine complex, involved TMDs 1, 3, 6, 10, and 11. In another study, the homology model of SERT was constructed using the BuildModel macro of ICM (Gabrielsen et al., 2012a). Tryptamine derivatives (including 5-HT) and SSRI were docked into putative substrate binding sites. In a further study, five classes of SERT inhibitors were docked into the outward-facing SERT homology model using a new 4D ensemble protocol (Gabrielsen et al., 2012b). 3-D computational models of LeuT-based monoamine transporters have been reviewed (Manepalli et al. 2012). Details regarding construction of the 3-D models previously published have been summarized in this review, which pointed out that computational models have guided elucidation of ligand binding sites, substrate translocation pathways, inter- and intramolecular interactions, and potential transporter conformations. Structure-based virtual screening for novel ligands is yielding leading compounds toward the development of new medications for neuronal disorders.

4   Interaction of GAT with TCAs

Recently, we investigated the potency of various TCAs in inhibiting mouse BGT1 compared with other GAT subtypes in cell cultures heterologously expressing mouse GAT subtypes (Gerile et al., 2012). In this section, we have described the interaction of GAT with TCAs based on our recent studies. Furthermore, we compared amino acid sequences between mouse GATs, rat SERT, and LeuT at regions predicted as antidepressant- and substrate-binding sites.

4.1   GAT Subtypes and their Genes

GAT subtypes are members of the SLC6 gene family. The nomenclature used for mice denotes the transporter as GAT1-4, whereas the corresponding transporters in rats and humans have been named GAT1 (SLC6A1), betaine/GABA transporter ((BGT)1), (SLC6A12), GAT2 (SLC6A13), and GAT3 (SLC6A11) (HUGO nomenclature) (Table 1). The human and rat nomenclatures are used in this review. They have 12 hydrophobic TMDs, a large extracellular loop between TMD3 and TMD4 with multiple glycosylation sites, and intracellular N- and C-termini (Amara & Kuhar, 1993) (Figure 1). GAT1 is preferentially localized on neuronal elements with lower expression levels on astrocytes. GAT2 and GAT3 are preferentially expressed in glial cells and BGT1 is expressed in glial cells and astrocytes (White et al., 2002). Furthermore, GATs are heterogeneously expressed in different brain regions and GAT1 is highly abundant within the CNS, whereas GAT3 is exclusively expressed in the brain. GAT2 and BGT1 have been found in many other organs (Yamauchi et al., 1992; Borden et al., 1995; Borden, 1996).

4.2   Pharmacology of GAT Subtypes

Since GABA is the major inhibitory neurotransmitter in the mammalian central nervous system, GATs may be an attractive target for therapies of CNS disorders associated with the GABAergic system, such as sleep disturbances, epilepsy, and various forms of pain (Dalby, 2003; Madsen et al., 2010). The inhibition of GATs in the brain increases synaptic GABA levels and thereby represents a way to stimulate overall GABAergic neurotransmission. Recent research focused on GAT inhibitors suggests novel pharmacological profiles and therapeutic benefits. The GAT1 selective inhibitor tiagabine is a drug used clinically for the treatment of partial seizures associated with epilepsy. In contrast, there are no selective ligands for the three other GAT subtypes reported so far. Previous reports demonstrated a functional role of mouse BGT1 (mBGT1) in the control of neuronal excitability and suggested the possible utility of BGT1-selective inhibitors for the treatment of epilepsy (Schousboe et al., 2004). The search for new selective GABA-uptake inhibitors for GAT subtypes, a very useful target for new drugs, is important.

4.3   Differential Sensitivity of GAT Subtypes to Antidepressants

TCAs, known as the inhibitors of monoamine neurotransmitter transporters, especially the transporters for SERT and NET (Langer & Schoemaker, 1998), are therapeutically useful ligands for the treatment of depression (Eshlemen et al., 1999). Since TCAs have been known to exert inhibitory effects on various targets including channels and transporters, which might be involved in neuropathic pain (Mico et al., 2006), it would be useful to evaluate the potency of TCAs in inhibiting GABA uptake through each GAT subtype including BGT1. To support this idea, Nakashita et al. (1997) reported the inhibitory effects of various antidepressants on the three subtypes of rat GAT (rGAT1 - GAT3). rGAT1 interacts with TCAs at concentrations similar to those of the functional investigation of antidepressant-residue interactions. We analyzed the potency of various TCAs in inhibiting mouse BGT 1 (mBGT1) in comparison with other GAT subtypes using [^{3}H]GABA uptake assays in cell cultures heterologously expressing mouse GAT (mGAT) subtypes. Furthermore, we selected three typical TCAs to evaluate the mode of inhibition by examining the kinetics of transport.

All antidepressants tested here inhibited [³H]GABA uptake through mBGT1 and mGATs in a rank order of potency of mBGT1 > mGAT1-3. Kinetic analyses for maprotilline, mianserine, and trimipramine revealed that they inhibited mBGT1 and mGAT1 noncompetitively, except for mianserine, which competitively inhibited mBGT1. These results provided a clue to investigate the structure-function relationship of mBGT1 using antidepressants as a tool, leading to the identification of potential candidates for the selective and specific inhibition of mBGT1 (Gerile *et al.*, 2012).

4.4   Predicted TCA Binding Site

SLC6 family members have a primary binding site (S1) in the center of the membrane, called the central site (Figure 2) (Yamashita *et al.*, 2005; Skovstrup *et al.*, 2010; Nyola *et al.*, 2010). In the case of LeuT, two Na⁺ ions bind together with the substrate in this site. A subsequent study reported a secondary substrate binding (S2) site in the vestibule, extracellular to the central site (Shi *et al.*, 2008). However, the existence and exact role of this binding site remains controversial (Piscitelli *et al.*, 2010). This extracellular vestibule (S2) is an important interim binding site and the same site at which TCAs and SSRIs molecules had been shown to bind (Zhou *et al.*, 2007; Singh *et al.*, 2007). Our previous results have suggested candidate amino acids interacting with TCA, which may result in the different sensitivity to TCA between mBGT1 and mGAT1 (Gerile *et al.*, 2010). The K448 of mGAT1 and the Q463 of mBGT1, corresponding to the D401 of LeuT, which was suggested to be located in the extracellular vestibule for TCA binding, are the most attractive candidates for possible sites involved in the TCA interaction, since the desipramine molecule was shown to be held in place by a salt bridge it formed with residue D401 (Zhou *et al.*, 2007). Therefore, the Q463 of mBGT1 was suggested to produce higher sensitivity to TCA than mGAT1.

In a previous report, the K490 of human SERT (hSERT), corresponding to the D401 of LeuT, was mutated into a threonine as found in rat SERT and human NET (hNET). The K490 of hSERT has been shown to be involved in the effects of TCA, and the mutant hSERT K490T also exhibited a higher degree of inhibition with desipramine. Gain-of-function mutagenesis findings demonstrated that desipramine bound to the same site in both hSERT and hNET as it does in LeuT (Zhou *et al.*, 2007). In another report, the K448 of rat GAT1, corresponding to the D401 in LeuT, was substituted with glutamate or aspartate and exhibited higher sensitivity to desipramine (Cherubino *et al.*, 2009). The stronger effect of desipramine may have been caused by a salt bridge between the charged tail of the amino group and the negatively charged aspartate or glutamate introduced by the mutation. On the other hand, the substitution of a negative charge in place of K448 caused an increase in sensitivity only to desipramine, while the other TCAs and SSRIs showed the same degree of inhibition as that in the wild type and K448A mutant (Cherubino *et al.*, 2009). They suggested that the mutant with the longer lateral chain, K448E, resulted in being the most inhibited by desipramine, which indicates that not only the charge, but also the steric effects influence this interaction.

I67, A310, Q313, and C413 of mBGT1 are also interesting candidates, whose counterparts are A61, G297, L300, and T400 of mGAT1, and A22, S256, F259, and I359 of LeuT, respectively (Figure 2). These were suggested to be located in the central substrate-binding site, indicating the possibility that these residues are responsible for the difference in sensitivity, not only for substrate transport, but also for the TCA interaction. Since mianserine exhibited the competitive inhibition of mBGT1, but noncompetitive inhibition of mGAT1, it is of interest to investigate the role of these residues in their interaction with TCA.

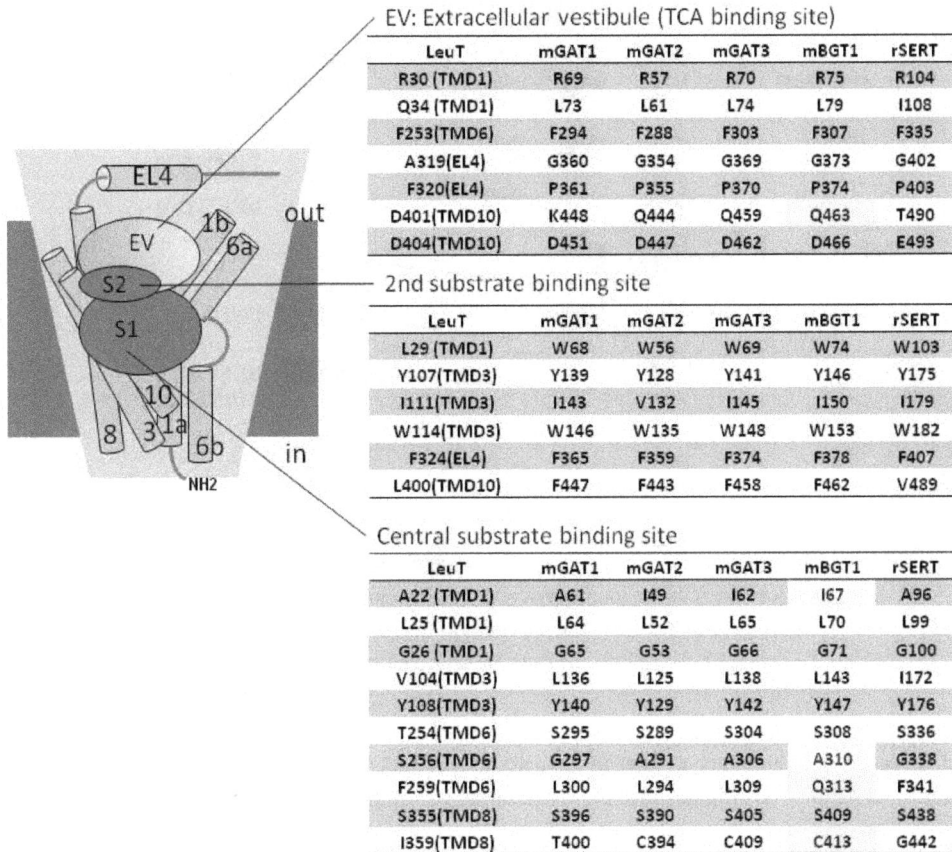

EV: Extracellular vestibule (TCA binding site)

LeuT	mGAT1	mGAT2	mGAT3	mBGT1	rSERT
R30 (TMD1)	R69	R57	R70	R75	R104
Q34 (TMD1)	L73	L61	L74	L79	I108
F253(TMD6)	F294	F288	F303	F307	F335
A319(EL4)	G360	G354	G369	G373	G402
F320(EL4)	P361	P355	P370	P374	P403
D401(TMD10)	K448	Q444	Q459	Q463	T490
D404(TMD10)	D451	D447	D462	D466	E493

2nd substrate binding site

LeuT	mGAT1	mGAT2	mGAT3	mBGT1	rSERT
L29 (TMD1)	W68	W56	W69	W74	W103
Y107(TMD3)	Y139	Y128	Y141	Y146	Y175
I111(TMD3)	I143	V132	I145	I150	I179
W114(TMD3)	W146	W135	W148	W153	W182
F324(EL4)	F365	F359	F374	F378	F407
L400(TMD10)	F447	F443	F458	F462	V489

Central substrate binding site

LeuT	mGAT1	mGAT2	mGAT3	mBGT1	rSERT
A22 (TMD1)	A61	I49	I62	I67	A96
L25 (TMD1)	L64	L52	L65	L70	L99
G26 (TMD1)	G65	G53	G66	G71	G100
V104(TMD3)	L136	L125	L138	L143	I172
Y108(TMD3)	Y140	Y129	Y142	Y147	Y176
T254(TMD6)	S295	S289	S304	S308	S336
S256(TMD6)	G297	A291	A306	A310	G338
F259(TMD6)	L300	L294	L309	Q313	F341
S355(TMD8)	S396	S390	S405	S409	S438
I359(TMD8)	T400	C394	C409	C413	G442

Figure 2: Comparison of the amino acid sequences between mGATs, rat SERT, and LeuT at the regions predicted for antidepressant- and substrate-binding sites.

5   Membrane Trafficking Motif Determined by Site-directed Mutagenesis: A Case for the C-terminal Splice Variants of NET

In this section, we have described our recent study (Sogawa *et al.*, 2007) in which we constructed mutants. We characterized the two major isoforms of human NET, hNET1, which has seven C-terminal amino acids encoded by exon 15, and hNET2, which has 18 amino acids encoded by exon 16, by site-directed mutagenesis in combination with NA uptake assays and cell surface biotinylation. PCR-based mutagenesis was used to delete the various regions encoding exon 14 and exon 15, and to selectively replace amino acids using the overlapping primers in which mutated nucleotides were introduced (Figure 3).

5.1   NET isoforms produced by alternative splicing

Alternative splicing of the neurotransmitter transporters has been reported as a way to regulate their expression and function. We and other laboratories have reported the various NET splice variants in different species including human NET (hNET) (Pacholczyk *et al.*, 1991; Kitayama & Dohi, 2004). These NET variants produced by alternative splicing at the 3'-region were shown to possess different carboxy-

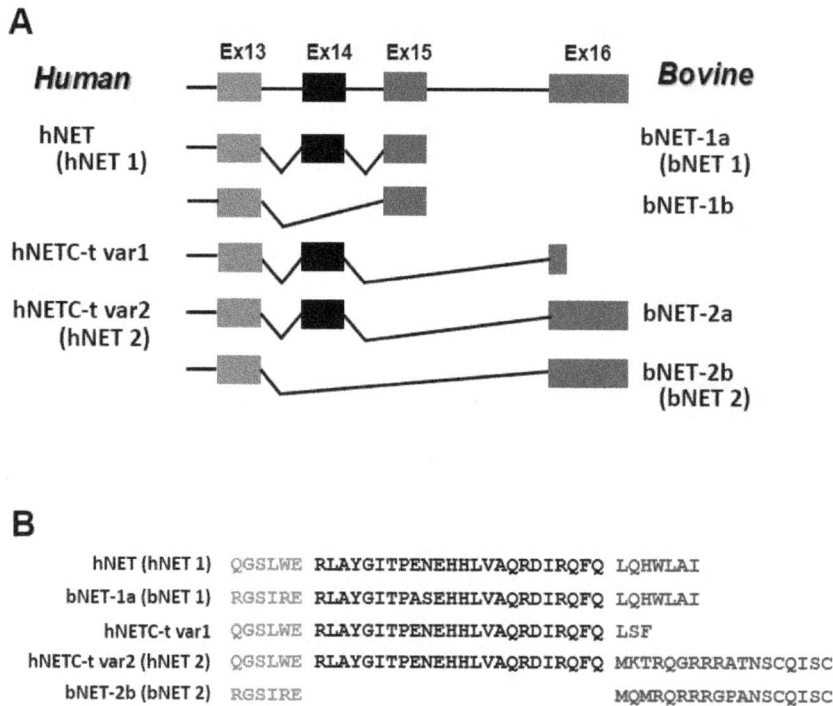

A

Human   Bovine

Ex13 Ex14 Ex15   Ex16

hNET
(hNET 1)   bNET-1a
                                                        (bNET 1)

                                                        bNET-1b

hNETC-t var1

hNETC-t var2   bNET-2a
(hNET 2)

                                                        bNET-2b
                                                        (bNET 2)

B

hNET (hNET 1)   QGSLWE RLAYGITPENEHHLVAQRDIRQFQ LQHWLAI
bNET-1a (bNET 1)   RGSIRE RLAYGITPASEHHLVAQRDIRQFQ LQHWLAI
hNETC-t var1   QGSLWE RLAYGITPENEHHLVAQRDIRQFQ LSF
hNETC-t var2 (hNET 2) QGSLWE RLAYGITPENEHHLVAQRDIRQFQ MKTRQGRRRATNSCQISC
bNET-2b (bNET 2)   RGSIRE   MQMRQRRRGPANSCQISC

Figure 3: (A) Summary of the NET isoforms produced by alternative splicing in the C-terminal region. (B) Alignment of the C-terical region of the NET isoforms.

termini, and had different characteristics of cell surface expression and transport activity (Burton *et al.*, 1998; Pörzgen *et al.*, 1998; Kitayama *et al.*, 1999; Kitayama *et al.*, 2001; Kitayama *et al.*, 2002; Distelmaier *et al.*, 2004).

Two laboratories independently reported homologous bovine (bNET) cDNAs that encoded different C-terminal tails (Lingen *et al.*, 1994; Jursky *et al.*, 1994). bNET1, reported by Lingen *et al.* (1994), was shown to be homologous to human NET (hNET) (Pacholczyk *et al.*, 1991), whereas bNET2, reported by Burton *et al.* (1998), had a different C-terminal tail from hNET and bNET1. Therefore, these isoforms may be produced by alternative pre-mRNA splicing. Analyses of hNET gene organization by Pörzgen *et al.* (1998) demonstrated differences in alternative splicing between human and bovine NET isoforms. They found two additional NET transcripts, designated hNET C-t var1 and hNET C-t var2, which were produced using a different 3'-acceptor site of exon 16 for splicing. These results indicated that the hNET C-t var1 C-terminal encoded by exon 16 had three amino acids, while that of hNET C-t var2 had 18 amino acids. The latter amino acid sequence was homologous to that of bNET2 (Burton *et al*, 1998) (Figure 3). bNET2 skipped both exons 14 and 15 and its c-terminal was homologous to the 18 amino acids of hNET C-t var2 (Figure 3).

We identified bovine NET mRNA expression in the brain and adrenal medulla by RT-PCR and found two additional transcripts produced by alternative splicing (Kitayama *et al.*, 2002). These were produced by the different uses of exon 13, exon 14, exon 15, and exon 16: a newly identified transcript consisting of exon 13-14-16, designated bNET2a, and because the inclusion of exon 14 differed from bNET2 (Jursky *et al.*, 1994); therefore, we designated bNET2 as bNET2b. bNET2a is a homologous counterpart of hNET C-t Var2. Another transcript, designated bNET1b, was shown to consist of exons 13-15 in contrast to exons 13-14-15 of bNET1 (Lingen *et al.*, 1994), with skipping of exon 14; thus, we designated bNET1 as bNET1a. We failed to find a homologous counterpart of hNET C-t var1 in bovine NET transcripts (Figure 3).

5.2   C-terminal Splice Variants: Function and Expression

Pörzgen *et al.* (1998) first demonstrated the expression of hNET splice variant mRNA in SK-N-SH cells, a human neuroblastoma cell line, from which they cloned NET variant cDNAs. NET is known to exist not only in the central nervous system, but also in peripheral neuronal and non-neuronal tissues. The expression of variant NET mRNA was also found in non-neuronal peripheral tissues, such as the placenta and adrenal medulla (Pörzgen *et al.*, 1998; Kitayama *et al.*, 2001).

Kitayama *et al.* (2002) demonstrated the expression of bNET splice variant mRNA in the bovine brain and adrenal medulla by reverse transcriptase-polymerase chain reaction (RT-PCR). All variants including bNET1a, bNET1b, bNET2a, and bNET2b were present in these tissues at possibly different levels. bNET1a appeared to be more abundant than bNET1b in these tissues, while bNET2b appeared to be more abundant than bNET2a (Kitayama *et al.*, 2002, unpublished observation).

At present, there is no useful probe (antibody) to specifically identify NET splice variant proteins. Burton *et al.* (1998) first demonstrated the different intracellular localization of bNET1 (bNET1a) and bNET2 (bNET2b) proteins in stably transfected cells using an antibody that recognizes both isoforms. bNET1a was localized in the plasma membrane, while bNET2b remained mainly within the cytosol.

Kitayama *et al.* (2001) demonstrated the expression of hNET (hNET1), hNET C-t var1, and hNET C-t var2 (hNET2) in transiently transfected COS-7 cells using an immunocytochemical approach. hNET1 and hNET2 were localized in the plasma membrane, whereas hNET2 appeared to be mainly localized in the cytosol, unlike hNET. hNET C-t var1 immunoreactivity was not observed in the plasma membrane. The schematic presentation of the transcriptional and post-transcriptional regulation of hNET was shown in Figure 4.

In addition to the different subcellular localization of NET isoforms as mentioned above, functional analysis of these variants showed different transport activity and pharmacology. Functional expression was only observed with hNET1/bNET1a and hNET2/bNET2a. Furthermore, both hNET2 and bNET2a were associated with a robust uptake of substrates with higher affinities and lower initial velocities than hNET and bNET1a. These results suggested the importance of the C-terminal in the transport activity of NET. The functional importance of the C-terminal region in catecholamine transporters was suggested by the results of investigations performed using site-directed mutagenesis and chimeras between DAT and NET (Bauman & Blakely, 2002; Buck & Amara, 1994; Giros *et al.*, 1994).

5.3   Determination of the motif that controls membrane trafficking

5.3.1   Deletion mutants

Recent studies on the expression and function of the neurotransmitter transporters in model cell expression systems demonstrated that the C-terminal region plays an important role in the cellular regulation of transporter trafficking to the plasma membrane. A candidate exists within the region encoded by exon 14, since we identified bovine NET splice variants skipping exon 14 to exon 15 (bNET1b) or to exon 16

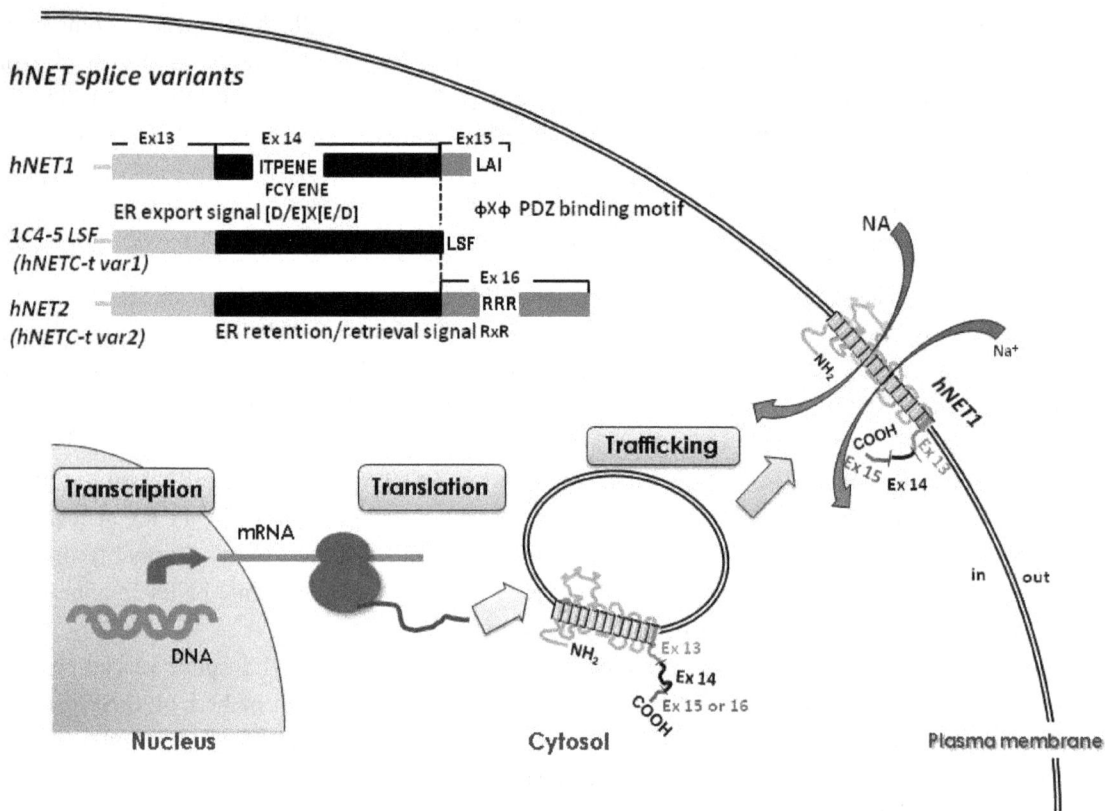

Figure 4: C-terminal structure of hNET splice variants and a schematic presentation of the transcriptional and post-transcriptional regulation of hNET. The important motifs examined are indicated.

(bNET2b), both of which displayed no [³H]noradrenaline transport activity or [³H]nisoxetine binding when expressed in COS-7 cells (Kitayama *et al.*, 2002). We constructed the hNET homologues to bNET1b and bNET2b, hNET lacking exon 14, and hNET2 lacking exon 14, respectively, by truncating the region encoded by exon 14, and examined its impact on the function and expression of NET. To explore the importance of the region encoded by exon 14 further, we constructed deletion mutants in which each of eight amino acids were deleted sequentially or additionally. Mutants lacking either one third or more of the 24 amino acids encoded by exon 14 revealed neither cell surface expression nor NE uptake activity in both isoforms, except that the mutant lacking the last 8 amino acids in hNET2 revealed expression and NE uptake patterns similar to those of the wild-type.

5.3.2   Substitution of Amino Acids Predicted for the Motif

To further address the motif important for the expression of NET variants, we focused on a candidate motif for the ER export signal lying in the C2 cassette within exon 14, ENE, corresponding to the known motif FCYENE observed in K channels (Tejani-Butt, 1992) or D(E)xE(D), the more general motif for trafficking (Figure 5A). We performed consecutive triple-alanine substitutions of these amino acids within this region of hNET1 and hNET2 and compared the results with those obtained from truncation mu-

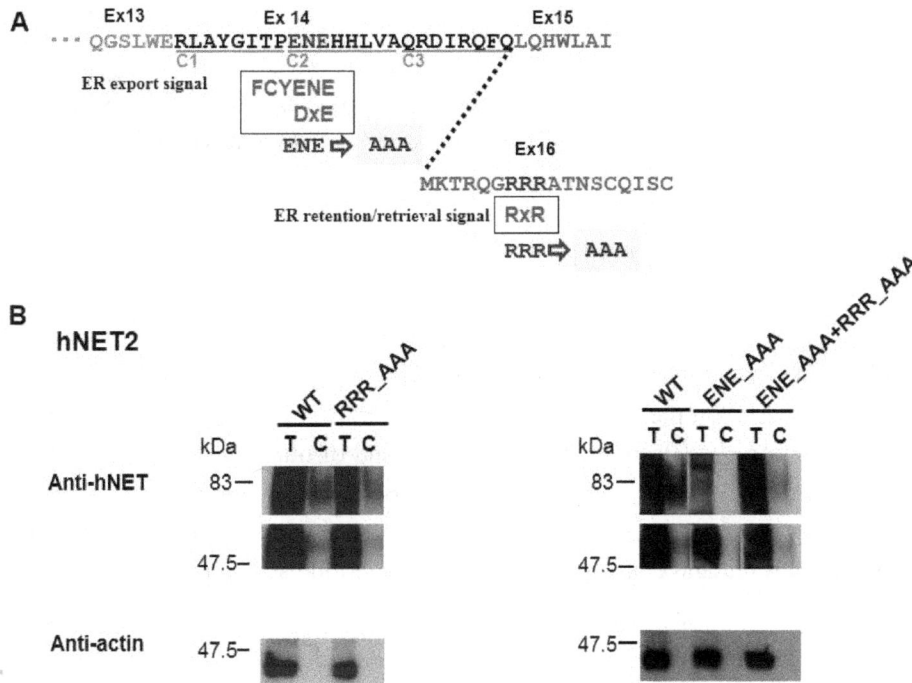

Figure 5: (A) The amino acid sequence in the C-terminal region and truncated and amino acid-substituted mutants of the hNET isoforms. (B) Western blot analyses of the hNET2 WT and mutants of hNET2 by cell surface biotinylation assays. COS-7 cells were transfected with the WT or substitution mutants of hNET2, and subjected to biotinylation assays, as described in section 6. This research was originally published in Biochemical Journal. C. Sogawa *et al*, C-terminal region regulates the functional expression of human noradrenaline transporter splice variants. Biochemical Journal, 2007; 401: 185-195 the Biochemical Society copyright holder.

tants. Triple alanine substitution of the candidate motif (ENE) in this region mimicked the influences of the cassette C2-truncation. The findings that the substitution of alanine for ENE residues caused a marked reduction in cell surface expression, together with a decrease in NE transport activity for both NET1 and NET2, support this possibility.

In addition, the C-terminal region of hNET2 encoded by exon 16 contains residues RRR (617-619), a RxR motif for the ER retrieval signal, suggesting that this may cause lower levels of cell surface expression of hNET2 than hNET1 (Kitayama *et al*., 2001; Bauman & Blakely, 2002; Distelmaier *et al*., 2004, and the present study). Therefore, we decided to perform an alanine substitution of this motif (RRR_AAA) in combination with the ENE_alanine substitution (ENE_AAA). An alanine substitution of RRR, an ER retention motif, in the C-terminus of hNET2 by itself revealed similar expression and function to that of the wild type, while it partly recovered the effects of ENE substitution (Figure 5B). These results suggest that, in addition to the function of the individual C-terminus, the common proximal region encoded by exon 14 differently regulates the functional expression of each splice variant, such as hNET1 and hNET2.

6   Protocols

The following protocols were used for our investigations (Sogawa *et al.*, 2007) as mentioned in section 5. We herein described the methods of DNA constructs, mutagenesis, and functional assays for hNET splice variants.

6.1   Vectors and Site-directed Mutagenesis

6.1.1   Vector Construction

The full-length cDNAs encoding hNET1 and hNET2 were isolated from SK-N-SH cells by RT-PCR with specific primers based on the sequences of human NET cDNA at the 5'-region upstream of the ATG translation initiation site (Pacholczyk *et al.*, 1991) and of our previously isolated clones by 3'-RACE (DDBJ accession numbers, AB022846 and AB022847). These were subcloned into the mammalian expression plasmid vector, pcDNA3 (Invitrogen). Every sixteen clones from each PCR amplification were analyzed and confirmed for correct nucleotide sequences.

6.1.2   Site-directed Mutagenesis

PCR-based mutagenesis was used to delete the various regions encoded by exons 14 and 15, and to selectively replace amino acids using overlapping primers, in which mutated nucleotides were introduced. The C-terminal-truncated mutants of hNET1 were created by introducing stop codons into the coding region of NET. After mutagenesis, these products were subcloned into the pGEM-T Easy TA cloning vector (Promega), and the results were verified by automated sequencing. Restriction fragments containing mutated sequences were digested with appropriate restriction enzymes, and subcloned into pcDNA3.

6.2   Cell Preparation and Transfection

6.2.1   Cell Culture

COS-7 cells (RIKEN Cell Bank, Tsukuba, Japan) were maintained in Dulbecco's modified Eagle's medium supplemented with 10% (v/v) fetal calf serum at 37°C in a 5% CO_2/95% air atmosphere.

6.2.2   Transfection

Transient transfections were performed using electroporation or liposomes. COS-7 cells at subconfluence were harvested and transfected with cDNA ($10\mu g/10^7$ cells) by electroporation for uptake assays. A parallel transfection with the pcDNA3 vector alone was performed each time as a negative control. After electroporation, cells were diluted in the cultured medium, plated in 24- or 48-well culture plates, and cultured for 2-3 days. Cells at subconfluence in 60mm diameter culture dishes (for immunoblotting) or in 4-well culture slides (for immunocytochemical analysis) were transfected with cDNA ($0.2\mu g/cm^2$ for culture plastic ware) for immunological analysis using FuGENE6[TM] transfection reagent (Roche Diagnostics, Mannheim, Germany) according to the manufacturer's instructions.

6.3   Analysis of Function and Expression

6.3.1   Uptake Assay

Cells were washed three times with oxygenated KRH (Krebs-Ringer Hepes-buffered solution; 125mM NaCl, 5.2mM KCl, 1.2mM $CaCl_2$, 1.4mM $MgSO_4$, 1.2mM KH_2PO_4, 5mM glucose, and 20mM Hepes, pH 7.3 ± 0.1) and incubated for 10min at 37°C with [^{3}H] labeled substrate in the presence of 0.1mM ascorbate and 50μM pargyline, as described previously (Kitayama et al., 2001). After the removal of excess radioligands, the cells were rapidly washed three times with ice-cold KRH and any radioactivity remaining in the cells was extracted with NaOH and measured by liquid scintillation spectrometry (RI Research Center, Okayama University Dental School, Okayama, Japan). Non-specific uptake was determined in the mock-transfected cells and also in each plate in the presence of specific inhibitors.

6.3.2   Binding Assay

Binding of nisoxetine, a specific ligand for NET, to plasma membrane NET was evaluated using radiolabeled nisoxetine and intact cells on ice. Transfected COS cells were washed with ice-cold KRH and incubated with 2 nM [^{3}H]nisoxetine in KRH for 2h on ice. Nonspecific binding was examined in the presence of 10 μM nisoxetine. Cells were incubated in KRH containing 2 nM [^{3}H]nisoxetine and 1-1000 nM cold nisoxetine for cold saturation analysis. Cells were incubated with 0.1-100 nM [^{3}H]nisoxetine in the presence or absence of 10 μM nisoxetine for hot saturation analysis (Kitayama et al., 1999).

6.3.3   Cell Surface Biotinylation and Western Blot Analysis

Cells grown in culture dishes 60mm in diameter were washed with ice-cold PBS, and then incubated for 120 min at 4°C with 1 mg/ml sulfo-NHS-SS-biotin under gentle agitation. Cells were then washed three times with ice cold PBS, collected with and solubilized in RIPA buffer [PBS containing 1% (v/v) Nonidet P40, 0.5% sodium deoxycholate, and 0.1% SDS], and then incubated at 4°C for 30 min. Non-lysates were removed by centrifugation for 20min at 20,000 g, and the biotinylated proteins were precipitated with NeutrAvidin^{TM} beads by incubating overnight at 4°C with gentle shaking. The precipitated proteins were then washed five times with RIPA buffer, and denatured by heating the beads in sample buffer at 95°C for 5min. Samples were analyzed by SDS-PAGE (5-20% gel, BioRad, Tokyo Japan), and transferred onto a PVDF membrane (GE Healthcare Biosciences, Buckinghamshire, UK). Western blotting was performed with a monoclonal mouse antibody to hNET (NET17-1) followed by a secondary antibody conjugated to horseradish peroxidase, and bands were detected by ECL (enhanced chemiluminescence; GE Healthcare Biosciences) on autoradiographic film (GE Healthcare Biosciences).

6.3.4   Immunocytochemistry

Cells were grown on Biocoat culture slides for immunostaining experiments. Cells were initially rinsed with Ca^{2+}- and Mg^{2+}-containing PBS, then fixed in 4% (w/v) paraformaldehyde. After washing three times with PBS, they were permeabilized in PBS containing 0.1% Triton X-100 for 10min and incubated in blocking solution [5% (v/v) goat serum] for 1h. The cells were incubated with a mouse anti-hNET monoclonal antibody (diluted 1:100) for 1h at room temperature (20-22°C) followed by incubation with a FITC-conjugated goat anti-mouse secondary antibody. They were then washed three times with PBS, and the filter containing the cells was excised from its support and mounted on a slide with Perma Fluor aqueous mounting medium (Thermo Shandon, Pittsburg, PA, USA). Immunofluorescent images were generated using a Zeiss LSM510 laser scanning confocal microscope (Central Research Laboratory, Okayama University Medical School, Okayama, Japan).

7   Concluding Remarks

Neurotransmitter transporters terminate neurotransmission by reuptaking, and thus clearing neurotransmitters from the synaptic cleft. They belong to solute carrier (SLC) gene families and Na^+/Cl^--dependent neurotransmitter transporters (neurotransmitter sodium symporters: NSSs), referred to as the SLC6 gene family. This family is the largest and includes transporters for monoamines, amino acids, osmolytes and energy metabolites. It also plays critical roles in regulating neurotransmission and homeostasis by mediating the uptake of released neurotransmitters. Neurotransmitter transporters, especially NSSs, are the targets of therapeutic drugs used in the treatment of psychiatric diseases including depression and psychostimulants such as cocaine and amphetamines. Cloning of their cDNAs has facilitated understanding of the structure-function relationship of these transporters. The recent success of X-ray crystallographic studies on the bacterial homolog of the mammalian NSS, LeuT, further advanced this field. However, difficulties are still associated with determining the structure of mammalian transporters, which prompted us to address this issue and investigate their structure-function relationships.

In this review, we summarized recent progress in the application of site-directed mutagenesis to determining the structure-function relationships of NSSs. When this was combined with functional assays of the mutant, this method allowed us to identify the unique structural motifs interacting with ligands (including substrates and drugs such as antidepressants and psychostimulants) within the transporters. These mutations sometimes caused loss-of-function mutations due to the absence of expression at the cell surface. Therefore, it remains difficulties to conclude the role of particular amino acid residues in functional properties. To facilitate methodological considerations, molecular biological and protein engineering techniques were additionally introduced by comparing their benefits and limitations. The major goals of transporter research are to understanding how the transporter works at the molecular level, how ligand binding and Na^+/Cl^- binding couple, and what determines the stoichiometry of ligand binding. X-ray crystallography of mammalian NSSs has emphasized the exact nature of the transporter interacting with ligands. However, in the absence of atomic resolution structures for these transporters other molecular tools need to be used. Differences in the pharmacological profiles of LeuT and mammalian neurotransmitter transporters, combined with site-directed mutagenesis, have been used as a rational strategy to localize domains and residues critical for ligand interactions. Furthermore, a combination of site-directed mutagenesis and computer modeling has also been a helpful approach adopted by many researchers. These techniques will be beneficial in future studies to advance understanding of the structure-function relationships of various proteins including neurotransmitter transporters.

Rusmussen *et al.* recently succeeded in obtaining an agonist-bound, active-state β_2-adrenoceptor crystal structure. They identified a camelid antibody fragment (nanobody) that exhibited G protein-like behavior towards the β_2-adrenoceptor (Rusmussen *et al.*, 2011a). They also elucidated the crystal structure of the active state ternary complex composed of an agonist-occupied monomeric β_2-adrenoceptor and nucleotide-free Gs heterotrimer (Rusmussen *et al.*, 2011b). Krishnamurthy and Gouaux mutated residues and used conformation-specific antibody fragments to stabilize the substrate-free and inward-open states in order to analyze the X-ray structure of LeuT. Regarding future studies on neurotransmitter transporters, X-ray crystallography of mammalian transporters according to the strategy of β_2-adrenoceptor and LeuT has emphasized the exact nature of the transporter interacting with ligands such as antidepressants and psychostimulants including cocaine. This achievement has also facilitated understanding of the structure-function relationship of the transporter in collaboration with different approaches including site-directed mutagenesis, functional assays, and novel X-ray crystallography techniques.

References

Amara, S.G. & Kuhar, M.J. (1993). Neurotransmitter transporters: Recent progress. Annual Review of Neuroscience, 16, 73-93.

Axelrod, J., Whitby, L. G. & Hertting, G. (1961). Effect of psychotropic drugs on the uptake of H^3-norepinephrine by tissues. Science, 133, 383-384.

Barker, L. B., Kimmel, L. H. & Blakely, D. R. (1995). Chimeric human and rat serotonin transporters reveal domains involved in recognition of transporter ligands. Molecular Pharmacology, 48, 799-807.

Bauman, P. A. & Blakely R. D. (2002). Determinants within the C-terminus of the human norepinephrine transporter dictate transporter trafficking, stability, and activity. Archives of Biochemistry and Biophysics, 404, 80-91.

Beurming, T., Shi, L., Javitch, J. A. & Weinstein, H. (2006). A comprehensive structure-based alignment of prokaryotic and eukaryotic neurotransmitter/Na^+ symporters (NSS) aids in the use of the LeuT structure to probe NSS structure and function. Molecular Pharmacology, 70, 1630-1642.

Blakely, R. D., Berson, H. E., Fremeau, R. T., Jr., Caron M. G., Peek, M. M. & Prince, H. K. (1991). Cloning and expression of a functional serotonin transporter from rat brain. Nature, 354, 66-70.

Borden, L. A., Smith, K. E., Harting, P. R., Bramchek, T. A. & Weinshank, R. L. (1992). Molecular heterogeneity of the gamma-aminobutyric acid (GABA) transport system. Cloning of two novel high affinity GABA transporters from rat brain. Journal of Biological Chemistry, 267, 21098-21104.

Borden, L. A., Smith, K. E, Gustafson, E.L., Branchek, T.A. & Weinshank, R.L. (1995). Cloning and expression of a betaine/GABA transporter from human brain. Journal of Neurochemistry, 64, 977-984.

Borden, L. A. (1996). GABA transporter heterogeneity: pharmacology and cellular localization, Neurochemistry International, 29, 335-356.

Bröer, S. & Gether, U. (2012). The solute carrier 6 family of transporters. British Journal of Pharmacology, 167, 256-278.

Buck, J. K. & Amara, S. G. (1995). Structural domains of catecholamine transporter chimeras involved in selective inhibition by antidepressants and psychomotor stimulants. Molecular Pharmacology, 48, 1030-1037.

Burton, L.D., Kippenberger, A.G., Lingen, B., Brüss, M., Bönisch, H., & Christie, D.L. (1998). A variant of the bovine noradrenaline transporter reveals the importance of the C-terminal region for correct targeting to the membrane and functional expression. Biochemical Journal, 330, 909-914.

Chen, J. G., Sachpaatzidis, A. & Rudnick, G. (1997). The third transmembrane domain of the serotonin transporter contains residues associated with substrate and cocaine binding. Journal of Biological Chemistry, 272(45), 28321-28327.

Cherubino, F., Miszner, A., Renna, M.D., Sangaletti, R., Giovannardi, S. & Bossi, E. (2009). GABA transporter lysine 448: a key residue for tricyclic antidepressants interaction. Cellular and Molecular Life Sciences, 66, 3797-3808.

Dalby, N.O. (2003). Inhibition of γ-aminobutyric acid uptake: anatomy, physiology and effects against epileptic seizures. European Journal of Pharmacology, 479, 127-137.

Distelmaier, F. Wiedemann, P. Brüss, M. & Bönisch, H. (2004). *Functional importance of the C-terminus of the human norepinephrine transporter. Journal of Neurochemistry, 91, 537-546.*

Eshleman, A. J., Carmolli, M., Cumbay, M., Martens, C., Neve, K. A. & Janowsky, A. (1997). *Characteristics of Drug interactions with recombinant biogenic amine transporters expressed in the same cell type. The Journal of Pharmacology and Experimental Therapeutics, 289, 877-885.*

Fremeau, R. T., Caron, M. G., & Blakely, R. D. (1992). *Molecular cloning and expression of a high affinity L-proline transporter expressed in putative glutamatergic pathways of rat brain. Neuron, 8, 915-926.*

Gabrielsen, M., Ravna, A. W., Kristiansen, K. & Sylte, I. (2012a). *Substrate binding and translocation of serotonin transporter studied by docking and molecular dynamics simulations. Journal of Molecular Modeling, 18, 1073-1085.*

Gabrielsen, M., Kurczab, R., Ravna, A. W., Kufareva, I., Abagyan, R., Chilmonczyk, Z., Bojarski, A. J. & Sylte, I. (2012b). *Molecular mechanism of serotonin transporter inhibition elucidated by a new flexible docking protocol. European Journal of Medicinal Chemistry, 47, 24-37.*

Gerile, Sogawa, C., Ohyama, K., Masuko, T., Kusama, T., Morita, K., Sogawa, N. & Kitayama, S. (2010). *Inhibitory action of antidepressants on mouse betaine/GABA transporter (BGT1) heterologously expressed in cell cultures. International Journal of Molecular Sciences, 13, 2578-2589.*

Gether, U., Andersen, P. H., Larsson, O. M. & Schousboe, A. (2006). *Neurotransmitter transporters: molecular function of important drug targets. Trends in Pharmacological Sciences, 27, 375-383.*

Giros, B., Wand, Y-M., Suter, S., Mcleskey, B.S., Pifi, C. & Caron, G. M. (1994). *Delineation of discrete domains for substrate, cocaine, and tricyclic antidepressant interactions using chimeric dopamine-norepinephrine transporters. Journal of Biological Chemistry, 269, 15985-15988.*

Giros, B., Jaber, M., Jones, S.R., Wightman, R.M. & Caron, M.G. (1996). *Hyperlocomotion and indifference to cocaine and amphetamine in mice lacking the dopamine transporter. Nature, 379, 606–612.*

Gu, H., Wall, S. C. & Rudnick, G. (1994). *Stable expression of biogenic amine transporters reveals differences in inhibitor sensitivity, kinetics, and ion dependence. Journal of Biological Chemistry, 269, 7124-7130.*

Gu, H., Wall, S. & Rudnick, G. (1996). *Ion soupling stoichiometry for the norepinephrine transporter in membrane vesicles from stably transfected cells. Journal of Biological Chemistry, 271, 6911-6916.*

Guastella, J., Nelson, N., Nelson, H., Czyzyk, L., Keynan, S., Miedel, M. C., Davidson, N., Lester, H. A. & Kanner, B. I. (1990). *Cloning and expression of a rat brain GABA transporter. Science, 249, 1303-1306.*

Guastella, J., Brecha, N., Weigmann, C., Lester, H. A. & Davidson, N. (1992). *Cloning, expression, and localization of a rat brain high-affinity glycine transporter. Proceedings of National Academy of Sciences of USA, 89, 7189-7193.*

Iversen, L. L. (1971). *Role of transmitter uptake mechanisms in synaptic neurotransmission. British Journal of Pharmacology, 41, 571-591.*

Jardetzky, O. (1996). *Simple allosteric model for membrane pumps. Nature, 211, 969-970.*

Javitch, J. A. (1998). *Probing structure of neurotransmitter transporters by substituted-cysteine accessibility method. Methods in Enzymology, 296, 331-346.*

Jeschke, G. (2013). *A comparative study of structures and structural transitions of secondary transporters with the LeuT fold. European Biophysics Journal, 42, 181-197.*

Jursky, F., Tamura, S., Tamura, A., Mandiyan, S., Nelson, H. & Nelson, N. (1994). *Structure, function and brain localization of neurotransmitter transporters. Journal of Experimental Biology, 196, 283-295.*

Kanner, B. I. (1994). *Sodium-coupled neurotransmitter transporters: structure, function and regulation. Journal of Experimental Biology, 196, 237-249.*

Keshet, G. I., Bendahan, A., Su, H., Mager, S., Lester, H. A. & Kanner, B. I. (1995). *Glutamate-101 is critical for the function of the sodium and chloride-coupled GABA transporter GAT-1. FEBS Letter, 371, 69-42*

Kilty, J. E., Lorang, D. & Amara S. G. (1991). *Cloning and expression of cocaine-sensitive rat dopamine transporter. Science, 254, 578-279.*

Kitayama, S., Shimada, S., Xu H., Markham L., Donovan D. M. & Uhl G. R. (1992). *Dopamine transporter site-directed mutations differentially alter substrate transport and cocaine binding. Proceedings of National Academy of Sciences of USA, 89, 7782-7785.*

Kitayama, S. & Dohi, T. (2003). *Norepinephrine transporter splice variants and their interaction with substrates and blockers. European Journal of Pharmacology, 479, 65-70.*

Kitayama, S., Ikeda, T., Mitsuhata, C., Sato, T., Morita, K. & Dohi, T. (1999). *Dominant negative isoform of rat norepinephrine transporter produced by alternative RNA splicing. Journal of Biological Chemistry, 274, 10731-10736.*

Kitayama, S., Morita, K. & Dohi, T. (2001). *Functional characterization of the splicing variants of human norepinephrine transporter. Neuroscience Letter, 312, 108-112.*

Kitayama, S., Kumagai, K., Morita, K. & Dohi, T. (2002). *Identification and functional characterization of the novel isoforms of bovine norepinephrine transporter produced by alternative splicing. Brain Research, 934, 152-156*

Krishnamurthy, H. & Gouaux, E. (2012). *X-ray structures of LeuT in substrate-free outward-open and apo inward-open states. Nature, 481, 469-474.*

Langer, Z. S. & Schoemaker, H., (1988). *Effects of antidepressants on monoamine transporters. Progress in Neuro-psychopharmacology & Biological Psychiatry, 12, 193-216.*

Lee, S. H., Chang, M. Y., Lee, K. H., Park, B. S., Lee, Y. S., Chin, H. R. & Lee Y. S. (2000). *Important of valine at position 152 for the substrate transport and 2beta-carbomethoxy-3beta-(4-fluorophenyl) tropane binding of dopamine transporter. Molecular Pharmacology, 57, 883-889.*

Lingen, B., Brüss, M. & Bönisch, H. (1994). *Cloning and expression of the bovine sodium-and chloride-dependent noradrenaline transporter. FEBS Letters, 342, 235-238.*

Liu, Q. R., Lopez-Corcuera, B., Nelson, H., Mandiyan, S. & Nelson, N. (1992a). *Cloning and expression of a cDNA encoding the transporter of taurine and beta-alanine in mouse brain. Proceedings of the National Academy of Sciences of USA, 89, 12145-12149.*

Liu, Q. R., Nelson, H., Mandiyan, S., Lopez-Corcuera, B., & Nelson, N. (1992b). *Cloning and expression of a glycine transporter from mouse brain. FEBS Letter, 305, 110-114.*

Manepalli, S., Surratt, C. K., Madura, J. D. & Nolan, T. L. (2012). *Monoamine transporter structure, function, dynamics, and drug discovery: a computational perspective. The AAPS Journal, 14, 820-831.*

Madsen, K.K., White, H.S., & Schousboe, A. (2010). *Neuronal and non-neuronal GABA transporters as targets for antiepileptic drugs. Pharmacology and Therapeutics, 125, 394-401.*

Mayser, W., Schloss, P., & Betz, H. (1992). *Primary structure and functional expression of a choline transporter expressed in the rat nervous system. FEBS Letter, 305, 31-36.*

Mico, J.A., Ardid, D., Berrocoso, E., & Eschalier, A. (2006). *Antidepressants and pain. TRENDS in Pharmacological Science, 27, 348-354.*

Mitrovic, A. D., Amara, S. G., Johnston, G. A. R. & Vandenberg, R. J. (1998). *Identification of functional domains of the human glutamate transporters EAAT1 and EAAT2. Journal of Biological Chemistry, 273 (24), 14698-14706.*

Nakashita, M., Sasaki, K., Sakai, N., & Saito, N., (1997). *Effects of tricyclic and tetracyclic antidepressants on the three types of GABA transporter. Neuroscience Research, 29, 87-91.*

Nyola, A., Karpowich, N. K., Zhen, J., Marden, J., Reith, M.E. & Wang, D-N. (2010). *Substrate and drug binding sites in LeuT. Current Opinion Structural Biology, 20, 415-422.*

Pacholczyk, T., Blakely, R.D. & Amara, S.G. (1991). *Expression cloning of a cocaine- and antidepressant-sensitive human noradrenaline transporter. Nature, 350, 350-354. P*

Piscitelli, C., Krishnamurthy, H. & Gouaux, E. (2010), Neurotransmitter / sodium symporter orthologue LeuT has a single high-affinity substrate site. Nature, 468, 1129-1132.

Pörzgen, P., Bönisch, H., Hammermann, R. & Brüss, M. (1998). The human noradrenaline transporter gene contains multiple polyadenylation sites and two alternatively spliced C-terminal exons. Biochimica Biophysica Acta, 1398, 365-370.

Radian, R., Bendahan, A. & Kanner, B. I. (1986). Purification and identification of the functional sodium- and chloride-coupled γ-aminobutyric acid transport glycoprotein from rat brain. Journal of Biological Chemistry, 261, 15437-15441.

Ravna, A. W., Sylte I. & Dahl, S. G. (2009). Structure and localization of drug binding sites on neurotransmitter transporters. Journal of Molecular Modeling, 15, 1155-1164.

Rusmussen, S. G., Choi, H-J., Fung J. J., Pardon, F., Casarosa, P., Chae, P. S., DeVree, B. T., Rosenbaum, D. M., Thian, F. S., Kobilka, T. S., Schnapp, A., Konetzki, I., Sunahara, R. K., Gellman, S. H., Pautsch, A., Steyaert, J., Weis, W. I. & Kobilka, B. K. (2011a). Structure of a nanobody-stabilized active state of the β2-adrenoceptor. Nature, 469, 175-180.

Rusmussen, S. G., DeVree, B. T., Zou, Y., Kruse, A. C., Chung, K. Y., Kobilka, T. S., Thian, F. S., Chae, P. S., Pardon, E., Calinski, D., Mathiesen, J. M., Shah, S. T. A., Lyos, J. A., Caffrey, M., Gellman, S. H., Steyaert, J., Skiniotis, G., Weis, W. I., Sunahara, R. K. & Kobilka, B. K. (2011b). Crystal structure of the β2 adrenergic receptor-Gs protein complex. Nature, 477, 549-555.

Schousboe, A., Larsson, O.M., Sarup, A., & White, H.S. (2004). Role of the betaine/GABA transporter (BGT-1/GAT2) for the control of epilepsy. European Journal of Pharmacology, 500, 281-287.

Seal, R. P. & Amara, S. G., (1998). A reentrant loop domain in the glutamate carrier EAAT1 participates in substrate binding and translocation. Neuron, 21, 1487-1498.

Shi, L., Quick, M., Zhao, Y., Weinstein, H. & Javitch, J. A. (2008). The mechanism of a neurotransmitter:Ssodium symporter-inward release of Na+ and substrate in triggerd by substrate in second binding site. Molecular Cell, 30, 667-677.

Singh, S. K., Yamashita, A. & Gouaux, E. (2007). Antidepressant binding site in a bacterial homolog of neurotransmitter transporters. Nature, 448, 952-956.

Singh, S. K., Piscitelli, C. L., Yamashita, A. & Gouaux, E. (2008). A Competitive inhibitor traps LeuT in an open-to out conformation. Science, 322, 1655-1661.

Skovstrup, S., Taboureau, O., Brauner-Osborne, H., Jorgensen, F. S. (2010). Homology modeling of the GABA transporter and analysis of tiagabine binding. Chem Med Chem, 5, 986-1000.

Smicun, Y., Campbell, S. D., Chen, M. A., Gu, H. & Rudnick, G. (1999). The role of external loop regions in serotonin transport. Journal of Biological Chemistry, 274, 36058-36064.

Smith, K. E., Borden, L. A., Harting, P. R., Branchek, T. & Weinshank, R. L. (1992). Cloning and expression of a glycine transporter reveal colocalization with NMDA receptors. Neuron, 8, 927-935.

Sogawa, C., Kumagai, K., Sogawa, N., Morita, K., Dohi, T. & Kitayama, S. (2007). C-terminal region regulates the functional expression of human noradrenaline transporter splice variants. Biochemical Journal, 401, 185-195.

Tejani-Butt, S. M. (1992). [³H]Nisoxetine: a radioligand for quantitation of norepinephrine uptake sites by autoradiography or by homogenate binding. Journal of Pharmacology and Experimental Therapeutics, 260, 427-436.

Valenstein, E. S. (2005). The war of the soups and the sparks: the discovery of neurotransmitters and the dispute over how nerves communicate. Columbia University Press.

White, H. S., Sarup, A., Bolving, T., Kristensen, A. S., Petersen, G., Nelson, N., Pickering, D. S., Larsson, O. M., Frølund, B., Krogsgaard-larsen, P. & Schousboe, A. (2002). Correlation between anticonvulsant activity and inhibitory action on glial γ-minobutyric acid uptake of the highly selective mouse γ-aminobutyric acid transporter 1 inhibitor 3-hydroxy-4-amino-4,5,6,7-tetrahydro-1,2-benzisoxazole and its N-alkylated analogs. The Journal of Pharmacology and Experimental Therapeutics, 302 (2), 636-644.

Yamauchi, A., Uchida, S., Kwon, H.M., Preston, A. S., Robey, R. B., Garcia-Perez, A., Burg, M.B. & Handler, J.S. (1992). Cloning of a Na$^+$- and Cl$^-$-dependent betaine transporter that is regulated by hypertonicity. Journal of Biological Chemistry, 267, 649-652.

Yamashita, A., Singh, S.K., Kawate, T., Jin, Y. & Gouaux, E. (2005). Crystal structure of a bacterial homologue of Na$^+$/Cl$^-$ dependent neurotransmitter transporters. Nature, 437, 215-223.

Zhou, Z., Zhen, J., Karpowich, N. K., Goetz, R. M., Law, C. J., Reith, M. E. A. & Wang, D.N. (2007). LeuT-desipramine structure reveals how antidepressants block neurotransmitter reuptake. Science, 317, 1390-1393.

The Use of Peptides Derived from G Protein-Coupled Receptors and Heterotrimeric G Proteins in the Study of their Structures and Functions

Alexander O. Shpakov
Department of Biochemistry
Sechenov Institute of Evolutionary Physiology and Biochemistry
Russian Academy of Sciences, St. Petersburg, Russia

Elena A. Shpakova
Department of Chemistry of Biologically Active Polymers
Institute of Macromolecular Compounds
Russian Academy of Sciences, St. Petersburg, Russia

1 Introduction

The transduction of hormonal signal from the surface receptor to the intracellular effector proteins controlling the fundamental cellular processes requires coordinated functioning of many signal proteins and is realized via both G protein-dependent and G protein-independent signaling cascades (Patel et al., 2004; Marty & Ye, 2010; George et al., 2012). The initial step of signal transduction is recognition and further specific binding of ligand with extracellular domains of sensor protein, such as G protein-coupled receptor (GPCR) that seven times penetrates the plasma membrane or the tyrosine kinase receptor having a single transmembrane region and a largest intracellular domain possessing the intrinsic tyrosine kinase activity.

A classical G protein-dependent signaling system involves GPCR, heterotrimeric G protein and, as a third component, the enzyme, generator of second messengers, or the G protein-regulated ionic channel. The superfamily of GPCR comprises a large group of cell surface receptors capable of binding a wide diversity of molecules, including amino acids and their derivatives, nucleotides, peptides, proteins, odorants, as well as photons and ions (Luttrell, 2006; Heitzler et al., 2009; George et al., 2012). GPCR are involved in the regulation and modulation of growth, differentiation, metabolism, neurotransmission, cell communication, and many other physiological events (Lohse & Hoffmann, 2009). All members of the GPCR superfamily share the same architecture and contain seven helical transmembrane regions (TM1–TM7) forming a transmembrane channel, an extracellular amino-terminal domain (NTD), an intracellular carboxy-terminal domain (CTD), three extracellular (ECL1–ECL3) and three intracellular loops (ICL1–ICL3). In a majority of GPCR, the ECL contain regions involved in the recognition and low-affinity binding of ligand, while a transmembrane channel and ECL/TM interfaces form a high-affinity ligand-binding site (Schwartz et al., 2006). The ICL and CTD are responsible for specific interactions with heterotrimeric G proteins and other intracellular proteins including the RGS (Regulators of G protein Signaling) proteins, arrestins, PDZ domain-containing proteins, G protein-coupled receptor kinases (Bockaert et al., 2008).

The heterotrimeric G proteins, an ancient family of membrane-attached regulatory proteins composed of three types of subunits, α, β and γ, transduce signal from GPCR to G protein-dependent effector proteins such as adenylyl cyclases (AC), phosphoinositide-specific phospholipases Cβ (PLCβ), cyclic nucleotide-specific phosphodiesterases, phosphatidylinositol 3-kinases, and some types of G protein-regulated ion channels (Offermanns, 2003; Birnbaumer, 2007; Smrcka, 2008; Woehler & Ponimaskin, 2009). G proteins consist of guanine nucleotide-binding Gα subunit that binds and hydrolyzes GTP and of closely associated G$\beta\gamma$ complex, both participating in hormonal signaling and interacting with specific targets in cell. G proteins fall into four main families based on the sequence similarity of Gα subunits: G$_{s/olf}$ proteins mediating activation of AC followed by an increase of intracellular cAMP level; G$_{i/o}$ proteins mediating AC inhibition and/or modulation of a number of Ca^{2+} and K$^+$ channels (via G$\beta\gamma$ complex) and the related G$_t$ proteins expressed in retina and mediating phototransduction via regulation of phosphodiesterase-γ activity; G$_{q/11,14,15/16}$ proteins mediating activation of PLCβ; and G$_{12/13}$ proteins mediating regulation of Rho guanine nucleotide exchange factors, which results in activation of small GTPase RhoA. The activation of GPCR by appropriate agonists induces a conformational change in GDP-bound Gα subunit and promotes the exchange of GDP for GTP, thereby leading to dissociation of the GTP-bound Gα subunit and the G$\beta\gamma$ complex. Binding of GTP gives rise to structural rearrangement within three segments of Gα subunit referred to as "switch" regions I–III due to their interaction with γ-phosphate of the bound GTP, this leads to conformational changes in the Gα subunit and allows specific recognition of downstream effector proteins. The cycle is terminated by the hydrolysis of GTP due to GTPase activity of Gα subunit. Then the GDP-bound Gα subunit reassociates with Gβγ dimer to enter another activation cycle (Johnston & Siderovski, 2007; Zheng *et al.*, 2010).

The regions of GPCR and G proteins participating in their interaction and responsible for transfer of hormonal signal to intracellular effector proteins are rather short and usually contain 8–25 amino acid residues (Shpakov & Pertseva, 2007; Parker *et al.*, 2011; Thaker *et al.*, 2012). Inducing minimal conformational changes in these regions, the replacement and the structural modification of amino acids can drastically influence the functional activity of signal proteins, disrupt the signal transduction and induce pathological alteration in the organs and tissues (Spiegel, 2007; Vassart & Costagliola, 2011). As was shown by several authors, synthetic peptides corresponding to these regions are able to trigger signaling cascades in the absence of hormonal stimulus, modulate protein–protein interaction and influence the functional activity of signal proteins induced by changes in their regulatory and catalytic sites (Wess, 1997; Covic *et al.*, 2007; Shpakov & Pertseva, 2007; Miller *et al.*, 2009; Dimond *et al.*, 2011; Shpakov, 2011a, 2011b; Tressel *et al.*, 2011; O'Callaghan *et al.*, 2012a). This allows a suggestion that a majority of functionally important regions in GPCR and G proteins are stabilized by relatively short-range interactions responsible for stabilization of conformation of rather small peptides mimicking these regions. It should be also taken into account that the interaction of peptide with the complementary regions of signal protein or with hydrophobic membrane surface can induce conformational changes in peptide molecule and make its three-dimensional (3D) structure close to that of the homologous region in full-size protein. Thus, the study of peptides, derivatives of GPCR and G proteins, has been used as an excellent tool to establish the 3D structure of these signal proteins and their functional domains and to make the mapping of functionally important sites in them. It should be noted at this point that the synthetic peptides derived from GPCR, including bacterial and mammalian rhodopsins, opioid and thromboxane receptors, were shown to adopt 3D structure similar to those observed by X-ray crystallography (Yeagle & Albert, 1998; Yeagle *et al.*, 2001; Choi *et al.*, 2002; Zhang *et al.*, 2002; Wu *et al.*, 2003; Fadhil *et al.,* 2004). Furthermore, the structural analysis of full-length GPCR was strongly limited by the difficulties in expression, purification, and their *in vitro* stability. Consequently, GPCR-peptides are a good alternative for studying the structure and dynamics of GPCR activation and signaling as compared with full-size receptor proteins (Britton *et al.*, 2012). The present review is devoted to the application of peptides, derivatives of GPCR and heterotrimeric G proteins, in the study of structural-functional organization and folding of these signal proteins, as well as to the achievements and perspectives of the use of peptides as probes to study the molecular mechanisms of signal transduction and for developing novel regulators of G protein-dependent signaling systems.

2   G Protein-coupled Receptors

2.1   Extracellular Domains

The 3D modeling of the ligand-binding site and detection of the molecular determinants responsible for recognition of ligand and specific interaction with it in the ECL and TM regions are today actual problems of molecular endocrinology and pharmacology (Katritch *et al.*, 2012; Mason *et al.*, 2012; Park, 2012). The solution of these problems is unavoidable for the development of highly selective and effective regulators and modulators of physiological functions. In structural investigations and functional mapping of hydrophilic ECL in full-size GPCR there arise some difficulties, because their conformation is very labile and strongly dependent on the microenvironment and the presence of ligand. Moreover, even in the case of extracellular domains that are stabilized by intra- and inter-loop disulfide bonds and form the extracellular extensions of helical TM, the 3D structure of ECL varies greatly depending on the receptor state, free or ligand-occupied, and on various physical-chemical factors.

According to the two-step model of interaction between GPCR and ligand, the ECL are responsible for the recognition and low-affinity binding of the ligand and for translocation of the latter into the transmembrane channel to the high-affinity binding site. The data obtained with the synthetic peptides corresponding to the ECL and the ECL/TM interfaces demonstrate a good applicability of ECL-derived peptides to establish the 3D structure of the ECL in full-length receptor and their conformational flexibility in free and ligand-occupied states, and is very consistent with that obtained using other approaches (Table 1). A similarity between the structural organization of ECL-peptide and the corresponding loop in intact receptor is due to the fact that the 3D structure of ECL in GPCR is stabilized by relatively short-range interactions between the amino acids and their clusters localized in N- and C-terminal segments of this loop and in the ECL/TM interfaces. Besides, it seems likely that at least some of ECL may contribute to structural stability and folding of the intact receptor protein during its synthesis and post-translational modification.

GPCR, localization	Amino acid sequence and its modifications	Method	Secondary structure and/or three-dimensional organization	References
ECL-, TM- and ECL/TM-peptides				
Bacteriorhodopsin *Halobacterium halobium*; ECL2 (1), ECL3 (2)	GALTKVYSYRFVWWA[119–133] (1); SAYPVVWLIGSEGAGIVPLN IETL[177–200] (2)	NMR	Each peptide forms helix-turn-helix structure	(Katragadda *et al.*, 2000)
Rhodopsin; NTD (1), ECL1 (2), ECL2 (3), ECL3 (4)	MNGTEGPNFYVPFSNKTGV VRSPFEAPQYYLAEPWNFS ML[1–40] (1); TTTLYTSLHGYFVFGPTGCN LEGFFATLGGEI[92–123] (2); LVGWSRYIPEGMQCSCGID YYTPHEETNNESFVI[172–205] (3); YAGVAFYIFTHQGSDFGPIF MTIPAF[268–293] (4)	NMR	The peptides show ordered structure, each peptide from ECL1-ECL3 (2–4) exhibits a turn in the central region, the ends of the peptides show an unwinding of TM to form this turn. Peptide 1 forms a compact domain consisting of α-helical regions with breaks and bands at proline residues	(Yeagle *et al.*, 2000)
Ste2 receptor of pheromonal α-factor; ECL1	Cyclic and linear analogs; SNYSSVTYALTGFPQFISRG DVHVYGATN[103–132]	CD; NMR	Each peptide is highly flexible in water and forms N-terminal helix in TFE and in the presence of DPC micelles	(Sen *et al.*, 1997; Naider *et al.*, 2005)
CCK receptor, the type 1; END (1); C-TM6/ECL3/N-T M7 (2)	MDVVDSLLVNGSNITPPCEL GLENETLFCLDQPRPSKEW QPAVQILL[1–47] (1); IFSANAWRAYDTASAERRL SGTPISFILLL[329–357] (2)	NMR	Peptide 1 has N- and C-terminal α-helices separated by a disulfide stabilized β-sheet; peptide 2 is composed of three α-helices	(Giragossian & Mierke, 2003)
CCK receptor, the type 2; C-TM6/ECL3/N-T	ANTWRAFDGPGAHRALSG APISFIHLLS[352–379]	NMR	Peptide consists of three α-helices corresponding to TM6/ECL3 and ECL3/TM7 interfaces and the entire	(Giragossian & Mierke, 2003)

			ECL3	
M7 Thromboxane A$_2$ receptor, ECL3	RNPPAMSPAGQLSRTTEKE^2$^{71-289}$	NMR	Peptide forms β turn 278–281, the distance between the ends of the N and C termini is close to that obtained using other approaches	(Wu et al., 2003)
Angiotensin II receptor, the subtype IA; ECL1	TAMEYRWPFGNYL$^{88-100}$	CD; NMR	The region WPFG$^{94-97}$ forms a type-II β-turn and undergoes Trp-Pro peptide bond cis-trans isomerization	(Nicastro et al., 2003)
GnRH receptor; ECL3	Cyclic CG-PEMLNRVSEP^{293-}^{302}-GC	CD; NMR	Peptide predominantly forms unordered structure, but β-hairpin with the turn 296–298 is also possible	(Petry et al., 2002)
δ-Opioid receptor; ECL3	IFVIVWTLVDIDRRDPLVVA A$^{279-299}$	CD; NMR	Peptide has a well defined helical conformation within the N-terminal part	(Fadhil et al., 2004)
Parathyroid hormone receptor; ECL1	DAVLYSGATLDEAERLTEE ELRAIAQAPPPPATAAAGY AGBRVAV$^{241-285}$	NMR	Peptide forms three α-helices in the presence of DPC micelles	(Piserchio et al., 2000)
CB$_1$-cannabinoid receptor; TM7/N-CTD(ICL4)	TVFAFCSMLCLNSTVNPIIY ALRSKDLRHAFRSMFPSCE^3$^{77-416}$	NMR	The regions corresponding to TM7 and to the entire contiguous helix 8 (ICL4) parallel to the membrane surface have helical conformation	(Tiburu et al., 2009)
Chemokine receptor CCR5; TM4/N-ECL2	VFASLPGIIFTRSQKEGL$^{157-174}$	CD; NMR; FRET	Peptide has two helical structures, whereas the C-terminal part remains unstructured	(Miyamoto & Togiya, 2011)
Chemokine receptor CCR3; NTD	VFTFGTTSYYDDVGLL$^{8-23}$	NMR	Phosphorylation of Tyr^{16} and Tyr^{17} alters free- and ligand-binding conformation of peptide	(Zhu et al., 2011)
5-HTR, the type 6; TM1–TM7 (1–7)	GSGWVAAALCVVIALTAA ANSLLIALICTQ$^{25-54}$ (1); SNFFLVSLFTSDLMVGLVV MPPAMLNALYG$^{61-90}$ (2), ARGLCLLWTAFDVMCCSAS ILNLCLISLDR$^{95-124}$ (3), RALALVLGAWSLAALASFL PLLLGWHE$^{142-168}$ (4), RLLASLPFVLVASGLTFFLP SGAICFTY$^{181-208}$ (5), CLKASLTLGILLGMFFVTW LPFFVANIVQ$^{264-291}$ (6), DCISPGLFDVLTWLGYCNST MNPIIYPLFMRD$^{294-326}$ (7)	FRET	The TM-peptides spontaneously assemble into liposomes in conformation that mimics native structure	(Lee et al., 2009)
A$_{2A}$-Adenosine receptor; TM1–TM7 (1–7)	KKKVYITVELAIAVLAILGN VLVCYA$^{8-30}$KKKK (1) KKKFVVSLAAADIAVGVLAI PYAITI$^{44-66}$KKKK (2) KKKLFIACFVLVLTQSSIFSL LAIAIDRY$^{78-103}$KKK (3) KKKRAKGIIAICWVLSFAIG	CD; NMR; FRET	Each of seven TM peptides forms thermally stable, independent α-helical structures both in micelles and vesicles; four peptides (TM3, TM4, TM5, TM7) exhibit very high-helical structure, and TM2- and TM6-peptides display low	(Thévenin & Lazarova, 2008)

	LTPMLGY[120–142]*KKKK* (4) *KKK*MNYMVYFNFFACVLV PLLLMLGVYLR[174–199]*KKK* (5) *KKK*LAIIVGLFAL*A*WLPLHII NCFTFF*A*PD[235–261]*KK* (6) *KKK*LWLMYLAIVLSHTNSV VNPFIYAYRIRE[267–294]*K* (7)		α-helicity	
ICL-peptides				
β₂-AR; C-ICL3	RRSSKFCLKEKKALK[259–273]	CD; NMR	In TFE solution the peptide forms α-helix located in the C-terminal part	(Okuda *et al.*, 2002)
5-HTR, the type 1A; C-ICL3	AKRKMALARERKTVKTL[330–346]	CD	Peptide has the helical structure in TFE	(Varrault *et al.*, 1994)
5-HTR, the type 6; C-ICL3	KHSRKALKASL[258–268]-KA (1); KHSRKALKASL[258–268]-K(Pal)A (2)	CD	Each peptide in neutral and acidic media has predominantly in the antiparallel β-sheet and disordered conformation; peptide 2 in the alkaline medium and in 40–80 % TFE has 12–14 % of α-helicity	(Shpakova *et al.*, 2012b)
Prostaglandin EP3α receptor; N-ICL3	TIKALVSRCRAKAAV[252–264]	NMR	Peptide forms α-helical structure with positively charged surface	(Kikkou *et al.*, 2006)
GABA_B receptor; ICL3	ETKSVSTEKINDHR[728–741]	NMR	Peptide forms α-helical structure and a positively charged cluster at the C terminus	(Kikkou *et al.*, 2008)
Prostacyclin receptor; ICL1	SARRPARPSAFAV[39–51]	NMR	Peptide forms two turns 41–44 and 45–49	(Zhang *et al.*, 2006)
Thromboxane A₂ receptor; ICL2 (1), ICL3 (2)	ERYLGITRPPFSRPAVASQR RA[129–149] (1); ATLCHVYHGQEAAQQRPR DSEVEMMAQ[220–246] (2)	NMR	Peptide 1 consists of a large turn structure formed by three bends; peptide 2 has N- and C-terminal α-helices with a turn located at residues QRPR[214–217]	(Wu *et al.*, 2008)
APG1 receptor, derived from human homologous *methuselah* gene; ICL3	RNGKRSNRTLREE[1050–1062]	NMR	Peptide forms an α-helical structure at the C terminal site and a positive charge cluster at the N-terminal site	(Kikkou *et al.*, 2007)
CB₁- and CB₂-cannabinoid receptors; CTD: CB₁ (1), CB₂ (2)	IYALRSKDLRHAFRSMFPSC EG[397–418] (1); IYALRSGEIRSSAHHCLAHW KK[298–319] (2)	NMR	Each peptide forms TM7/CTD interface helix and are parallel to the juxtamembrane helix separated by L-shaped turn	(Xie & Chen, 2005)
V₂-vasopressin receptor; ICL3	Cyclic QVLIFREIHASLVPGPSERA GRRRRGRRTGSPSEGAHVS AAMAKTVRMT[225–273]	CD; NMR	Peptide forms a left-twisted α-helical hairpin structure consisting of 225–243 and 254–271 helices	(Bellot *et al.*, 2009)
Angiotensin II receptor, the type 1; N-ICL-3, (1), C-ICL-3 (2)	TSYTLIWKALKKAYEIQKN[213–231] (1); EIQKNKPRNDDIFRII[227–242] (2)	CD; NMR	Peptide 1 has a stable α-helix; peptide 2 has α-helix 9–15 and poorly defined N terminus structure	(Franzoni *et al.*, 1999)

Chemokine receptor CCR5; full-size ICL3	LRCRNEKKRHRAVRLIFTI[22] 2-240	CD; NMR; FRET	Peptide has a helical structure in the C-terminal region (13-16), whereas the N-terminal part remains unstructured	(Miyamoto et al., 2010)
Receptor of luteinizing hormone; C-ICL3	QKDTKIAKK(Nle)A$^{562-572}$ (1); QKDTKIAKK(Nle)A$^{562-572}$-K(Pal)A(2)	CD	Each peptide at pH 2 and 7 has predominantly the antiparallel β-sheet and disordered structure; peptide 2 at pH 11and in the presence of 40–80 % TFE has 14–27 % of α-helicity.	(Shpakov et al., 2011)

Table 1: The secondary structure of GPCR-peptides studied by NMR, CD spectroscopy and the fluorescence resonance energy transfer (FRET) measurements

The data on the peptides corresponding to the ECL of bacterial rhodopsins, heptahelical receptor proteins that are similar to eukaryotic GPCR in topology and structural-functional organization, give strong evidences for similarity of the 3D structure of ECL-peptides and the corresponding region in full-size receptor. The 3D structure of peptides 119–133 and 177–200, derivatives of ECL2 and ECL3 of light-sensitive bacteriorhodopsin from *Halobacterium halobium*, obtained using NMR had a remarkable similarity with the structure of the loops revealed by X-ray crystallography of intact rhodopsin. In both cases the segments 119–133 and 177–200 formed a helix-turn-helix motif (Katragadda et al., 2000).

The helix-turn-helix structures are typical of ECL-peptides, derivatives of eukaryotic GPCR, such as mammalian rhodopsin, κ-opioid receptor and thromboxane A$_2$ receptor (Yeagle et al., 2000; Ruan et al., 2001; Zhang et al., 2002). Peptide 196–228 corresponding to the entire ECL2 and neighboring segments of TM4 and TM5 of κ-opioid receptor contained a well-defined helical structure Val^{201}-Cys^{210} analogous to that formed by similar regions in the native receptor, a β-turn formed by the D^{217} and D^{218} residues and two helical turns in TM4/ECL2 and ECL2/TM5 interfaces (Zhang et al., 2002). Based on crystallographic studies of κ-opioid receptor the distance between Val^{201} and Cys^{210} is 7.08 Å (Wu et al., 2012), which is very close to calculated for peptide 196–228 using NMR approach. The bovine rhodopsin peptide 92–123 corresponding to ECL1 exhibited a helix-turn-helix motif with short helices on each side of the turn likely to be extracellular extensions of TM2 and TM3 helices in the intact receptor. Peptide 172–205 corresponding to ECL2 of rhodopsin also showed a helix-turn-helix structure stabilized by hydrophobic interaction between the side chains of Trp^{175}, Ile^{179}, Ile^{189}, and Tyr^{191} located in N- and C-terminal helices (Yeagle et al., 2000).

The ECL-peptides corresponding to the NTD and the ECL of some receptors, e.g. receptors of cholecystokinin (CCK) and parathyroid hormone, contained three or more α-helices (Piserchio et al., 2000; Giragossian & Mierke, 2003). ECL1-peptide 241–285 of parathyroid hormone receptor in dodecylphosphocholine (DPC), a molecule inducing formation of membrane-mimicking micelles, formed two α-helices 241–244 and 275–284 corresponding to the end and the beginning of TM2 and TM3, and, additionally, the helix 256–264 that was localized in the middle of peptide and specifically interacted with hormone (Piserchio et al., 2000). Using NMR it was shown that peptides 329–357 and 352–379, derivatives of ECL3 of CCK receptors of the types 1 and 2, were composed of three helices corresponding to TM6/ECL3 and ECL3/TM7 interfaces and the entire region of ECL3 (Giragossian & Mierke, 2003).

Some ECL-peptides have an unordered conformation with a few minor contributions of β-sheet structure (Petry *et al.*, 2002). At the N and C termini of these peptides there are, as a rule, no segments as the extensions of helical TM regions that would correspond to ECL/TM interfaces. The latter interact with each other; this leads to stabilization of the cyclic structure of ECL of intact receptor and increases contribution of the ordered structure, the helical in particular. It was found that modification of ECL-peptides with segments corresponding to ECL/TM interfaces and with other hydrophobic moieties as well as their cyclization using disulphide or amide bonds gives peptides with high-ordered structure.

To stabilize the conformation of ECL-peptide and to make it be similar to that in full-size receptor, the construction of cyclic and pseudo cyclic structures were used, as was well demonstrated with peptides that correspond to ECL1 of sphingosine 1-phosphate receptor of the type 4 and contain ligand-recognizing site (Pham *et al.*, 2007). To achieve similarity in the structural organization of peptides and the ECL1 in intact receptor, the authors used three approaches based on the construction of different cyclic ECL1-mimicking structures. One approach consisted in introduction of cysteine residues in the TM2/ECL1 and ECL1/TM3 interfaces and the construction of the cyclic structure by forming the internal disulfide bond between these residues. Another one was based on the replacement of hydrophobic helical segments corresponding to extracellular ends of TM2 and TM3 by the sequences capable of forming coiled-coil structures, which promotes the interaction between N- and C-terminal helices of peptide and gives the pseudo cyclic structure. A third approach was combination of the two others. It was shown that cyclic ECL1-mimetic peptides adopted a helical hairpin share with helical segments at the N- and C-termini. The cyclization markedly stabilized the helical hairpin conformation. It is illustrated by the fact that cyclic ECL1-peptide in 20 % 2,2,2-trifluoroethanol (TFE), an organic solvent known to preferentially induce formation of α-helical conformation, showed the same content of the ordered structure as its acyclic analog in 50 % TFE. The ability to form the coiled-coil structures adopted partially helical structure in 20 % TFE with a highly ordered helix within the N-terminal segment and a shorter, less ordered helix within the C-terminal segment of peptide. A cyclic peptide stabilized by the disulphide bond and having coiled-coil structure specifically bound to phosphoethanolamine, selective agonist of type 4 sphingosine 1-phosphate receptor, and in this binding both charged and hydrophobic residues, in particular Glu[122] that forms sphingosine 1-phosphate-binding surface of the receptor and is essential for its activation, were involved. Acyclic analog of the peptide was not effective in this respect. Thus, the combination of coiled-coil extension replacing N- and C-terminal segments, derivatives of the adjacent TM regions, and interhelical disulfide bonds is a general design approach promoting native-like biologically active structure of the ECL (Pham *et al.*, 2007).

The cyclization was used by Ruan and coworkers for the design of peptides mimicking the ECL of prostacyclin receptor, thromboxane A_2 receptor and the type 3 prostaglandin E_2 receptor, belonging to the prostanoid receptors family (Ruan *et al.*, 2001, 2003, 2004, 2005; So *et al.*, 2003; Wu *et al.*, 2003; Chillar *et al.*, 2008). The study of ECL-peptides made it possible to establish the localization of disulfide bond connecting ECL1 and ECL2 of thromboxane A_2 receptor which form the ligand-recognition pocket (Ruan *et al.*, 2001; So *et al.*, 2003; Wu *et al.*, 2003). The cyclic ECL2-peptide 173–193 containing N- and C-terminal homocysteines added for peptide cyclization interacted more effectively with ligand as compared to its linear analog. This demonstrates that cyclization of ECL-peptides mimics a highly ordered structure similar to that in the intact receptor and enhances the biological activity of peptides. Using NMR and fluorescence spectroscopy it was found that the residues Val[176], Leu[185], Thr[186] and Leu[187] located in this peptide were involved in receptor recognition of thromboxane A_2. A similar constrained peptide corresponding to ECL2 of prostacyclin receptor homologous to thromboxane A_2

receptor effectively bound to iloprost, selective agonist of prostacyclin receptor, and this binding involved multiple interactions, e.g. between positively charged Arg^{173} and negatively charged C-1 carboxylate of iloprost, between the hydrophobic residues Ala^{172}, Met^{174}, Leu^{177} and hydrophobic radical of iloprost, and between the polar residues Gln^{172} and Gln^{178} of peptide and the C-11 and C-15 hydroxyl groups of this agonist (Ruan et al., 2003, 2005). Studying cyclic peptide 189–227 corresponding to ECL2 of the type 3 prostaglandin E_2 receptor, it was found that two residues, Ser^{211} and Arg^{214}, located in the non-conserved region of ECL2 were involved in ligand recognition (Chillar et al., 2008). As it follows from the data concerning the localization of the ligand-recognition site in ECL2 of prostanoid receptors, it differs from the high affinity ligand-binding site located in receptor transmembrane channel. Studying cyclic forms of ECL2-peptides of prostanoid receptors the results were obtained allowing creation of a two-step model of ligand binding to a prostanoid receptor involving the low-affinity binding of ligand with extracellular regions of the receptor and the subsequent deposition of ligand into the transmembrane channel towards final, high-affinity, ligand-binding site (Ruan et al., 2004). Thus, ECL-peptides corresponding to extracellular regions of GPCR appear to be excellent probes for modeling ligand-recognition and ligand-binding sites and identification of amino acid residues responsible for specific recognition of ligand. Furthermore, there is a good agreement between the structure of cyclic peptides and the corresponding loops in the full-size receptor, making it possible to use ECL-peptides for studying the 3D structure of the receptor domains. Thus, a distance between the N- and C-terminal residues in the cyclic peptide 271–289 corresponding to ECL3 of human thromboxane A_2 receptor is 9.45 Å, which agrees with the distance between the two residues at the ends of TM6 and TM7 connecting this loop in the thromboxane A_2 receptor working model generated using molecular modeling, based on the crystal structure of bovine rhodopsin (Wu et al., 2003).

ECL-peptides were widely used for identification of molecular determinants in the extracellular domains of GPCR and for the study of ligand–ECL interaction. It has been already mentioned that in the prostanoid receptors hydrophobic and ionic interactions were both involved in ligand recognition. A similar picture was observed with GPCR activated by peptide hormones, the role of ionic interactions being, however, more important and usually participating in these interactions are two or more charged amino acids (Ferguson et al., 2000; Petry et al., 2002; Zhang et al., 2002; Underwood et al., 2010). Depending on the charge of ligand-recognition site, peptide hormone-activated GPCR can be divided into two groups. One includes the chemokine receptors, nociceptin receptor, gonadotropin-releasing hormone (GnRH) receptor, neurokinin-1 receptor, and glucagon-like peptide-1 (GLP-1) receptor having a negatively charged ligand-recognizing region in ECL that interacts with positively charged sites of hormonal molecule (Clubb et al., 1994; Mizoue et al., 1999; Skelton et al., 1999; Ye et al., 2000; Petry et al., 2002; Ulfers et al., 2002; Runge et al., 2008; Vincent et al., 2008; Underwood et al., 2010). The other group includes types 1 and 2 CCK receptors and δ-opioid receptor with positively charged ligand-recognizing region interacting with negatively charged peptide hormone (Giragossian & Mierke, 2003; Fadhil et al., 2004).

It was found that the cyclic peptide 189–214 mimicking ECL2 of nociceptin receptor belonging to the family of opioid receptors specifically interacted with nociceptin, and this interaction involved an ionic contact of two positively charged motifs of nociceptin (RK^{8-9} and RK^{12-13}) and acidic residues of ECL2-peptide, and a hydrophobic contact of N-terminal segment of nociceptin and aromatic cluster of the peptide corresponding segment $YW^{210-211}$ at the beginning of TM5 (Vincent et al., 2008). The cyclic peptide 293–302 corresponding to the ECL3 of mouse GnRH receptor with a disulfide bridge formed by N- and C-terminal cysteine residues introduced additionally specifically bound GnRH and significantly inhibited GnRH-induced activation of G_q protein-coupled GnRH receptor. The negatively charged Glu[301] of peptide 293–302 interacted with positively charged Arg[8] of GnRH, inducing a folded configuration of GnRH and stabilizing β-hairpin structure of ECL3-peptide. This is the evidence that the interaction between ECL3 and GnRH induces conformational changes both in the receptor and the ligand. The results obtained with ECL3-peptide 293–302 were consistent with the previous data that the substitution of Arg[8] in GnRH and the replacement of Glu[301] in mouse GnRH receptor or Asp[302] in human GnRH receptor by neutral amino acids led to 10- to 100-fold decrease in binding affinity of mutant receptors (Flanagan *et al.*, 1994; Fromme *et al.*, 2001). The peptide corresponding to the NTD of GLP-1 receptor bound GLP-1 with low affinity and exendin-4(9–39), competitive antagonist of the receptor, with high affinity (IC_{50}, 6 nM) (Runge *et al.*, 2007). The difference in affinity can be accounted for by the fact that GLP-1 had only one positively charged residue (Lys[26]) interacting with negatively charged Glu[128] located in the NTD, while exendin-4(9–39) had two positively charged residues, Arg[20] and Lys[27] interacting with negatively charged Glu[128] and Glu[127] of the NTD, respectively (Runge *et al.*, 2008). It was also established that the hydrophobic face of α-helical region 13–33 of GLP-1 interacted with receptor NTD. For example, the alkyl radical of Val[33] made hydrophobic contacts with aromatic ring of Tyr[69] and alkyl radical Leu[123] (Underwood *et al.*, 2010).

Numerous studies show that peptides corresponding to the negatively charged NTD of chemokine receptors specifically bind to cognate polycationic chemokines (Clubb *et al.*, 1994; Skelton *et al.*, 1999; Mayer & Stone, 2000; Ye *et al.*, 2000; Veldkamp *et al.*, 2008; Simpson *et al.*, 2009; Zhu *et al.*, 2011). Peptide 1–35 corresponding to the NTD of CCR3-chemokine receptor and its truncated fragment 8–23 specifically bound to CCR3-agonist eotaxin and induced conformational changes in hormonal molecule (Ye *et al.*, 2000; Simpson *et al.*, 2009). On the other hand, peptides corresponding to ECL1 and ECL3 of CCR3-chemokine receptor did not interact with eotaxin, and both the linear and the disulfide-cyclized ECL2-peptides bound to eotaxin with lower affinity (Ye *et al.*, 2000). The central region of NTD rich in negatively charged amino acids (Glu[9], Asp[18], and Asp[19]) was involved in the specific binding with positively charged eotaxin having isoelectric point at 9.9. The increase of negative charge of NTD due to sulfation of Tyr[16] and Tyr[17] residues led to an increase in selectivity and in affinity of binding of the sulfated peptide 8–23 with eotaxin (Simpson *et al.*, 2009; Zhu *et al.*, 2011). The nonsulfated peptide 8–23 bound to the three chemokines, namely eotaxin-1/CCL11, eotaxin-2/CCL24, and eotaxin-3/CCL26, with approximately equal affinity, sulfation of Tyr[16] gave rise to 9–16-fold selectivity for eotaxin-1 over the other two chemokines, sulfation of Tyr[17] also increased the selectivity for eotaxin-1, but to a lesser extent, and the doubly sulfated peptide selectively bound to both eotaxin-1 and eotaxin-3 approximately 10-fold more tightly than to eotaxin-2. It was also shown that as a result of sulfation of Tyr[17] in peptide 8–23 the affinity for eotaxin-1 was enhanced 7-fold, and sulfation of Tyr[16] or both tyrosine residues induced more than 28-fold increase of it (Simpson *et al.*, 2009). This indicates that the influence of tyrosine sulfation on chemokine binding affinity and selectivity is substantial and dependent on the position of tyrosine residue, the target of sulfation. The nonsulfated, Tyr[21]-sulfated, and triply sulfated (Tyr[7], Tyr[12], and Tyr[21]) peptides corresponding to 1–38 region of the NTD of CXCR4-chemokine receptor specifically bound to a cross-linked dimeric form of chemokine stromal cell-derived factor 1. Each chemokine dimer bound to two CXCR4-peptides in a symmetric fashion, and sulfotyrosines Tyr[7] and Tyr[12] of CXCR4-peptide occupied positively charged clefts on opposing chemokine subunits (Veldkamp *et al.*, 2008). Tyr[21] bound with the positively charged crevice between the N-loop and the β3-strand, the site equivalent to that identified for binding of sulfated CCR3-peptides to eotaxin-1, -2, and -3. The data obtained with sulfated peptides, derivatives of NTD of chemokine receptors, shows that the tyrosine sulfation of this domain is an effective mechanism for regulating the chemokine affinity and responsiveness of chemokine receptors, which agrees with the genetic data showing that mutations of tyrosine residues in the NTD of chemokine receptors CCR5, CCR8, CXCR3, CXCR4, and CX3CR1 lead to decrease of binding and activation of the receptors by the cognate chemokines (Farzan *et al.*, 2002; Gutierrez *et al.*, 2004; Colvin *et al.*, 2006). Thus, the peptide strategy based on the use of ECL-peptides is a substantial contribution to the understanding of the functional and structural consequences of tyrosine sulfation of GPCR.

In some receptors, e.g. CCK and δ-opioid receptors, the positively charged residues localized in the extracellular regions interact with negatively charged peptide ligand (Giragossian, Mierke, 2003; Fadhil *et al.*, 2004). Peptides 1–47 and 329–357 of the NTD and ECL3 of type 1 CCK receptor and peptide 352–379 corresponding to the ECL3 of type 2 CCK receptor specifically interacted with CCK-8 and sulfated CCK-15 (Giragossian, Mierke, 2003). The C-terminal Asp^{32} of CCK-8 interacted with Arg^{336} and Arg^{345} located in N-terminal part of the ECL3, minimizing repulsive interaction between the positively charged arginines and inducing conformational changes in the ligand-binding site of the receptors. Alongside with electrostatic interactions, the hydrophobic contacts were also involved in the effective binding of hormone and ECL-peptide. It was shown that the hydrophobic residues Tyr^{27} and Met^{28} of CCK interacted with Trp^{39} of NTD-peptide, and the hydrophobic residues Trp^{30} and Met^{31} of hormone with Ala^{334} and Asn^{333} of ECL3-peptide. In respect to peptide 279–299 of the ECL3 of δ-opioid receptor and its short analogs, positively charged Arg^{291} and aromatic Trp^{284} of receptor were found to interact respectively with anionic Glu^{4} and aromatic Phe^{3} of selective δ-agonist deltorphin II (Fadhil *et al.*, 2004). Hydrophobic interactions between Leu^{295}, Val^{296}, and Val^{297} of peptide 281–297 and the C-terminal segment of deltorphin, Val^{5} and Val^{6} in particular, were identified. This data coincides with the results obtained using the other approaches where it was shown that the negative charge associated with Glu^{4}, the size and hydrophobic nature of Phe^{3} of deltorphin are critical determinants of selective binding to δ-opioid receptor, while Arg^{291} as well as the hydrophobic segment 295–300 of the receptor are important for specificity of δ-agonist binding (Bryant *et al.*, 1997; Pepin *et al.*, 1997).

As was shown in the case of peptides, derivatives of ECL2 of the κ-opioid receptor, the hydrophobic, unlike electrostatic, interactions were very important for the ligand binding by ECL2 of the receptor (Ferguson *et al.*, 2000; Zhang *et al.*, 2002). Peptide 196–228 corresponding to ECL2 and N- and C-terminal segments of TM4 and TM5 of the κ-opioid receptor in the presence of DPC micelles formed the amphiphilic α-helix Val^{201}–Ala^{210} and a β-turn around the anionic cluster $DD^{217-218}$ similar to ECL2 in full-size receptor (Zhang *et al.*, 2002). The helix Val^{201}–Ala^{210} interacted with helix $GFLRRIR^{3-9}$ of dynorphin A-(1–17), and this interhelical structure was stabilized by hydrophobic interaction because neutralization of negative charge of ECL2-peptide had very little or no influence on the binding of dynorphin (Ferguson *et al.*, 2000). This furnishes evidence for multiple mechanisms of ligand recognition and binding to be responsible for selection of a suitable ligand among the myriads of molecules contacting with extracellular surface of GPCR.

The fact that short extracellular regions of GPCR selectively bind to a ligand specific to this receptor makes it possible to use peptides corresponding to these regions to identify ligand-recognition and ligand-binding sites in the ECL and to model the ligand-receptor interaction. The use of these peptides opens way for new technologies for screening synthetic and natural compounds as potential candidates for the role of regulators of hormonal functions, as well as for new approaches in designing novel GPCR agonists and antagonists and to study their binding characteristics, owing to the ability of ligand to induce conformational changes in ECL-peptides. This finds confirmation in the data on the interaction between peptide 279–299, a derivative of ECL3 of the δ-opioid receptor, and selective δ-agonist, deltorphin II (Fadhil *et al.*, 2004). In the deltorphin-binding state the helical conformation of peptide 279–299 was significantly destabilized by the changes in conformation of Phe^{280} and Trp^{284} residues. Upon binding of selective μ-agonists endomorphin-1 and endomorphin-2 containing, like deltorphin II, Tyr-Xxx-Phe/Trp motif the helicity of peptide 279–299 was also decreased, but not significantly. Selective κ-agonist dynorphin A-(1–13) lacking Tyr-Xxx-Phe/Trp motif interacted weakly with the peptide but not like deltorphin II and induced to a little extent stabilization of the helical conformation. These data are in good agreement with the affinity of opioid peptides mentioned above to the δ-opioid receptor. It should be noted in this connection that low molecular weight non-peptidic κ-agonist U-50488 that interacts directly with the ligand-binding cavity located within transmembrane channel of the receptor does not elicit a conformational change in peptide 279–299 (Fadhil *et al.*, 2004). It is also important that ECL-peptides can be used for the study of structural organization of a ligand-binding site, as their conformation is very close to that of homologous regions in the full-size receptor. Indeed, the distance between the residues Trp^{284} and Arg^{291} in ECL3 of the δ-opioid receptor (3.95 Å) calculated on the basis of the crystal structure of this receptor (PDB ID: 4EJ4; Granier *et al.*, 2012) was very close to that in peptide 279–299 (4.7 Å).

ECL-peptides are a promising tool to be used in the study of pathogenesis of some diseases, because the production of autoantibodies against ECL of GPCR has an important role in the development of cardiomyopathy, complex regional pain syndrome, chronic Chagas' disease, cognitive dysfunctions, as well as Sjögren's syndrome and primary biliary cirrhosis often associated with this syndrome (Berg *et al.*, 2010; Kohr *et al.*, 2011; Segovia *et al.*, 2012). Autoantibodies against ECL2 of β1-adrenergic receptor (β1-AR) were identified in 30–40 % of patients with idiopathic dilated cardiomyopathy and in 89 % of patients with periodontitis associated with cardiac dysfunctions (Magnusson *et al.*, 1994; Iwata *et al.*, 2001; Jahns *et al.*, 2006; Segovia *et al.*, 2012). In periodontitis these autoantibodies inhibited primary cell-specific growth and induced over-expression of pro-inflammatory mediators, but additionally, bound to the β1-AR in the myocardium, acting as partial β1-AR agonists, and modified cardiac contractility, which led to heart failure (Segovia *et al.*, 2012). The immunization of animals with peptides, derivatives of β1-AR ECL2, induced cardiomyopathy (Iwata *et al.*, 2001; Jahns *et al.*, 2004; Buvall *et al.*, 2007). Monoclonal β1-AR–ECL2 autoantibodies induced endoplasmic reticulum stress and apoptosis in isolated cardiomyocytes (Staudt *et al.*, 2003). These antibodies bound with high specificity to native β1-AR, impaired its radioligand binding, acted as full or partial agonists, and did not interact with β2-AR and other GPCR, which indicates their high receptor specificity (Jahns *et al.*, 2000; Matsui & Fu, 2006; Jane-wit *et al.*, 2007). In addition to modeling cardiovascular diseases, the β1-AR ECL-peptides can be also used to prevent them. The immunosorbents obtained by immobilization of peptides corresponding to ECL1 (125–133) and ECL2 (206–218) of β1-AR were used for removing β1-AR autoantibodies from the plasma of patients with dilated cardiomyopathy (Sidorova *et al.*, 2009).

Autoantibodies against peptide, derivative of ECL2 of m2-muscarinic acetylcholine receptor (m2-MChR), recognized by immunoglobulins from patients with chronic Chagas' disease significantly increased the affinity of m2-MChR to acetylcholine and enhanced the activation of the receptor by agonists (Hernandez *et al.*, 2008). The molecular mechanism of action of the m2-MChR ECL2-antibodies is in that they specifically interacted with m2-MChR and cross-linked them into functionally active di- and oligomeric complexes (Beltrame *et al.*, 2011). ECL2-peptide and m2-MChR allosteric antagonist gallamine blocked these effects of autoantibodies, which indicates that m2-MChR–ECL2 antibodies specifically interacts with a common allosteric site and has a positive cooperative effect on acetylcholine action. Autoantibodies against the ECL2 of human m_1- and m_3-MChR detected in the serum of 40 % of patients with Sjogren syndrome interacted with the cognate receptors of cerebral frontal cortex membranes inhibiting the binding of non-selective muscarinic antagonist quinuclidinyl benzilate to MChR and stimulated the hydrolysis of phosphoinositides acting as agonists (Reina et al., 2004). Autoantibodies, such as immunoglobulin G directed against peptide sequences of ECL2 of β_2-AR and m_2-MChR, were identified in serum samples from patients with complex regional pain syndrome, a painful condition affecting one or more extremities of the body (Kohr et al., 2011). The antibodies against peptide corresponding to ECL2 of 5-hydroxytryptamine receptor of the type 4 (5-HT$_4$R) specifically recognized 5-HT$_4$R; at concentrations 50 and 500 pM they decreased AC stimulating effect of serotonin but at 5 pM increased it, all this speaks in favor of the fact that 5HT$_4$R–ECL2 monoclonal antibody functions as high-affinity modulator of 5-HT$_4$R (Kamel et al., 2005). The preparation of monoclonal antibodies against ECL-peptides opens a new avenue for the production of non-hormonal regulators that not only mimic the action of hormones and, in addition, are able to regulate the functional activity of GPCR and G protein-coupled signaling systems. The advantage of such regulators consists in that they are able to interact only with one or, at the most, a few types of receptors that have highly homologous ECL.

ECL-peptides can also be used to inhibit binding of infectious agents, such as viruses, to the cell membrane. Peptide 1–27 derived from the NTD of GPR1 receptor and the antibodies against the peptide blocked the infection induced by HIV-1 that uses GPR1 as a co-receptor, or by X4, R5 and R5X4 viruses that have quite different co-receptors (Jinno-Oue et al., 2005). The peptide directly interacted with X4 envelope glycoprotein gp120 and competitively inhibited the interaction of gp120 with GPR1 receptor on the surface of target cell membrane. Peptide 1–27 with tyrosine residues Tyr^{15}, Tyr^{17}, Tyr^{21}, Tyr^{22} substituted by alanines did not bind to gp120 and, as a result, did not inhibit HIV-1 infection, which suggests tyrosine residues contribute to the interaction of GPR1 receptor with gp120 protein, making it more effective and have a crucial role in inhibition of HIV-1 infection.

2.2   Transmembrane Domains

The peptides corresponding to hydrophobic TM helices are widely used to study folding, assembly, stability, and conformational flexibility of GPCR in the membrane, as well as the mechanisms of ligand binding and G protein coupling. The use of TM-derived peptides in the study of structural organization and architecture of GPCR is based on the two-state model of membrane protein assembly. According to this model, the final structure of the transmembrane channel results from the accretion of smaller elements, such as TM helices, each of which has reached thermodynamic equilibrium with the lipid and aqueous phases before packing (White & Wimley, 1999; Popot & Engelman, 2000; Topiol & Sabio, 2009). TM-peptide first interacts with membrane-lipid polar head groups to come into the hydrophobic interface of the membrane, forms α-helical structure to be spontaneously inserted into the bilayer core, and then α-helical peptide specifically interacts with the other TM and assembles into the 3D structure of the transmembrane channel or a related structure. The complexes between TM-peptides are formed by van der Waals packing forces, electrostatic interactions and hydrogen bonds. The results obtained with TM-peptides, derivatives of different GPCR, are in good agreement with this two-state model and prove it to be correct.

It was found that the interaction between TM-peptides is specific and similar to that in full-size receptor. The peptides corresponding to each of the seven TM of A_{2A}-adenosine receptor had stable contacts in sodium dodecyl sulphate (SDS) micelles and formed only certain pairs (Thévenin et al., 2005,

2008). TM3-peptide interacted preferably with four peptides corresponding to the TM2, TM4, TM6, and TM7, TM6-peptide with three other peptides, TM5- and TM7-peptides with two peptides, while TM1-, TM2- and TM4-peptides with only one counterpart, which correlates very well with the results obtained using the other approaches, like in the case of GPCR structurally resembling A_{2A}-adenosine receptor. The content of α-helical conformation is very important for translocation of TM-peptide into membrane and for interaction with the other peptides. It should be noted as this point that TM6-peptide had a low α-helicity and when alone could not be properly inserted in detergent micelles and lipid bilayer. However, in the presence of TM5-peptide the α-helicity of TM6-peptide increased significantly due to helix-helix interaction and TM6-peptide was able to fold properly and to be inserted into the membrane. This resembles the case of TM2-peptide that also had a low α-helicity and required a highly helical TM3-peptide. Thus, high-helical TM-peptides are required for peptides with low α-helicity to be inserted into the membrane and form the appropriate transmembrane structures. These findings show that the interaction between TM-peptides is likely to precede their insertion in the membrane. This is confirmed by the results of fluorescence resonance energy transfer (FRET) measurements of the interaction between the peptides corresponding of TM5 and TM6, or TM2 and TM3 of A_{2A}-adenosine receptor in the presence of SDS (Thévenin et al., 2008). It was also found that the formation of a stable homodimeric complex containing two molecules of peptide, a derivative of TM5, may contribute to the formation of the dimeric complex of A_{2A}-adenosine receptor. A similar picture was observed with peptide corresponding to TM6 of α-factor receptor Ste2p of yeasts Saccharomyces cerevisiae, showing a high tendency to aggregate even in denaturing conditions (Arshava et al., 2002).

The insertion of peptides corresponding to single TM into membrane or membrane-mimicking media induced their folding into the biologically relevant conformation (Zheng et al., 2006; Lee et al., 2009; Neumoin et al., 2009; Tarasov et al., 2011). However, the conformation of peptides was similar to that in intact receptor only when using two and more TM-peptides or their constructs linked by the ECL or other cross-linking sequences, as was shown for different composition of peptides corresponding to single TM as well as for peptide constrains of the TM–ECL–TM or the ECL–TM–ICL types (Fowler et al., 2004; Kerman & Ananthanarayanan, 2005, 2007; Zou et al., 2008; Lee et al., 2009; Neumoin et al., 2009; Britton et al., 2012). It follows that the specific interactions between TM-peptides are of prime importance in stabilizing the appropriate conformation of the peptides that were inserted in the liposome and detergent micelles or placed in helix-promoting solvents. It was found that peptide that includes ECL3, TM7 and the membrane-proximal region of CTD of A_{2a}-adenosine receptor adopted α-helical structure similar to those in the intact receptor (Britton et al., 2012). The topologically similar peptide corresponding to sequence 271–326 of human type 2 cannabinoid receptor, comprising ECL3, TM7 and juxtamembrane region of CTD, in digitonin and Brij58 micelles adopted more than 75 % of α-helical structure, with the remainder having β-strand structure (Zhang & Xie, 2008). The peptide constrain which included ECL1, TM2 and TM3 of μ-opioid receptor in helix-promoting solvent TFE had 78 % of α-helicity, which was very close to the predicted α-helicity using homology modeling (Kerman & Ananthanarayanan, 2005, 2007). The use of detergents with long alkyl chain, 14 carbons or more, also increased the α-helicity of constrain, suggesting that hydrophobic interactions were responsible for stabilization of the helical structure of TM-peptides. These data speak in favor of the fact that detergents with long fatty-acid chains can be used for refolding protocols where single TM may be important intermediates of protein folding.

Using peptides, derivatives of single TM, it is possible to construct and study the ligand-binding site located within the transmembrane channel, this is illustrated by the data on the peptides corresponding to seven individual TM regions of 5-HT$_6$R (Lee *et al.*, 2009). The peptides reconstituted in liposomes selectively bound to free serotonin and serotonin-conjugated magnetic beads, yielding a K$_d$ of 0.84 μM. The affinity of such ligand-binding site to serotonin was, however, much lower compared with the affinity of native 5-HT$_6$R in the membranes, likely due to the lack of ECL connecting TM helices, which provides stabilization of the assembled structure of seven TM in the native receptor. The interaction of TM-peptides reconstituted in liposome with the ligand was specific. The preincubation of liposomes containing TM-peptides with 5-methoxy-*N,N*-dimethyltryptamine, agonist of 5-HT$_6$R, led to a significant decrease of fluorescence intensity induced by serotonin covalently linked to magnetic beads; this shows that the reconstituted TM-peptides in liposomes possessed specific binding affinity to ligand, and supports the notion that the peptides reconstituted in liposomes adopted a native-like conformation. The ease of preparation and purification of synthetic TM-peptides and their ability to assemble and specifically bind ligands may offer a good alternative to screening and identification of selective agonists and antagonists of GPCR, especially in the cases when the binding and functional characteristics of receptors are difficult to study (Lee *et al.*, 2009).

The specificity of action of TM-peptides on the cognate receptor suggests novel approaches for their use as functional probes for studying the structure, stability and functions of the oligomeric receptor complexes (Hebert *et al.*, 1996, Ng *et al.*, 1996; George *et al.*, 2003; Tarasov *et al.*, 2011). Peptides, derivatives of the TM of the D$_2$-dopamine receptor, induced the dissociation of homodimer complex to monomeric form of the receptor, but did not have any influence on the stability of dimeric complexes formed by other receptors, such as the D$_1$-dopamine receptor, 5-HT$_{1B}$R and β$_2$-AR (Hebert *et al.*, 1996; Ng *et al.*, 1996; George *et al.*, 2003). The peptide corresponding to TM6 of the β$_2$-AR significantly reduced the amount of β$_2$-AR dimeric complexes in the Sf9 membranes, and this was accompanied by a concomitant increase of the level of monomer (Hebert *et al.*, 1996).

TM-peptides demonstrate the biological activity *in vitro* and *in vivo* specifically interacting with the cognate receptor (Hebert *et al.*, 1996; George *et al.*, 2003). Peptides, derivatives of TM of the D$_2$-dopamine receptor, induced dissociation of the homodimer complex of receptor and altered its activation by selective agonists. This action of peptides was very specific, since they did not have any influence on the same complexes formed by D$_1$-dopamine receptor or 5-HT$_{1B}$R (George *et al.*, 2003). The peptide corresponding to TM6 of β$_2$-AR induced the dissociation of the homodimeric complex and decreased agonist-stimulated AC activity (Hebert *et al.*, 1996). *In vivo* the injection of peptide corresponding to TM7 of the D$_2$-dopamine receptor into the caudate nucleus of apomorphine-treated rats caused the ipsilateral asymmetric body rotation, like in the treatment with selective D$_2$-antagonists. The administration of peptide, derivative of TM7 of the α$_1$-AR, led to a reduction of systolic and diastolic pressure, to the rise in the heart rate, the same as in the case of α$_1$-AR antagonist treatment, and prevented the elevation of blood pressure induced by α$_1$-AR agonists. The injection of β$_1$-AR TM7-peptide was followed by a short-lived but marked retardation of the heart rate with a selective drop in diastolic pressure. The administration of TM7-peptide of the V$_2$-vasopressin receptor induced a slight increase in urine output, suggesting the antagonism of the effects of vasopressin (George *et al.*, 2003).

Peptides derived from TM of the chemokine receptor CXCR4 specifically abolished signaling induced by CXCR4-agonist stromal cell-derived factor-1. The 24-mer TM2-peptide with two additional aspartic acid residues at C-termini being the most potent antagonist completely blocked agonist effects at 0.2 μM concentration (Tarasova *et al.*, 1999). TM2-, TM4 and TM7-peptides of the CXCR4 receptor inhibited the functional activity of this receptor participating in HIV-1 entry into host cells and, thus, prevented the replication of virus. The inhibitory effect of these peptides was selective, as they had no influence on signal transduction via the CCR5 chemokine receptor CCR5 also involved in HIV-1 entry. Peptide derived from TM2 of CCR5 receptor completely abolished stimulation of the receptor by agonist RANTES (Regulated on Activation Normal T cell ExpreSsed) but had no effect on CXCR4-signaling. These data indicate new approaches in designing antiviral drugs on the basis of TM-peptides derived from chemokine receptors (Tarasova *et al.*, 1999).

2.3   Intracellular Domains

At present, a large number of peptides and their derivatives corresponding to ICL of bacterial and eukaryotic rhodopsins and the receptors of the biogenic amines, peptide and protein hormones, prostaglandins, fatty acids and cannabinoids were synthesized and their structural and functional characteristics were described (Wess, 1997; Shpakov & Pertseva, 2005, 2007; Shpakov, 2011a, 2011b). Note that ICL contain the regions responsible for selective binding and activation of different types of the heterotrimeric G proteins and for specific interaction with a variety of the regulatory and adaptor proteins, RGS proteins in particular. The multiplicity of intracellular proteins functionally interacting with the ICL of ligand-bound GPCR and the differences in the molecular mechanisms of the interactions between them lead to a considerable variability of structural-functional organization of ICL. At the same time, many of G protein-binding and G protein-activating regions of GPCR have some structural features in common, such as the ability to form amphipathic helices and the segments rich in positively charged amino acids that form BBXXB and the related motifs, where B is a basic amino acid, usually lysine or arginine.

It should be pointed out here that the use of ICL-derived peptides in the study of the 3D structure of intracellular domains, their molecular dynamics and involvement in the interaction with G protein and other intracellular targets encounters some problems along the way. One is due to the fact that membrane-proximal intracellular regions in native receptor are cytoplasmic extension of helical TM and are associated with the cytoplasmic surface of the membrane, which strongly influences their secondary structure and increases the content of the ordered structures, mainly α-helical conformation (Naider *et al.*, 2005). Synthetic ICL-peptides lacking the hydrophobic portion corresponding to the cytoplasmic segments of neighboring TM helices are usually characterized by low content of ordered structure. The modification of ICL-peptides with the hydrophobic radical simulating the TM leads, as a rule, to an increase of the content of ordered structure, the latter, however, may differ from that in intact protein, as instead of the helical TM segments fatty acid radicals are commonly used for modification. Using CD spectroscopy, we showed significant differences between the secondary structure of peptides, derivatives of the ICL3 of 5-HT$_6$R and luteinizing hormone receptor (LHR), and their analogs modified by palmitoyl radical at the C-terminal lysine residue in the presence of TFE and at high pH (Shpakov *et al.*, 2011; Shpakova *et al.*, 2012b). The content of α-helical conformation in the presence of 40–80 % TFE increased to 14 % in the both palmytoylated peptides, in alkaline pH to 27 % in LHR-peptide, and to 12 % in 5-HT$_6$R-peptide, while unmodified analogs under similar conditions did not show α-helicity at all.

Another problem is that ICL in full-size receptor have a pseudo cyclic structure, while a majority of ICL-peptides are not cyclic. A promising approach to solve this problem is to create the cyclic or the pseudo cyclic ICL-peptides, similar to cyclic forms of ECL-peptides. At present, there are few investigations describing the cyclic analogs of ICL-peptides, and they all are devoted to ICL3 of the type 2 vasopressin receptor. It was shown that cyclic peptide corresponding to region 224-274 formed a hairpin stabilized by a disulfide bond between its N- and C-terminal segments and mimicked the native structure of ICL3 in the full-length vasopressin receptor (Bellot *et al.*, 2011). Peptide 225–273 with the cyclic structure formed by amide bond between the N-terminal glycine and C-terminal *S*-carboxymethyl cysteine had the same hairpin conformation (Granier *et al.*, 2004). In the presence of DPC and 50 % TFE the content of α-helical conformation in the case of cyclo-225–273 increased to 22 and 36 %, respectively, which points to a tendency for helical structures to be formed in helix-promoting conditions.

The study of hydrophilic non-cyclic ICL-peptides showed a wide variety of their secondary structures and a rather high content of randomized structures (Table 1). The proportion of ordered and disordered structures strongly depends on the pH, dielectric constant and the polarity of the medium, the presence of detergents and micelle-forming compounds and the proteins capable of interacting with the peptides.

Many hydrophilic peptides in the presence of TFE, SDS and DPC were able to form the helical structures as demonstrated for peptides corresponding to membrane-proximal regions of ICL3 of the 5-HT$_{1A}$R, β_2-AR, GABA$_B$ receptor, prostaglandin EP3α receptor, the type 1A angiotensin II receptor, thromboxane A$_2$ receptor, CCK receptor of the type CCR5 and APG1 receptor (Varrault *et al.*, 1994; Franzoni *et al.*, 1999; Okuda *et al.*, 2002; Kikkou *et al.*, 2006, 2007, 2008; Wu *et al.*, 2008; Bellot *et al.*, 2009; Miyamoto *et al.*, 2010). Using CD spectroscopy it was shown that peptide corresponding to C-terminal region 330–346 of 5-HT$_{1A}$R ICL3 had 37 % of helicity in 50 % TFE (Varrault *et al.*, 1994). Peptide 259–273 corresponding to C-terminal portion of the ICL3 of β_2-AR in the TFE solution had helical conformation and, according to NMR spectroscopy, consisted of a positively charged cluster KEKKALK at the C-termini (Okuda *et al.*, 2002). Peptides, derivatives of C-terminal region of ICL3 of GABA$_B$ receptor and N-terminal region of the same loop of prostaglandin EP3α receptor, were structurally related to peptide 259–273 of β_2-AR, and in the presence of SDS formed the α-helices rich in positively charged amino acid residues, Lys[3], Lys[9], His[13], and Arg[14] in GABA$_B$ receptor-peptide, and Lys[3], Arg[8], Arg[10], and Lys[12] in prostaglandin EP3α receptor, all located on one side of the helix (Kikkou *et al.*, 2006, 2008). Peptide corresponding to ICL3 of APG1 receptor protein derived from *APG1* gene, a human homolog of *mth* gene, in SDS micelles also formed a helix with five basic amino acid residues, such as Arg[1], Lys[4], Arg[5], Arg[8], and Arg[11], located on one side of the helix (Kikkou *et al.*, 2007). These peptides were active and selectively interacted with heterotrimeric G proteins functionally coupled with GPCR homologous to them. With the increase of α-helicity of the peptides their biological activity also increased, and substitution of amino acids leading to reduction of α-helicity and to alteration in the distribution of positively charged amino acids led to its decrease (Kikkou *et al.*, 2006, 2008). Using NMR spectroscopy, it was shown that in 30 % TFE two overlapping peptides mapping the entire ICL3, interacting with purified G proteins, had high content of helical conformation (Franzoni *et al.*, 1999). Peptide 213–231 corresponding to the N-terminal half of ICL3 of the rat angiotensin II AT$_{1A}$ receptor adopted a stable amphipathic α-helix extending over almost the entire peptide, while peptide 227–242 corresponding to its C-terminal half showed a more flexible conformation with α-helix spanning from Asn[9] to Ile[15] and a poorly defined N-terminus. According to CD and NMR data, peptide corresponding to juxtamembrane region 300–320 of NTD of the same receptor, which was critical for the G protein coupling, in acidic water and in the presence of TFE, also formed helical structures that, depending upon experimental conditions, presented various extension in the stretch Leu[6]–Tyr[20] (Franzoni *et al.*, 1997). Within α-helix 6–20, hydrophilic residues Lys[8], Lys[9], Lys[11], Lys[12], Lys[19], and Gln[16] were located on one side of the peptide molecule, while hydrophobic residues Leu[6], Phe[10], Phe[14], Leu[17], and Leu[18] on the other.

As is seen, positively charged helices formed by membrane-proximal intracellular regions of GPCR might play a crucial role in activation of G proteins. It should be mentioned in this connection that the polycationic helical peptides, non-homologous to GPCR, are also able to activate G-proteins, though with lower selectivity and efficiency compared with GPCR-peptides (Shpakov, 2010; Shpakov et al., 2010b). Mastoparan, a cationic amphiphilic tetradecapeptide toxin isolated from wasp venom, taken at micromolar concentrations stimulated functional activity of G_i and G_o proteins and mimicked membrane-proximal intracellular regions of GPCR (Higashijima et al., 1990). The region 3–14 in mastoparan and in the structurally related mastoparan-X (INWKGIAAMAKKLL), like the membrane-proximal region of GPCR, had the α-helical conformation, and all the positively charged amino acids were localized on the hydrophilic side of the helix (Higashijima et al., 1983; Todokoro, 2006). Stabilization of the helical conformation was reached when polycationic MP-X interacted with negatively charged GPCR-interacting regions of $G\alpha_{i/o}$ subunit. It follows that of prime importance for this interaction was positively charged hydrophilic side of the helix (Kusunoki et al., 1998). The addition of two positively charged lysine residues at positions 5 and 8, which together with Lys^4 located on the hydrophilic side of amphiphilic helix of mastoparan and forming the BBXXB-motif, and the addition of lysine residue at position 10 in $[Lys^{10}, Leu^{13}]$-mastoparan gave analogs with the activity higher compared to mastoparan (Mukai et al., 2007). The peptide corresponding to the membrane-proximal region 646–658 of intracellular tyrosine kinase domain of epidermal growth factor receptor one time penetrating the membrane and, like GPCR, coupled with heterotrimeric G proteins also formed polycationic amphipathic helix (Sun et al., 1995). This peptide stimulated GTP-binding and GTPase activities of G_s protein coupled to this receptor. The phosphorylation of residue Thr^{654} led to destabilization of the helical conformation and, as a result, its ability to activate G_s protein vanished.

The helicity and polycationic nature of G protein-binding and G protein-activating regions of GPCR are important in receptor–G protein interaction because the extreme C-terminal segment of α-subunit of G protein, responsible for its effective and selective interaction with these regions of ligand-activated GPCR, is negatively charged (Lambright et al., 1996). Thus, the C-terminal segment of Gα-subunit binds with polycationic regions of GPCR and also interacts with the synthetic GPCR-peptides corresponding to these regions. Activated GPCR uses this segment as a "latch" to alter the conformation of the α5 helix of Gα subunit, which induces change in the conformation of the β6/α5 loop, destabilizes its contacts with the guanine ring of GDP and allows GDP/GTP exchange in guanine nucleotide-binding site of Gα subunit (Van Eps et al., 2006). As evidence for a direct contact between polycationic helical peptides with Gα subunit serve the data on the decrease of α-helicity of $G\alpha_{i/o}$-subunit as a result of its binding with mastoparan. This is followed by conformational change in guanine nucleotide-binding site, by acceleration of the GDP/GTP exchange and thus by the activation of $G_{i/o}$ protein (Tanaka et al., 1998).

It seems quite likely assume that the polycationic GPCR-peptides may influence the stability of di- and oligomeric GPCR complexes, which are formed by electrostatic interactions and hydrogen bonds between the positively and negatively charged regions of the ICL. Cyclic peptide 225–273 constructed on the basis of a full-size ICL3 of the V_2-vasopressin receptor and adopted a left-twisted α-helical hairpin structure inhibited vasopressin-induced AC stimulation and decreased specific binding of vasopressin due to the transition of the receptor high-affinity to low-affinity state (Granier et al., 2004). The inhibitory influence of this peptide was observed in the presence of non-hydrolysable GTP analog preventing the coupling of receptor to G protein. Therefore, there are reasons to say that cyclic peptide 225–273 interacted directly with the V_2-vasopressin receptor and did not influence the receptor–G_s protein coupling. This peptide induced a significant inhibition of the bioluminescence resonance energy-transfer signal between constrains V_2-vasopressin receptor–luciferase and V_2-vasopressin receptor–yellow fluorescent protein, indicating that it alters the distance and/or orientation between these constrains engaged in dimeric complex formation. The influence of peptide on the conformation and stability of the receptor dimeric complex led to a loss of high affinity binding site of V_2-vasopressin receptor (Granier *et al.*, 2004). Note that the same peptide also interacted with gC1qR protein, a potential chaperone of GPCRs, and this interaction induced conformational changes in cyclic peptide 225–273, which in the case of intact receptor is expected to lead to the alteration in the ligand-binding site (Bellot *et al.*, 2009). It was found that in agreement with this conformational rearrangement, binding of gC1qR to the full-length receptor changed the intrinsic tryptophan fluorescence binding curves of V_2-vasopressin receptor to antagonist.

Peptides, derivatives of ICL, specifically interact with the cognate receptor and other signal proteins coupled with it and trigger intracellular signaling cascades mimicking hormone-activated receptor (Shpakov, 2011a, 2010b). There are many publications showing that the peptides, derivatives of ICL3 of receptors of biogenic amines, peptide and glycoprotein hormones, prostaglandin and sphingolipid, specifically regulate the activity of hormonal signaling systems and their influence on them is receptor-, G protein- and tissue-specific (Shirai *et al.*, 1995; Megaritis *et al.*, 2000; Mukhopadhyay & Howlett, 2001; Bavec *et al.*, 2003; Zhang *et al.*, 2006; Shpakov *et al.*, 2007, 2010a, 2011, 2012; Shpakov & Shpakova, 2011; Shpakova *et al.*, 2012a).

The biological activity and selectivity of GPCR-peptides were markedly increased due to their modification by hydrophobic C_{12}–C_{18} acyl or steroid radicals or TM fragments, and these peptides having hydrophobic radicals were designated as pepducins (Covic *et al.*, 2002a, 2002b). Pepducins are able to penetrate through the plasma membrane, rapidly gain access to intracellular targets, and effectively interact with complementary regions of the cognate GPCR and, although less likely, with receptor-binding regions of other signal proteins. Pepducins anchor in lipid matrix of the membrane and form stable complexes with GPCR. This increases pepducin concentration at the perimembranous interface where the targets of pepducin action are localized. It is assumed that the hydrophobic tail of pepducin penetrates into GPCR transmembrane channel while its hydrophilic portion, usually positively charged, is localized in the cytoplasm. Pepducin interacts with complementary regions of the receptor, inducing change of their conformation and, as a result, of the entire G protein-interacting surface. Depending on the changes, pepducin acts either as agonist or as antagonist, strengthening or weakening the signal transduction via the cognate receptor. It was shown in the last few years that pepducins, derivatives of different types of GPCR, are active not only *in vitro*, but also *in vivo*, which possible to create highly effective pepducin-based drugs, regulators of physiological functions of humans and animals (Covic *et al.*, 2007; Miller *et al.*, 2009; Dimond *et al.*, 2011; Tressel *et al.*, 2011; O'Callaghan *et al.*, 2012a).

Cell-penetrating pepducins corresponding to intracellular regions of a large number of GPCR, e.g. protease-activated receptors PAR1, PAR2, and PAR4, chemokine receptors CXCR1, CXCR2, CXCR4, and CCR5, the sphingosine-1-phosphate receptor, the relaxin receptor RXFP1, the receptors of luteinizing hormone and thyroid-stimulating hormone (TSH), α_{1B}-AR, 5-HT$_{1B}$R and 5-HT$_6$R, function as intracellular allosteric agonists, antagonists or modulators of their cognate receptors, their action is realized at the stage of specific interaction between the receptor and G protein (Covic *et al.*, 2002a, 2002b, Licht *et al.*, 2003; Kaneider *et al.*, 2005; Shpakov *et al.*, 2005, 2007, 2010a, 2011; Shpakova *et al.*, 2012a; Kubo *et al.*, 2006; Swift *et al.*, 2006; Janz *et al.*, 2011). Pepducins can be used as suppressors of arterial thrombosis, inhibitors of tumor survival and metastasis, regulators of angiogenesis and hematopoiesis, and in the treatment of potentially debilitating inflammatory diseases (Kaneider *et al.*, 2005; Leger *et al.*, 2006; Remsberg *et al.*, 2007; Agarwal *et al.*, 2008; Miller *et al.*, 2009; Tchernychev *et al.*, 2010; Cisowski *et al.*, 2011; Dimond *et al.*, 2011; Sevigny *et al.*, 2011; Tressel *et al.*, 2011; Abdel-Latif & Smyth, 2012; O'Callaghan *et al.*, 2012a, 2012b; Zhang *et al.*, 2012). Below are given some examples of possible application of proteins in practice.

Pepducin ATI-2341 corresponding to ICL1 of chemokine receptor CXCR4 induced CXCR4- and G protein-dependent signaling, receptor internalization, and chemotaxis in CXCR4-expressing cells, but when systemically administered intravenously in mice and monkeys the same pepducin acted as functional antagonist and dose-dependently mediated the release of granulocyte/macrophage progenitor cells from the bone marrow. The conclusion was made that ATI-2341 is a potent and efficacious mobilizer of bone marrow polymorphonuclear neutrophils and also of hematopoietic stem and progenitor cells; it can be used for the recruitment of these cells before autologous bone marrow transplantation (Tchernychev *et al.*, 2010). Pepducin P2pal-18S, derivative of ICL3 of PAR2, a cell surface receptor for trypsin-like proteases, *in vitro* completely suppressed trypsin and mast cell tryptase signaling mediated via PAR2 in neutrophils and colon cancer cells, and *in vivo* blocked with high efficiency PAR2-dependent inflammatory response in mice. In PAR2-deficient and mast-cell-deficient mice pepducin had no effect, which indicates the specificity of its action (Sevigny *et al.*, 2011). Pepducins, derivatives of ICL1 and ICL3 of PAR1, strongly inhibited PAR1-driven cell migration in the primary and the established cell lines, and ICL3-, unlike ICL1-pepducins, effectively inhibited PAR1-mediated extracellular regulated kinase 1/2 activation and tumor growth. Comparable in efficacy with Bevacizumab, monotherapy with PAR1 ICL3-pepducin P1pal-7 provided 75 % inhibition of lung tumor growth in nude mice (Cisowski *et al.*, 2011). Pepducins corresponding to ICL1 and ICL3 of chemokine receptor CXCR4 completely abrogated CXCL12-mediated cell migration of lymphocytic leukemias and lymphomas, and the treatment of mice bearing disseminated lymphoma xenografts with the pepducins alone or in combination with rituximab, a chimeric monoclonal antibody against protein CD20, significantly increased their survival (O'Callaghan *et al.*, 2012b). Palmitoylated peptide 612–627-KA, derivative of N-terminal portion of ICL3 of TSH receptor, *in vitro* effectively stimulated AC activity and G_s protein GTP binding capacity in thyroidal membranes and decreased TSH-induced stimulating effects on AC system, while *in vivo* when systemically administered intranasally to rats it significantly increased the level of thyroxin and inhibited the stimulating influence of thyroliberin, a hypothalamic TSH-releasing factor, on TSH and thyroxin secretion (Shpakova *et al.*, 2012a).

3   Heterotrimeric G proteins

In the case of heterotrimeric G-proteins, unlike the integral receptor proteins, there are numerous data on their 3D structure and conformational rearrangements have been obtained using X-ray analysis, NMR, FRET and other techniques. Therefore, the structural investigations of peptides derived of G protein subunits primarily are very important in the study of the molecular mechanisms and the molecular dynamics of G protein-mediated signal transduction and in comparative analysis of the conformation of peptide and the region homologous to it in the full-size proteins. A large number of investigations are devoted to peptides corresponding to the C-terminal segment of Gα-subunits, unique for each subunit type and responsible for specific interaction with activated GPCR (Table 2). The segment in receptor-interacting state promotes the changes in the guanine nucleotide-binding site of the Gα-subunit, inducing the GDP/GTP exchange.

Peptide 340–350 corresponding to C-terminal segment of transducin, Gα$_t$ subunit, and its analog with Lys[341] replaced by leucine interacted with photoactivated form of light-activated receptor rhodopsin, meta-II-rhodopsin, stabilized its active conformation, thus mimicking the effects of transducin (Hamm *et al.*, 1988; Angel *et al.*, 2006). This peptide also bound to meta-Ib-rhodopsin, another intermediate of light-activated rhodopsin, forming a complex with inactive GDP-bound transducin, and with opsin, the ligand-free form of rhodopsin (Morizumi *et al.*, 2003; Scheerer *et al.*, 2008).

Gα subunit, localization	Amino acid sequence	Specific activity	References
Gα$_t$, C-terminal region	IKENLKDCGLF[340–350]	Peptide stabilizes the active state of opsin, meta-II-rhodopsin and meta-Ib-rhodopsin	(Hamm *et al.*, 1988; Morizumi *et al.*, 2003; Angel *et al.*, 2006; Scheerer *et al.*, 2008)
Gα$_s$, C-terminal region	RVFNDARDIIQRMHLR QYELL[374–394] and its short analogs	These peptides selectively inhibit transduction of hormonal signal via G$_s$ protein-coupled receptors	(Mazzoni *et al.*, 2000)
Gα$_s$, Switch I (1) and II (2) regions	RCRVLTSGIFETKFQVD K[199–216] (1); FDVGGQRDERRKWIQ CFNDVTAIIFV[222–247] (2)	The peptides increase the basal and forskolin-stimulated AC2 and AC6 activities; inhibit Gα$_s$-stimulated activity of both AC isoforms; behave as partial agonist	(Chen *et al.*, 2001)
Gα$_s$, α3-β5 region	EALNLFKSIWNNRWL-RTIS[268–286]	Peptide inhibits the basal and forskolin-stimulated activities of AC2 and AC6; decreases the Gα$_s$-mediated stimulation of AC activity	(Chen *et al.*, 2001)

Table 2: The biological activity of peptide, the derivatives of α subunits of heterotrimeric G proteins

Studying the molecular mechanisms of interaction of C-terminal peptide 340–350 and its analogs with G protein-bound opsin it was found that the peptide had contacts with the inner segments of the TM5, TM6, and TM7 regions and with the N-terminus of the additional helix 8 (Acharya *et al.*, 1997; Koenig *et al.*, 2002). The interaction between peptide 340–350(K[341]L) and rhodopsin led to destruction of hydrogen bond network which includes the side chains of residues Arg[135] and Glu[134] forming the conserved E(D)RY motif that is localized in the TM3/ICL2 interface and the side chains of residues Glu[247] and Thr[251] located in the inner segment of TM6 region. These events provoke the outward movement of the TM6 region and the formation of TM5–TM6 pair stabilized by new interactions between the Glu[247] and Thr[251] of this region, which releases Arg[135] and Lys[231] of the TM5 region (Van Eps *et al.*, 2010). The contacts with inner segments of the TM5 and TM6 regions induce α-helical conformation of peptide 340–350(K[341]L) with a C-terminal reverse turn. The carbonyl groups in the reverse turn constitute the center of a hydrogen bond network which links the two receptor regions containing the E(D)RY motif and the conserved NPxxY(x)$_{5,6}$F motif connecting the TM7 region and the helix 8.

The stabilization of meta-II-rhodopsin can be achieved by cross-linking C-terminal peptide 340–350(K[341]L) to native reactive cysteines, Cys[140] and Cys[316], located on the intracellular surface of receptor.

Using synthetic peptides with cross-linking group localized either at the N-terminus or the C-terminus of peptide 340–350(K^{341}L), it was shown that the N-terminus of peptide analog M-23S was cross-linked to Cys^{140} and the C-terminus of peptide analog B23S-IA to Cys^{316}, and both modifications were required for stabilization of meta-II-rhodopsin (Angel *et al.*, 2006). At the same time, peptide B23S-IA stabilized the more compact meta-IIa-rhodopsin conformation, whereas peptide M-23S stabilized meta-IIb-rhodopsin, protonation form of meta-II-rhodopsin capable of activating the G protein. It was shown that negatively charged residues Glu^{342} and Asp^{346} of peptide 340–350 of $G\alpha_t$ participated in specific binding with positively charged intracellular regions of rhodopsin (Fahmy, 1998). The elimination of the N-terminal NH_2-group of peptide 340–350, delocalization of positive charge replacing lysines by arginines and the substitution of Lys by Leu increased the affinity of modified peptide for meta-II-rhodopsin, whereas elimination of the C-terminal COOH-group, on the contrary, reduced it (Martin *et al.*, 1996; Aris *et al.*, 2001).

The efficiency of the interaction between $G\alpha$-subunit-derived C-terminal peptides and GPCR, and their influence on the hormonal signal transduction via G_s protein are strongly depend on the similarity of the 3D structure of the peptides and homologous to them regions in the full-length $G\alpha$-subunit. Studying the $G\alpha_s$ subunit crystal structure, the evidence was obtained that the α5-helix responsible for effective interaction with the receptors involves the region from Asp^{368} to Leu^{394} (Sunahara *et al.*, 1997). The peptides 378–394(C^{379}A), 376–394(C^{379}A) and 374–394(C^{379}A) of $G\alpha_s$, 17 to 21 residues long, had a stronger propensity to assume α-helical conformation and showed high specific activity, stimulating specific binding of selective agonist CGS21680 to the G_s-coupled A_{2A}-adenosine receptor in the rat brain membranes both in the presence and in the absence of GTPγS uncoupling G proteins from receptors (Mazzoni *et al.*, 2000). Using NMR data a suggestion was put forward that 21-mer peptide 374–394(C^{379}A) in hexafluoroacetone/water, a mixture with structure stabilizing properties, demonstrated a marked propensity to form the longest α-helix spanning region from Asp^{381} to Leu^{394}. The peptide 384–394 in the same conditions formed the shortest α-helix between Arg^{389} and Leu^{394} and was less active compared with 17–21-mer peptides (Mazzoni *et al.*, 2000; Albrizio *et al.*, 2004). The conjugation of 21-mer peptide 374–394(C^{379}A) with 16-mer membrane-permeable sequence of penetratin giving the 37-mer constrain did not interfere with the ability to form an extended helix within $G\alpha_s$ sequence (D'Ursi *et al.*, 2006). The NMR analysis showed that the segment 375-393 in this constrain formed amphipathic helix with a polar surface lined by Asp^{378}, Arg^{390}, Asp^{381}, and Arg^{385} and two hydrophobic surfaces formed by less polar residues Ile^{382}, Ile^{383}, Met^{386}, His^{387}, Tyr^{391}, and Leu^{393}. Penetratin fragment also possessing α-helical structure encompassing sequence 3-10 had hydrophobic and hydrophilic residues forming clustered surfaces at the N-terminus and in the center of the fragment, and was responsible for internalization of peptide 374–394(C^{379}A) by endocytosis. Constrain penetratin-374–394(C^{379}A) significantly inhibited A_{2A}-adenosine receptor- and β-AR-mediated regulation of AC activity in different cell lines, suggesting that it competed with $G\alpha_s$ for the interaction with G_s-coupled GPCR; but did not directly modulate AC activity, nor did it affect G_i- and G_q-coupled receptor signaling. Thus, in all probability the specific target for peptide is the receptor G_s-binding and -activating surfaces (D'Ursi *et al.*, 2006).

The strong evidences for the key role of the C-terminal segment of $G\alpha$ subunits in their selective interaction with GPCR were obtained with the minigene strategy based on the expression of plasmid vectors encoding 11-mer C-terminal segments of $G\alpha_i$, $G\alpha_o$, $G\alpha_q$, $G\alpha_{12}$ and $G\alpha_{13}$ subunits (Gilchrist *et al.*, 1999, 2001; Vanhauwe *et al.*, 2002). The vector expressing the $G\alpha_{i1/2}$ C-terminal peptide inhibited the stimulation of inwardly rectifying K^+ channel activity mediated via $G_{i1/2}$-coupled m_2-MChR, the vectors expressing the $G\alpha_o$ and $G\alpha_q$ C-terminal peptides decreased thrombin-stimulated intracellular Ca^{2+} level and inhibited the stimulatory effects of thrombin on PLC activity mediated via the human thromboxane A_2 receptor coupled with G_o and G_q proteins, and the vectors expressing the $G\alpha_{12}$ and $G\alpha_{13}$ C-terminal peptides decreased thrombin-stimulated stress fiber formation that is mediated via $G_{12/13}$ protein family. A minigene encoding mutated C-terminal sequence of G_q protein in which two C-terminal residues, Ala and Val, were replaced by the Thr and Lys residues, had a little effect on thrombin-induced PLC activity (Gilchrist et al., 2001). Thus, the action of minigenes is very specific, it is realized provided hormonal responses are mediated via the cognate G proteins, which can be used as a powerful tool to study participation of different types of G proteins in GPCR-mediated signal transduction.

The strategy based on $G\alpha$-derived peptides can be used to study the molecular mechanisms of interaction between G proteins and the effector enzymes on the one hand and the selectivity of this interaction on the other. The influence of three peptides 199–216, 222–247, 268–286 of $G\alpha_s$ subunit corresponding to AC-interacting regions and, as was found in crystallographic investigations, having a direct contact with the enzyme on the activity of the types 2 and 6 AC was studied (Chen et al., 2001). Peptide 199–216 including the Switch I region of $G\alpha_s$ stimulated the basal and forskolin-stimulated activity of AC2 and AC6 and significantly inhibited their activity stimulated by GTP-bound $G\alpha_s$, thus functioning as a partial agonist. Peptide 199–216 with the substitutions $G^{206}P$, $I^{207}D$, $E^{209}K$, and $K^{211}A$ had no effect on the enzyme activity, which agrees with the data that the residue Ile^{207} of $G\alpha_s$ had contact with AC while the residues Gly^{206}, Glu^{209} and Lys^{211} were responsible for appropriate conformation of the Switch I region. Peptide 222–247 including the Switch II region also stimulated the basal and forskolin-stimulated activity of both AC isoforms and inhibited $G\alpha_s$-stimulated AC activity. The effects of peptides 199–216 and 222–247 on AC2 activity were additive at lower, but not at saturating concentrations. At the same time, peptide 222–247 lowered the stimulating effect of peptide 199–216 on AC6 activity. In the case of AC2 the stimulating effect of peptide 199–224 was stronger compared with peptide 222–247, while in the case of AC6 predominating was the effect of peptide 222–247. These data indicate that the molecular mechanisms underlying interaction of the Switch regions of $G\alpha_s$ with different AC isoforms are not all alike. Peptides 199–224 and 204–229 corresponding to the Switch II regions of the $G\alpha_i$ and $G\alpha_q$ subunits, respectively, were very similar to the Switch II region of $G\alpha_s$, nevertheless they were not capable of stimulating the AC activity. Peptide 268–286 that corresponds to $G\alpha_s$ subunit $\alpha3$-$\beta5$ region interacting with both central and C-terminal cytoplasmic domains of the enzyme inhibited the basal and forskolin-stimulated activity of AC2 and AC6 and, in addition, significantly decreased their $G\alpha_s$-stimulated activity, which shows the involvement of $\alpha3$-$\beta5$ region in stabilization of the appropriate conformation of the Switch regions required for stimulation of AC activity. The replacement of highly conservative residues Trp^{277} and Trp^{280} by Arg and Lys led to the loss of biological activity of the peptide (Chen et al., 2001). These data allowed us to identify functionally important sites and single amino acid residues in $G\alpha$ subunits responsible for activation of effectors.

4   Conclusion

The comprehensive analysis of the data on the synthetic peptides corresponding to functionally important regions of GPCR and $G\alpha$ subunits would facilitate the study of the structure and function of GPCR and G proteins, which is very important for the development of new approaches and technologies to be used in control and regulation of G protein-dependent signaling systems. The screening of the pair interactions between TM-peptides contributes to the understanding of the architecture of GPCR transmembrane channel having a key role in the ligand binding and stabilization of di- and oligomeric receptor complexes and participating in formation of G protein-binding and G protein-interacting surfaces. The use of TM-peptides to construct the model of ligand-free transmembrane channel and the peptides chemically cross-linked to ligands or forming a complex with them to obtain the model of ligand-regulated channels made it possible for us to study the molecular dynamics of ligand-binding pocket of the receptor and to identify single amino acid residues and their clusters involved in the formation of hydrogen bond network that connects the ligand-binding site of GPCR, its ICL regions and the guanine nucleotide-binding site of $G\alpha$ subunit. The use of ECL-peptides and their cyclic and pseudo cyclic constrains provides opportunities to identify the molecular determinants in ECL responsible for recognition and binding of hormonal molecules and to reveal their structural features critical for formation of the productive ligand–receptor complex. Promising prospects expected in the application of peptides to study ligand binding and subsequent transduction of hormonal signal into cell come from the fact that the conformation of the ECL- and ICL-derived peptides is often very similar to that of the corresponding loops in the intact receptor, especially in the case of ECL- and ICL-peptides with the cyclic structure formed by disulfide, amide and other covalent bonds between N- and C-terminal amino acid residues or with the pseudo cyclic structure stabilized due to interaction between TM/ECL- and TM/ICL-interfaces and artificial amino acid sequences forming interhelical contacts. ICL-peptides and $G\alpha$ protein-peptides are functional probes to be used in the study of structural-functional organization of receptor-G protein binding interaction, identification of molecular determinants responsible for the selectivity and efficiency of the interaction. They can be used for development of a new generation of regulators and modulators of hormonal signaling systems.

GPCR- and $G\alpha$ protein-peptides can be used for isolation and identification of GPCR and their endogenous and artificial ligands, G protein subunits and signal proteins interacting with GPCR and G proteins. The gold-chemisorbed peptides 218–230 and 361–373, derivatives of the ICL3 of G_i-coupled α_2-AR, bound with high specificity to the G_i protein and did not interact with other G proteins (Vahlberg *et al.*, 2006). The preparation of mixed monolayers of ICL3-peptides and GGGC-peptide induced the increase of G protein absorption capability and selectivity, being a perspective approach for the improvement of binding characteristics of adsorbents with immobilized GPCR-peptides (Balau *et al.*, 2007).

A better knowledge of the structure and the use of peptides as functional probes to study signaling cascades give grounds for the development of a new generation of peptide-based therapeutic agents that can be widely applied in pharmacy and clinical medicine. There is a good reason to expect such drugs to exert influence on the initial stages of signal transduction, ligand-induced receptor activation, and on post-receptor stages, including GPCR–G protein coupling and regulation of a wide spectrum of effector proteins. Even small structural modifications of GPCR- and $G\alpha$ protein-peptides, as in the case of pepducins, can lead to significant changes in their therapeutic potential. This allows creation of a large set of homologs with different pharmacological characteristics (Dimond *et al.*, 2011). Thus, there are good prospects for these signal protein-peptides to be applied in future both in fundamental science and in medical practice in the treatment of many diseases having various etiology and pathogenesis.

References

Abdel-Latif, A. & Smyth, S.S. (2012). Preventing platelet thrombosis with a PAR1 pepducin. Circulation, 126, 13–15.

Acharya, S., Saad, Y. & Karnik, S.S. (1997). Transducin-α C-terminal peptide binding site consists of C-D and E-F loops of rhodopsin. Journal of Biological Chemistry, 272, 6519–6524.

Agarwal, A., Covic, L., Sevigny, L.M., Kaneider, N.C., Lazarides, K., Azabdaftari, G., Sharifi, S. & Kuliopulos, A. (2008). Targeting a metalloprotease-PAR1 signaling system with cell-penetrating pepducins inhibits angiogenesis, ascites, and progression of ovarian cancer. Molecular Cancer Therapeutics, 7, 2746–2757.

Albrizio, S., D'Ursi, A., Fattorusso, C., Galoppini, C., Greco, G., Mazzoni, M.R., Novellino, E. & Rovero, P. (2004). Conformational studies on a synthetic C-terminal fragment of the α subunit of Gₛ proteins. Biopolymers, 54, 186–194.

Angel, T.E., Kraft, P.C. & Dratz, E.A. (2006) Metarhodopsin-II stabilization by crosslinked Gtₜ C-terminal peptides and implications for the mechanism of GPCR–G protein coupling. Vision Research, 46, 4547–4555.

Aris, L., Gilchrist, A., Rens-Domiano, S., Meyer, C., Schatz, P.J., Dratz, E.A. & Hamm, H.E. (2001). Structural requirements for the stabilization of metarhodopsin II by the C terminus of the α subunit of transducin. Journal of Biological Chemistry, 276, 2333–2339.

Arshava, B., Taran, I., Xie, H., Becker, J.M. & Naider, F. (2002). High resolution NMR analysis of the seven transmembrane domains of a heptahelical receptor in organic-aqueous medium. Biopolymers, 64, 161–176.

Balau, L.S., Vahlberg, C., Petoral, R.M. & Uvdal, K. (2007). Mixed monolayers to promote G-protein adsorption: α_{2A}-adrenergic receptor-derived peptides coadsorbed with formyl-terminated oligopeptides. Langmuir, 23, 8474–8479.

Bavec, A., Hallbrink, M., Langel, U. & Zorko, M. (2003). Different role of intracellular loops of glucagon-like peptide-1 receptor in G-protein coupling. Regulatory Peptides, 111, 137–144.

Bellot, G., Granier, S., Bourguet, W., Seyer, R., Rahmeh, R., Mouillac, B., Pascal, R., Mendre, C. & Demene, H. (2009). Structure of the third intracellular loop of the vasopressin V_2 receptor and conformational changes upon binding to gC1qR. Journal of. Molecular Biology, 388, 491–507.

Beltrame, S.P., Auger, S.R., Bilder, C.R., Waldner, C.I. & Goin, J.C. (2011). Modulation of M_2 muscarinic receptor-receptor interaction by immunoglobulin G antibodies from Chagas' disease patients. Clinical and Experimental Immunology, 164, 170–179.

Berg, C.P., Blume, K., Lauber, K., Gregor, M., Berg, P.A., Wesselborg, S. & Stein, G.M. (2010). Autoantibodies to muscarinic acetylcholine receptors found in patients with primary biliary cirrhosis. BMC Gastroenterology, 10, 120.

Birnbaumer, L. (2007). Expansion of signal transduction by G proteins. The second 15 years or so: from 3 to 16 α subunits plus βγ dimers. Biochimica et Biophysica Acta, 1768, 772–793.

Bockaert, J., Marin, P., Dumuis, A. & Fagni, L. (2003). The "magic tail" of G protein-coupled receptors: an anchorage for functional protein networks. FEBS Letters, 546, 65–72.

Britton, Z.T., Hanle, E.I. & Robinson, A.S. (2012). An expression and purification system for the biosynthesis of adenosine receptor peptides for biophysical and structural characterization. Protein Expression and Purification, 84, 224–235.

Bryant, S.D., Guerrini, R., Salvadori, S., Bianchi, C., Tomatis, R., Attila, M. & Lazarus, L.H. (1997). Helix-inducing alpha-aminoisobutyric acid in opioid mimetic deltorphin C analogues. Journal of Medicinal Chemistry, 40, 2579–2587.

Buvall, L., Tang, M.S., Isic, A., Andersson, B. & Fu, M. (2007). Antibodies against the β_1-adrenergic receptor induce progressive development of cardiomyopathy. Journal of Molecular and Cellular Cardiology, 42, 1001–1007.

Chen, Y., Yoo, B., Lee J.B., Weng, G. & Iyengar, R. (2001). The signal transfer regions of Gαₛ. Journal of Biological Chemistry, 276, 45751–45754.

Chillar, A., Wu, J., So, S.P. & Ruan, K.H. (2008). Involvement of non-conserved residues important for PGE2 binding to the constrained EP3 eLP2 using NMR and site-directed mutagenesis. FEBS Letters, 582, 2863–2868.

Choi, G., Landin, J., Galan, J.F., Birge, R.R., Albert, A.D. & Yeagle, P.L. (2002). Structural studies of metarhodopsin II, the activated form of the G-protein coupled receptor, rhodopsin. Biochemistry, 41, 7318–7324.

Cisowski, J., O'Callaghan, K., Kuliopulos, A., Yang, J., Nguyen, N., Deng, Q., Yang, E., Fogel, M., Tressel, S., Foley, C., Agarwal, A., Hunt, S.W. 3rd, McMurry, T., Brinckerhoff, L. & Covic, L. (2011). Targeting protease-activated receptor-1 with cell-penetrating pepducins in lung cancer. The American Journal of Pathology, 179, 513–523.

Clubb, R.T., Omichinski, J.G., Clore, G.M. & Gronenborn, A.M. (1994). Mapping the binding surface of interleukin-8 complexed with an N-terminal fragment of the type 1 human interleukin-8 receptor. FEBS Letters, 338, 93–97.

Colvin, R.A., Campanella, G.S., Manice, L.A. & Luster, A.D. (2006). CXCR3 requires tyrosine sulfation for ligand binding and a second extracellular loop arginine residue for ligand-induced chemotaxis. Molecular and Cellular Biology, 26, 5838–5849.

Covic, L., Gresser, A.L., Talavera, J., Swift, S. & Kuliopulos, A. (2002a). Activation and inhibition of G protein-coupled receptors by cell-penetrating membrane-tethered peptides. Proceedings of the National Academy of Sciences of the United States of America, 99, 643–648.

Covic, L., Misra, M., Badar, J., Singh, C. & Kuliopulos, A. (2002b). Pepducin-based intervention of thrombin-receptor signaling and systemic platelet activation. Nature Medicine, 8, 1161–1165.

Covic, L., Tchernychev, B., Jacques, S. & Kuliopulos, A. (2007). Pharmacology and in vivo efficacy of pepducins in hemostasis and arterial thrombosis. Handbook of Cell-Penetrating Peptides, Taylor & Francis, New York, 245–257.

Dimond, P., Carlson, K., Bouvier, M., Gerard, C., Xu, L., Covic, L., Agarwal, A., Ernst, O.P., Janz, J.M., Schwartz, T.W., Gardella, T.J., Milligan, G., Kuliopulos, A., Sakmar, T.P. & Hunt, S.W. 3rd. (2011). G protein-coupled receptor modulation with pepducins: moving closer to the clinic. Annals of the New York Academy of Sciences, 1226, 34–49.

D'Ursi, A.M., Giusti, L., Albrizio, S., Porchia, F., Esposito, C., Caliendo, G., Gargini, C., Novellino, E., Lucacchini, A., Rovero P. & Mazzoni M.R. (2006). A membrane-permeable peptide containing the last 21 residues of the $G\alpha_s$ carboxyl terminus inhibits G_s-coupled receptor signaling in intact cells: correlation between peptide structure and biological activity. Molecular Pharmacology, 69, 727–736.

Fadhil, I., Schmidt, R., Walpole, C. & Carpenter, K.A. (2004). Exploring deltorphin II binding to the third extracellular loop of the delta-opioid receptor. Journal of Biological Chemistry, 279, 21069–21077.

Fahmy, K. (1998). Binding of transducin and transducin-derived peptides to rhodopsin studies by attenuated total reflection-Fourier transform infrared difference spectroscopy. Biophysical Journal, 75, 1306–1318.

Farzan, M., Babcock, G. J., Vasilieva, N., Wright, P. L., Kiprilov, E., Mirzabekov, T. & Choe, H. (2002). The role of post-translational modifications of the CXCR4 amino terminus in stromal-derived factor 1R association and HIV-1 entry. Journal of Biological Chemistry, 277, 29484–29489.

Ferguson, D.M., Kramer, S., Metzger, T.G., Law, P.Y. & Portoghese, P.S. (2000). Isosteric replacement of acidic with neutral residues in extracellular loop-2 of the κ-opioid receptor does not affect dynorphin A (1-13) affinity and function. Journal of Medicinal Chemistry, 43,1251–1252.

Flanagan, C.A., Becker, I.I., Davidson, J.S., Wakefield, I.K., Zhou, W., Sealfon, S.C. & Millar, R.P. (1994). Glutamate 301 of the mouse gonadotropin-releasing hormone receptor confers specificity for arginine 8 of mammalian gonadotropin-releasing hormone. Journal of Biological Chemistry, 269, 22636–22641.

Fowler, C.B., Pogozheva, I.D., Lomize, A.L., LeVine, H. & Mosberg, H.I. (2004). Complex of an active mu-opioid receptor with a cyclic peptide agonist modeled from experimental contrains. Biochemistry, 43, 8700–8710.

Franzoni, L., Nicastro, G., Pertinhez, T.A., Oliveira, E., Nakaie, C.R., Paiva, A.C., Schreier, S. & Spisni A. (1999). Structure of two fragments of the third cytoplasmic loop of the rat angiotensin II AT_{1A} receptor. Implications with respect to receptor activation and G-protein selection and coupling. Journal of Biological Chemistry, 274, 227–235.

Franzoni, L., Nicastro, G., Pertinhez, T.A., Tato, M., Nakaie, C.R., Paiva, A.C., Schreier, S. & Spisni, A. (1997). Structure of the C-terminal fragment 300-320 of the rat angiotensin II AT_{1A} receptor and its relevance with respect to G protein coupling. Journal of Biological Chemistry, 272, 9734–9741.

Fromme, B.J., Katz, A.A., Roeske, R.W., Millar, R.P. & Flanagan, C.A. (2001). Role of aspartate[7.32(302)] of the human gonadotropin-releasing hormone receptor in stabilizing a high-affinity ligand conformation. Molecular Pharmacology, 60, 1280–1287.

George, L., Arnau, C. & Leonardo, P. (2012). The G-protein coupled receptor family: actors with many faces. Current Pharmaceutical Design, 18, 175–185.

George, S.R., Ng, G.Y., Lee, S.P., Fan, T., Varghese, G., Wang, C., Deber, C.M., Seeman, P. & O'Dowd, B.F. (2003). Blockade of G protein-coupled receptors and the dopamine transporter by a transmembrane domain peptide: novel strategy for functional inhibition of membrane proteins in vivo. The Journal of Pharmacology and Experimental Therapeutics, 307, 481–489.

Gilchrist, A., Bunemann, M., Li, A., Hosey, M.M. & Hamm, H.E. (1999). A dominant-negative strategy for studying roles of G proteins in vivo. Journal of Biological Chemistry, 274, 6610–6616.

Gilchrist, A., Vanhauwe, J.F., Li, A., Thomas, T.O., Voyno-Yasenetskaya, T. & Hamm, H.E. (2001). Gα minigenes expressing C-terminal peptides serves as specific inhibitors of thrombin-mediated endothelial activation. Journal of Biological Chemistry, 276, 25672–25679.

Giragossian, C. & Mierke, D.F. (2003). Determination of ligand-receptor interactions of cholecystokinin by nuclear magnetic resonance. Life Sciences, 73, 705–713.

Granier, S., Manglik, A., Kruse, A.C., Kobilka, T.S., Thian, F.S., Weis, W.I. & Kobilka, B.K. (2012). Structure of the δ-opioid receptor bound to naltrindole. Nature, 485, 400–404.

Granier, S., Terrillon, S., Pascal, R., Demene, H., Bouvier, M., Guillon, G. & Mendre, C. (2004). A cyclic peptide mimicking the third intracellular loop of the V_2 vasopressin receptor inhibits signaling through its interaction with receptor dimer and G protein, Journal of Biological Chemistry, 279, 50904–50914.

Gutierrez, J., Kremer, L., Zaballos, A., Goya, I., Martinez, A. C. & Marquez, G. (2004). Analysis of post-translational CCR8 modifications and their influence on receptor activity. Journal of Biological Chemistry, 279, 14726–14733.

Hamm, H.E., Deretic, D., Arendt, A., Hargrave, P.A., Koenig B. & Hofmann, K.P. (1988). Site of G protein binding to rhodopsin mapped with synthetic peptides from the α subunit. Science, 241, 832–835.

Hebert, T.E., Moffett, S., Morello, J.P., Loisel, T.P., Bichet, D.G., Barret, C. & Bouvier, M. (1996). A peptide derived from a $β_2$-adrenergic receptor transmembrane domain inhibits both receptor dimerization and activation. Journal of Biological Chemistry, 271, 16384–16392.

Heitzler, D., Crepieux, P., Poupon, A., Clement, F., Fages, F. & Reiter, E. (2009). Towards a systems biology approach of G protein-coupled receptor signalling: challenges and expectations. Comptes Rendus Biologies, 332, 947–957.

Hernandez, C.C., Nascimento, J.H., Chaves, E.A., Costa, P.C., Masuda, M.O., Kurtenbach, E., Campos, D.E., Carvalho, A.C. & Gimenez, L.E. (2008). Autoantibodies enhance agonist action and binding to cardiac muscarinic receptors in chronic Chagas' disease. Journal of Receptor and Signal Transduction Research, 28, 375–401.

Higashijima, T., Burnier, J. & Ross, E.M. (1990). Regulation of G_i and G_o by mastoparan, related amphiphilic peptides and hydrophobic amines, Journal of Biological Chemistry, 265, 14176–14186.

Higashijima T., Wakamatsu K., Takemitsu M., Fujino M., Nakajima T. & Miyazawa T. (1983). Conformational change of mastoparan from wasp venom on binding with phospholipid membrane. FEBS Letters, 152, 227–230.

Iwata, M., Yoshikawa, T., Baba, A., Anzai, T., Nakamura, I., Wainai Y., Takahashi, T. & Ogawa, S. (2001). Autoimmunity against the second extracellular loop of β1-adrenergic receptors induces β-adrenergic receptor desensitization and myocardial hypertrophy in vivo. Circulation Research, 88, 578–586.

Jahns, R., Boivin, V., Hein, L., Triebel, S., Angermann, C.E., Ertl, G. & Lohse, M.J. (2004). Direct evidence for a β_1-adrenergic receptor-directed autoimmune attack as a cause of idiopathic dilated cardiomyopathy. The Journal of Clinical Investigation, 113, 1419–1429.

Jahns, R., Boivin, V., Krapf, T., Wallukat, G., Boefe, F. & Lohse, M.J. (2000). Modulation of β_1-adrenoceptor activity by domain-specific antibodies and heart failure-associated autoantibodies. Journal of the American College of Cardiology, 36, 1280–1287.

Jahns, R., Boivin, V. & Lohse, M.J. (2006). β_1-Adrenergic receptor-directed autoimmunity as a cause of dilated cardiomyopathy in rats. International Journal of Cardiology, 112, 7–14.

Jane-wit, D., Altuntas, C.Z., Johnson, J.M., Yong, S., Wickley, P.J., Clark, P., Wang, Q., Popović, Z.B., Penn, M.S., Damron, D.S., Perez, D.M. & Tuohy, V.K. (2007). β_1-Adrenergic receptor autoantibodies mediate dilated cardiomyopathy by agonistically inducing cardiomyocyte apoptosis. Circulation, 116, 399–410.

Janz, J.M., Ren, Y., Looby, R., Kazmi, M.A., Sachdev, P., Grunbeck, A., Haggis, L., Chinnapen, D., Lin, A.Y., Seibert, C., McMurry, T., Carlson, K.E., Muir, T.W., Hunt, S. 3rd & Sakmar, TP. (2011). Direct interaction between an allosteric agonist pepducin and the chemokine receptor CXCR4. Journal of the American Chemical Society, 133, 15878–15881.

Jinno-Oue, A., Shimizu, N., Soda, Y., Tanaka, A., Ohtsuki, T., Kurosaki, D., Suzuki, Y. & Hishino, H. (2005). The synthetic peptide derived from the NH_2-terminal extracellular region of an orphan G protein-coupled receptor, GPR1, preferentially inhibits infection of X4 HIV-1. Journal of Biological Chemistry, 280, 30924–30934.

Johnston, C.A. & Siderovski, D.P (2007). Receptor-mediated activation of heterotrimeric G-proteins: current structural insights. Molecular Pharmacology, 72, 219–230.

Kamel, R., Eftekhari, P., Garcia, S., Berthouze, M., Berque-Bestel, I., Peter, J.C., Lezoualc'h, F. & Hoebeke, J. (2005). A high-affinity monoclonal antibody with functional activity against the 5-hydroxytryptaminergic (5-HT4) receptor. Biochemical Pharmacology, 70, 1009–1018.

Kaneider, N.C., Agarwal, A., Leger, A.J. & Kuliopulos A. (2005). Reversing systemic inflammatory response syndrome with chemokine receptor pepducins. Nature Medicine, 11, 661–665.

Katragadda, M., Alderfer, J.L. & Yeagle, P.L. (2000). Solution structure of the loops of bacteriorhodopsin closely resembles the crystal structure. Biochimica et Biophysica Acta, 1466, 1–6.

Katritch, V., Cherezov, V. & Stevens, R.C. (2012). Diversity and modularity of G protein-coupled receptor structures. Trends in Pharmacological Sciences, 33, 17–27.

Kerman, A. & Ananthanarayanan, V.S. (2005). Expression and spectroscopic characterization of a large fragment of the mu-opioid receptor. Biochimica et Biophysica Acta, 1747, 133–140.

Kerman, A. & Ananthanarayanan, V.S. (2007). Conformation of a double-membrane-spanning fragment of a G protein-coupled receptor: effects of hydrophobic environment and pH. Biochimica et Biophysica Acta, 1768, 1199–1210.

Kikkou, T., Matsumoto, O., Ohkubo, T., Kobayashi, Y. & Tsujimoto, G. (2006). NMR structure of an intracellular loop peptide derived from prostaglandin EP3α receptor. Biochemical and Biophysical Research Communications, 345, 933–937.

Kikkou, T., Matsumoto, O., Ohkubo, T., Kobayashi, Y. & Tsujimoto, G. (2007). NMR structure of a human homologous Methuselah gene receptor peptide. Biochemical and Biophysical Research Communications, 352, 17–20.

Kikkou, T., Matsumoto, O., Ohkubo, T., Kobayashi, Y. & Tsujimoto, G. (2008). NMR structure of an intracellular third loop peptide of human GABA$_B$ receptor. Biochemical and Biophysical Research Communications, 366, 681–684.

Koenig, B.W., Kontaxis, G., Mitchell, D.C., Louis, J.M., Litman, B.J. & Bax, A. (2002). Structure and orientation of a G protein fragment in the receptor bound state from residual dipolar couplings. Journal of Molecular Biology, 322, 441–461.

Kohr, D., Singh, P., Tschernatsch, M., Kaps, M., Pouokam, E., Diener, M., Kummer, W., Birklein, F., Vincent, A., Goebel, A., Wallukat, G. & Blaes, F. (2011). Autoimmunity against the β₂ adrenergic receptor and muscarinic-2 receptor in complex regional pain syndrome. Pain, 152, 2690–2700.

Kubo, S., Ishiki, T., Doe, I., Sekiguchi, F., Nishikawa, H., Kawai, K., Matsui, H. & Kawabata, A. (2006). Distinct activity of peptide mimetic intracellular ligands (pepducins) for proteinase-activated receptor-1 in multiple cells/tissues. Annals of the New York Academy of Sciences, 1091, 445–459.

Kusunoki, H., Wakamatsu, K., Sato, K., Miyazawa, T. & Kohno, T. (1998). G protein-bound conformation of mastoparan-X: heteronuclear multidimensional transferred nuclear overhauser effect analysis of peptide uniformly enriched with ^{13}C and ^{15}N. Biochemistry, 37, 4782–4790.

Lambright, D.G., Sondek, J., Bohm, A., Skiba, N.P., Hamm, H.E. & Sigler, P.B. (1996). The 2.0 A crystal structure of a heterotrimeric G protein. Nature, 379, 311–319.

Lee, W.K., Han, J.J., Jin, B.S., Boo, D.W. & Yu, Y.G. (2009). Functional reconstitution of the human serotonin receptor 5-HT(6) using synthetic transmembrane peptides. Biochemical and Biophysical Research Communications, 390, 815–820.

Leger, A.J., Jacques, S.L., Badar, J., Kaneider, N.C., Derian, C.K., Andrade-Gordon, P., Covic, L. & Kuliopulos A. (2006). Blocking the protease-activated receptor 1–4 heterodimer in platelet-mediated thrombosis. Circulation, 113, 1244–1245.

Licht, T., Tsirulnikov, L., Reuveni, H., Yarnitzky, T. & Ben-Sasson, S.A. (2003). Induction of pro-angiogenic signaling by a synthetic peptide derived from the second intracellular loop of S1P3 (EDG3). Blood, 102, 2099–2107.

Lohse, M.J. & Hoffmann, C. (2009). GPCR and G proteins: drug efficacy and activation in live cells. Molecular Endocrinology, 23, 590–599.

Luttrell, L.M. (2006). Transmembrane signaling by G protein-coupled receptors. Methods in Molecular Biology, 332, 3–49.

Magnusson, Y., Wallukat, G., Waagstein, F., Hjalmarson, A. & Hoebeke, J. (1994). Autoimmunity in idiopathic dilated cardiomyopathy: characterization of antibodies against the β₁-adrenoreceptor with positive chronotropic effect. Circulation, 89, 2760–2767.

Martin, E.L., Rens-Domiano, S., Schatz, P.J. & Hamm, H.E. (1996). Potent peptide analogues of a G protein receptor-binding region obtained with a combinatorial library. Journal of Biological Chemistry, 271, 361–366.

Marty, C. & Ye, R.D. (2010). Heterotrimeric G protein signaling outside the realm of seven transmembrane domain receptors. Molecular Pharmacology, 78, 12–18.

Mason, J.S., Bortolato, A., Congreve, M. & Marshall, F.H. (2012). New insights from structural biology into the druggability of G protein-coupled receptors. Trends in Pharmacological Sciences, 33, 249–260.

Matsui, S. & Fu, M.L. (2006). Pathological importance of anti-G-protein coupled receptor autoantibodies. International Journal of Cardiology, 112, 27–29.

Mayer, K.L. & Stone, M.J. (2000). NMR solution structure and receptor peptide binding of the CC chemokine eotaxin-2. Biochemistry, 39, 8382–8395.

Mazzoni, M.R., Taddei, S., Giusti, L., Rovero, P., Galoppini, C., D'Ursi, A., Albrizio, S., Triolo, A., Novellino, E., Greco, G., Lucacchini. A. & Hamm, H.E. (2000). A Gαₛ carboxyl-terminal peptide prevents Gₛ activation by the A₂ₐ adenosine receptor. Molecular Pharmacology, 58, 226–236.

Megaritis, G., Merkouris, M. & Georgoussi, Z. (2000). Functional domains of δ- and μ-opioid receptors responsible for adenylyl cyclase inhibition. Receptors & Channels, 7, 199–212.

Miller, J., Agarwal, A., Devi, L.A., Fontanini, K., Hamilton, J.A., Pin, J.P., Shields, D.C., Spek, C.A., Sakmar, T.P., Kuliopulos, A. & Hunt, S.W. (2009). Insider access: pepducin symposium explores a new approach to GPCR modulation. Annals of the New York Academy of Sciences, 1180, E1–E12.

Miyamoto, K. & Togiya, K. (2011). Solution structure of LC4 transmembrane segment of CCR5. PloS One [electronic resource], 6, e20452.

Miyamoto, K., Togiya, K., Kitahara, R., Akasaka, K. & Kuroda, Y. (2010). Solution structure of LC5, the CCR5- derived peptide for HIV-1 inhibition. Journal of Peptide Science, 16, 165–170.

Mizoue, L.S., Basan, J.F., Johnson, E.C. & Handel, T.M. (1999). Solution structure and dynamics of the CX3C chemokine domain of fractalkine and its interaction with an N-terminal fragment of CX3CR1. Biochemistry, 38, 1402–1414.

Morizumi, T., Imai, H. & Shichida, Y. (2003). Two-step mechanism of interaction of rhodopsin intermediates with the C-terminal region of the transducin α-subunit. Journal of Biochemistry, 134, 259–267.

Mukai, H., Kikuchi, M., Suzuki, Y. & Munekata, E. (2007). A mastoparan analog without lytic effects and its stimulatory mechanisms in mast cells. Biochemical and Biophysical Research Communications, 362, 51–55.

Mukhopadhyay, S. & Howlett, A.C. (2001). CB1 receptor–G protein association: subtype selectivity is determined by distinct intracellular domains. European Journal of Biochemistry, 268, 499–505.

Naider, F., Khare, S., Arshava, B., Severino, B., Russo, J. & Becker, J.M. (2005). Synthetic peptides as probes for conformational preferences of domains of membrane receptors. Biopolymers, 80, 199–213.

Neumoin, A., Cohen, L.S., Arshava, B., Tantry, S., Becker, J.M., Zerbe, O. & Naider, F. (2009). Structure of a double transmembrane fragment of a G-protein-coupled receptor in micelles. Biophysical Journal, 96, 3187–3196.

Ng, G.Y., O'Dowd, B.F., Lee, S.P., Chung, H.T., Brann, M.R., Seeman, P. & George, S.R. (1996). Dopamine D2 receptor dimmers and receptor-blocking peptides. Biochemical and Biophysical Research Communications, 227, 200–204.

Nicastro, G., Peri, F., Franzoni, L., de Chiara, C., Sartor, G. & Spisni, A. (2003). Conformational features of a synthetic model of the first extracellular loop of the angiotensin II AT1A receptor. Journal of Peptide Science, 9, 229–243.

O'Callaghan, K., Kuliopulos, A. & Covic, L. (2012a). Turning receptors on and off with intracellular pepducins: new insights into G-protein-coupled receptor drug development. Journal of Biological Chemistry, 287, 12787–12796.

O'Callaghan, K., Lee, L., Nguyen, N., Hsieh, M.Y., Kaneider, N.C., Klein, A.K., Sprague, K., Van Etten, R.A., Kuliopulos, A. & Covic, L. (2012b). Targeting CXCR4 with cell-penetrating pepducins in lymphoma and lymphocytic leukemia. Blood, 119, 1717–1725.

Offermanns, S. (2003). G-proteins as transducers in transmembrane signalling. Progress in Biophysics and Molecular Biology, 83, 101–130.

Okuda, A., Matsumoto, O., Akaji, M., Taga, T., Ohkudo, T. & Kobayashi, Y. (2002). Solution structure of intracellular signal-transducing peptide derived from human β2-adrenergic receptor, Biochemical and Biophysical Research Communications, 291, 1297–1301.

Park, P.S. (2012). Ensemble of G protein-coupled receptor active states. Current Medicinal Chemistry, 19, 1146–1154.

Parker, M.S., Park, E.A., Sallee, F.R. & Parker, S.L. (2011). Two intracellular helices of G-protein coupling receptors could generally support oligomerization and coupling with transducers. Amino Acids, 40, 261–268.

Patel, T.B. (2004). Single transmembrane spanning heterotrimeric g protein-coupled receptors and their signaling cascades. Pharmacological Reviews, 56: 371–385.

Pepin, M.C., Yue, S.Y., Roberts, F., Wahlestedt, C. & Walker, P. (1997) Novel "restoration of function" mutagenesis strategy to identify amino acids of the delta-opioid receptor involved in ligand binding. Journal of Biological Chemistry, 272, 9260–9267.

Petry, R., Craik, D., Haaima, G., Fromme, B., Klump, H., Kiefer, W., Palm, D. & Millar, R. (2002). Secondary structure of the third extracellular loop responsible for ligand selectivity of a mammalian gonadotropin-releasing hormone receptor. Journal of Medicinal Chemistry, 45, 1026–1034.

Pham, T.C., Kriwacki, R.W. & Parrill, A.L. (2007). Peptide design and structural characterization of a GPCR loop mimetic. Biopolymers, 86, 298–310.

Piserchio, A., Bisello, A., Rosenblatt, M., Chorev, M. & Mierke, D.F. (2000). Characterization of parathyroid hormone/receptor interactions: structure of the first extracellular loop. Biochemistry, 39, 8153–8160.

Popot, J.L. & Engelman, D.M. (2000). Helical membrane protein folding, stability, and evolution. Annual Review of Biochemistry, 69, 881–922.

Reina, S., Sterin-Borda, L., Orman, B. & Borda, E. (2004). Autoantibodies against cerebral muscarinic cholinoreceptors in Sjogren syndrome: functional and pathological implications. Journal of Neuroimmunology, 150, 107–115.

Remsberg, J.R., Lou, H., Tarasov, S.G., Dean, M. & Tarasova, N.I. (2007). Structural analogues of smoothened intracellular loops as potent inhibitors of Hedgehog pathway and cancer cell growth. Journal of Medicinal Chemistry, 50, 4534–4538.

Ruan, K.H., So, S.P., Wu, J., Li, D., Huang, A. & Kung, J. (2001). Solution structure of the second extracellular loop of human thromboxane A_2 receptor. Biochemistry, 40, 275–280.

Ruan, C.H., Wu, J. & Ruan, K.H. (2005). A strategy using NMR peptide structures of thromboxane A2 receptor as templates to construct ligand-recognition pocket of prostacyclin receptor. BMC Biochemistry [electronic resource], 6, doi:10.1186/1471-2091-6-23.

Ruan, K.H., Wu, J., So, S.P. & Jenkins, L.A. (2003). Evidence of the residues involved in ligand recognition in the second extracellular loop of the prostacyclin receptor characterized by high resolution 2D NMR techniques. Archives of Biochemistry and Biophysics, 418, 25–33.

Ruan, K.H., Wu, J., So, S.P., Jenkins, L.A. & Ruan, C.H. (2004). NMR structure of the thromboxane A2 receptor ligand recognition pocket. European Journal of Biochemistry, 271, 3006–3016.

Runge, S., Thøgersen, H., Madsen, K., Lau, J. & Rudolph, R. (2008). Crystal structure of the ligand-bound glucagon-like peptide-1 receptor extracellular domain, Journal of Biological Chemistry, 283, 11340–11347.

Scheerer, P., Park, J.H., Hildebrand, P.W., Kim, Y.J., Krauss, N., Choe, H.W., Hofmann, K.P. & Ernst O.P. (2008). Crystal structure of opsin in its G-protein-interacting conformation. Nature, 455, 497–502.

Schwartz, T.W., Frimurer, T.M., Holst, B., Rosenkilde, M.M. & Elling, C.E. (2006). Molecular mechanism of 7TM receptor activation – a global toggle switch model. Annual Review of Pharmacology and Toxicology, 46, 481–519.

Segovia, M., Ganzinelli, S., Reina, S., Borda, E. & Sterin-Borda, L. (2012). Role of anti-β1 adrenergic antibodies from patients with periodontitis in cardiac dysfunction. Journal of Oral Pathology & Medicine, 41, 242–248.

Sen, M., Shah, A. & Marsch, L. (1997). Two types of α-factor receptor determinants for pheromone specificity in the mating-incompatible yeasts S. cerevisiae and S. kluyveri. Current Genetics, 31, 235–240.

Sevigny, L.M., Austin, K.M., Zhang, P., Kasuda, S., Koukos, G., Sharifi, S., Covic, L. & Kuliopulos, A. (2011). Protease-activated receptor-2 modulates protease-activated receptor-1-driven neointimal hyperplasia. Arteriosclerosis, thrombosis, and vascular biology, 31, e100–106.

Shirai, H., Takahashi, K., Katada, T. & Inagami, T. (1995). Mapping of G protein coupling sites of the angiotensin II type 1 receptor. Hypertension, 25, 726–730.

Shpakov, A.O. (2010). Natural and synthetic cationic peptides as regulators of hormone-sensitive signaling systems and molecular mechanisms of their action. Current Topics in Peptide & Protein Research, 11, 1–30.

Shpakov, A.O. (2011a). GPCR-based peptides: structure, mechanisms of action and application. Global Journal of Biochemistry, 2, 96–123.

Shpakov, A.O. (2011b). Signal protein-derived peptides as functional probes and regulators of intracellular signaling. Journal of Amino Acids, 2011, DOI:10.4061/2011/656051

Shpakov, A.O., Gur'yanov, I.A., Kuznetsova, L.A., Plesneva, S.A., Shpakova, E.A., Vlasov, G.P. & Pertseva, M.N. (2007). Studies of the molecular mechanisms of action of relaxin on the adenylyl cyclase signaling system using synthetic peptides derived from the LGR7 relaxin receptor. Neuroscience and Behaviour Physiology, 37, 705–714.

Shpakov, A.O. & Pertseva, M.N. (2005). Use of the peptide strategy to study mechanisms of transferring the hormone signal to the cell. Journal of Evolutionary Biochemistry & Physiology, 41, 389–403.

Shpakov, A.O. & Pertseva, M.N. (2007). The peptide strategy as a novel approach to the study of G protein-coupled signaling systems. Signal Transduction Research Trends (Grachevsky N.O., ed.), Nova Science Publishers, Inc., New York, 45–93.

Shpakov, A.O., Pertseva, M.N., Gur'ianov, I.A. & Vlasov, G.P. (2005). The influence of the peptides, derivatives of the third cytoplasmic loop of type 1 relaxin receptor, on the stimulation of GTP binding activity of the G proteins by relaxin. Biological Membranes, 22, 435–442. (in Russian).

Shpakov, A.O. & Shpakova, E.A. (2011). Development of non-hormonal regulators of the adenylyl cyclase signaling system based on the peptides, derivatives of the third intracellular loop of somatostatin receptors. Biochemistry (Moscow), Suppl. Ser. B: Biomedical Chemistry, 5, 246–252.

Shpakov, A.O., Shpakova, E.A., Tarasenko, I.I. & Derkach, K.V. (2012). Receptor and tissue specificity of the effect of peptides corresponding to intracellular regions of the serpentine type receptors. Biochemistry (Moscow), Suppl. Ser. A: Membrane and Cell Biology, 64, 16–25.

Shpakov, A.O., Shpakova, E.A., Tarasenko, I.I., Derkach, K.V., Chistyakova, O.V., Avdeeva, E.A. & Vlasov, G.P. (2011). The influence of peptides corresponding to the third intracellular loop of luteinizing hormone receptor on basal and hormone-stimulated activity of the adenylyl cyclase signaling system. Global Journal of Biochemistry, 2, 59–73.

Shpakov, A.O., Shpakova, E.A., Tarasenko, I.I., Derkach, K.V. & Vlasov, G.P. (2010a) The peptides mimicking the third intracellular loop of 5-hydroxytryptamine receptors of the types 1B and 6 selectively activate G proteins and receptor-specifically inhibit serotonin signaling via the adenylyl cyclase system. International Journal of Peptide Research and Therapeutics, 16, 95–105.

Shpakov, A.O., Tarasenko, I.I., Shpakova, E.A., Guryanov, I.A., Derkach, K.V. & Vlasov, G.P. (2010b). Molecular mechanisms of action of G protein-coupled receptor (GPCR)-derived and non-GPCR cationic peptides on adenylyl cyclase signaling system. Current Topics in Peptide & Protein Research, 11, 49–65.

Shpakova, E.A., Shpakov, A.O., Chistyakova, O.V., Moyseyuk, I.V. & Derkach, K.V. (2012a). Biological activity in vitro and in vivo of peptides corresponding to the third intracellular loop of thyrotropin receptor. Doklady. Biochemistry and Biophysics, 443, 64–67.

Shpakova, E.A., Skvortsova, E.A., Tarasenko, I.I. & Shpakov, A.O. (2012b). The secondary structure of peptides derived from the third intracellular loop of the serpentine type receptors and its interrelation with their biological activity. Tsitologiia, 54, 119–129. (In Russian).

Sidorova, M.V., Pal'keeva, M.E., Molokoedov, A.S., Az'muko, A.A., Sekridova, A.V., Ovchinnikov, M.V., Levashov, P.A., Afanas'eva, O.I., Berestetskaia, Y.V., Afanas'eva, M.I., Razova, O.A., Bespalova, Zh.D. & Porkovskii, S.N. (2009). Synthesis and properties of a new conformational antigen modeling an extracellular region of β1-adrenoreceptor. Bioorganicheskaia Khimiia, 35, 311–322. (In Russian).

Simpson, L.S., Zhu, J.Z., Widlanski, T.S. & Stone, M.J. (2009). Regulation of chemokine recognition by site-specific tyrosine sulfation of receptor peptides. Chemistry & Biology, 16, 153–161.

Skelton, N.J., Quan, C., Reilly, D. & Lowman, H. (1999). Structure of a CXC chemokine-receptor fragment in complex with interleukin-8. Structure, 7, 157–168.

Smrcka, A.V. (2008). G protein βγ subunits: central mediators of G protein-coupled receptor signaling. Cellular and Molecular Life Sciences, 65, 2191–2214.

So, S.P., Wu, J., Huang, G., Huang, A., Li, D. & Ruan, K.H. (2003). Identification of residues important for ligand binding of thromboxane A_2 receptor in the second extracellular loop using the NMR experiment-guided mutagenesis approach. Journal of Biological Chemistry, 278, 10922–10927.

Spiegel, A.M. (2007). Inherited endocrine diseases involving G proteins and G protein-coupled receptors. Endocrine Development, 11, 133–144.

Staudt, A., Mobini, R., Fu, M., Grosse, Y., Stangl, V., Stangl, K., Thiele, A., Baumann, S. & Felix, S.B. (2001). β1-adrenoreceptor antibodies induce positive inotropic response in isolated cardiomyocytes. European Journal of Pharmacology, 423, 115–119.

Sun, H., Seyer, J.M. & Patel, T.B. (1995). A region in the cytosolic domain of the epidermal growth factor receptor antithetically regulates the stimulatory and inhibitory guanine nucleotide-binding regulatory proteins of adenylyl cyclase. Proceedings of the National Academy of Sciences of the United States of America, 92, 2229–2233.

Sunahara, R.K., Tesmer, J.J., Gilman, A.G. & Sprang, S.R. (1997). Crystal structure of the adenylyl cyclase activator $G_{s\alpha}$. Science, 278, 1943–1947.

Swift, S., Leger, A.J., Talavera, J., Zhang, L., Bohm, A. & Kuliopulos, A. (2006). Role of the PAR1 receptor 8th helix in signaling: the 7-8-1 receptor activation mechanism. Journal of Biological Chemistry, 281, 4109–4116.

Tanaka, T., Kohno, T., Kinoshita, S., Mukai, H., Itoh, H., Ohya, M., Miyazawa, T., Higashijima, T. & Wakamatsu, K. (1998). α helix content of G protein α subunit is decreased upon activation by receptor mimetics. Journal of Biological Chemistry, 273, 3247–3252.

Tarasov, S.G., Gaponenko, V., Howard, O.M., Chen, Y., Oppenheim, J.J., Dyba, M.A., Subramaniam, S., Lee, Y., Michejda, C. & Tarasova, N.I. (2011). Structural plasticity of a transmembrane peptide allows self-assembly into biologically active nanoparticles. Proceedings of the National Academy of Sciences of the United States of America, 108, 9798–9803.

Tarasova, N.I., Rice, W.G. & Michejda, C.J. (1999). Inhibition of G-protein-coupled receptor function by disruption of transmembrane domain interactions. Journal of Biological Chemistry, 274, 34911–34915.

Tchernychev, B., Ren, Y., Sachdev, P., Janz, J.M., Haggis, L., O'Shea, A., McBride, E., Looby, R., Deng, Q., McMurry, T., Kazmi, M.A., Sakmar, T.P., Hunt, S. 3rd & Carlson, K.E. (2010). Discovery of a CXCR4 agonist pepducin that mobilizes bone marrow hematopoietic cells. Proceedings of the National Academy of Sciences of the United States of America, 107, 22255–22259.

Thaker, T.M., Kaya, A.I., Preininger, A.M., Hamm, H.E. & Iverson, T.M. (2012). Allosteric mechanisms of G protein-coupled receptor signaling: a structural perspective. Methods in Molecular Biology, 796, 133–174.

Thévenin, D. & Lazarova, T. (2008). Stable interactions between the transmembrane domains of the adenosine A_{2A} receptor. Protein Science, 17, 1188–1199.

Thévenin, D., Roberts, M.F., Lazarova, T. & Robinson, C.R. (2005). Identifying interactions between transmembrane helices from the adenosine A_{2A} receptor. Biochemistry, 44, 16239–16245.

Tiburu, E.K., Bowman, A.L., Struppe, J.O., Janero, D.R., Avraham, H.K. & Makriyannis, A. (2009). Solid-state NMR and molecular dynamics characterization of cannabinoid receptor-1 (CB1) helix 7 conformational plasticity in model membranes. Biochimica et Biophysica Acta, 1788, 1159–1167.

Todokoro, Y., Yumen, I., Fukushima, K., Kang, S.W., Park, J.S., Kohno, T., Wakamatsu, K., Akutsu, H. & Fujiwara, T. (2006). Structure of tightly membrane-bound mastoparan-X, a G-protein-activating peptide, determined by solid-state NMR. Biophysical Journal, 91, 1368–1379.

Topiol, S. & Sabio, M. (2009). X-ray structure breakthroughs in the GPCR transmembrane region, Biochemical Pharmacology, 78, 11–20.

Tressel, S.L., Koukos, G., Tchernychev, B., Jacques, S.L., Covic, L. & Kuliopulos, A. (2011). Pharmacology, biodistribution, and efficacy of GPCR-based pepducins in disease models. Methods in Molecular Biology, 683, 259–275.

Ulfers, A.L., Piserchio, A. & Mierke, D.F. (2002). Extracellular domains of the neurokinin-1 receptor: structural characterization and interactions with substance P. Biopolymers, 66, 339–349.

Underwood, C.R., Garibay, P., Knudsen, L.B., Hastrup, S., Peters, G.H., Rudolph, R. & Reedtz-Runge, S. (2010). Crystal structure of glucagon-like peptide-1 in complex with the extracellular domain of the glucagon-like peptide-1 receptor. Journal of Biological Chemistry, 285, 723–730.

Vahlberg, C., Petoral, R.M., Lindell, C., Broo, K. & Uvdal, K. (2006). α_{2A}-adrenergic receptor derived peptide adsorbates: A G-protein interaction study. Langmuir, 22, 7260–7264.

Van Eps, N., Anderson, L.L., Kisselev, O.G., Baranski, T.J., Hubbell, W.L. & Marshall, G.R. (2010). Electron paramagnetic resonance studies of functionally active, nitroxide spin-labeled peptide analogues of the C-terminus of a G-protein α subunit. Biochemistry, 49, 6877–6886.

Vanhauwe, J.F., Thomas, T.O., Minshall, R.D., Tiruppathi, C., Li, A., Gilchrist, A., Yoon, E.J., Malik, A.B. & Hamm, H.E. (2002). Thrombin receptors activate G_o protein in endothelial cells to regulate intracellular calcium and cell shape changes. Journal of Biological Chemistry, 277, 34143–34149.

Varrault, A., Le Nguyen, D., McClue, S., Harris, B., Jouin, P. & Bockaert, J. (1994). 5-Hydroxytryptamine1A receptor synthetic peptides. Mechanisms of adenylyl cyclase inhibition. Journal of Biological Chemistry, 269, 16720–16725.

Vassart, G. & Costagliola, S. (2011). G protein-coupled receptors: mutations and endocrine diseases. Nature reviews. Endocrinology, 7, 362–372.

Veldkamp, C.T., Seibert, C., Peterson, F.C., De la Cruz, N.B., Haugner, J.C. 3rd, Basnet, H., Sakmar, T.P. & Volkman, B.F. (2008). Structural basis of CXCR4 sulfotyrosine recognition by the chemokine SDF-1/CXCL12. Science Signalling [electronic resource], 1, ra4.

Vincent, B., Mouledous, L., Bes, B., Mazarguil, H., Meunier, J.C., Milon, A. & Demange, P. (2008). Description of the low-affinity interaction between nociceptin and the second extracellular loop of its receptor by fluorescence and NMR spectroscopies. Journal of Peptide Science, 14, 1183–1194.

Wess, J. (1997). G-protein-coupled receptors: molecular mechanisms involved in receptor activation and selectivity of G-protein recognition. FASEB Journal, 11, 346–354.

White, S.H. & Wimley, W.C. (1999). Membrane protein folding and stability: physical principles, Annual Review of Biophysics and Biomolecular Structure, 28, 319–365.

Woehler, A. & Ponimaskin, E.G. (2009). G protein-mediated signaling: same receptor, multiple effectors. Current Molecular Pharmacology, 2, 237–248.

Wu, H., Wacker, D., Mileni, M., Katritch, V., Han, G.W., Vardy, E., Liu, W., Thompson, A.A., Huang, X.P., Carroll, F.I., Mascarella, S.W., Westkaemper, R.B., Mosier, P.D., Roth, B.L., Cherezov, V. & Stevens, R.C. (2012). Structure of the human κ-opioid receptor in complex with JDTic. Nature, 485, 327–332.

Wu, J., Feng, M. & Ruan, K.H. (2008). Assembling NMR structures for the intracellular loops of the human thromboxane A_2 receptor: implication of the G protein-coupling pocket. Archives of Biochemistry and Biophysics, 470, 73–82.

Wu, J., So, S.P. & Ruan, K.H. (2003). Solution structure of the third extracellular loop of human thromboxane A_2 receptor. Archives of Biochemistry and Biophysics, 414, 287–293.

Xie, X.-Q. & Chen, J.-Z. (2005). NMR structural comparison of the cytoplasmic juxtamembrane domains of G-protein-coupled CB_1 and CB_2 receptors in membrane mimetic dodecylphosphocholine micelles. Journal of Biological Chemistry, 280, 3605–3612.

Ye, J., Kohli, L.L. & Stone, M.J. (2000). Characterization of binding between the chemokine eotaxin and peptides derived from the chemokine receptor CCR3. Journal of Biological Chemistry, 275, 27250–27257.

Yeagle, P.L. & Albert, A.D. (1998). Structure of the G-protein-coupled receptor, rhodopsin: a domain approach. Biochemical Society Transactions, 26, 520–531.

Yeagle, P.L., Choi, G. & Albert, A.D. (2001). Studies on the structure of the G-protein-coupled receptor rhodopsin including the putative G-protein binding site in unactivated and activated forms. Biochemistry, 40, 11932–11937.

Yeagle, P.L., Salloum, A., Chopra, A., Bhawsar, N., Ali, L., Kuzmanovski, G., Alderfer, J.L. & Albert, A.D. (2000). Structures of the intradiskal loops and amino terminus of the G-protein receptor rhodopsin. Journal of Peptide Research, 55, 455–465.

Zhang, L., Bastepe, M., Juppner, H. & Ruan, K.H. (2006). Characterization of the molecular mechanisms of the coupling between intracellular loops of prostacyclin receptor with the C-terminal domain of the $G\alpha_s$ protein in human coronary artery smooth muscle cells. Archives of Biochemistry and Biophysics, 454, 80–88.

Zhang, L., DeHaven, R.N. & Goodman, M. (2002). NMR and modeling studies of a synthetic extracellular loop II of the κ opioid receptor in a DPC micelle. Biochemistry, 41, 61–68.

Zhang, P., Gruber, A., Kasuda, S., Kimmelstiel, C., O'Callaghan, K., Cox, D.H., Bohm, A., Baleja, J.D., Covic, L. & Kuliopulos, A. (2012). Suppression of arterial thrombosis without affecting hemostatic parameters with a cell-penetrating PAR1 pepducin. Circulation, 126, 83–91.

Zhang, Y. & Xie, X.Q. (2008). Biosynthesis, purification, and characterization of a cannabinoid receptor 2 fragment (CB2(271-326)). Protein Expression and Purification, 59, 249–257.

Zheng, H., Loh, H.H. & Law, P.Y. (2010). Agonist-selective signaling of G protein-coupled receptor: mechanisms and implications. International Union of Biochemistry and Molecular Biology Life, 62, 112–119.

Zheng, H., Zhao, J., Sheng, W. & Xie, X.Q. (2006). A transmembrane helix-bundle from G-protein coupled receptor CB2: biosynthesis, purification, and NMR characterization. Biopolymers, 83, 46–61.

Zhu, J.Z., Millard, C.J., Ludeman, J.P., Simpson, L.S., Clayton, D.J., Payne, R.J., Widlanski, T.S. & Stone, M.J. (2011) Tyrosine sulfation influences the chemokine binding selectivity of peptides derived from chemokine receptor CCR3. Biochemistry, 50, 1524–1534.

Zou, C., Naider, F. & Zerbe, O. (2008). Biosynthesis and NMR-studies of a double transmembrane domain from the Y4 receptor, a human GPCR. Journal of Biomolecular NMR, 42, 257–269.

Solid-Phase Derivatization: Application to Phosphoprotein Structural Characterization

Heinz Nika
Department of Developmental and Molecular Biology
Laboratory for Macromolecular Analysis and Proteomics
Albert Einstein College of Medicine, USA

David H. Hawke
Department of Pathology
MD Anderson Cancer Center, USA

Ian M. Willis
Department of Biochemistry
Albert Einstein College of Medicine, USA

Ruth Hogue Angeletti
Department of Developmental and Molecular Biology
Laboratory for Macromolecular Analysis and Proteomics
Albert Einstein College of Medicine, USA

1   Introduction

Protein phosphorylation is recognized as a critical event in modulation of cellular processes including cellular signaling, cell cycle progression and differentiation (Helmbrecht *et al.*, 2000). Existing approaches to map this important post-translational modification rely predominately on the use of mass spectrometry methods to identify and sequence the peptide of interest (Annan & Carr, 1996; Liao *et al.*, 1994; Annan *et al.*, 2001; Tholey *et al.*, 1999). Matrix-assisted laser desorption/ionization mass spectrometry (MALDI-TOF MS) is commonly employed to detect phosphopeptides by monitoring the indicative metastable post-source decay (PSD) products or the characteristic mass shift after alkaline phosphatase treatment (Annan *et al.,* 1996; Liao *et al.*, 1994). Various strategies utilizing electro-spray ionization (ESI) tandem mass spectrometry coupled to liquid chromatography are often used, including precursor ion and neutral loss scanning for diagnostic ions generated under the conditions of collisionally-induced dissociation (CID) (Annan *et al.*, 2001; Tholey *et al.*, 1999). However, these methods are often challenged by the ionization inefficiency of the phosphopeptides, their low stoichiometry relative to the unphosphorylated counterparts and the limited information content of the MS/MS spectra due to the intrinsic lability of the phosphate group upon CID. Immobilized metal ion affinity chromatography (IMAC) is a frequently reported technique to address these problems by phosphopeptide enrichment (Posewitz & Tempst, 1999). However, in many instances this approach had been ineffective due to co-adsorption of non-phosphorylated (acidic) peptides that contaminate the IMAC fractions and is further complicated by variability of phosphopeptide elution. Phosphopeptide enrichment by titanium dioxide (TiO_2) chromatography is currently widely used but this technique also suffers from non-specific peptide adsorption, and has been shown to poorly enrich phosphopeptides derived from basophilic kinase substrates (Larsen *et al.*, 2005; Klemm *et al.*, 2006). MALDI-matrix additives such as ammonium salts or phosphoric acid have been shown to promote phosphopeptide ionization during MALDI-MS (Yang *et al.*, 2004; Stensballe & Jensen, 2004). Although the above strategies may afford improved phosphopeptide detection, issues still persist with regard to neutral loss of phosphate because, as the favored fragmentation event, it dominates over peptide backbone cleavage. Subjecting the resultant neutral loss product ion from the MS/MS spectrum to a further cycle of fragmentation (MS/MS/MS) may improve the peptide sequence information content and thus aid in phosphorylation site determination (Beausoleil *et al.*, 2004). Electron transfer dissociation (ETD) of phosphopeptides has emerged as a viable method to minimize phosphate gas-phase β-elimination. The method proved informative on large, multiply protonated peptides, predominantly contained in endopeptidase Lys-C protein digests and has been used more recently in combination with CID in a complementary fashion (Molina *et al.*, 2007).

Chemically-induced β-elimination of phosphate from serine and threonine residues coupled with Michael addition provides a chemical strategy to afford improved MS/MS sequence information by precluding neutral loss of phosphate. One approach advocates the use of ethanethiol as nucleophile for concurrent β-elimination/Michael addition (Jaffe *et al.*, 1998). The derivatization proved to enhance ionization of the modified peptides during liquid chromatography mass spectrometry (LC-MS) analysis and afforded improved MS/MS spectral information. As applied to digests of protein kinase A, this advantage has been exploited to completely map the phosphorylation sites of the protein in a single LC-MS/MS experiment (Shen *et al.* 2004). In contrast; multiple experiments were required for each of the optional techniques employed in this study to provide complementary data. However, the relatively stringent conditions employed in these protocols raised concerns about chemical contamination, peptide bond hydrolysis and unwanted chemistry side reactions. Typically, sodium hydroxide in high concentrations is utilized as elimination reagent, fortified with organic solvents and the mixtures are incubated for several hours or overnight, conditions known to promote protein degradation. Reagent excess is commonly removed by ultra-filtration, dialysis or precipitation, manipulations known to incur substantial, adsorptive sample loss which may limit the general usefulness of these methods. Several approaches employing the β-elimination/Michel addition reaction have been advocated to detect phosphopeptides by signal enhancement (Molloy & Andrews, 2001; Ahn *et al.*, 2007; Chen *et al.*, 2010). The MALDI-TOF response of phosphoseryl and phosphothreonyl peptides after reaction with alkanethiols of increasing carbon chain length was examined of which octanethiol proved most effective to promote phosphopeptide signal enhancement (Molloy & Andrews, 2001). Improved MALDI-TOF detection was demonstrated employing guanidinoethanethiol as Michael addition reagent (Ahn *et al.*, 2007). The signal-enhancing effect observed in the MALDI-MS spectra was most noticeable for the two lysine-terminated phosphorylated peptides contained in tryptic digests of α-S1 casein. However, the tag proved to be only partially stable upon MALDI-TOF/TOF fragmentation. Recently, (2-mercaptoethyl) trimethylammonium hydrochloride has been used as Michael donor in the addition reaction resulting in markedly enhanced detection of a model phosphopeptide during electro spray mass spectrometry (Chen *et al.*, 2010). This label was also susceptible to fragmentation during CID thereby complicating MS/MS data interpretation.

Noticeably milder reaction conditions were reported that employ barium hydroxide as elimination reagent and 2-aminoethanethiol as Michael donor, eliminating the use of sodium hydroxide and organic solvent mixtures and allowing the reaction to proceed in pure aqueous solution (Thompson *et al.*, 2003). Barium hydroxide has been reported to preferentially catalyze the β-elimination of phosphoserine (Byford, 1991). With these developments, the chemistry became amenable to solid phase adaptation, as demonstrated employing ZipTip$_{C18}$ pipette tips as analyte sorbent for the in-situ reaction (Nika *et al.*, 2004; Nika *et al.*, 2012). This derivatization format offers several compelling advantages over the classical in-solution based methods, the predominant sample preparation technique in current proteomic studies. Samples are cleaned up in-situ eliminating interfering matrix components and excess reagent. The process inherently concentrates the analyte providing for completeness of reaction, improved throughput and efficient use of dilute samples and is highly amenable to automation. However, application of this technique for protein characterization had been scarce and focused on *in situ* protein digestion with trypsin using C4, C8 and C18 bonded-phase silica supports for protein concentration (Pavel *et al,* 2002; Docette *et al*, 2003). Since the introduction of this sample handling format to phosphoprotein characterization (Nika *et al.*, 2004), its' apparent benefits have been exploited in only a few proteomics studies aimed at the facilitation of *de novo* sequence interpretation. Lysine-containing peptides bound to Cleanup C$_{18}$ Pipette Tips were reacted to completion with 2-methoxy-4,5-dihydro-1*H*-imidazole at a 3-fold faster reaction rate (Cindric *et al.*, 2006). Near quantitative solid-phase peptide amino group sulfonation employing 3-sulfopropionic acid N-hydroxysuccinimide ester was accomplished in less than 3 min whereas the analogous solution-phase reaction typically required up to 30 min for completion (Conrotto & Hellman, 2005). More recently, an automated high throughput pre-column peptide dimethylation method has been developed coupled with tandem mass spectrometry to study differences in composition between purified protein complexes (Raijmakers *et al,* 2008). In a recent report, we have demonstrated the utility of ZipTip$_{C18}$ pipette tips for peptide *in situ* permethylation (Farmar *et al*, 2009).

It should be noted here that modern analytical sample preparation techniques are almost exclusively based on derivatization on various sorbents packed into solid-phase extraction cartridges (SPE) for off-line applications or on pre-columns coupled on-line with chromatographic separation and spectroscopic/mass spectrometric detection systems, and have in these applications found widespread use for automated trace analysis of bioorganic compounds contained in pharmaceutical, environmental and biological samples (Rosenfeld, 1999; Johnson & Carpenter, 2005). In these comprehensive reviews, several general considerations for the application of these highly advantageous techniques were discussed including sorbent selection, reagent selection, reaction conditions and analyte pre-concentration on the stationary supports.

We have shown that the solid-phase chemical strategy afforded improved phosphoseryl peptide detection in unfractionated digest from model proteins and experimental samples (Nika et al., 2012). The conversion products were readily recognized in the MALDI-TOF spectra of unfractionated digests by the resultant signal enhancement and their characteristic mass shifts. In addition, sequencing upon CID proved to be substantially more informative than for the corresponding chemically unmodified peptides. Experimental samples examined included tryptic digests of α-catenin immunoprecipitated from epidermal growth factor (EGF)-stimulated A431 human epidermoid carcinoma cells, and tryptic digests of the yeast Maf1 transcriptional repressor protein that had been expressed in E. coli and subsequently phosphorylated in vitro. Human α-catenin (UniProtKB accession code: P35221) is a hydrophilic protein of 906 amino acids in length with an isoelectric point of 5.95 and a molecular mass of 99.8 kDa. The protein's cDNA comprises 21 243 base pairs. EGF stimulation of A431 human epidermoid carcinoma cells results in disruption of the α-catenin/β-catenin intercellular adhesion complex promoting β-catenin transactivation. This finding was the starting point for comprehensive biochemical studies to reveal α-catenin's role in the intercellular adhesion complex and its correlation to tumor cell invasion (Ji et al., 2009). The solid-phase strategy provided evidence of a phosphorylation event localized at serine 641 that is implicated in the protein's dissociation from the adhesion complex. Yeast Maf1 (UniProtKB accession code: P41910) is a hydrophilic protein of 395 amino acids in length with an isoelectric point of 5.15 and a molecular mass of 44.7 kDa. The protein's cDNA contains 1185 base pairs. Phosphorylation of yeast Maf1 on consensus protein kinase A (PKA) sites regulates its distribution between the cytoplasm and the nucleus, and simultaneous mutation of serine residues 90, 101, 177, 178, 209 and 210 at the PKA consensus sites (6SA mutant) leads to nuclear accumulation. Relocation of MAF1 from the cytoplasm to the nucleus is thought to provide one level of control over its inhibitory interaction with RNA polymerase III (Moir et al., 2006). The solid-phase protocol enabled unambiguous identification of five phosphorylated fragments that could be mass matched to the known protein sequence. These fragments were contiguous with or contained PKA recognition sites and allowed identification of two previously assigned and two novel sites of phosphorylation.

The current communication includes a more detailed discussion of several critical aspects of the solid-phase method and of representative results so far achieved. Additional data presented here highlight the advantage of the solid-phase strategy to perform serial chemical reactions which are in general perceived as problematic because of the high potential of adsorptive samples loss incurred during the requisite intermittent sample purification. In our sequential solid-phase protocol reagents are exchanged directly on the support eliminating the need for sample transfer between the reaction steps, thereby allowing the chemistries to proceed with minimal sample loss. As shown in our study, the utility of this technique was exploited to prepare peptides for phosphorylation site determination by chemical targeted proteolysis (Rusnak et al., 2002; Knight et al., 2003). In this alternative approach to phosphorylation site determination, the tagged peptides are selectively cleaved by lysine endopeptidase C-terminally to the site of the chemical modification. This strategy exploits the finding that S-2-aminoethylcysteine and β-methyl- S-2-aminoethylcysteine derivatives are recognized by the enzyme as structural analogs of lysine. The phosphorylation site is determined by mass matching the predicted cleavage products to the known protein sequence and/or by Edman degradation. The initial acetylation reaction in this sequential reaction scheme ensures for the selectivity of proteolysis of the lysine analog. Moreover, the amine blocking step renders the amino group in subsequently formed thiol adducts the sole targets for further chemical manipulation. In pilot experiments, we have exploited this reaction sequence to introduce via amino group *in situ* thiolation an affinity tag into phosphoprotein digests providing a means to isolate the selectively modified analyte by covalent chromatography on activated Thiol Sepharose. This strategy is anticipated to expand the scope of the solid-phase analytical platform to purification of substoichiometric amounts of phosphopeptides from complex protein digests, and is expected in a scaled-up format to be utilized to prepare prefractionated proteomics samples for LC-MS/MS-based large-scale phosphoproteome profiling (Villen & Gygi, 2008; Dephoure & Gygi, 2011).

2   Materials

Trifluoroacetic acid (TFA), Bond Breaker TCEP solution (0.5M), hydroxylamine hydrochloride, urea (sequenal grade), Zebra Desalt Spin Columns (0.5 mL resin bed) and GelCode Blue Stain Reagent were obtained from Pierce (Rockford, IL). Formic acid, 2-aminoethanethiol hydrochloride and barium hydroxide octahydrate were from Aldrich (Milwaukee, WI). Ammonium hydrogen carbonate and sodium phosphate dibasic dodecahydrate were purchased from Fluka (Ronkonkoma, NJ). *N*-octyl glucoside (OGS) was obtained from Roche Diagnostics (Indianapolis, IN). Methanol and acetonitrile was from Burdick & Jackson (Muskegon, MI). Bis(2-mercaptoethylsulfone) (BMS) was obtained from Calbiochem (La Jolla, CA). Isopropyl-1-thio-β-D-galactopyranoside was from United States Biochemical (Cleveland, OH). Tris (hydroxymethyl)aminomethane, magnesium chloride, sodium chloride, sodium fluoride and dithiothreitol (DTT), iodoacetamide, sodium carbonate, sodium phosphate monobasic monohydrate, angiotensin I human acetate salt hydrate, human serum albumin, horse heart myoglobin, β-lactoglobulin from bovine milk, carbonic anhydrase form bovine erythrocytes, ovalbumin, bovine α-S1 casein, bovine β-casein, anhydrous methanol and anhydrous, deuterated methanol (CD_3OD) were purchased from Sigma-Aldrich (St. Louis, MO). GelCode Blue Stain Reagent was from Pierce (Rockford, IL). Ni^{2+}-NTA-agarose beads were obtained from Qiagen (La Jolla, CA). *E. coli* Rosetta 2 (DE3) and pET-30a (+) were purchased from Novagen (San Diego, CA). The protease inhibitors leupeptin and pepstatin were obtained from Roche (Indianapolis, IN). Resource Q resin, [γ-^{32}] adenosine 5'-triphosphate (ATP) and unlabeled ATP were from GE Healthcare (Piscataway, NJ). Recombinant murine protein kinase A was purchased from New England Biolabs (Ipswitch, MA). ZipTip$_{C18}$ pipette tips (0.6μl bed volume) and ZipTip$_{μ-C18}$ pipette tips (0.2 μl bed volume) were purchased from Millipore Corp. (Billerica, MA). α-cyano-4-hydroxycinnamic acid (α-CHCA) was from Agilent Technologies (Palo Alto, CA). Polyacrylamide gels (Criterion Precast gel, 1mm, 10%) were from Bio-Rad (Hercules, CA). The following model phosphopeptides were synthesized in-house and purified by HPLC: P1, RAD**pS**HEGEVA, *m/z* 1150.4; P2, SHNSALY**pS**QVQK, *m/z* 1441.2; P3, GIKSHN**pS**ALYSQVQK, *m/z* 1739.3; P4, TATG**pS**GIK-SHNSAL, *m/z* 1423.6; P5, RGA**pS**PVE, *m/z* 795.5; P6, RRQ**pS**PVA, *m/z* 835.5; P7, KR**pT**IRR, *m/z* 909.9. The following phosphopeptides were purchased from AnaSpec Inc. (San Jose, CA): β-casein phosphopeptide T6: FQ**pS**EEQQQTEDELQDK; *m/z* 2061.8. Protein kinase A (PKA) regulatory subunit II substrate phosphopeptide: DLDVPIPGRFDRRV**pS**VAAE; *m/z* 2192.4. UOM9, protein kinase C (PKC) substrate-3 phosphopeptide: KRP**pS**QRHGSKY amide; *m/z* 1422.5. DAM1, outer kinetochore protein DAM1 phosphopeptides: SFVLNPTNIGM**pS**KSSQGHVTK; *m/z* 2312.6. Myristoylated alanine-rich C kinase substrate (MARCKS) phosphopeptide: KKKKKRF**pS**FKK**pS**FKLSGF**pS**FKKNKK, *m/z* 3321.7. The phosphorylated cholecystokinin fragment; residue 10-20: IKNLQ**pS**LDPSH, *m/z* 1331.4 was obtained from Protea Biosciences Inc. (Morgantown, WV). Trypsin (modified sequencing grade) was purchased from Promega (Madison, WI). Pepsin from porcine gastric mucosa was purchased from Sigma-Aldrich (St. Louis, MO). Materials used to generate and purify phosphorylated α-catenin were as recently described (Ji *et al.*, 2009).

3   Methods

3.1   Maf1 Protein Purification and *in vitro* Phosphorylation

A full length cDNA clone of *Saccharomyces cerevisiae* Maf1 was inserted into pET-30a (+) to yield a C-terminal hexahistidine tagged protein. The plasmid was transformed into *E. coli* Rosetta 2(DE3) and protein expression induced by adding 0.1mM isopropyl-1-thio-β-D-galactopyranoside at 15°C followed by incubation overnight. The protein was purified under native conditions using Ni^{2+}-NTA-agarose according to the manufacturer's recommendations. Maf1 in 50 mM Tris-HCl (pH:7.0), 75 mM NaCl, 10% glycerol, 1 mM DTT and protease inhibitors (leupeptin and pepstatin, each at 1 μg/ml) was further purified by liquid chromatography at a flow rate of 0.5 ml/min using a Resource Q column (7x114mm). A linear gradient from 75 mM to 1 M NaCl was employed and the protein eluted at 300 mM NaCl. The Maf1 concentration of pooled fractions was determined by absorbance measurement at 280 nm using a molar extinction co-efficient calculated from the protein sequence. Aliquots of Maf1 were stored at –70 °C until use. *In vitro* phosphorylation of native recombinant Maf1 (5μg) was performed with recombinant murine protein kinase A (PKA, 1.25 units) in a 50 μl reaction volume following the manufacturer's recommendations. The reaction mixture containing 50 mM Tris-HCl (pH:7.5), 10 mM $MgCl_2$, 10 mM NaF and 1 mM [γ-^{32}P] ATP (22 dpm/pmol) or 1 mM cold ATP was incubated at 30 °C for 30 min and an aliquot analyzed by SDS-polyacrylamide electrophoresis. After staining with GelCode Blue Stain Reagent, the gel was dried and exposed to a phosphor storage screen together with aliquots of [γ-^{32}P] ATP spotted on filter paper as a standard. Signal intensities of labeled Maf1 and ATP standard were quantified using ImageQuant software obtained from Molecular Dynamics (Sunnyvale, CA). The stoichiometry of phosphorylation as observed in separate experiments ranged from 2-3 moles of phosphate incorporated per mole of Maf1. Phosphorylated protein prepared in parallel reactions with unlabeled ATP was stored at -70°C until use. Methods used to generate and purify phosphorylated α-catenin were as recently described (Ji *et al.*, 2009).

3.2   Protein In-Gel Carboxamidomethylation and In-Gel Proteolytic Digestion

GelCode blue stained bands from 5- 50 pmoles of protein loaded onto the gels were excised and destained twice with 200 μL of 25 mM ammonium bicarbonate in 50% aqueous acetonitrile for 30 min at 37 °C. Bands were then briefly dried in a SpeedVac and then incubated for 15 min at 37 °C in 100 μL of 2 mM BMS/25 mM ammonium bicarbonate; the supernatant was removed. The gel bands were incubated in 100 μL of 20 mM iodoacetamide in 25 mM ammonium bicarbonate for 30 min at 37 °C; the supernatant was then discarded. The gel bands were washed three times with 200 μL of 25 mM ammonium bicarbonate for 15 min and subsequently dried. Bands were dehydrated for 10 min in 100 μL of acetonitrile, briefly dried in a SpeedVac. Dried gel bands were swollen at room temperature in 20 μl of 25mM ammonium bicarbonate/0.01% OGS or in 20 µL of 10mM hydrochloric acid/0.01% OGS supplemented with Promega-modified trypsin or pepsin, respectively to an enzyme to substrate ratio of 1 to 10 (w/w). After 20 min, 40 µl of 25mM ammonium bicarbonate or 40 µL of 10 mM hydrochloric acid/0.01% OGS was added and the digestion continued for 18 hours at 37°C. After incubation, 50 µL of 0.1% TFA was added. The supernatant was removed and another 50 µL of 0.1% TFA was added. The gel bands were incubated for 30 min at 37°C. The combined extracts were reduced in volume to 35 µL, acidified by addition of 5 µL of 10 % TFA and immobilized on ZipTip$_{C18}$ pipette tips as described below.

3.3   Protein In-Solution Proteolytic Digestion

In-solution tryptic digestion of 2 -20 pmoles of protein was performed in 35 µL of 50 mM ammonium bicarbonate/ 0.005% OGS at an enzyme to substrate ratio of 1 to 100 (w/w). After 18 hours at 37˚C, the digests were acidified by addition of 5 µL of 10% TFA to and immobilized on ZipTip$_{C18}$ pipette tips as described below. Protein can be reduced and carboxamidomethylated prior to digestion as follows: Protein samples are reconstituted in 40 µL of 10mM sodium phosphate /1M urea/0.005% OGS (pH 8.0) supplemented with 2.5 mM TCEP. After 20 min incubation at 55 °C, 10 uL of a 150 mM iodoacetamide solution prepared in 10 mM sodium phosphate/1M urea/0.005% OGS is added to a final concentration of 30 mM and the incubation continued for 30 min at 37 °C in the dark. The samples are subjected to buffer exchange into 50 mM ammonium bicarbonate/1M urea/ 0.005% OGS on Zebra Desalt Spin Columns according to the manufactures recommendations. After sample adsorption, 10 µL of buffer is applied to the resin bed followed by centrifugation. The recovered fractions (60 µL) are supplemented with trypsin to an enzyme to substrate ratio of 1 to 50 (w/w). After 18 hours incubation at 37 °C, the digests are acidified to a final concentration of 1.25% TFA and immobilized on ZipTip$_{C18}$ pipette tips as described below.

3.4   Sample Immobilization

ZipTip$_{C18}$ pipette tips or ZipTip$_{u-C18}$ pipette tips were wetted six times with 10µL of methanol followed by six washes with 10 µL of 0.1% TFA. Model peptides (2-20 pmoles) were loaded from 10 µL aliquots of 0.2 % TFA/0.01% OGS solutions onto ZipTip$_{C18}$ pipette tips and subjected to ten sample load/dispense cycles. The ZipTip$_{C18}$ pipette tips were then washed three times with 10 µL of 0.1% TFA. For high volume sample enrichment (40 uL), peptides (0.125-20 pmoles) were sequentially loaded in 10 µL aliquots onto ZipTip$_{C18}$ pipette tips or ZipTip$_{u-C18}$ pipette tips and dispensed into a 0.5 ml microfuge tube. The sample was then transferred back in this step-wise mode to the original collection tube. This alternating load/dispense enrichment cycle was repeated five times. The ZipTip pipette tips were then washed five times with 10 µL of 0.1% TFA. Optionally, 200 µL disposable pipette tips can be press-fitted into ZipTip$_{u-C18}$ pipette tips or ZipTip$_{C18}$ pipette tips, as suggested by the manufacturer and operated with a 200 µL pipettor to pass the sample slowly ten times over the resin. Up to 200 µL of sample can be processed for binding in this manner.

3.5   On-Resin β-Elimination and β-Elimination with Concurrent Michael Addition

An aqueous 66 mM barium hydroxide solution was used for β-elimination (7.49mg/mL). A 2/1 mixture of aqueous 100 mM barium hydroxide (31.54 mg/mL) and aqueous 100 mM 2-aminoethanethiol hydrochloride (11.36 mg/mL) [66 mM barium hydroxide /33 mM 2-aminoethanethiol hydrochloride, pH 12.1] was used for β-elimination with concurrent Michael addition. Barium hydroxide was finely ground to facilitate dissolution. Residuals, mainly carbonates were removed by centrifugation (1 min at 13 000 rpm). Freshly prepared solutions of the elimination base and of the nucleophile were used for each experiment. The analyte was bound to ZipTip$_{C18}$ pipette tips or ZipTip$_{\mu\text{-}C18}$ pipette tips which were then flushed twice to waste with 10 μL of the reagents. 10 μL of the reagents were then loaded onto the solid supports from 60 μL that had been placed into 0.5 ml microcentrifuge tubes. Alternatively, the incubation was carried out in 1 ml capped microcentrifuge tubes that had been loaded with 80 μL of the reagents. The samples were incubated in the tubes for predetermined times at 37 °C or 55 °C while immersed in the reagent solutions. After incubation, the tips were washed with 100 μL of 0.1% TFA passed over the resin in 10 μL aliquots. Peptides were eluted in 5-10 μL of 50% acetonitrile/0.1% TFA/0.01% OGS and combined with matrix containing 0.1% TFA in a 1/1 ratio. 1 μL aliquots of the mixtures were used for MALDI-MS analysis. In some experiments, ZipTip$_{\mu\text{-}C18}$ pipette tips were directly eluted in 1 μL of matrix containing 0.1% TFA onto the MALDI plate.

3.6   In-Solution β-Elimination and β-Elimination with Concurrent Michael Addition

For in-solution derivatization, 40 μL aliquots of solutions containing 50 fmol/μL of peptide were taken to complete dryness by SpeedVac evaporation. The peptides were then resuspended in 40 μL of 66mM barium hydroxide/33 mM 2-aminoethanethiol hydrochloride or in 66 mM barium hydroxide and incubated for predetermined times at 55 °C. After derivatization, the preparations were acidified with 2 μL of 20% TFA and submitted to ZipTip$_{\mu\text{-}C18}$ pipette tip purification. Peptides were eluted onto the target in 1 μL of matrix containing 0.1% TFA.

3.7   Differential Peptide Mapping

In-gel digests were prepared in replicates from equimolar amounts of protein loaded onto the gel. Model peptides used for method optimization and in-solution digests were split into equal fractions. Samples were immobilized on ZipTip$_{C18}$ pipette tips or ZipTip$_{\mu\text{-}C18}$ pipette tips. One set of ZipTips were loaded with 10 μL of 0.1% TFA, left immersed in solvent and set as controls. The other set of ZipTips was processed for derivatization. Unmodified and derivatized material was eluted from the ZipTip$_{C18}$ pipette tips typically in 5-10 μL of 50% acetonitrile/0.1% TFA/0.01% OGS. Eluates were combined with matrix containing 0.1% TFA in a 1/1 ratio. 1μL portions of the mixtures were used for MALDI analysis. ZipTip$_{\mu\text{-}C18}$ pipette tips were directly deposited in 1μL of matrix containing 0.1% TFA onto the MALDI plate. Comparison of the MALDI-MS maps enables semiquantitative assessment of derivatization efficiency as well as identification of phosphopeptides in unfractionated digest as discussed later in the text.

For optimal use of low level samples, the analyte may be recovered from MALDI spots for subsequent derivatization according to a previous procedure with minor modifications (Larsen et al., 2001). In this strategy, the protein digest (<2 pmoles) enriched from dilute solutions onto a ZipTip$_{\mu\text{-}C18}$ pipette tip, is deposited in 1 μL of α-CHCA matrix supplemented with 0.1% TFA onto the MALDI plate. After MALDI-TOF analysis, the plate is removed from the instrument. 4 -5 μL of 0.5% TFA is placed onto the MALDI spot. The solubilized analyte is then concentrated on a preconditioned ZipTip$_{\mu\text{-}C18}$ pipette tip directly from the droplet using ten load/dispense cycles. The ZipTip$_{\mu\text{-}C18}$ pipette tip is washed ten times with 10 μL of 0.1% TFA to remove the matrix. The sample is then subjected to the chemical treatment, desalted and deposited in matrix onto the sample stage. In this simple manner, only a single sample needs to be committed to differential mass mapping.

3.8   On-Resin Acetylation

A 20 mM sodium phosphate buffer (pH 8.0) was supplemented with 20 mM sulfo-NHS acetate. ZipTip$_{C18}$ pipette tip-bound peptides were flushed three times with the reagent, incubated in 10 µL of reagent for 20 min at 55°C while left immersed in the solution. The Tips were then washed ten times with 10 µL 0.1% TFA. Sample processing for MALDI-TOF was as described above. The reagent was prepared fresh for daily use.

3.9   On-Resin Deacylation

This procedure was combined with acetylation to reverse unwanted O-acylation. Peptides were acetylated and desalted as described above. The desalted ZipTip$_{C18}$ pipette tips were then flushed three times to waste with 10 µL of 1M sodium carbonate supplemented with 2% hydroxylamine hydrochloride (pH 9.4). 10 µL of the reagent was loaded on the supports which were then incubated immersed in reagent for 15 min at 37 °C, and subsequently washed ten times with 10 µL of 0.1% TFA and the five times with 10 µL of water. Sample processing for MALDI-TOF was as described above.

3.10   Preparation of Substrates for Chemoenzymatic Phosphosite Determination

Phosphopeptides (2-20 pmoles) were subjected to on-column acetylation as described above. The post-reaction desalting step was omitted. Instead, the Tips were flushed three times to waste with 10 µL of the 33 mM 2-aminoethanethiol/ 66 mM barium hydroxide followed by aspiration of 10 µL of the reagent mixture. After 60 min incubation at 37 ° C, the tips were processed for MALDI-TOF as described above. ZipTip$_{u-C18}$ pipette tips were used to derivatize 2 pmoles or lower amounts of peptide. The Tips were eluted in matrix directly onto the target.

3.11   ZipTip$_{C18}$ Pipette Tip Alkali Compatibility Evaluation

The efficiency of relative peptide recovery of peptide from the silica-based reversed phase support before and after the alkali treatment was assessed using the isotope dilution procedure. Methanolic HCl solutions were prepared freshly by drop-wise adding 40 µL of acetyl chloride to 250 µL of methanol or deuterated methanol kept on ice. Aliquots of the model peptide angiotensin I (2 nmoles) were taken to dryness in a SpeedVac followed by addition of 25 µL of the methanolic HCl reagents. After 90 min incubation at 12 °C, the reaction mixtures were dried. The methyl-d_0-esterified peptide and the methyl-d_3-esterified peptide were dissolved in 50% acetonitrile/0.1% TFA and stored at -21°C prior to use. The methyl-d_0-esterified preparation was used as a reference peptide after appropriate dilution.

Efficiency and reproducibility of relative peptide recovery from the support was assessed as follows: aliquots of angiotensin I solutions in 0.2% TFA/0.01% OGS containing 50 pmoles of peptide were subjected to ten sample load/dispense cycle. The ZipTip$_{C18}$ pipette tips were then washed three times with 10 µL of 0.1% TFA to remove unbound material and eluted twice with 10 µL of 50% acetonitrile/0.1% TFA/0.01% OGS. Eluates were dried in a SpeedVac, dissolved in 25 µL of the isotopically labeled methanolic HCl, incubated for 90 min at 12°C and subsequently dried. The methyl-d_3-esterified peptides were then dissolved in 10 µL of 50% acetonitrile/0.1% TFA and 5 µL of the peptide solutions were mixed with 5 µL of the methyl-d_0-esterified reference peptide followed by addition of 10 µL of MALDI matrix. 1 µL of the final mixture was then applied to the MALDI target for subsequent relative quantitation of the eluted peptides.

To assess the potential impact of silica alkali exposure on peptide recovery, 50 pmoles of peptide was immobilized in replicates as described above. The ZipTip$_{C18}$ pipette tips were rinsed three times with 10 μL of 0.1% TFA, flushed three times with 33 mM 2-aminoethanethiol/66 mM barium hydroxide, and then loaded with 10 μL of the reagent. The concurrent reaction was allowed to proceed for 1 h at 55 °C. The ZipTips were washed by passing 100 μL of 0.1% TFA in 10 μL aliquots over the resin and eluted twice with 10 μL of 50% acetonitrile/0.1% TFA/0.01% OGS. The eluates were dried and methyl-d$_3$-esterified under the conditions described above. The methyl-d$_3$-esterified peptides were then dissolved in 10 μL of 50% acetonitrile/0.1% TFA and 5 μL of the peptide solutions were mixed with 5 μL of the methyl-d$_0$-esterified reference peptide followed by addition of 10 μL of MALDI matrix. 1 μL of the final mixture was then applied to the MALDI target for subsequent relative quantitation of the eluted peptides. Potential alkali-induced sample loss from the reversed-phase support was determined by measuring the ratio of the relative abundance of the methyl-d$_3$ and methyl-d$_0$-esterified peptides in the mass spectra.

3.12   Mass Spectrometry

A Voyager-DE STR (Applied Biosystems, Foster City, CA) was used and operated in the reflector mode at an accelerating voltage of 20kV. Laser intensity was typically set at 1690-2400 and spectra were acquired using 100- 200 laser shots/spectrum. The data shown are based on three accumulated acquisitions sampled from three spot positions. Some spectra were obtained in the linear mode using 80 laser shots/spectrum and 5-10 spectra acquired from the spots at different positions were averaged. For peptide fragmentation, a 4700 Proteomics Analyzer was used and operated in the MS and MS/MS modes; typical laser power for MS was about 3700, for MS/MS, about 4500. Usually 1000-2000 shots were acquired for MS, 2000-20000 for MS/MS.

4   Results and Discussion

4.1   Sample Handling

4.1.1   Solid-Phase Derivatization

The β-elimination with concurrent Michael addition chemistry using barium hydroxide as elimination base and 2-aminoethanethiol as nucleophile is schematically depicted in Figure 1A. The reactions involve base-induced abstraction of the proton from the α-carbon atom with subsequent release of phosphate, carbamidothiolate or O-glycan from the β-carbon atom. The resultant α.β-unsaturated derivative (dehydroalanine) is concurrently attacked by the nucleophilic sulfur resulting in adduct formation. The solid-phase adaptation of the chemistry is exceedingly simple in implementation (Figure 1B). Peptides or protein digests are bound to ZipTip$_{C18}$ pipette tips or ZipTip$_{μ-C18}$ pipette tips followed by a brief solvent wash to remove contaminants from the support that may interfere with the reaction. The ZipTips are then loaded with the reagent and left immersed in the reagent during the subsequent incubation. The ZipTips are desalted prior to product elution. As further depicted in Figure 1B, solid-phase derivatization can be readily expanded to accommodate serial reaction schemes. In this sample handling format, reagents are exchanged directly on the support eliminating sample transfer between the reaction steps.

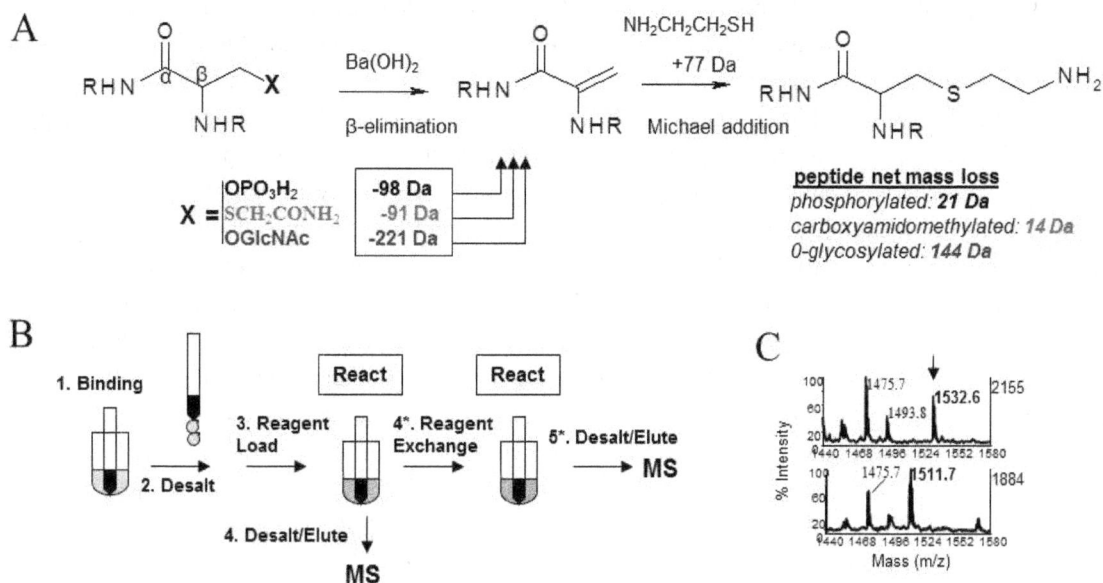

Figure 1: Solid-phase strategy for phosphopeptide identification in protein digests. (A) Representation of the chemical reactions using barium hydroxide as β-elimination base and 2-aminoethanethiol as nucleophile. Note that the reactions in the applications occur concurrently. The differential β-elimination-induced mass loss from phospho-,carboxyamidomethylated cysteinyl-, and OGlcNAc peptides is indicated in a box. The peptide net mass loss after concurrent incorporation of the nucleophile (M$_r$ 77 Da) and the corresponding spectral mass shifts, providing distinction between these peptides, are highlighted in italics. OGlcNAc denotes O-linked β-N-acetylglucosamine. (B) Schematic representation of the sample handling steps using ZipTip$_{C18}$ pipette tips as reaction bed. The sample is bound to the ZipTip (1) and desalted (2). The tip is then loaded with reagent and left immersed in the reagent solution during incubation (3). The tip is desalted and eluted prior to MALDI-MS analysis (4). For serial derivatization, reagents are exchanged directly on the solid phase (4 *). After incubation, the tip is desalted followed by elution of the final reaction product (5*). (C) Application of the strategy to a tryptic digest of yeast Maf1. A section of the MALDI-MS spectra produced before (upper spectrum) and after derivatization (lower spectrum) is shown. Arrow indicates the phosphopeptide at m/z 1532.6 identified by the mass shift of 21 Da relative to its tagged counterpart at m/z 1511.7 (see Figure 7 for expanded spectra).

4.1.2   Solid-Phase Derivatization Advantages

The solid-phase derivatization format offers some notable advantages over the classical in-solution based methods, the predominant sample preparation technique in current proteomic studies, as follows: (1) The process of sample adsorption inherently concentrates the analyte on the support allowing the chemistry to take place in an environment which is essentially free of reagent dilution. As a result, the reaction proceeds *in situ* at higher efficiency and faster kinetics than in solution as demonstrated by the experiments described below. (2) The digests can be effectively enriched on the solid phase from dilute solutions in which chemical reactions inherently proceed at slow reaction rates. In these sample limited situations, ZipTip$_{\mu-C18}$ pipette tip are preferentially used enabling product elution directly onto the target in as little as 0.5 μL of matrix with consequent improved mass detection. (3) The solid-phase strategy obviates the need for sample dry-down commonly practiced in proteomics studies to concentrate peptide mixtures prior to derivatization in solution. As noted for low-level samples (<2 pmole), this sample handling step can cause substantial adsorptive peptide loss ranging up to 50% or more of the starting solution (Speicher *et al.*, 2000). (4) The solid-phase procedure should be readily amenable to automation on ZipTip$_{C18}$ pipette and ZipTip$_{\mu\text{-C18}}$ pipette tip compatible liquid handling stations. (5) For optimal use of low level samples, the starting material can be recovered after the initial mass analysis from the MALDI-TOF sample spot on the reversed phase support for subsequent derivatization (see Materials and Methods). In addition, after MALDI MS and MALDI MS/MS analysis, the remainder of derivatized sample may be recovered from the MALDI spot and analyzed by nano LC-MS/MS to obtain complementary sequence data.

As demonstrated in our report and in an earlier communication (Nika *et al.*, 2005), the solid-phase format proved particularly advantageous for combining distinct chemistries into serial reaction schemes. Once the peptides are bound to the support and processed for the initial derivatization, subsequent sample handling is confined to reagent exchanges *in situ* and elution of the final derivatives (Figure 1B). Thus, intermittent sample purification as practiced during in-solution derivatization that may incur significant, cumulative adsorptive sample loss is avoided (Speicher *et al.*, 2000; Rusnak *et al.*, 2002; Knight *et al.*, 2003). Accordingly, the high efficiency of the individual *in situ* reactions can be fully exploited to ensure optimal recovery of the final derivatives providing a significant advantage in sample limited situations.

4.1.3   Use of *N*-octyl Glucoside

As has been reported, inclusion of trace amounts of the non-ionic detergent OGS in the in-gel digestion buffers affords improved peptide recovery by enhancing peptide solubility and minimizing peptide adsorption associated with sample handling (Katayama *et al.*, 2001). The detergent proved highly compatible with MALDI-TOF analysis and with liquid chromatography mass spectrometry owing to its strong retention on reversed phase columns (Katayama *et al.*, 2004). To take advantage of this favorable effect, in-gel and in-solution protein digestion was performed in the presence of the additive and test peptide solutions evaluated in this study were supplemented with OGS prior to immobilization.

4.2   On-Resin β-Elimination and β-Elimination with Concurrent Michael Addition

4.2.1   Reaction with Model Peptides

A panel of peptides phosphorylated at serine and at serine C-terminally adjoined by proline were used to define the experimental conditions for efficient β-elimination and β-elimination with concurrent Michael addition. The analysis of phosphopeptides containing the phosphoserine/proline sequence feature is a special interest since a significant portion of cellular phosphorylation events are regulated by proline-directed kinases (Ubersax & Ferrell, 2007). Representative MALDI-TOF data from the derivatization experiments are shown in Figures 2 and 3. A mixture of the phosphoseryl peptides P2 (SHNSALY**p**-SQVQK), P3 (GIKSHN**pS**ALYSQVQK) and T6 (FQ**pS**EEQQQTEDELQDK) was subjected β-elimination, or to β-elimination with concurrent Michael addition for 1 hour at 37 °C. As semiquantitatively assessed by MALDI-MS the peptides were effectively converted to their dehydroalanine and S-2-aminoethylcysteine counterparts, respectively (Figure 2A, B, C) as were the additional phosphoseryl peptides listed in Materials and Methods with the exception of the model peptide P2 that partially remained in its β-eliminated form. The data are consistent with the perception that the chemistry can be subject to

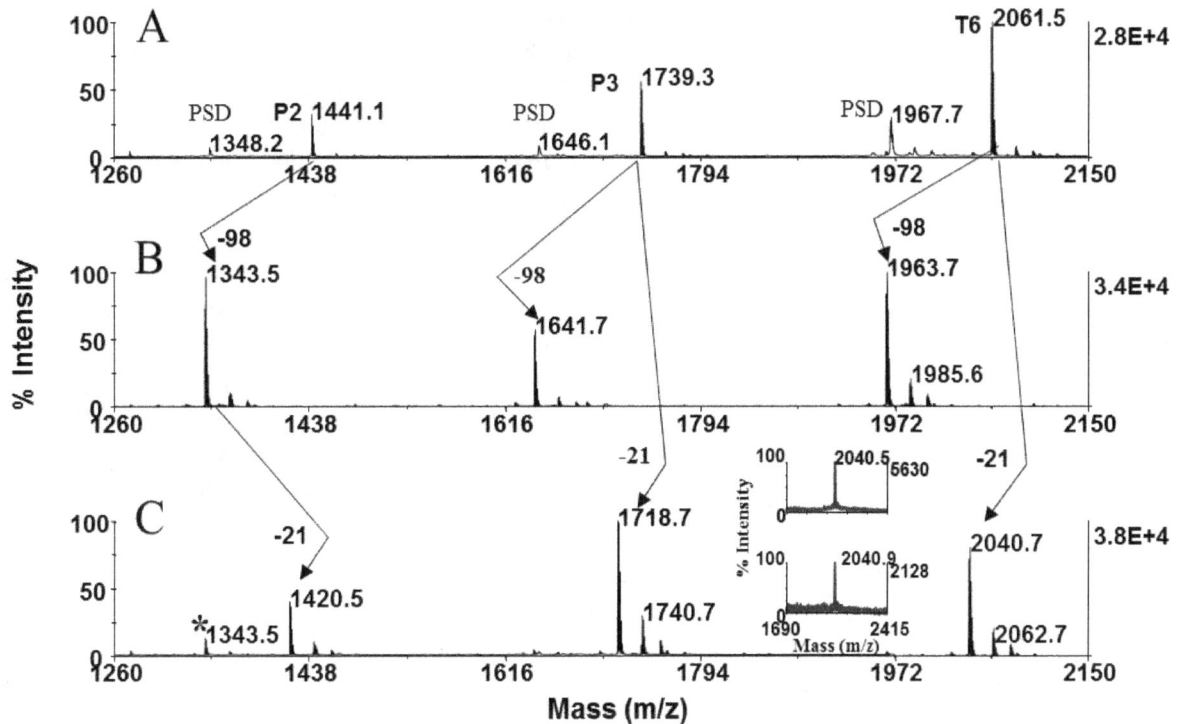

Figure 2: Solid-phase β-elimination and β-elimination with concurrent Michael addition of phosphoseryl peptides. The mixture composed of the model peptides P2 (SHNSALY**pS**QVQK), P3 (GIKSHN**pS**ALYSQVQK) and T6 (FQ**pS**EEQQQTEDELQDK) was bound to ZipTip$_{C18}$ pipette tips and incubated with 66 mM barium hydroxide or the barium hydroxide/2-aminoethanethiol reaction mixture composed of 66 mM base and 33 mM nucleophile. After 1 h at 37 °C the reactions were terminated by a solvent wash. MALDI-TOF spectra of 2 pmoles of (A) unmodified peptides; (B) after β-elimination; (C) after β-elimination with concurrent Michael addition. Cross arrows indicate the characteristic mass shift of 98 Da per eliminated phosphate and the 21 Da mass shift arising from the loss of phosphate and the concurrent incorporation of the nucleophile (M_r 77 Da). Asterisk denoted residual β-elimination product. Low intensity ions in B and C represent sodium and potassium adducts. PSD denotes post source decay products. Inset in C shows the MALDI mass spectra of the Michael addition products of T6 at sample loads of 250 fmole (upper panel) and 125 fmole (lower panel). Samples were derivatized on ZipTipμ-$_{C18}$ pipette tips and directly eluted in matrix onto the target. These spectra were acquired in the linear mode.

some degree to reactivity modulation by amino acids flanking the site of phosphorylation. As indicated in Figure 2, β-elimination-induced removal of the phosphate group imparted as mass shift 98 Da onto the naïve peptides (Figure 2A, B) whereas the concurrent reaction was accompanied by a mass shift of 21 Da, arising from the nucleophilic addition of 2-aminoethanethiol (M_r 77 Da) to the dehydroalanyl residues (Figure 2A, C) (see Figure 1A). These characteristic mass signatures provide a means to identify phosphopeptides in the MALDI mass maps of unfractionated protein digests, as discussed later in the text. We note here that moderately reduced reactivity of phosphopeptides, such as noted for the model peptide P2, should not detract from the utility of the method to scan for phosphopeptides in protein digests. In fact, residual β-elimination products, recognized by the mass signature of 98 Da, provide complementary evidence for the presence of a phosphopeptide in a mixture.

Under the mild reaction conditions, shown effective to convert phosphoseryl residues, a substantial portion of the peptide P5 (RGApSPVE) in which the phosphoseryl residue is adjoined by proline remained in its dehydroalanyl form (Fig. 3B, inset, asterisk). The slower reaction kinetics of the addition reaction is expected, since proline shields the residue's β-carbon from the nucleophilic attack. Similar results were obtained with the phosphothreonyl peptide P7 (KRpTIRR) which is consistent with the common perception that the residue's methyl group protects the β-carbon from nucleophilic attack (Byford, 1991) (data not shown). Conversion yields improved when the peptides were incubated at increased temperatures. As shown by Figure 3 B, the S-2-aminoethylcysteine derivative of P5 was efficiently formed after 1 h incubation at 55 °C. Comparable results were obtained with P6 (RRQpSPVA) (results not shown) and, as would be expected, with the phosphoseryl peptides listed in Materials and Methods. Under these more stringent reaction conditions, the phosphothreonyl peptide P7 (KRpTIRR) was efficiently converted to its β-methyl-S-2-aminoethylcysteine derivative (Figure 3D).

At the same temperature, the β-elimination product of this peptide was fully formed on the solid-phase already after 30 min incubation indicating that the concurrent addition phase limits the rate of the overall reaction (Figure 3C, inset). This trend became considerably more pronounced when the same reaction was performed in solution (see below).

4.2.2   Effect of Sample Preconcentration on Reaction Kinetics

In the experiments, 40 μL aliquots of the phosphothreonine peptide solution (50 fmol/μL) were processed for binding on ZipTipμ-c$_{18}$ pipette tips providing for approx. 200-fold analyte enrichment on the 200 μL sorbent beds. The resultant locally increased peptide concentration should, in principle, allow the chemistry to proceed more efficiently and faster on the solid-phase than in solution. To test the validity of this notion, we subjected the phosphothreonyl peptide P7 (KRpTIRR) to in-solution concurrent β-elimination with Michael addition. In this procedure, aliquots of the phosphopeptide solution were subjected to SpeedVac evaporation followed by addition of 40 μL of the alkaline nucleophile reagent to reconstitute the dried peptide to its original concentration. After incubation for 1 h at 55 °C, the in-solution preparations were purified on ZipTip$_{μ-C18}$ pipette tips and deposited directly in matrix onto the MALDI plate. The MALDI-TOF spectra of the samples revealed that the β-elimination product was accumulated to near completion whereas the concurrent addition reaction was markedly retarded (Figure 3D, inset). Similarly, under conditions that afforded complete β-elimination on the solid-phase (Figure 3C, inset), approx. 50% of the peptide remained intact when the treatment was performed in solution, and an additional 30 min incubation was needed to complete the reaction (results not illustrated). The comparison data clearly identified the peptide preconcentration effect on the solid-phase as critical determinant of the accelerated reaction rate and of the relatively high efficiency of the overall reaction. We note that the moderate reactivity of phosphothreonine upon in-solution reaction at elevated temperatures has been recognized in earlier studies using 2-aminoethanethiol or other nucleophiles, and has been addressed in these protocols by prolonged incubation (> 4 h) (Molloy & Andrews, 2001; Rusnak et al., 2002). However, experimentation to optimize the in-solution protocol was not pursued in our study. Our data are in general accord with those reported in proteomics studies exploiting accelerated in situ peptide amine-directed chemical modification to facilitate de novo sequence interpretation (Conrotto & Hellman, 2005; Cindric et al., 2006).

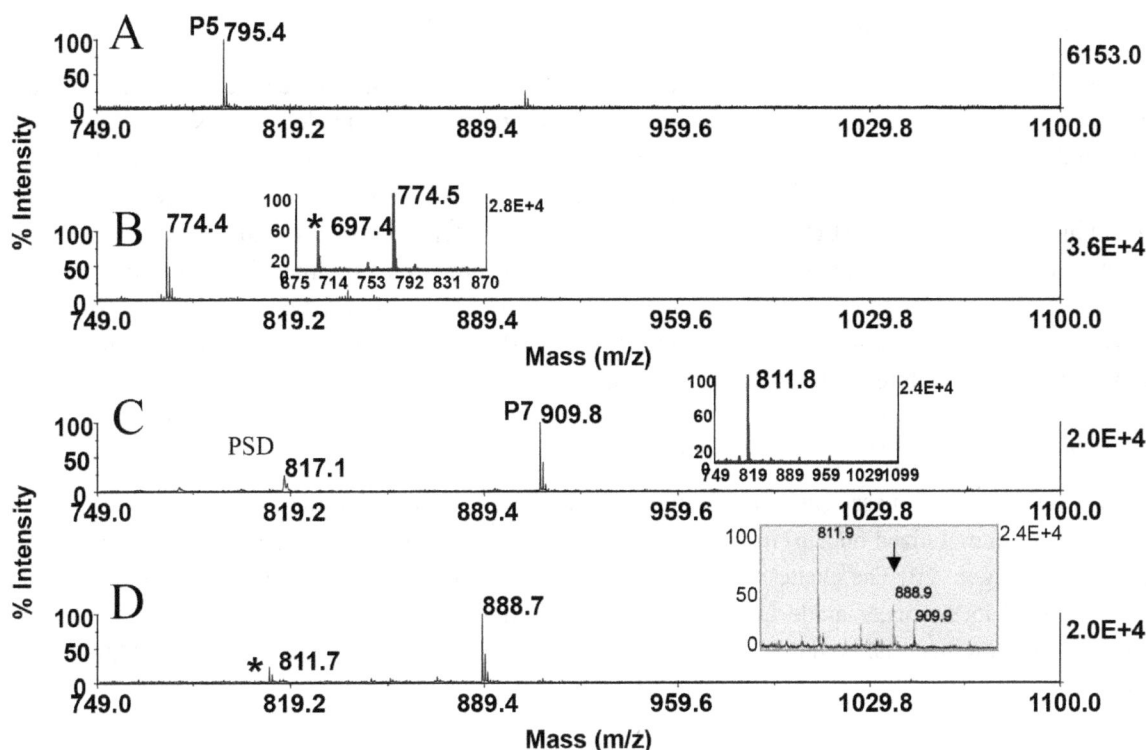

Figure 3: Solid-phase β-elimination with concurrent Michael addition of phosphoseryl /proline- and phosphothreonyl-containing peptides. Model peptides P5 (RGApSPVE) and P7 (KRpTIRR) were enriched on ZipTipµ-C18 pipette tips from 40 µL aliquots of a 50 fmol/µL solution and incubated in the 66 mM barium hydroxide/33 mM 2-aminoethanethiol for 1h at 55 °C. In parallel, P7 was incubated in 66 mM barium hydroxide for 30 min at 55 °C. Equimolar amounts of P7 were taken to dryness, reacted for 1 h at 55 °C in 40 µL of the alkaline nucleophile solution followed by ZipTipµ-C18 pipette tip purification. The samples were eluted in matrix onto the target. MALDI-TOF spectra of (A) unmodified peptide P5; (B) after the concurrent reaction; (C) unmodified peptide P7; (D) after the concurrent reaction. Note efficiency of solid-phase reactions. Inset in B shows the MALDI-TOF spectrum of P5 after solid-phase reaction for 1 h at 37 °C. Asterisk designates residual β-elimination product. Note incompleteness of Michael addition. Inset in C shows the MALDI-TOF spectrum of P7 after 30 min solid-phase β-elimination. Inset in D shows MALDI-TOF spectrum of P7 after concurrent in-solution derivatization. Note incompleteness of thiol adduct formation (arrow). PSD denotes post source decay product. PSD in C and asterisk in D denote post source decay and residual β-elimination product, respectively.

With these developments, MALDI-TOF maps prepared from digest before and after derivatization can be scanned for both serine and threonine phosphorylation, as discussed later in the text. However, we recognize the need for an expanded data set to demonstrate the general utility of the method for derivatization of phosphothreonyl peptides, and have to this purpose in recent work extended the evaluation of the solid-phase chemical strategy to a panel phosphothreonyl peptides including phosphothreonyl peptides adjoined by proline. A manuscript detailing the optimized derivatization conditions is currently in preparation.

4.3   Reliability of Derivatization

The reliability of derivatization at low sample levels was assessed in a semiquantitative mode with the synthetic β-casein peptide T6 (data not shown). 1 pmole of peptide was loaded from 40 µl aliquots of a 25 fmole/µl peptide solution onto 8 separate ZipTip$_{\mu\text{-}C18}$ pipette tips and subjected to β-elimination/Michael addition under the conditions described in Figure 1. The samples were then directly eluted in matrix onto the MALDI plate. Eighty laser shots were typically required to obtain stable signals. A total of 640 laser shots sampled from 8 different spot positions were summed for each spectrum. The spectra were devoid of signal from the unmodified species and signal variations observed between the individual spectra were at most 15%. The comparable MALDI response observed in the spectra was interpreted to reflect high reliability of derivatization.

4.4   Derivatization of Peptide at the Femtomole Level

To explore the overall mass sensitivity of the method, aliquots from serial dilutions of the β-casein peptide T6 were immobilized on ZipTip$_{\mu\text{-}C18}$ pipette tips and converted to the Michael addition analogues as described in Figure 2B. The eluates were directly deposited in matrix onto the MALDI plate and spectra were acquired in the linear mode from eight different positions. As illustrated in Figure 2C, inset, 125 fmoles of starting material could be effectively carried through the β-elimination/Michael addition reaction.

4.5   ZipTip$_{C18}$ Pipette Tip Alkali-Compatibility Evaluation

Alkali-induced silica resin decomposition has been reported to diminish to a minor extent the retention of the silane-bonded stationary phase during long-term C18 reversed-phase column testing (> 1 week) with mobile phases at pH 9-12.3 (Kirkland *et al.*, 1995). This effect was attributed to mechanical attrition around the covalently attached silanes eventually causing splitting off of the bonded organic phase, and could therefore potentially reduce the analyte recovery from the silica-based reaction bed. However, our data show that peptides in general exhibited comparable signal intensities in the MALDI spectra prepared from the derivatized and the untreated samples suggesting that the analyte was efficiently retained on the solid-phase when exposed to the alkaline reaction conditions (see Figure 5 and 6). In support of this interpretation, we assessed the relative recovery of a model peptide (angiotensin I) from ZipTips before and after the chemical treatment using a stable isotope dilution technique. In support of this observation, we assessed the relative recovery of the model peptide angiotensin I (DRVYIHPFHL, *m/z* 1296.6) from ZipTips before and after the chemical treatment using a stable isotope dilution technique. To this purpose, the peptide (2 nmoles) was treated with methanolic HCl or with deuterated methanolic HCl. The differentially labeled peptide stock solutions were adjusted to a concentration of 1 pmole/µl, mixed in equimolar amounts and applied to the MALDI target. The spectra showed that the methyl-d_0 and methyl-d_3 esterified peptides were observed at nearly equal abundance, and there were no chemistry side reactions (data not illustrated). The methyl-d_0 esterified preparation was then used as internal reference in the experiments described below for relative peptide quantitation.

We first accessed the recovery of peptide from untreated reversed-phase support. To this purpose, 50 pmoles of peptide were immobilized in replicates, washed to remove unbound material, eluted, methyl-d_3-esterified and mixed with the methyl-d_0-esterified internal reference peptide. As estimated from the spectral abundance ratio calculated for the replicates, an average of 80 % of peptide was reproducibly recovered in the eluted fractions (Figure 4A). The reproducibility and high efficiency of peptide recovery from untreated resin noted here is in accord with an earlier evaluation of ZipTipc$_{18}$ pipette tips using ^{14}C-accelerator mass spectrometry for peptide quantitation (Palmblad & Vogel, 2005).

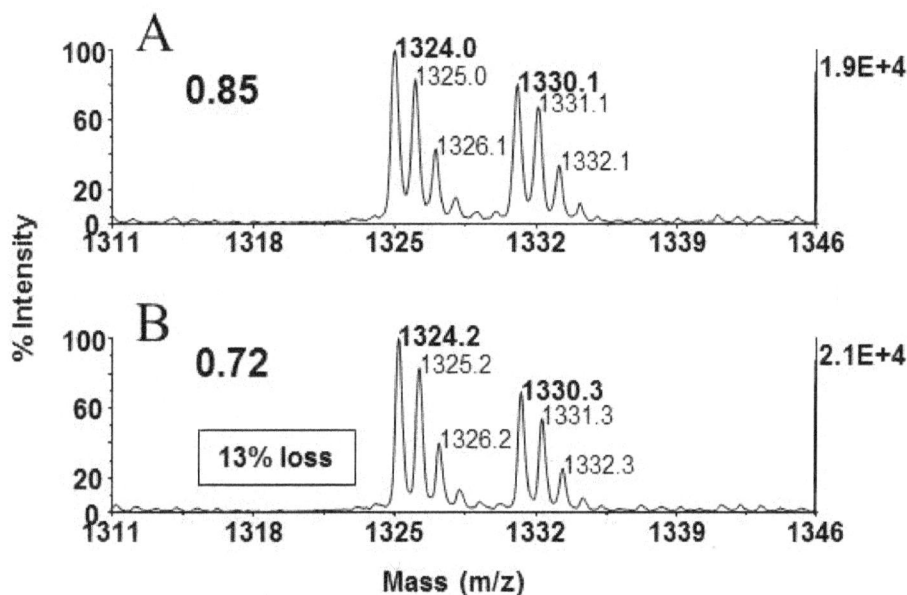

Figure 4: ZipTipC18 pipette tip alkali-compatibility evaluation. Angiotensin I; DRVYIHPFHL at m/z 1296.5 (50 pmoles) was immobilized on a ZipTipC18 pipette tips which were briefly washed to remove unbound material. The tips were then exposed to the β-elimination/Michael conditions as described in Figure 3, or left untreated. Peptides with and without incubation were desorbed, methyl-d$_3$-esterified and mixed in equimolar amounts with the methyl-d$_0$-esterified reference peptide. Experiments were in triplicate. MALDI-TOF spectra were acquired using 400 laser shots/spectrum accumulated from 5 different spot positions. MALDI-TOF spectra of (A) methyl-d$_3$-esterified peptide from untreated sample mixed with methyl-d$_0$-esterfied internal reference peptide; (B) methyl-d$_3$-esterified peptide from alkali-exposed sample mixed with methyl-d$_0$-esterified internal reference peptide. Labels in A and B designate the relative peptide abundance ratios. The alkali-induced minor sample loss is highlighted with a box. Approximately 0.5 pmoles of peptides were applied to the target.

To assess the potential impact of the alkali treatment on peptide retention, ZipTip$_{C18}$ pipette tips were loaded with 50 pmoles of peptide and briefly washed. Samples were then carried through the concurrent β-elimination/Michael addition reaction scheme as described in Figure 3, desalted and eluted. The eluates were methyl-d$_3$-esterified, reconstituted and mixed with the methyl-d$_0$ esterified peptide internal reference. As estimated from the spectral abundance ratio calculated for the replicates, an average of 70 % of peptide could be reproducibly recovered from the chemically treated supports (Figure 4B). The comparison data show that a small fraction of the sample (av. 10 %) could not be retrieved from the support after the alkali exposure or was lost from the support due to silica leakage during the post-reaction sample purification. Taken together, the overall benefits gained from this sample preparation format as demonstrated in the report including ease of operation and completeness of the serial reactions well compensate for this minor sample loss.

4.6   Phosphopeptide Detection/Identification by Signal Enhancement

4.6.1   Application to Protein Digests

In these experiments, 2 picomoles of a resin-bound tryptic digest of β-casein, enriched from 50 femtomole/μL solutions onto ZipTip$_{C18}$ pipette tips were subjected to β-elimination and to β-elimination with concurrent Michael addition for 1 h at 37 °C. An equimolar amount of the digest was immobilized and left untreated as a control. Comparison of the MALDI-MS spectra prepared from these samples revealed the formation of a prominent ion at *m/z* 3038.6 representing the thiol adduct of the tetraphosphorylated peptide at theoretical *m/z* 3122.2 (RELEELNVPGEIVE**pSL**p**SpSpS**EESITR, residues 1-25) that was undetectable in its native form (arrow in Fig. 5A). In contrast, the monophosphorylated peptide observed at *m/z* 2061.8 (FQ**pS**EEQQQTEDELQDK), residues 33-48) exhibited a decreased signal intensity after concurrent derivatization (Figure 5C, filled arrowhead). As semiquantitatively assessed by MALDI-MS, a marked increase in relative signal intensity was observed for the substoichiometrically, monophosphorylated peptide at *m/z* 1660.7 (VPQLEIVPN**pS**AEER, residues 121-134) in the mass maps of an in-gel tryptic digest of α-S1 casein after β-elimination and β-elimination with concurrent Michael addition, respectively (Figure 5 D-F). An equally prominent signal enhancement was noted for the tryptic peptide at m/z 2088.8 (EVVG**pS**AEAGVDAASVSEEFR, residues 240-359) derived from an in-gel digest of ovalbumin (data not shown). Using the autolytic fragment of trypsin at m/z 906.7 as internal standard, a 3.6-fold enhancement in relative ionization intensity was noted for the phosphopeptide at m/z 2239.0 (TPEELDD**pS**DFETEDFDVR, residues 634-651) recovered from an in-gel digest of α-catenin (Figure 6A, B). The results validate the utility of the on-resin derivatization strategy to facilitate phosphopeptide detection/identification in unfractionated digests. We note here that ions corresponding to residual β-elimination products that would indicate incomplete Michael addition were not observed in the data set. No ions were observed that correspond to residual starting material.

4.6.2   Peptide Structure Modulation Effect on Signal Enhancement

The signal enhancement noted in our study appears to be attributable to the replacement of the negatively charged phosphate by the S-2-aminoethyl group which incorporates a protonatable hydrophobic moiety into the peptides, consistent with the observation that basic and hydrophobic residues in peptides tend to enhance the desorption/ionization process (Baumgart *et al.*, 2004). The enhanced MALDI response upon derivatization of the digests was found most prominent with phosphopeptides containing a high proportion of glutamic and/or aspartic residues (Figure 5D-F, and Figure 6) and with multiple phosphorylated species (Figure 5A-C). In contrast, phosphopeptides bearing multiple basic residues such as derived from the basophilic kinase substrates of Maf1 (e.g. RD**pS**NSFWEDK) were moderately enhanced by the nucleophilic substitution. Evidently, the additional protonatable moiety had only a minor impact on the favorable ionization behavior of these highly basic peptides. Accordingly, the native peptides and their modified counterparts appeared in the spectra with similar high abundance enabling facile identification of the phosphorylated species by interrogating the MALDI-mass maps for the characteristic derivatization

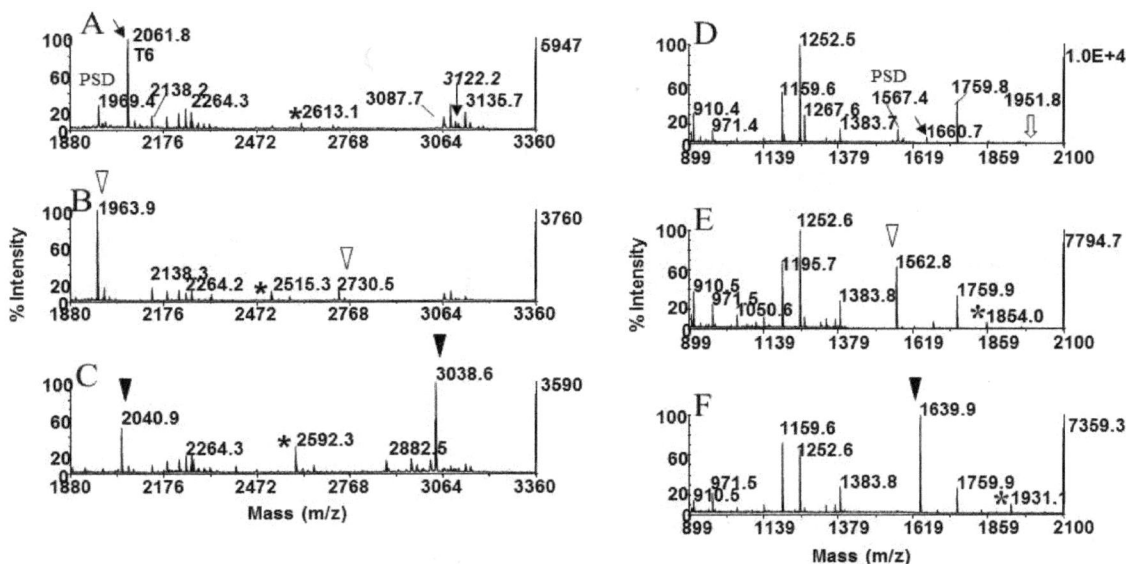

Figure 5: Phosphopeptide detection by signal enhancement. In-solution tryptic digests of β-casein (2 pmoles) immobilized onto ZipTip$_{C18}$ pipette tips were subjected to β-elimination and to β-elimination with concurrent Michael addition under the conditions described in Fig. 2. Expanded MALDI-TOF spectra of 400 fmoles of (A) untreated digest; (B) after β-elimination; (C) after β-elimination with concurrent Michael addition. Note the prominent ion at *m/z* 3038.6 corresponding to thiol adduct of the tetraphosphorylated species (RELEELNVPGEIVE**pSL**p**S**p**S**p**S**SEESITR) (filled arrowhead). The native counterpart at theoretical *m/z* 3122.2 was undetectable in A (arrow). Open arrowhead in B designates its dehydroalanyl derivative. Asterisks in A, B and C designate unidentified singly phosphorylated fragment and enhanced reaction products, respectively. Note diminished ionization response of T6 (FQ**pS**EEQQQTEDELQDK) after concurrent reaction. In-gel tryptic digests of α-casein S1 (20 pmoles) bound to ZipTip$_{C18}$ pipette tips were subjected to β-elimination and β-elimination with concurrent Michael addition as described in Fig. 2. MALDI-TOF spectra of (D) untreated digest; (E) after β-elimination; (F) after β-elimination with concurrent Michael addition. Arrow, open arrowhead and filled arrowhead indicate the phosphoserine peptide at *m/z* 1660.7 (VPQLEIVPN**pS**AEER), its dehydroalanyl derivative at *m/z* 1562.8 and its thiol adduct at m/z 1639.9, respectively. Note prominent ionization efficiency of the reaction products relative to the native counterpart. Asterisks in B and C denote the β-elimination product at *m/z* 1854.0 and the thiol adduct at *m/z* 1931.1, respectively, of the miscleavage product (YKVPQLEIVPN**pS**AEER) at theoretical *m/z* 1951.8 undetectable in A (open arrow). PSD denotes post source decay product.

mass shift of 21 Da per phosphoamino acid (see Figure 7). In addition, this mass signature provides information on the status of phosphorylation. In contrast to these basic phosphopeptides, phosphorylated fragments bearing multiple acidic amino acid residues such as contained in the digest of α-S1 casein and ovalbumin became undetectable at low sample level (<2 pmoles) but were clearly discernible as their tagged counterparts, and as such distinguishable from the non-phosphorylated peptides. In this situation, the tagged fragments are selected for MS/MS analysis which effectively reveals the identity of the peptides. Multiply phosphorylated species, as noted above, (*e.g.*, the tetraphosphorylated peptide of β-casein) are often detectable only after derivatization.

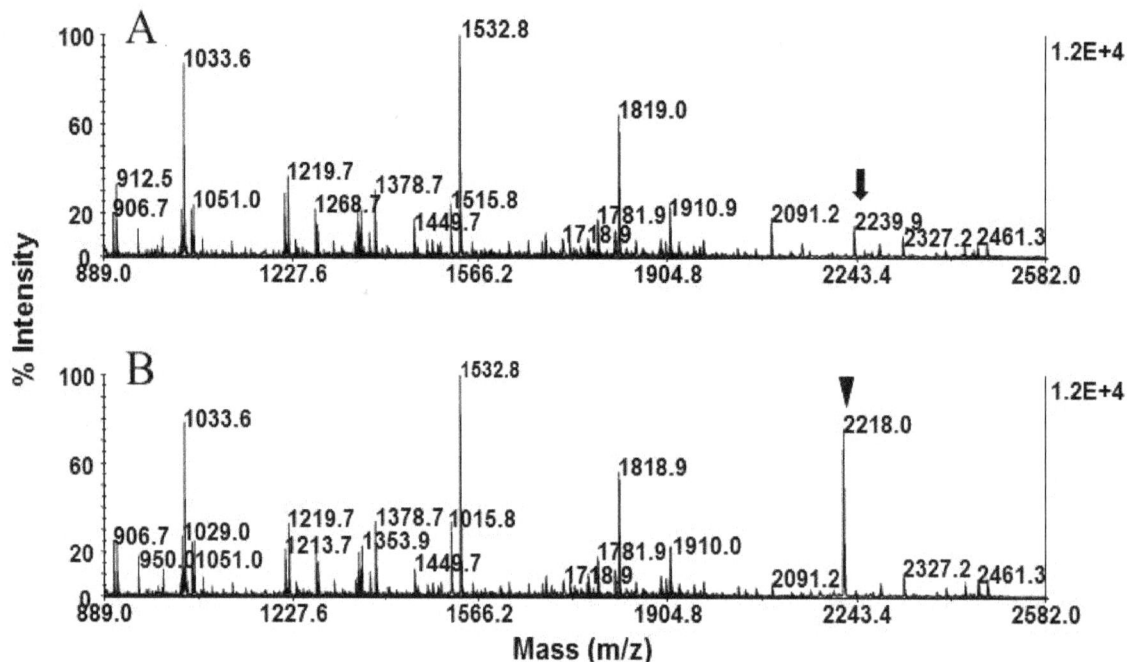

Figure 6: Phosphopeptide identification in proteolytic digests of α-catenin immunoprecipitated from EGF-stimulated A431 cells. Tryptic in-gel digests of α-catenin (M_r 99.8 kDa; pI 5.95), derived from 20 pmoles of protein loaded onto the gels were bound to ZipTipC18 pipette tips and subjected to β-elimination with concurrent Michael addition for 1h at 37 °C. One-tenths of the eluates were applied to the target. Experiment was in duplicate. MALDI-TOF spectra of (A) untreated tryptic digest; (B) after β-elimination with concurrent Michael addition. Arrow and arrowhead denote the phosphopeptide at m/z 2239.0 and its thiol adduct at m/z 2218.0, respectively. Using the autolytic tryptic fragment at m/z 906.7 as internal standard, a 3.6-fold signal enhancement was assessed for the native species recognized by the diagnostic mass signature of 21 Da as a monophosphorylated species. In-silico analysis revealed the corresponding tryptic fragment TPEELDDSDFETEDFDVR spanning residue 634 to 651 containing three kinase targets. Since conversion of phosphothreonine is markedly disfavored under the described, mild reaction conditions, serine 641was tentatively assigned as the site of phosphorylation (Byford, 1999). This differential reactivity-based phosphorylation site assignment was confirmed by MALDI-TOF/TOF MS/MS.

4.6.3   Limitations of the Solid-Phase Approach for Phosphopeptide Detection in Complex Mixture

We recognize that highly complex peptide mixtures with phosphopeptides present at substoichiometrically levels (<10%) can be difficult to analyze by this method because of the signal suppression effect that may compromise the mass spectral detection of the species of interest. Phosphopeptide enrichment on TiO_2 supports, preceding the reactions, would address this challenge by reducing the abundant, undesired background. However, this procedure has been shown to poorly enrich for phosphopeptides from basophilic kinase substrates, thereby excluding this class of functionally relevant phosphopeptides from analysis (Klemm et al., 2006). Fractionation of the digest before and after derivatization by nano-flow reversed phase chromatography coupled with on-target fraction collection using an automated eluent/matrix dispensing device should thus offer a preferred means to alleviate the signal suppression problem. In pre

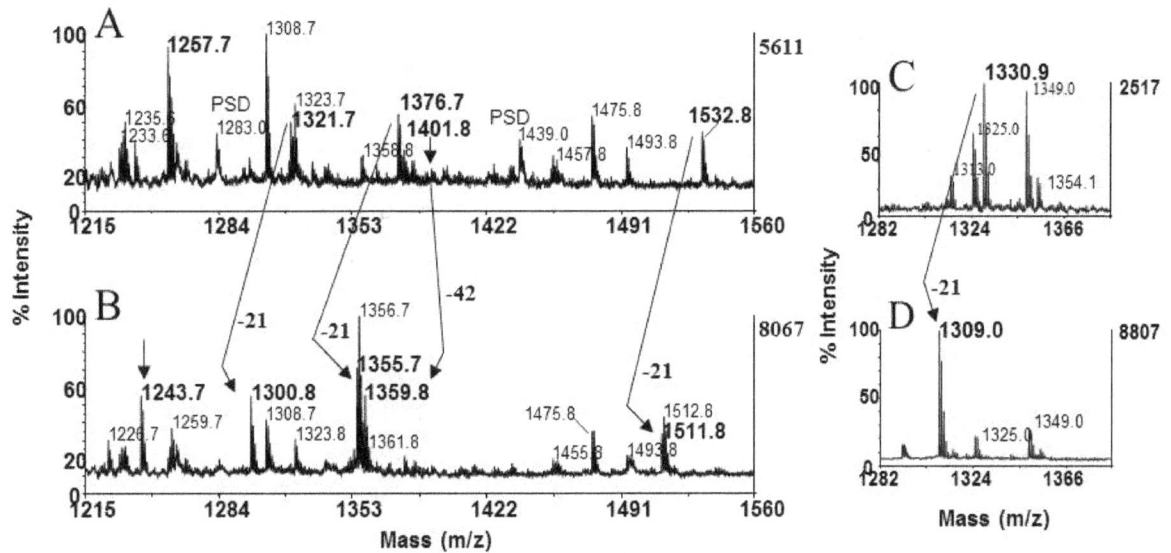

Figure 7: Phosphopeptide identification in proteolytic digests of Maf1. Tryptic and peptic in-gel digests of Maf1 (M_r 44.7 kDa; pI 5.15), derived from 15 pmoles of protein loaded onto the gels were bound to ZipTipC18 pipette tips and subjected to β-elimination with concurrent Michael addition under the conditions described in Fig. 2. Experiments were in duplicate. Expanded MALDI-TOF spectra of one-tenths of the eluates of (A) untreated tryptic digest; (B) after derivatization; (C) untreated peptic digest; (D) after derivatization. Cross arrows indicate fragments recognized as phosphorylated by the characteristic mass shift of 21 Da per phosphoamino acid. Monophosphorylated tryptic peptides identified correspond to RR**pS**SSSSISSFK at m/z 1321.7, RD**pS**NSFWEQK at m/z 1376.7 and RD**pS**NSFWEQKR at m/z 1532.8. The doubly phosphorylated peptide corresponds to RR**p-SpS**SSSISSFK at theoretical m/z 1401.8 marked by arrow. Note that this peptide was detectable solely as its thiol adduct at m/z 1359.8. The monophosphorylated peptic peptide at m/z 1330.9 corresponds to WEQKRR**IpSF**. Phosphorylated residues are indicated in bold with novel sites highlighted in red. The peptide identified as a carbamidomethylated species by the unique mass shift of 14 Da corresponds to VAYLYLI**Cam**SR at m/z 1257.7. The thiol adduct is marked by arrow. Cam denotes carbamidomethylated cysteinyl residue. PSD denoted post source decay products.

liminary experiments, we begun to explore the potential of this technique with model systems, and found that low-level synthetic phosphopeptides spiked into abundant backgrounds of non-phosphorylated peptides could be readily detected in the MALDI-TOF spectra of the collected fractions. We note that this technique is especially attractive since the LC-separation and MS analyses are decoupled and each step can be separately optimized. In addition, the predominant formation of singly charged ions in MALDI alleviates in isotope-coded proteomics studies the assignment of isotopomer (Chenau *et al.*, 2008).

Furthermore, we have been exploring the solid-phase derivatization platform in an effort to render phosphopeptides amenable to purification by covalent chromatography (McLachlin & Chait, 2003). In this strategy, all amino groups in the digest are blocked by acetylation prior to β-elimination/Michael addition making the amino group of S-2-aminoethylcysteine/β-S-2-aminoethylcysteine the sole target for subsequent N-thiolation. Pilot experiments with low level amounts of a model phosphopeptide spiked into a tryptic digest of HSA showed that the analyte could be selectively retrieved from the affinity support. The isolates by virtue of the nucleophilic substitution precluding neutral loss of phosphate proved highly suitable for phosphorylation site determination by CID. Application of this enrichment strategy in a scaled-up solid-phase format to fractionated proteome digests (Villen & Gygi, 2008; Dephoure & Gygi, 2011) has the potential to serve as a viable means to condition complex proteolytic mixtures derived from fractionated cell lysates for LC-MS/MS-based large-scale phosphoproteome profiling. We note here that covalent affinity enrichment of phosphopeptides from complex mixtures has been recently demonstrated using the well-known phosphoramidate chemistry (PAC) (Bodenmiller *et al.*, 2007). However, the method regenerates the original phosphopeptides rendering site mapping subject to ambiguity due to phosphate neutral loss under the conditions of CID.

4.7   Chemistry Side Reactions

Alkali-catalyzed peptide bond hydrolysis is of concern since it could introduce unwanted complexity into the spectra confounding phosphopeptide identification. This side reaction has been studied in some detail and the amide bonds in model peptides most susceptible at pH 12.6 were identified as those linking glycine or serine N-terminally to glycine (Noll *et al.*, 1974). As assessed by MALDI-TOF, UOM9, protein kinase C (PKC) substrate-3 phosphopeptide KRP**pS**QRH**GS**KY amide, containing this sequence feature, remained intact when exposed to elimination base (pH 12.7) or the elimination/addition reagent mixture (pH 12.1) for 1 h at 37°C or 55°C (data not illustrated). To examine a wide range of peptides, we prepared a tryptic digest from an equimolar mixture of human serum albumin, bovine carbonic anhydrase, bovine lactoglobulin and bovine myoglobin. Inspection of the resultant complex tryptic mass maps generated from the untreated sample and after the incubations revealed only minor ion intensity changes in the spectral profiles indicating that the peptides were unaffected by the chemical treatment (data not shown). It has been reported that under base-catalyzed conditions a small fraction (1.7%) of serine or threonine may convert to dehydro-derivatives by elimination of water which can react with nucleophiles (McLachlin & Chait, 2003). Although our reaction conditions were similar to those reported, we have not observed this side reaction in our dataset. However, should this reaction occur, it would not confound the phosphopeptide identification as the derivatization results in net mass shift of 59 Da arising from the loss of water from the native peptide and concurrent incorporation of the nucleophile (M_r 77 Da). Derivatization of carbamidomethylated cysteinyl-peptides imparts a mass shift of 14 Da to the native species dictated by the nominal mass of the eliminated moiety (91 Da) whereas a mass shift of 144 Da is observed after derivatization of O-linked *β-N*-glucosamine (OGlcNAc)-modified peptides which β-eliminate with a mass loss of 220Da (Rusnak *et al.*, 2002). Consequently, these unique mass signatures can be exploited to distinguish these peptides from each other in a mixture (see Figure 1A). Ions corresponding to water addition across the double bond of the β-eliminated residues which would regenerate the hydroxyl amino acid residues were not observed in the spectra. This potential side reaction, known to proceed at slow reaction rate, is effectively arrested by the endogenous nucleophile (Thompson *et al.,* 2003).

4.8   Identification of Phosphopeptides in Proteolytic Digests from Real-Life Protein Samples

4.8.1   Application to α-Catenin Immunoprecipitated from Carcinoma Cells

As reported recently, EGF stimulation of A431 human epidermoid carcinoma cells results in disruption of the α-catenin/β-catenin complex, which subsequently promotes β-catenin transactivation (Ji *et al.*, 2009). In the early stage of this study we examined whether dissociation of α-catenin from β-catenin involves a possible unknown posttranslational modification on α-catenin. To this purpose, we applied our method to in-gel tryptic digests of α-catenin immunoprecipitated from EGF-stimulated A431 cells. In the experiments, digest immobilized on ZipTip$_{C18}$ pipette tips was subjected to β-elimination with concurrent Michael addition at 37 °C for 1 h, and analyzed by MALDI-TOF (Figure 6A, B). These reactions resulted in a prominent signal at m/z 2218.0 representing the Michael addition product. The unique mass signatures of 21 Da, accompanying the concurrent reactions identified the presence of a single phosphoamino acid in a peptide recognized at *m/z* 2239.0 in its native form, therefore providing evidence of the nature of the post-translational modification. The phosphopeptide peptide mass matched to a tryptic fragment within the known protein sequence spanning residues 634-651 (**T**PEELDD**S**DFE**T**EDFDVR) containing the phosphorylatable serine 641, threonine 634 and threonine 645. Since this peptide was effectively derivatized under mild reaction condition known to selectively effect phosphoseryl conversion, serine 641 was assigned as the most likely kinase target (Byford, 1991). The assignment was confirmed by MALDI-TOF MS/MS and LC-MS/MS analysis (Ji et al., 2009). Subsequent biochemical studies revealed casein kinase α-subunit II (CK2$_α$) as the protein kinase involved in phosphorylation of α-catenin at serine 641 and that this phosphorylation event disrupts the α-catenin/β-catenin complex and consequently promotes β-catenin transactivation

4.8.2   Application to Recombinant Yeast Maf1

We next applied the chemical strategy to preparations of recombinant yeast Maf1 that had been expressed in *E. coli* under native conditions and phosphorylated *in vitro* by recombinant murine PKA. The Maf1 amino acid sequence contains six PKA recognition motifs that render the protein susceptible to modification at serine 90, 101, 177, 178, 209 and 210 (Moir *et al.*, 2006). Of these, serine 90, 177, 209 and 210 have been previously assigned as phosphorylated by LC-MS/MS during large scale phosphoproteome mapping of *Saccharomyces cerevisiae* (Chi *et al.*, 2007; Li *et al.*, 2007; Albuquerque *et al.*, 2008). In our experiments, in-gel tryptic or peptic digests of Maf1 bound to ZipTip$_{C18}$ pipette tips were subjected to β-elimination with concurrent Michael addition, and subsequently analyzed by MALDI-TOF along with untreated digests as a control (Figure 7). This reaction results in a mass shift of 21 Da per phosphoamino acid and was accompanied by a moderate signal enhancement of the native peptides. Accordingly, the tryptic peptides at *m/z* 1321.7, *m/z* 1376.7 and *m/z* 1532.8 in Figure 7A and the peptic peptide at *m/z* 1330.0 (Figure 7C) were identified as monophosphorylated species. Of these, the peptic peptide at *m/z* 1330.0 could be mass matched by data base search to the sequence WEQKRRI**pSF** (residues 94-102) and hence the sole serine in position 101 was assigned as a novel site of phosphorylation. This result highlights the potential of the method to locate sites of phosphorylation in known protein sequences solely on the basis of peptide mass measurement alone. The tryptic peptide at *m/z* 1376.7 mass matched to a pair of isobaric fragments spanning residues 88 to 97 or residues 89-98. MALDI-TOF/TOF analysis of this peptide selected the former sequence as produced by the enzyme corresponding to RD**pS**NSFWEQK and unambiguously assigned serine 90 as the site of phosphorylation (data not shown). Serine 90 has been identified as a modification site in a large scale phosphoproteome profiling study of *Saccharomyces cerevisiae* (Albuquerque *et al.*, 2008). The presence of the N-terminal arginine in this peptide was expected because of the neighboring aspartic acid which is known to inhibit trypsin cleavage.

As illustrated in Figure 7A and B, the tryptic peptide at *m/z* 1359.8 recognized as a doubly phosphorylated species was detectable solely as the Michael addition product in contrast to its monophosphorylated counterpart at *m/z* 1321.7. This fragment mass matched to RR**pSpS**SSISSFK (residues 175 to 185), aligns with the corresponding larger fragment NDERIRRR**pS**SSSISSFK (residues 169-185) that had been sequenced earlier to localize serine 177 as the site of modification (Chi *et al.*, 2007). Assignment of serine 178 as a likely novel site of phosphorylation relies on the presence of PKA recognition motifs overlapping each other and the fact that recombinant PKA was employed for *in vitro* phosphorylation of Maf1. As noted above, the doubly phosphorylated peptide was observed only after derivatization highlighting the benefit of the method to reveal this class of peptides for subsequent structural characterization. Charge neutralization by intra-peptide salt bridge formation between the oppositely charged proximal residues can be invoked as the most likely cause to account for the native peptide's ionization inefficiency (Hider *et al.*, 1985).We note that phosphorylation at adjacent serines, induced by PKA as well as by other members of the AGC kinase family (e.g. ribosomal protein S6 kinase) has been shown to play a pivotal role in modulation of a variety physiological processes such as neuronal excitability and cardiac muscle contractility (McDonald *et al.*, 1998; Zhang *et al.*, 1995). A potential physiological significance of phosphorylation at the proximal serine residues 177 and 178 in Maf1 in context with this protein's inhibitory interaction with RNA polymerase III warrants future investigation (Moir *et al.*, 2006).

As further illustrated in Figure 7, the peptide at *m/z* 1257.7 was identified as a carboxamidomethylated species by the characteristic mass shift of 14 Da arising from the β-elimination-induced mass loss of -91 Da and concurrent addition of the 2-aminoethanethiol (M_r 77 Da), and as such, is clearly distinguishable from the phosphopeptide counterparts (See Figure 1A). This fragment mass matched to VAYLYLICSR (residues 333 to 342) in the known protein sequence. The result was in contrast with earlier reports (Byford, 1999; Simpson *et al.*, 1972).

4.9   Phosphorylation Site Mapping by MALDI TOF-TOF MS/MS Analysis

We next explored the potential of the on-resin protocol for phosphorylation site mapping. In the experiments, model peptides (2 pmoles) and their Michael addition products were subjected to MALDI-tandem sequence analysis. Representative data obtained from the tryptic phosphoseryl peptide P2 (SHNSALY**p**-**S**QVQK, *m/z* 1441.8) are illustrated in Figure 8. The MALDI-MS/MS spectrum of the underivatized species showed a predominant ion at m/z 1344.0 formed by neutral loss of phosphate as the primary mode of fragmentation (Figure 8A).The product spectrum is complicated by the presence of diverse, low intensity ions and was thus of limited informative value rendering phosphorylation site determination subject to ambiguity. In contrast, the thiol adduct at *m/z* 1420.8 fragmented to a noticeably higher extent (Figure 8B). This is expected since the nucleophilic substitution precludes neutral loss as major fragmentation pathway (Thompson *et al.*, 2003; Nika *et al.*, 2012). As exemplified by the product ion spectrum of the thiol adduct, a nearly uninterrupted b and y ion series was produced in high abundance including y5 and b8 representing the first y and b ions that retain the modification as well as y4 and b7 that are contiguous to the modification. The location of the modification could be readily identified by its unique residue mass (146 Da) and hence serine in position 7 as the site of phosphorylation. It is noteworthy that the S-2-aminoethyl group specifying the site of phosphorylation remained stable upon CID aiding facile MS/MS data interpretation. Similarly, β-elimination with concurrent Michael addition of a tryptic digest of ovalbumin using 2-aminoethanethiol provided significantly more sequence information from the tagged phosphopeptide at *m/z* 2067.8 than from its unmodified counterpart. While both spectra shared y15 as a prominent ion, the product ions y16, y17, y18 and y19 that retained the modification, and thus afforded unambiguous phosphorylation site assignment of serine 345 were only observed after derivatization (data not shown). The data show that our derivatization protocol provides material highly suitable for unambiguous phosphorylation site determination. Collectively, the solid-phase sample preparation method addresses the need for high-confidence phosphoprotein characterization which can be a challenging task using mass spectrometric-based approaches alone.

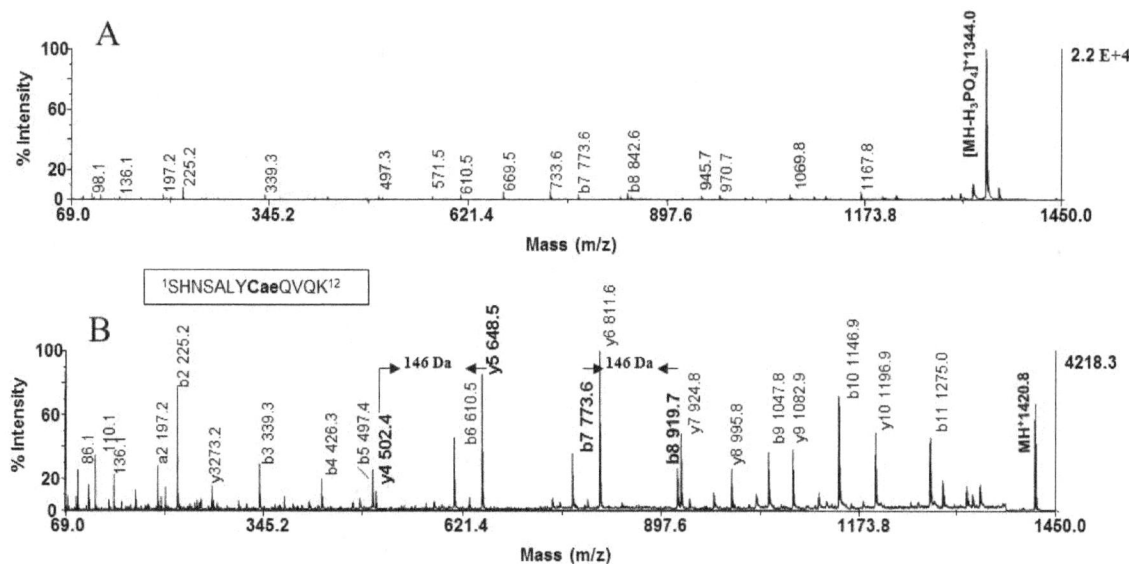

Figure 8: Phosphorylation site mapping by MALDI-tandem MS. The model peptide P2 (SHNSALY**pS**QVQK, *m/z* 1441.8) adsorbed on ZipTip$_{C18}$ pipette tips was subjected to β-elimination with concurrent Michael addition as described in Figure 2. MALDI-TOF/TOF spectra of (A) unmodified peptide; (B) S-2-aminoethylcysteine derivative. Note that the nucleophilic substitution markedly increased peptide backbone fragmentation yielding a nearly uninterrupted b and y-type ion series and discriminates the site of phosphorylation as the unique residue mass of 146 Da. The product ions retaining this unique mass signature are indicated in bold as are those which are contiguous to the modification. The presence of these ion pairs afforded unambiguous assignment of serine in position 7 as the site of phosphorylation. Cae denotes 2-aminoethylcysteine.

4.10   Sample Preparation for Chemoenzymatic Phosphosite Determination

In this approach, the 2-aminoethyl/β-2-aminoethyl cysteine residue incorporated into digests since mimicking a lysine residue is C-terminally cleaved by lysyl endopeptidase (Lys-C). The MALDI-mass map is then interrogated for the phosphorylation site-specific cleavage products whose masses can be predicted from the known protein sequence. To confine the proteolysis to the lysine analog, internal lysine residues that may occur in proteolytic fragments need to be blocked, and guanidination or N-acetylation prior to the nucleophilic phosphate substitution are most commonly employed for this purpose (Rusnak *et al.*, 2002; Knight *et al,* 2003). In these in-solution serial derivatization procedures, the derivatives were intermittently purified by micro dialysis or reversed-phase chromatography followed by Speed concentration of the desalted samples, transfer manipulations well-known to incur substantial, adsorptive sample loss (Speicher *et al.*, 2000). In our solid-phase adaptation of this serial reaction scheme described below, the sample handling of the immobilized analyte is minimal since confined to reagent exchanges in situ, thereby abrogating the need for intermittent sample purification.

4.10.1   Evaluation of the Solid-Phase Sample Preparation Method

To evaluate the efficiency of the N-acetylation reaction on the solid-phase support, the synthetic fragment of cholecystokinin phosphorylated at serine (IKNLQ**pS**LDPSH, *m/z* 1331.4) containing an internal lysine was to bound to ZipTip$_{C18}$ pipette tips, exposed to a phosphate-buffered 20 mM sulfo-NHS acetate solution (pH 8.0) for 20 min at 55 °C, and subsequently subjected to β-elimination with concurrent Michael addition under the conditions as described in Figure 2. The two-step serial derivatization procedure was halted by a solvent wash prior to MALDI-TOF of the final reaction products. The MALDI-TOF spectra prepared from this sample revealed that the acylation of the primary and ε-amino group in this peptides and the subsequent thiol adduct formation proceeded with high efficiency and that the reactions were accompanied by expected net mass addition of 63 Da (Figure 9 A and B). Additional model peptides examined with this method were P2 (SHNSALY**pS**QVQK, m/z 1441.5), the DAM1 phosphopeptides (SFVLNPTNIGM**pS**KSSQGHVTK, m/z 2312.6) and the MARCKS phosphopeptide (KKKKKRF-**pS**FKK**pS**FKLSGF**pS**FKKNKK, m/z 3321.7. As semiquantitatively assessed by MALDI-MS, the peptides were highly amenable to serial derivatization (data not illustrated). In separate experiments, the acetylation products of the model peptides were examined. The spectra showed that the peptides were impervious to *O*-acylation with the exception of the model peptide P2, which became fully *O*-acylated at its internal serine in position 4 because of the proximity of histidine, known to promote the NHS-ester reaction (Miller *et al.*, 1997). This side-reaction was rapidly reversed by ester bond hydrolysis under the basic condition of the β-elimination/Michael addition yielding the desired, doubly N-acetylated thiol adduct at m/z 1504.9 (data not shown). If the solid-phase N-acetylation were to be used as a selective amine-labeling method, the side-reaction can be readily reversed *in situ* via ester bond hydrolysis by a brief hydroxylamine treatment (Miller *et al.*, 1997). In our solid-phase adaptation of this dual reaction scheme, the acetylation reaction is terminated by a solvent wash. The ZipTips are then loaded with the alkaline 2% hydroxyl amine solution, reacted for 15 min at 37 °C, desalted and eluted. As applied to the model peptide P2, MALDI-MS revealed the desired doubly N-acetylated species at m/z 1525.6 as essentially the sole ion in the spectrum (data not shown). As an application, the method provides for a viable tool to make lysine-rich proteolytic fragments amenable to sequence determination by CID, and to differentiate this residue from isobaric glutamine (Biemann, 1990).

Phosphopeptides present in complex digest at substoichiometrically level (<10%) can be difficult to analyze with the chemoenzymatic approach because of the signal suppression effect that may compromise the mass spectral detection of the phosphospecific fragments. Fractionation of the proteolytic mixture after Lys-C digestion by nano-flow reversed phase chromatography coupled with on-target eluent/matrix dispensing, is anticipated to provide a means to alleviate this problem. Since N-acetylation blocks both α-and ε-amino groups, the Lys-C cleavage product released immediately C-terminal to the substituted phosphate becomes the sole peptide in the digest bearing a free amino group. Consequently, chemical sequencing by Edman degradation can be exploited to determine the site of phosphorylation in unfractionated, complex protein digests (Rusnak *et al.*, 2002) (see Figure 9B, inset). In this strategy, the phosphorylation site is ascertained by alignment of the Edman sequence tag with the known protein sequence. Sorting of Edman sequence readouts derived from peptides mixtures has been demonstrated using algorithms developed for this task, thus facilitating localization of individual phosphorylation sites separated from each other along the polypeptide chain (Henzel *et al*, 1999). Notably, Edman degradation inherently provides unambiguous sequence data. However, at least 1 pmoles of peptide is typically needed to obtain readily interpretable mid femto-mole level sequence data, and thus confining the method's capability to analyze substoichiometric phosphorylation events to proportionally higher sample levels.

Edman degradation coupled with accelerator mass spectrometry has been shown to generate sequence readouts of ten contiguous amino acid residues with as little as 1.8 fmoles of *in vitro* ^{14}C-labeled glutathione S-transferase (M_r 22.8 kDa) consumed for analysis. At sample loads of 100- 450 amoles, a

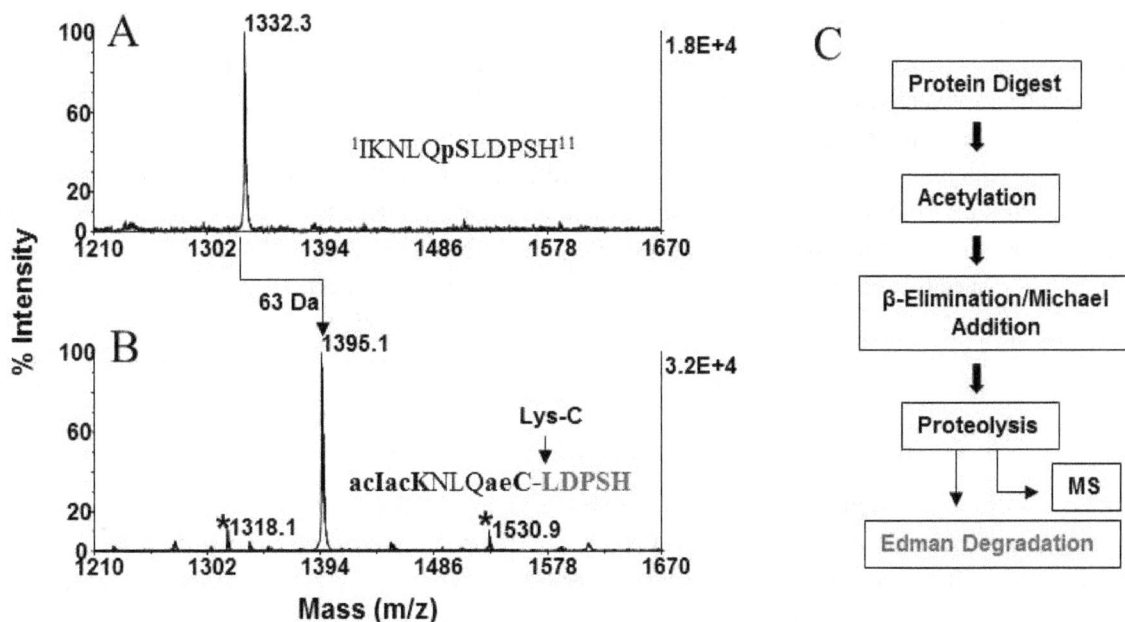

Figure 9: Preparation of substrates for phosphorylation site determination by chemical targeted proteolysis. The phosphorylated cholecystokinin fragment IKNLQpSLDPSH (2 pmoles) bound to ZipTipμ-C18 pipette tips was subjected to on-column N-acetylation for 20 min at 55 °C and subsequently to concurrent β-elimination with Michael addition as described in Figure 2. MALDI-TOF spectra of (A) unmodified peptide; (B) after N-acetylation and subsequent β-elimination with concurrent Michael addition. Cross arrow indicates the characteristic net mass addition 63 Da. Asterisks denote peptide synthesis by-products' adducts. Inset in B shows the sequence of the peptide's derivative with the Lys-C sensitive cleavage point indicated by arrow. aeC denotes 2-aminoethylcysteine residue, the lysine structural analog. ac denotes acetyl group. The Lys-C cleavage product bearing the free amino group is highlighted in red. Note that the initial N-acetylation step makes this peptide the sole target for Edman degradation. (C) schematic representation of the chemoenzymatic solid-phase workflow for post-reaction proteolysis and subsequent phosphorylation site determination by mass spectrometry and Edman degradation. Phosphorylation site determination relies on in silico mass matching of the liberated fragment and/ or by alignment of the Edman sequencing tag to the known protein sequence.

sequence of five contiguous amino acid residues could be determined with a limit of absolute quantification of 30 amole of identified amino acid residue (Miyashita *et al.*, 2001). In order to establish the general utility of this technique, further work is needed to adapt the chemical degradation to extrinsic ^{14}C-labeling. A miniaturized protein sequencer platform, accelerated Edman reaction schemes and high-throughput reversed-phase PTH separation protocols that would be highly suitable to this purpose had been devised more than a decade ago (Calaycay *et al.*, 1991; Nika *et al.*, 1992; Hihara, 1993). We believe that chemical sequencing in conjunction with accelerator mass spectrometry holds the promise to exploit in the near future the full potential of the chemoenzymatic strategy and to furnish unambiguous *de novo* sequence information from low abundance proteins that are not present in the public data bases.

Collectively, the results validate the utility of the on-resin sequential strategy to prepare phospho-protein digests for chemoenzymatic phosphorylation site determination by mass analysis and/or Edman degradation. Importantly, the completeness of the individual reaction steps afforded by the solid-phase approach and the ability of this sample handling format to carry the analyte through the sequential reaction scheme with minimal sample loss as demonstrated by the data fully meets the requirements for a serial chemical method to be useful for proteomics studies. Figure 9C depicts the schematic representation of the chemo enzymatic solid-phase workflow. We note here that the initial N-acetylation step can be optionally replaced by guanidination. However, the selectivity for Edman degradation is compromised by this method since N-terminal amino groups are unaffected by guanidination.

5   Conclusions

A method for β-elimination and β-elimination with concurrent Michael addition on C18 reversed phase supports has been developed using a panel of model phosphopeptides and protein digests to demonstrate the feasibility of the approach. The approach combines simplicity of operation with improved throughput and completeness of derivatization using equipment readily available in most biological laboratories. The reaction conditions proved highly compatible with the integrity of the samples. The protocol facilitates high-sensitivity mass spectrometric detection of phosphorylated peptides in unfractionated protein digests and enables facile assignment of phosphorylated residues from enhanced MS/MS sequencing information. The 2-aminoethyl group specifying the site of phosphorylation remained stable upon CID aiding MS/MS data interpretation Although MALDI-TOF tandem MS was employed in this study for phosphorylation site determination, ZipTip$_{C18}$ pipette tips or ZipTip$_{u-C18}$ pipette tips can be readily interfaced with nano spray mass spectrometry techniques or the eluates can be optionally analyzed by LC-MS/MS. As applied to α-catenin immunoprecipitated from EGF-stimulated A431 cells, the method provided evidence of a phosphorylation event localized at serine 641. As applied to Maf1, the method afforded conclusive identification of peptides as phosphorylated species containing known and novel PKA targets. Two novel phosphorylation sites could be assigned based on *in silico* data base search alone. The solid-phase derivatization strategy was readily expanded to prepare samples for phosphorylation site determination by chemical targeted proteolysis. The sample handling format proved in this and in a separate but unrelated application highly advantageous to carry the analyte at minimal sample loss through the sequential reactions, and is anticipated to accommodate additional chemistries for mass spectrometry-based protein structural characterization The solid phase method is its current configuration provides a simple and effective tool to prepare isolated proteins for high-fidelity phosphorylation site determination, which can be a challenging task using mass spectrometric-based approaches alone. The solid-phase sample handling format holds promise to serve as a platform for phosphopeptide affinity enrichment from complex protein digests with a future view to employ this technique as integral component for large-scale phosphoproteome profiling by tandem LC-MS/MS mass spectrometry.

Acknowledgments

This work was funded by NIH grant # R33CA101150 to R.H.A, NIH grant # GM427228 to I.M.W. and NCI grant # CA16672 to Dr. John Mendelsohn. The authors thank the U.T.-M.D. Anderson Cancer Center and the Einstein College for Medicine for its generous support, the U.T.-M.D. Anderson Proteomics Facility, Mr. Edward Nieves for helpful discussions and Ms. Junko Hihara for valuable editorial assistance in preparing the manuscript.

References

Annan, R. S., & Carr, S.A. (1996). Phosphopeptide analysis by matrix-assisted laser desorption time-of-flight mass spectrometry. Anal Chem, 68, 3413-3421.

Annan, R.S, Huddleston, M.J, Verma, R., Deshaies, R.J, & Carr S.A. (2001). A multidimensional electrospray MS-based approach to phosphopeptide mapping. Anal Chem, 73, 393-404.

Ahn, Y.H, Ji, E.S, Cho, K., & Yoo. J.S. (2007). Arginine-mimic labeling with guanidinoethanethiol to increase mass sensitivity of lysine-terminated phosphopeptides by matrix-assisted laser desorption/ionization time-of-flight mass spectrometry. Rapid Commun Mass Spectrom, 21, 2204-2210.

Albuquerque, C.P., Smolka, M.B., Payne, S.H., Bafna, V., Eng, J., & Zhou, H. (2008). A multidimensional chromatography technology for in-depth phosphoproteome analysis. Mol Cell Proteomics, 7, 1389-1396.

Biemann, K. (1990). Sequencing of peptides by tandem mass spectrometry and high-energy collision-induced dissociation. Methods Enzymol, 193, 455-479.

Byford, M.F. (1991). Rapid and selective modification of phosphoserine residues catalysed by Ba^{+2} ions for their detection during peptide micro sequencing. Biochem J, 280, 261-265.

Baumgart, S., Lindner, Y., Kuhne, R., Oberemm, A., Wenschu, H., & Krause, E. (2004). The contributions of specific amino acid side chains to signal intensities of peptides in matrix-assisted laser desorption/ionization mass spectrometry. Rapid Commun Mass Spectrom, 18, 863-868.

Beausoleil, S.A, Jedrychowki, M., Schwartz, D., Elias, J.E., Villen, J., Li, J., Cohn, L.C., & Gygi, S.P. (2004). Large-scale characterization of Hela cell nuclear phosphoproteins. Proc Natl Acad Sci USA, 101, 12130-12135.

Bodenmiller, B., Mueller, L.N., Pedrioli, P.G., Plieger, D., Junger, M.A., Eng, J.K., & Tao, W.A. (2007). An integrated chemical, mass spectrometric and computational strategy for phosphoproteomics: application to Drosophila melanogaster Kc167 cells. Mol Biosyst 3, 275-286.

Calaycay, J., Rusnak, M., & Shively, J.E. (1991). Microsequence analysis of peptides and proteins. An improved, compact, automated instrument. Anal Biochem, 192, 23-31.

Conrotto, P., & Hellman, U. (2005). Sulfonation chemistry as a powerful tool for MALDI TOF/TOF de novo sequencing and posttranslational modification analysis. J Biomol Tech, 16, 441-452.

Cindric, M., Cepo, T., Skrlin, A., Vuletin, M., & Bindila, L. (2006). Accelerated on-column lysine derivatization and cysteine methylation by imidazole reaction in a deuterated environment for enhanced product ion analysis. Rapid Commun Mass Spectrom, 20, 694-702.

Chi, A., Huttenhower, C., Geer, L.Y., Coon, J.J., Syka, J.E., Bai, D.L., Shabanowitz, J., Burke, D.J., Troyanskaya, O.G., & Hunt, D.F. (2007). Analysis of phosphorylation sites on proteins from Saccharomyces cerevisiae by electron transfer dissociation (ETD) mass spectrometry. Proc Natl Acad Sci USA, 104, 2193-2198.

Chenau, J., Michelland, S., Sidibe, J., & Seve, M. (2008). Peptide OFFGEL electrophoresis: a suitable pre-analytical step for complex eukaryotic samples fractionation compatible with quantitative iTRAQ labeling. Proteome Sci 6, 1-8.

Chen, M., Su, X., Yang, J., Jenkins, C.M., Cedars, A.M., & Gross, R.W. (2010). Facile identification and quantitation of protein phosphorylation via beta-elimination and Michael addition with natural and stable isotope labeled thiocholine. Anal Chem, 82, 163-171.

Docette, A., Craft, D., & Li, L. (2003). Mass spectrometric study of the effects on hydrophobic surface chemistry and morphology on digestion of surface-bound protein. J Am Soc Mass Spectrom 14, 203-214.

Dephoure, N., & Gygi, S.P. (2011). A solid phase extraction-based platform for rapid phosphoproteomic analysis. Methods, 54, 379-386.

Farmar, J.G., Nika, H., Che, F-Y., Weiss, L., & Hogue Angeletti, R. (2009). IVICAT for masses: an improved technique for permethylation of peptides. J Biomol, 20, 285-292.

Hider, R.C., Ragnarsson, U., & Zetterquist O. (1958). The role of phosphate group for the structure of phosphopeptide products of adenosine 3', 5'-cyclic mono phosphate-dependent protein kinase. Biochem J, 229, 485-489.

Hihara, J. (1993). Approaches to separation of PTH-TRP/DPU using accelerated PTH-elution gradients. 7th Symposium of the Protein Society, San Diego, CA, Applied Biosystems poster compilation, pp. 15-20.

Helmbrecht, K., Zeise, F., & Rensing, L. (2000). Chaperones in cell cycle regulation and mitotic signal transduction: a review. Cell Proliferation, 33, 341-356.

Henzel, W., Tropea, J., & Dupont, D. (1999). Protein identification using 20-minute Edman cycles and sequence mixture analysis. Anal Biochem, 267, 148-160.

Jaffe, H., Veeranna, & Harish, C.P. (1998). Characterization of serine and threonine phosphorylation in β-elimination/ethanethiol addition-modified proteins by electrospray tandem mass spectrometry and database searching. Biochemistry, 37, 16211-16224.

Johnson, M.E., & Carpenter, T.S. (2005). The use of solid-phase supports for derivatization in chromatography and spectroscopy. Applied Spectroscopy Reviews, 40, 391-412.

Ji, H., Wang, J., Nika, H., Hawke, D., Keezer, S., Ge, Q., Fang, B., Fang, X., Fang, D., Lichtfield, D.W., Aldape, K., & Lu, Z. (2009). EGF-induced ERK activation promotes CK2-mediated disassociation of α-catenin from β-catenin and transactivation of β-catenin. Mol Cell, 36, 547-559.

Kirkland, J.J., van Straten, M.A., & Claessens, H.A. (1995). High pH mobile phase effects on silica-based reversed-phase high-performance liquid chromatography. J Chromatog A, 691, 3-19.

Katayama, H., Nagasu, .T, & Oda, Y. (2001). Improvement of in-gel digestion protocol for peptide mass fingerprinting by matrix-assisted laser desorption/ionization time-of-flight mass spectrometry. Rapid Commun Mass Spectrom, 5, 1416-1421.

Katayama, H., Tabata, T., Ishihama, Y., Sato, T., Oda, Y., & Nagasu, T. (2004). Efficient in-gel digestion procedure using 5-cyclohexyl-1-pentyl-β-D-maltoside as an additive for gel-based membrane proteomics. Rapid Commun Mass Spectrom, 18, 2388-2394.

Knight, Z.A, Schilling, B., Row, R.H., Kenski, D.M, Gibson, B.W., & Shokat, K.M. (2003). Phosphospecific proteolysis for mapping sites of protein phosphorylation. Nat Biotech, 21, 1047-1054.

Klemm, C., Otto, S., Wolf, C., Haseloff, R.F., Beyermann, M., & Krause, E. (2006). Evaluation of the titanium dioxide approach for MS analysis of phosphopeptides. J Mass Spectrom, 41, 1623-1632.

Liao, P.C., Leykam, J., Andrews, P.C., Gage, D.A., & Allison, J. (1994). An approach to locate phosphorylation sites in a phosphoprotein: mass mapping by combining specific enzymatic degradation with matrix-assisted laser desorption/ionization mass spectrometry. Anal Biochem, 219, 9-20.

Larsen, M.R., Sorensen, G.L., Fey, S.J., Larsen, P.M., & Roepstorff, P. (2001). Phospho-proteomics: evaluation of the use of enzymatic de-phosphorylation and differential mass spectrometric peptide mass mapping for site specific phosphorylation assignment in proteins separated by gel electrophoresis. Proteomics, 1, 223-238.

Larsen, M.R., Thingholm, T.E., Jensen, O.N., Roepstorff, P., & Jorgensen, J.D. (2005). Highly selective enrichment of phosphorylated peptides from peptide mixtures using titanium dioxide micro columns. Mol Cell Proteomics, 4, 873-886.

Li, X., Gerber, S.A., Rudner, A.D., Beausoleil, S.A., Haas, W., Villen, J., Elias, J.E., & Gygi, S.P. (2007). Large-scale phosphorylation analysis of α-factor-arrested Saccharomyces cerevisiae. J Proteome Res, 6, 1190-1197.

Miller, B.T., Collins, T.J., Rogers, M.E., & Kurosky, A. (1997). Peptide biotinylation with amine-reactive esters: differential side chain reactivity. Peptides, 18, 1585-1595.

McDonald, B.J., Amato, A., Connolly, C.N., Benke, D., Modd, S.J., & Smart, T.G. (1998). Adjacent phosphorylation sites on GABA_A receptor β subunits determine regulation by cAMP-dependent protein kinase. Nat Neurosci, 1, 23-28.

Molloy, M.P., & Andrews, P.C. (2001). Phosphopeptide derivatization signatures to identify serine and threonine phosphorylated peptides by mass spectrometry. Anal Chem, 73, 5387-5394.

Miyashita, M., Presley, J.M., Buchholz, B.A., Lam, K.S., Lee, Y.M., Vogel, J.S., & Hammock, B.D. (2001). Attomole level protein sequencing by Edman degradation coupled with accelerator mass spectrometry. Proc Natl Acad Sci, 98, 4403-4408.

McLachlin, D.T., & Chait, B.T. (2003). Improved β-elimination-based affinity purification strategy for enrichment of phosphopeptides. Anal Chem 75, 6826-6836.

Moir, R.D, Lee, J.H, Haeusler, R.A, Desai, N., Engelke, D.R., & Willis, I.M. (2006). Protein kinase A regulates RNA polymerase III transcription through the nuclear localization of Maf1. Proc Natl Acad Sci USA, 103, 15044-15049.

Molina, H., Horn, D.M, Tang, N., Mathivanan, S., & Pandey, A. (2007). Global proteomic profiling of phosphopeptides using electron transfer dissociation tandem mass spectrometry. Proc Natl Acad Sci USA, 104, 2199-2204.

Noll, B.W., Jarboe C.J., & Hass, L.F. (1974). Kinetic studies on the alkali-catalyzed hydrolysis and epimerization of model alkyl and hydroxyalkyl di-and tripeptides. Biochemistry, 13, 5164-5169.

Nika, H., Tabanfar, S., & Mattaliano, R.J. (1992). An investigation of accelerated concepts using a modified 477A sequencer. 6th Symposium of the Protein Society, San Diego, CA, Abstr. M 96.

Nika, H., Hawke, D.H., & Kobayashi, R. (2004). Derivatization on reversed-phase supports for enhanced detection of phosphorylated peptides. 52nd ASMS Conf. on Mass Spectrometry & Allied Topics, Nashville, TN, Abstr ThPN 292.

Nika, H., Hawke, D.H, & Kobayashi, R. (2005). Derivatization on reversed phase supports for chemoenzymatic phosphorylation site determination. ABRF Biomolecular Technologies: Discovery to Hypothesis, Savannah, GA, Abstr. P75-T.

Nika, H., Lee, J.H., Willis, I.M., Angeletti, R.H, & Hawke, D.H. (2012). Phosphopeptide characterization by mass spectrometry using reversed-phase supports for solid-phase β-elimination/Michael addition. J Biomol Tech, 23, 2012-2302.

Posewitz, M.C, &Tempst, P. (1999). Immobilized gallium (III) affinity chromatography of phosphopeptides. Anal Chem, 71, 2883-2892.

Pavel, M., O'Donnel, P., Vassilovski, G., & Ashman, K. (2002). Automated, rapid solid-phase proteolytic cleavage and sample preparation for proteomics. J Biomol Tech, 13, 49-55.

Palmblad, M., & Vogel, J.S. (2005). Quantitation of binding, recovery and desalting efficiency of peptides and proteins in solid phase extraction micropipette tips. J Chromatogr. B, 814, 309-313.

Rosenfeld, J.M. (1999). Solid-phase analytical derivatization: enhancement of sensitivity and selectivity of analysis. J Chromatogr A, 843, 19-27.

Raijmakers, R., Berkers, C.R., de Jong, A., Ovaa, H., & Heck, A.J.R. (2008). Automated online sequential isotope labeling for protein quantitation applied to proteasome tissue-specific diversity. Mol Cell Proteomics, 7, 1755-1762.

Rusnak, F., Zhou, J., & Hathaway, G.M. (2002). Identification of phosphorylated and glycosylated sites in peptides by chemically targeted proteolysis. J Biomol Tech, 13, 228-237.

Simpson, D.L, Hranisavljevic, J., & Davidson, E.A. (1972). β-elimination and sulfite addition as a means of localization and identification of substituted seryl and threonyl residues in proteins and proteoglycans. Biochemistry, 11, 1849-1856.

Speicher, D.T, Kolbas, O., Harper, D., & Speicher, D.W. (2000). Systematic analysis of peptide recoveries from in-gel digestions for protein identifications in proteome studies. J Biomol Tech, 11, 74-86.

Stensballe, A., & Jensen, O.N. (2004) Phosphoric acid enhances the performance of Fe (III) affinity chromatography and matrix-assisted laser desorption/ionization tandem mass spectrometry for recovery, detection and sequencing of phosphopeptides. Rapid Commun Mass Spectrom, 18, 1721-1730.

Shen, J., Smith, R.A., Stoll, V.S., Edalji, R., Jacob, C., Walter, K., Gramling, E., Dorwin, S., Bartley, D., Gunasekera, A., Yang, J., Holzman, T., & Johnson, R.W. (2004). Characterization of protein kinase A phosphorylation: multi-technique approach to phosphate mapping. Anal Biochem, 324, 204-218.

Tholey, A., Reed, J., & Lehmann, W. (1999). Electrospray tandem mass spectrometric studies of phosphopeptides and phosphopeptide analogues. J Mass Spectrom, 34, 117-12.

Thompson, A.J., Hart, S.R., Franz, C., Barnouin, K., Ridley, A., & Cramer, R. (2003). Characterization of protein phosphorylation by mass spectrometry using immobilized metal ion affinity chromatography with on-resin β-elimination and Michael addition. Anal Chem, 75, 3232-3243.

Ubersax, J.A., & Ferrell, J.E. Mechanism of specificity in protein phosphorylation. (2007). Nat Rev Mol Cell Biol, 8, 530-541.

Villen, J., & Gygi, S.P. (2008). The SCX/IMAC enrichment approach for global phosphorylation analysis by mass spectrometry. Nat Protoc, 3, 1630-1638.

Yang, X., Wu, H., Kobayashi, T., Solaro, R.J., & van Breemen, R.B. (2004). Enhanced ionization of phosphorylated peptides during MALDI-TOF mass spectrometry. Anal Chem, 76, 1532-1536.

Zhang, R., Zhao, J., & Potter, J.D. (1995). Phosphorylation of both serine residues in cardiac troponin I is required to decrease the Ca 2+ affinity of cardiac troponin C. J Biol Chem, 270, 30773-30780.

Genetic Mechanisms of Cartilage Degradation in the Development and Osteoarthritis

Elena V. Tchetina
Research Institute of Rheumatology
Russian Academy of Medical Sciences, Russia

Luidmila A. Semyonova
Research Institute of Rheumatology
Russian Academy of Medical Sciences, Russia

1   Introduction

Osteoarthritis (OA) is the most common joint disease, which is associated with a risk of mobility disability. It affects approximately 12% of the aging Western population while a quarter of people aged over 55 have an episode of persistent knee pain (Hunter & Felson, 2009). The pathology of OA involves the whole joint and is associated with focal and progressive hyaline articular cartilage loss, concomitant sclerotic changes in the subchondral bone and the development of osteophytes. Soft tissue structures in and around the joint including synovium, ligaments and muscles are also involved (Abramson & Attur, 2006).

OA affects predominantly articular cartilage, which degrades by gradual loss of its extracellular matrix (ECM) composed mainly of aggrecan and type II collagen (the structure and function of the major extracellular matrix proteins are comprehensively discussed in (Poole, 2005; Heinegård, 2009; Eyre *et al.*, 2006). Loss of large proteoglycan aggrecan decreases cartilage compressive stiffness and precedes the damage to collagen fibrillar network, which is responsible for tensile properties of the tissue (Poole, 2005). Aggrecan degradation is associated with upregulation of aggrecanases ADAMTS (a disintegrin and metalloprotease with thrombospondin motifs)-4 and -5 as well as matrix metalloproteinases (MMPs) (the structure and function of the enzymes involved in extracellular matrix degradation are thoroughly discussed in (Troeberg & Nagase, 2012, Lin & Lin, 2010). The excessive cleavage of type II collagen in OA is caused by increased synthesis and activities of collagenases (Poole *et al.*, 2002, 2003, 2007), primarily MMP-13 (Wu *et al.*, 2002a; Billinghurst *et al.*, 1997; Dahlberg *et al.*, 2000). Presently it is believed that articular cartilage destruction in OA results from excessive loading, age-related changes and metabolic imbalance in the tissue (Aigner *et al.*,2007; Aigner & Gerwin, 2007; van der Kraan *et al.*, 2010).

OA also exhibits features of a systemic disease as it has been shown to involve vascular pathology (Find-lay, 2007; Ghosh & Cheras, 2001) as well as T-cell immune response (de Jong, 2010; Sakkas & Platsoucas, 2007) accompanied by upregulation of cytokines such as interleukin(IL)-β and tumor necrosis factor (TNF)α(Poole, 2005; Attur, 2011), which aggravate cartilage resorption (Kobayashi *et al.*, 2005a). As the mechanism of OA development is not completely understood, the disease manifestation, which is associated with cartilage resorption and inflammation, suggests a treatment involving inhibition of pro-inflammatory cytokines or MMP activity to prevent matrix destruction. However it does not result in disease modification and produces severe side effects (Little & Forsang, 2010).

Articular cartilage degeneration in OA is also associated with changes in chondrocyte phenotype (Tchetina *et al.*, 2005; Yagi *et al.*, 2005; van der Kraan *et al.*, 2010). Specifically these changes resemble those observed during chondrocyte differentiation in endochondral ossification and are characterized by cell cloning, expression of differentiation related genes such as parathyroid hormone related peptide (PTHrP) (Terkeltaub *et al.*, 1998a), type X collagen (von der Mark *et al.*,1996; Girkontaite *et al.*, 1996; Walker*et al.*, 1995), annexins and alkaline phosphatase (ALP) (Kirsch *et al.*, 2000; Pfander *et al.*, 2003), osteocalcin (Pullig *et al.*, 2000), matrix calcification (Karpouzas & Terkeltaub, 1999; Johnson & Terkeltaub, 2004), as well as apoptotic cell death of terminally differentiated chondrocytes (Blanco *et al.*, 1998; Robertson *et al.*, 2006). All these cellular changes including increased cleavage of type II collagen by MMP-13 are also associated with chondrocyte hypertrophy observed in the growth plate (Tchetina *et al.,* 2003). This suggests that, as articular cartilage shares a common embryological origin with the epiphyseal growth plate (Ham & Cormack, 1987), destruction of cartilage matrix in OA may involve some of the same cellular and regulatory mechanisms that govern normal chondrocyte terminal differentiation and ECM resorption in skeletal growth and repair (Tchetina *et al.*, 2005).

The aim of this review is to summarize current evidence supporting the involvement of molecular mecha-nisms observed in the course of chondrocyte progression through the growth plate in cartilage matrix destruction in OA.

2   Gene Expression in the Epiphyseal Growth Plate

A central process in endochondral bone formation is a progressive differentiation of proliferating matrix assembling chondrocytes to growth-arrested hypertrophic cells. This involves remodeling and mineraliza-tion of the cartilage matrix and leads eventually to its subsequent replacement by bone.

Primary mammalian growth plate physis is structurally organized and can be divided into zones namely, the resting, proliferative, and hypertrophic (Table 1). Resting zone chondrocytes show very limited cell division evidenced by low proliferating cell nuclear antigen (PCNA) expression (Yamane et al., 2007). They elaborate an extensive extracellular matrix, which is composed predominantly of type II collagen and proteoglycan aggrecan; however, it also contains other collagen types VI, IX, XI, link protein, and small leucine-rich proteoglycans (SLRPs) such as decorin and fibromodulin (Yamane et al., 2007). Ex-pression of several regulatory growth factors, such as bone morphogenetic proteins (BMP-) 3, 5, 7, fibro-blast growth factor (FGF-)2, and transforming growth factor (TGF)β1-3 has been detected in this zone as well (Yamane et al., 2007; Krejci et al., 2007; Nilsson et al., 2007; Anderson et al., 2000; Matsunaga et al., 1999; Damron et al., 2004; Verdier et al., 2001).

In contrast to resting zone, proliferative zone chondrocytes actively divide, which is evidenced by the expression of cyclins (Blanco et al., 1998; Beier et al., 2001) and the presence of PCNA positive cells (Roach et al., 2003). They produce long columns of flattened cells and express hyaline ECM similar to resting zone chondrocytes. The space for the cells newly formed in the course of cell division is generated by the matrix degrading activity of collagenases MMP-13, MT1-MMP (Mwale et al., 2000; Neuhold et al., 2001) and other MMPs such as MMP-3 (Armstrong et al., 2002), which activity is limited to the chondrocyte pericellular region. These cells also express proliferation-specific growth factors, namely TGFβ1-3, FGF-2 (Tchetina et al., 2003; Verdier et al., 2005; Wezeman & Bollnow, 1997; Horner et al.,1998), PTHrP, insulin growth factor (IGF-) I and II (Tchetina et al., 2003; Wang et al., 2006; de los Rios & Hill, 1999; Shinar et al., 1993), a cell death inhibitor that regulates apoptosis Bcl-2 (B-cell lym-phoma-2)(Ma et al., 2007), and transcription factors SRY-type high-mobility-group box transcription factor (Sox)9 (Tchetina et al., 2003; Akiyama et al., 2002). Sox9 is coexpressed with Sox5 and Sox6 (Lefebvre & Smits, 2005). Although PTHrP (Burton et al., 2005), TGFβ2 and FGF-2 (Uria et al., 1998; Borden et al., 1996) have been reported to stimulate MMP-13 expression in rodents, in the early prolifer-ative zone of the growth plate, their expression does not induce significant matrix loss probably due to the lack of gelatinase (MMP-2 and -9) expression (Tchetina et al., 2003; Haeusler et al., 2005).

Cessation of cell division in the growth plate is associated with upregulation of cell cycle inhibitors p18, p19 and p21 (Li et al.,1999), growth arrest and DNA damage-inducible (GADD) 45beta gene(Tsuchimochi et al., 2010; Ijiri et al., 2005], as well as apoptosis inhibitors Bcl2 and Bag1 (Bcl2-associated athanogen 1), a Bcl2 –binding protein capable of enhancing Bcl2 activity (Damron et al., 2004; Kinkel et al., 2004), and a marker of apoptosis caspase-3 (Anderson et al., 2000). At this point, chondrocytes partially resorb their extracellular matrix, enlarge, round up and finally mature into hyper-trophic cells, which express type X collagen (COL10A1), a marker of chondrocyte hypertrophy (von der Mark et al., 1992; Girkontaite et al., 1996). Alkaline phosphatase shows the most pronounced

Growth plate zones	Gene expression
Resting	Collagens type II,VI, IX, XI (Yamane *et al.*, 2007); Aggrecan (Yamane *et al.*, 2007); TGFβ 1-3 (Matsunaga *et al.*, 1999; Verdier *et al.*, 2005); BMP 3,-5,-7(Nillson *et al.*, 2007; Anderson *et al.*, 2000); PTHrP (Damron *et al.*,2004); FGF2 (Krejci *et al.*, 2007); Bcl2 (Damron *et al.*, 2004)
Proliferative	Collagens type II,VI, IX, XI (Yamane *et al.*, 2007); TGFβ 1-3(Verdier *et al.*, 2005; Horner *et al.*, 1998); FGF2(Tchetina *et al.*,2003; Wezeman & Bollnow, 1997); PTHrP (Tchetina *et al.*,2003); IGFI,-II (Wang *et al.*,2006); Sox9 (Akiyama *et al.*, 2002; Tchetina *et al.*,2003); MMP13 (Neuhold *et al.*, 2001); MMP3 (Armstrong *et al.*, 2002); CyclinB2 (Damron *et al.*, 2004); Bcl2 (Ma *et al.*, 2007); PCNA (Roach *et al.*, 2003)
Hypertrophic	COL10A1(von der Mark *et al.*, 1992; Girkontaite *et al.*, 1996); COL2A1 (Tchetina *et al.*,2003; Wang *et al.*, 2004); MMP13(Jimenez *et al.*, 1999); TGFβ 1-3 (Tchetina *et al.*,2003; Horner *et al.*, 1998); BMP2,-4,-6,-7 (Nillson *et al.*, 2007; Anderson *et al.*, 2000; Pogue & Lions, 2006; Wang *et al.*, 2004; Sakou *et al.*, 1999); CTGF (Fukunaga *et al.*, 2003); VEGF (Haeusler *et al.*, 2005; Alvarez *et al.*, 2005); Ihh (Tchetina *et al.*,2003; MacLean & Kronenberg, 2005; Kindblom *et al.*, 2002); Cbfa1 (Ducy *et al.*, 1997); Gadd45b (Tsuchimochi *et al.*, 2010; Ijiri *et al.*, 2005); p18,-19,-21 (Li *et al.*, 1999); ALP (Tuckermann *et al.*, 2000; Henson *et al.*, 1995); Osteocalcin (Pullig *et al.*, 2000); ANK (Wang *et al.*, 2005a); Annexin II, -V, VI (Wang *et al.*, 2003; Kirsch, 2005); Bag1 (Kinkel *et al.*, 2004); Bcl2 (Damron *et al.*, 2004; Beier *et al.*, 2001); Caspase 3 (Pucci *et al.*, 2007); IL-1 (Yamashita *et al.*, 1989);

Table 1: Zonal gene expression in the fetal growth plate.

expression also in hypertrophic chondrocytes (Tuckermann *et al.*,2000; Henson *et al.*,1995). This pheno-typic modification in growth plate chondrocytes is associated with dramatic alteration in regulatory gene expression, namely, upregulation of growth factors such as TGFβ1 and -3 (Tchetina *et al.*, 2003; Horner *et al.*, 1998), BMP-2, -4, -6, and -7(Nilsson *et al.*, 2007; Anderson *et al.*, 2000; Pogue & Lyons, 2006; Wang *et al.*, 2004; Sakou *et al.*,1999), connective tissue growth factor (CTGF) (Fukunaga *et al.*, 2003), vascular endothelial growth factor (VEGF)(Haeusler *et al.*, 2005; Alvarez *et al.*, 2005), and Indian hedgehog (Ihh) (Tchetina *et al.*, 2003; MacLean & Kronenberg, 2005; Kindblom *et al.*, 2002). Inflammation-related cytokine IL-1 expression also has been observed only in the hypertrophic chondrocytes (Yamashita *et al.*, 1989).

These regulatory growth factors are expressed in association with runt-related transcription factor(Runx)2, which is essential both for osteoblast differentiation (Ducy *et al.*, 1997) and chondrocyte maturation during endochondral ossification (van der Kraan *et al.*, 2009; Komori, 2000; Takeda *et al.*, 2001; Ueta *et al.*,2001; Porte *et al.*,1999), and is capable of inducing MMP-13 expression (Porte *et al.*, 1999; Jimenez *et al.*, 1999).

Expression of these growth and transcription factors is also associated with upregulation of matrix proteins, such as type II collagen (COL2A1) concomitantly with their degrading enzymes MMP-13 and gelatinases MMP-2 and -9 (Tchetina *et al.*, 2003; Wang *et al.*, 2004). At this time, overt type II collagen degradation occurs (Mwale *et al.*, 2000) indicating that genes for both matrix synthesis and degradation are co-regulated. However aggrecan remains retained in the tissue at that time (Poole, 2005).

In the lower hypertrophic zone, mineralization (or calcification) of residual matrix is initiated in discrete focal sites between collagen fibrils and rapidly radiates out of these centers (Poole, 2005). This involves deposition of hydroxyapatite mineral (Mwale *et al.*,2002). Mineralization process in the lower hypertrophic zone of the growth plate is associated with expression of osteocalcin, which is a marker of mature osteoblasts and is involved in chondrocyte mineralization and Ca^{+2} homeostasis (Pullig *et al.*, 2000). Upregulation of ankylosis protein (Ank), which is responsible for transport of intracellular inorganic pyrophosphate to the extracellular milieu, has been also observed in this zone (Wang *et al.*, 2005a). Mineralization is likely regulated by annexins II, V, and VI, which are highly expressed in the hypertrophic and terminally differentiated mineralizing growth plate chondrocytes and form calcium channels enabling formation of first mineral phase (Wang *et al.*,2003; Kirsch, 2005). For example, annexin V has been shown to be capable of upregulating annexins II, VI, osteocalcin, Runx2, and ALP as well as stimulating apoptotic activity in the lowest part of the growth plate (Wang *et al.*,2003; Wang *et al.*,2005b). In contrast TGFβ2, which is also expressed by lower hypertrophic chondrocytes (Tchetina *et al.*, 2003), is most probably involved in osteoblast formation (Gill*et al.*, 1998).

Therefore, chondrocyte maturation in the growth plate is associated with expression of stage-specific set of regulatory growth and transcription factors producing changes in cellular phenotype and synthesis of stage-specific extracellular matrix, which eventually degrades in the hypertrophic zone. All these cellular activities require careful and specific coordination.

3   Regulation of Endochondral Ossification in Mammals

Chondrocyte differentiation is initiated in the center of the cartilaginous bone rudiment and is thought to be induced by hypoxia and/or nutrient deficiency (Shapiro *et al.*,1995). The pace of chondrocyte differentiation is regulated by various agents including paracrine and autocrine growth factors and hormones (Poole, 2005; Olney *et al.*, 2004). They are responsible for specific regulatory molecule expression by chondrocytes in the course of their progression through the growth plate.

Growth factors secreted by fetal chondrocytes are in charge of mutually exclusive processes of chondrocyte proliferation and terminal differentiation. Thus, proliferation-related growth factors such as basic fibroblast growth factor and parathyroid hormone related peptide stimulate resting chondrocytes to proliferate and suppress terminal differentiation of hypertrophic chondrocytes (Hutchison *et al.*, 2007; Kronenberg, 2006; Li *et al.*, 2004a; Dong *et al.*, 2006; Kiepe *et al.*, 2006; Karaplis *et al.*, 1994; Amizuka *et al.*, 1994; Weir *et al.*, 1996). In addition, PTHrP in combination with Indian hedgehog, regulate chondrocyte differentiation through the establishment of a negative feedback mechanism, whereby Ihh and PTHrP can together suppress hypertrophy (Weir *et al.*, 1996; Vortkamp *et al.*, 1996; Yoshida *et al.*, 2001; St-Jacques *et al.*, 1999). Alternatively interactions of Ihh with syndecan-3, which serves a growth factor co-receptor, are important for restricting mitotic activity to the proliferative zone of mammalian growth plate (Pacifici *et al.*, 2005).

Transforming growth factor betas are multifunctional molecules regulating cellular proliferation, differentiation, and extracellular matrix function (van der Kraan *et al.*, 2009; Roberts & Sporn, 1993). TGFβ signals via heteromeric complexes of transmembrane type I and type II receptors. TGFβ binds to a type II receptor followed by phosphorylation of a type I receptor (activin receptor-like kinase, ALK). Upon type I receptor activation, intracellular signaling is initiated by phosphorylation of Sma and Mad Related Family (Smad) proteins (Studer *et al.*,2012). The Smad 1/5/8 activation mediated by ALK1, -2, -3, and -6 induces hypertrophy. Activation of the Smad2/3 pathway by ALK5 inhibits hypertrophy and stimulates chondrogenesis due to stabilization of the Sox9 transcription complex (Yang*et al.*, 2001). Moreover, TGFβ activation of Smad 3 produces repression of Runx2-inducible MMP-13 expression, while in the absence of Smad3, TGFβ signals to induce expression of this collagenase (Chen*et al.*, 2012). Both TGFβ1 (Serra *et al.*, 1999; Fergusson *et al.*, 2000; Ballock *et al.*, 1993) and TGFβ2 (Bohme *et al.*, 1995) each are able to suppress chondrocyte hypertrophy by coordinate inhibition of collagenase expression. This is partially associated with upregulation of PTHrP gene expression that exerts both PTHrP-dependent and PTHrP-independent effects on endochondral bone formation (Serra *et al.*, 1999; Bohme *et al.*, 1995; Pateder *et al.*, 2000; Terkeltaub *et al.*, 1998b).

FGF2 is a growth factor that exists in several isoforms differing in their N-terminal extensions, subcellular distribution and function. The smallest, an 18kDa FGF2 low molecular weight variant is released by cells and acts through activation of cell surface FGF-receptors, whereas a 34 kDa FGF2 is localized to the nucleus and signal independently of FGFR (Chlebova *et al.*, 2009). Extracellular signals from FGF-2 to the cells are transduced through one of four high affinity receptors (FGF receptor 1 – 4) (Ellman *et al.*, 2008). FGF2 binding to FGFR1 has been demonstrated to increase proliferation of growth plate chondrocytes, whereas FGF2 binding to FGFR3 inhibits proliferation and promotes differentiation (Wang *et al.*, 2009). TGFβ2 in synergy with FGF-2 has been also shown to suppress chondrocyte maturation and hypertrophy (Nagai *et al.*, 2002; Szuts *et al.*, 1998).

BMP signaling is also essential for chondrocyte progression through the growth plate (Pogue & Lyons, 2006). Zone specific expression of various BMPs suggests their involvement in chondrocyte phenotypic changes in the course of both proliferation and hypertrophy. Thus, BMP-2 and -6 have been shown to promote chondrocyte hypertrophy by upregulation of Ihh and type X collagen expression and downregulation of FGF signaling involving Runx2 (Wang *et al.*, 2007; Kobayashi *et al.*, 2005b; Yoon *et al.*, 2006; Stewart *et al.*, 2004; Zhang *et al.*, 2003; Grimsrud *et al.*, 1999). At the same time, BMP-2 and -9 augmented mitogenic effect of IGF-1, while BMP-5 increased cell proliferation and cartilage matrix synthesis (Takahashi *et al.*, 2007; Mailhot *et al.*, 2008).

IGF-1, a structural and functional analog of insulin, promotes chondrocyte proliferation and differentiation while inhibits apoptosis (Hutchison *et al.*, 2007; Kiepe *et al.*, 2006). It is also an important regulator of PTHrP-Ihh feedback loop. The lack of IGF results in downregulation of Ihh expression and upregulation of PTHrP (Wang *et al.*, 2006). IGF-1 favors chondrocyte hypertrophic development as it induces type X collagen and alkaline phosphatase in avian sternal chondrocytes (Bohme *et al.*, 1995; Szuts *et al.*, 1998). In addition, insulin and IGF-1 (Laron, 2001) both are strong stimulators of aggrecan and type II collagen synthesis (Hui *et al.*,2001).

Furthermore, chondrocyte differentiation in the growth plate is regulated by various transcription factors (Lefebvre & Smits, 2005). Transcription factors Sox9 and -4 have been shown to determine the rate of chondrocyte differentiation into hypertrophy and the expression of chondrocyte-specific matrix molecules including COL2A1, COL9A2, COL11A1, and aggrecan (Hattori *et al.*, 2010; Wuelling & Vortkamp, 2010; Zhao *et al.*, 1997; de Crombrugghe *et al.*, 2000; Ng *et al.*, 1997; Bi *et al.*, 2001; Reppe *et al.*, 2000). Sox5 and Sox6 are not absolutely required for chondrocyte differentiation; however, they are capable of potentiating Sox9 chondrogenic activity (Lefebvre & Smits, 2005). They are also required to prevent conversion of proliferating chondrocytes into hypertrophic chondrocytes (Akiyama *et al.*, 2002). The ratio of Sp1/Sp3 complex of transcription factors is suggested to be a general means controlling the expression of different collagen isotypes in the course of chondrocyte differentiation (Ghayor *et al.*, 2001), as Sp1-dependent activation of COL2A1 was counteracted by Sp3, while increased Sp3/Sp1 ration favored COL10A1 expression in hypertrophic chondrocytes (Magee *et al.*, 2005). Transcription factors Runx1-3 are the most important as they play a crucial role both in chondrocyte maturation and had been shown to induce MMP-13 expression (Takeda *et al.*, 2001; Jimenez *et al.*, 1999; Wuelling & Vortkamp, 2010; Soung *et al.*, 2007). Recently the involvement of several other transcription factors such as Shox/Shox2, Dlx5, and MEF2C has been shown to control skeletal growth that suggests their potential contribution in ectopic chondrocyte hypertrophy development (Solomon *et al.*, 2008; Drissi *et al.*, 2005). Wnt/beta-catenin signaling can also mediate chondrocyte hypertrophy as is capable of upregulating type X collagen, Runx2, alkaline phosphatase expression while inhibiting Sox9 and type II collagen expression (Dong *et al.*, 2006).

Prostaglandin E2 (PGE2), a potent lipid molecule that regulates a broad range of physiologic reactions, can inhibit growth plate chondrocyte differentiation by downregulation of differentiation-related genes COL10A1, VEGF, MMP-13, and alkaline phosphatase expression as well as their enzymatic activity (Li *et al.*, 2004b; Zhang *et al.*, 2004; Domowicz *et al.*, 2009). At the same time, low concentrations of this prostaglandin are capable of increasing proliferation of growth plate chondrocytes (Schwarz *et al.*,1998; Brochhausen *et al.*, 2006). In contrast, chemokine stromal sell-derived factor 1, annexin V, and Ank have been shown to stimulate hypertrophy, mineralization, and apoptosis, when are overexpressed in nonmineralizing growth plate chondrocytes (Wang *et al.*, 2005a; Wang *et al.*, 2005b; Wei *et al.*, 2010; Wang & Kirsch, 2006).

Extracellular matrix proteins produced by chondrocytes have also exhibited a capacity to regulate growth plate chondrocyte hypertrophy. Thus, type II collagen, aggrecan, and matrilin-3 are likely to inhibit hypertrophy as these matrix component deficiencies produced premature maturation in mutant chondrocytes (Domowicz *et al.*, 2009; van der Weyden *et al.*, 2006; Cancedda & Garofalo, 2003). Furthermore, downregulation of chondrocyte hypertrophy evidenced by suppression of type X collagen, Runx2, and MMP-13 expression is associated with inhibition of collagen cleavage activity in cultured hypertrophic growth plate chondrocytes treated with MMP-13 inhibitor (Wu *et al.*, 2002a; Borzi *et al.*, 2010). This indicates a functional link between chondrocyte hypertrophy and extracellular matrix degradation (van der Kraan & van den Berg, 2012).

It is necessary to note that variable effects of regulatory molecules are carefully coordinated to provide accuracy in the process of endochondral ossification. Thus, it has been demonstrated that growth plate chondrocyte progression to hypertrophy is a subject to negative control that can be arrested at various checkpoints (Szuts *et al.*, 1998). Accordingly, an early proliferative phenotype in avian fetal chondrocytes has been reassumed by treatment with TGFβ2, FGF-2 and insulin in combination, while increased Ihh expression was responsible for acquisition of the late proliferative phenotype in hypertrophic cells (Szuts *et al.*, 1998). In another study, the release of terminally differentiated hypertrophic chondrocytes from their environment also resulted in downregulation of type X collagen synthesis, activation of proliferation, and reinitiation of aggrecan synthesis (Chen *et al.*, 1995).

Therefore, chondrocyte differentiation is carefully regulated in the course of endochondral ossification. Eventually, epiphyseal chondrocytes give rise to articular cartilage, whose structural components and regulatory networks at least partially resemble that in the growth plate.

4   Gene Expression in the Healthy Articular Cartilage

Healthy articular cartilage is characterized by a very low expression of collagens type II, VI, IX, and XI (Buck-walter & Mankin, 1998), and relatively high turnover rate for aggrecan (Hardingham*et al.*, 1992). It is also characterized by expression of matrix turnover genes such as MMP-3 (Aigner *et al.*, 2003), occasionally detected MMP-1, -8, -13 (Tetlow *et al.*, 2001), and growth factors TGFβ1 (van den Berg, 1995) and PTHrP (Terkeltaub *et al.*, 1998a; Chen *et al.*, 2008). Antiangiogenic factor chondromodulin-1 (Hiraki *et al.*, 1997; Kitahara *et al.*, 2003), p16INK4α, and Gadd45α/β genes, the latter is associated with environmental and intrinsic stress (Ijiri *et al.*, 2008; Zhou*et al.*, 2004), CTGF (Omoto *et al.*, 2004), are expressed in all the cartilage zones. At the same time no expression of type I and X collagens (Aigner & McKenna, 2002; Poole, 2003), a complete lack of expression of TGFβ2, IGF-1, Ihh (Scharstuhl *et al.*, 2002; Bos *et al.*, 2001), annexin VIII (White *et al.*, 2002), and osteocalcin (Pullig *et al.*, 2000) was observed in healthy cartilage (Table 2).

Articular cartilage can be divided into superficial, mid-, and deep zones; the latter is followed by the calcified cartilage providing junction of the cartilage to the subchondral bone (Poole, 2003). These zones differ in expression of specific matrix molecules, their modifying enzymes, and regulatory growth factors, which are responsible for articular cartilage integrity and function. Although normal articular chondrocytes are less metabolically active than the growth plate chondrocytes, some similarity in gene expression pattern in the individual cartilage zones has been noted.

Superficial zone of healthy articular cartilage contains flattened chondrocytes surrounded by specialized extracellular matrix rich in thin collagen fibrils (Kempson *et al.*, 1973) and small leucine-rich proteoglycans – decorin and biglycan (Poole *et al.*, 1996). It also contains the lowest amount of predominant cartilage proteoglycan aggrecan compared to other zones of articular cartilage. This zone is rich in regulatory molecules such as TGFβ1 and -3, and BMP 1-6 (Yamane *et al.*, 2007; Anderson *et al.*, 2000). Proliferative potential of these cells is indicated by the expression of cyclin D2; however it may be suppressed by cell division inhibitors such as growth arrest specific protein (Gas)-1 and Gadd45α, which are also expressed in this cartilage zone (Yamane *et al.*, 2007). This is supported by the lack of superficial chondrocyte proliferative activity determined by PCNA staining (Pfander *et al.*, 2001). MMP-3 expression was observed in this cartilage zone more often than MMP-1, -8, and -13; however, these proteinases do not produce any matrix degradation and are likely involved in matrix turnover (Tetlow *et al.*, 2001; Wu *et al.*, 2002b). Expression of antiapoptotic Bcl2 and Bag1 genes was detected predominantly in this zone in old mice, while it was observed throughout the articular cartilage in the young animals (Kinkel *et al.*, 2004).

Cartilage zones	Normal	Early & moderate OA	Late OA
Superficial	Chondromodulin1 (Hiraku *et al.*, 1997; Kitahara *et al.*, 2003); TGFβ1-3 (Yamane *et al.*, 2007; van den Berg, 1995); PTHrP (Terkeltaub *et al.*, 1998a; Chen *et al.*, 2008); p16INK4a (Zhou *et al.*, 2004); Aggrecan (Hardingham *et al.*, 1992); Decorin (Poole *et al.*, 1996); Biglycan (Poole *et al.*, 1996); MMP1,-3,-8,-13 (Aigner *et al.*, 2003; Tetlow *et al.*, 2001); BMP1-6 (Anderson *et al.*, 2000); CyclinD2 (Yamane *et al.*, 2007); Gas1 (Yamane *et al.*, 2007]; Gadd45a (Yamane *et al.*, 2007; Ijiri *et al.*, 2008); PCNA (Pfander *et al.*, 2001); Bcl2 (Kinkel *et al.*, 2004); Bad1(Kinkel *et al.*, 2004); Collagens II,VI,IX,XI (Buckwalter &Mankin, 1998; Kempson *et al.*, 1973); CTGF (Omoto *et al.*, 2004)	COL10A1 (Tchetina *et al.*, 2007b); MMP13 (Tchetina *et al.*, 2007b); PCNA (Tchetina *et al.*, 2007b); Ki67 (Tchetina *et al.*, 2007b); Apoptotic activity (Tchetina *et al.*, 2007b); CTGF (Omoto *et al.*, 2004); IL-1β (Moldovan *et al.*, 2000)	Zonal organization is disturbed. Upregulated genes: PCNA (Pfander *et al.*, 2001); Syndecan (Pfander *et al.*, 2001); AnnexinVI (Zhao *et al.*, 1997); ALP (Pfander *et al.*, 2001); Apoptotic activity (Yatsugi *etal.*, 2000); Collagens I,II,III,IV,X (Bay-Jenson *et al.*, 2008; Pfander *etal.*, 1999; Lorenz & Richter, 2006); IL-1β (Tetlow *et al.*, 2001); TNFα (Tetlow *et al.*, 2001); CTGF (Omoto *et al.*, 2004); TGFβ1-3 (Blaney Davidson *etal.*, 2006; Gomez-Barrena *et al.*, 2004); Smad2 (Blaney Davidson *et al.*, 2006); BMP2 (Blaney Davidson *et al.*, 2006); P53 (Yatsugi *et al.*, 2000) P16INK4a (Zhou *et al.*, 2004); Ihh (Wei *et al.*, 2012); VEGF (Pufe *et al.*, 2001)
Middle	Chondromodulin1(Hiraku *et al.*, 1997; Kitahara *et al.*,2003); p16INK4a (Zhou *et al.*, 2004); FGF2 (Wezeman &Bollnow, 1997); CTGF (Omoto *et al.*, 2004); Collagens II,VI,IX,XI (Buckwalter &Mankin, 1998; Kempson *et al.*, 1973); Aggrecan (Hardingham *et al.*, 1992); Gadd45a (Yamane *et al.*, 2007; Ijiri *et al.*, 2008); PCNA(Pfander *et al.*, 2001); BMP1-7 (Anderson *et al.*, 2000)	COL10A1 (Tchetina *etal.*, 2007b); MMP13(Tchetina *et al.*, 2007b); PCNA (Tchetina *et al.*, 2007b); Ki67 (Tchetina *et al.*, 2007b); ALP (Pfander *et al.*, 2001); AnnexinVI (Pfander *et al.*, 2001)	Annexin VII (White *et al.*, 2002); Osteocalcin (Pullig *et al.*, 2000)
Deep	Chondromodulin1 (Hiraku *et al.*, 1997; Kitahara *et al.*,2003); MMP13 (Tetlow *et al.*, 2001); p16INK4a (Zhou *et al.*, 2004); COL10A1(Tuckermann *et al.*, 2000); Aggrecan (Buckwalter &Mankin, 1998; Maroudas *etal.*, 1980); BMP1-7 (Anderson *et al.*, 2000); Annexin VI (Pfander *et al.*, 2001);	IL-1β (Moldovan *et al.*, 2000); Annexin VI,VIII (White *et al.*, 2002)	Annexin VII (White *et al.*, 2002); Osteocalcin (Pullig *et al.*, 2000)

ALP(Tuckermann *et al.*, 2000); Apoptitic activity (Aigner *et al.*, 2001a; Kuhn *et al.*, 2004); CTGF (Omoto *et al.*, 2004); Gadd45a (Yamane *et al.*, 2007; Ijiri *et al.*, 2008); Collagens II,VI,IX,XI (Buckwalter &Mankin, 1998); SLRP (Poole *et al.*, 1996); Ihh (Semevolos *et al.*, 2005) MMP13(Tetlow *et al.*, 2001)		

Table 2: Zonal gene expression in normal and osteoarthritic articular cartilage

Mid zone chondrocytes are round in shape, surrounded by ECM composed of thick collagen fibrils and rich in aggrecan. Chondrocytes in this zone do not show any proliferative activity determined by PCNA staining similar to superficial zone cells (Pfander *et al.*, 2001). However, these cells are likely to possess a potential for proliferation, as FGF-2, capable of inducing proliferation in normal articular chondrocytes in culture (Quintavalla *et al.*, 2005), has been detected in the mid zone of mouse articular cartilage (Wezeman & Bollnow,1997). BMP1-7 expression was also observed in the mid zone of normal articular cartilage (Anderson *et al.*, 2000).

Deep zone chondrocytes are grouped in clusters and resemble hypertrophic chondrocytes of the growth plate (Poole, 2005). In this zone cartilage matrix has the highest content of aggrecan (Maroudas *etal.*, 1980), the lowest amounts of small leucine-rich proteoglycans (Poole *et al.*, 1996), and the largest diameter of collagen fibrils. Similar to hypertrophic zone of the growth plate BMP1-7 (Anderson *et al.*, 2000), Ihh expression (Semevolos *et al.*, 2005), and the highest amount of annexin VI-positive cells were observed in the deep zone of human articular cartilage (Pfander*et al.*, 2001). The lowest part of the deep zone, which is partly calcified, expressed a marker of chondrocyte hypertrophy type X collagen and is rich in alkaline phosphatase. MMP-13 expression (Tetlow *et al.*, 2001) and negligible activity of chondrocyte apoptosis was also sometimes observed here (Aigner *et al.*, 2001a; Kuhn*et al.*, 2004).

However, in spite of low activity of cellular and matrix turnover, healthy articular cartilage possesses a strong metabolic potential, whose activation is observed during development of pathological condition such as OA.

5   Early Osteoarthritic Changes in Articular Cartilage

Early OA changes in articular cartilage are associated with significant metabolic activation of articular chondrocytes. This involves sequential and zonal upregulation of chondrocyte differentiation related genes as well as an increase in the activity of the same MMPs, which are responsible for matrix degradation in the hypertrophic zone of the growth plate. Spatially these genes are upregulated in the mid- and superficial zones of articular cartilage, where lately the first signs of cartilage destruction occur (Table 2).

An early OA articular cartilage degeneration is observed focally. Spatial distribution of chondrocyte differentiation-related gene expression in the areas adjacent to and remote from the early lesion is also resembles that in the growth plate and is associated with increased collagenase cleavage of type II collagen. Thus, collagenases MMP-1, MMP-14 (MT1-MMP), and aggrecanase ADAMTS-5 (but not ADAMTS-4); cytokines IL-1α/β, and TNF-α; chondrocyte terminal differentiation-related genes COL10A1, MMP-13, MMP-9, Ihh, and caspase-3 were often upregulated in the vicinity of the lesion. Growth factors associated with growth plate chondrocyte proliferation, namely, FGF-2, PTHrP, and TGF β1/2, as well as the matrix molecules COL2A1 and aggrecan, were expressed adjacent to and remote from the lesion (Tchetina et al., 2005). In addition, a distinct spatial reorganization in human superficial chondrocytes in the remote area from early OA lesions has been recently reported (Rolauffs et al.,2010). However, of all genes only caspase-3 and ADAMTS-5 expression was exclusively seen in association with early lesions. Elevation of collagenase activity was associated with a frequent elevation of COL10A1, caspase-3, IL-1α/β, MMP-1, and ADAMTS-5 expression, and a decreased expression of Sox-9, TGF-β1, TGF-β2, TNF-α, and aggrecan (Tchetina et al., 2005).

For the assessment of articular cartilage damage associated with the disease severity a Mankin grading system has been developed (Mankin et al., 1971). For this purpose cartilage histological sections are stained by hematoxylin and eosin, and safranin-O-fast green and analyzed for abnormalities in structure, cell distribution and density, safranin-O stain distribution denotes polysaccharide content, and the integrity of the tidemark (Table 3). The scores in each of these subcategories are summed up for each sample. The total scores for different areas range from 1 to 13. The correlation demonstrated is that the higher the grade the greater the severity of the disease process. Although articular cartilage grading provides little information regarding the etiology or basic pathogenesis of the process, as well as no insight into the intermediary pathways, it offers a means for evaluation of biochemical and metabolic response of cartilage to the chronic stress of OA state.

			Grade				Grade
I.	**Structure**			**III.**	**Safranin-O staining**		
a.	Normal		0	a.	Normal		0
b.	Surface irregularities		1	b.	Slight reduction		1
c.	Pannus and surface irregularities		2	c.	Moderate reduction		2
d.	Clefts to transitional zone		3	d.	Severe reduction		3
e.	Clefts to radial zone		4	e.	No dye noted		4
f.	Clefts to calcified zone		5	**IV.**	**Tidemark integrity**		
g.	Complete disorganization		6	a.	Intact		0
II.	**Cells**			b.	Crossed by blood vessels		1
a.	Normal		0				
b.	Diffuse hypercellularity		1				
c.	Cloning		2				
d.	Hypocellularity		3				

Table 3: Mankin histological-histochemical grading (Mankin et al., 1971)

Mild OA changes (Mankin 1-4) are characterized by the loss of proteoglycans in the surface area (Pfander et al., 2001; Dumond et al., 2004; Fernandes et al., 1998). Although these changes were not accompanied by significant structural disturbances in the tissue, they were associated with increased type II collagen and aggrecan synthesis, upregulation of chondrocyte proliferation evidenced by increased PCNA and Ki67 staining and MMP-13 expression (Tchetina et al., 2007b; Lorenz et al., 2005;Matyas et al., 1999; 2002).

This was followed by the cellular changes similar to those observed in hypertrophic zone of the growth plate as indicated by type X collagen production, collagenase and alkaline phosphatase staining, and increased type II collagen cleavage activity in the mid-zone (Tchetina et al., 2007b; Appleton et al., 2007a). Later, chondrocyte activation extends to the superficial zone, where it is accompanied by CTGF upregulation and chondrocyte apoptosis evidenced by the presence of the cells carrying DNA nicks (Omoto et al., 2004; Tchetina et al., 2007b). IL-1β expression is also upregulated both in the superficial and deep cartilage zones in early OA (Moldovan et al., 2000). Similar to biphasic MMP-13 expression in the growth plate, upregulation of this collagenase in the articular cartilage was initially preceded and later accompanied by type X collagen and alkaline phosphatase expression (Tchetina et al., 2007b; Appleton et al., 2007a).

Moderate OA changes in the articular cartilage (Mankin 6-9), which are characterized by the lack of fib-rillations, some loss of superficial zone and some clustering of cells (Pfander et al., 2001; Fernandes et al., 1998), are associated with the increase of PCNA staining in the superficial zone, which is accompanied by intense CTGF staining in proliferating chondrocytes forming cell clusters (Omoto et al., 2004), as well as annexin VI and VIII antigen upregulation in the mid- and deep zones (White et al., 2002; Pfander et al., 2001; Miosge et al., 2004).

Therefore, articular chondrocyte activation in early OA, which is the most pronounced in the superficial and mid-zones, resembles that observed during chondrocyte maturation in the growth plate.

6   Gene Expression in the Late Osteoarthritic Cartilage

Severe OA (Mankin ≥ 10) is characterized by extensive fissuring, fibrillation, clustering of chondrocytes, and loss of cartilage (Pfander et al., 2001). Cartilage zonal organization is disturbed (Table 2). The superficial zone degradation produces rough fibrillated surface, fissures and cracks extending to the calcified zone. This is accompanied by severe proteoglycan loss followed by degradation of type II collagen (White et al., 2002; Hollander et al., 1995). Collagen degradation occurs around chondrocytes. At this time, upregulation of MMPs-13,-2,-11, ADAMTS as well as expression of collagens type I, II, III, VI, and X were observed near the articular surface (Aigner et al., 2001b, 2003; Poole et al., 1995; Gebauer et al., 2005; Bay-Jenson et al., 2008; Pfander et al., 1999; Veje et al., 2003; Lorenz & Richter, 2006; Blaney Davidson et al.,2006) and this was accompanied by strong expression of IL-1β and TNFα (Tetlow et al., 2001). At the same time, collagen replenishment is limited as COL2A N-propeptide, a marker of collagen synthesis, was detected only in the deep zone close to subchondral bone (Bay-Jenson et al., 2008). As it was stated above, all these gene activities have been also observed in the hypertrophic zone of the fetal growth plate.

Chondrocyte terminal differentiation-related gene expression is also observed in cell clusters located around fissures (Pfander et al., 1999; Veje et al., 2003). In these clusters, collagen type II and X synthesis (Lorenz & Richter, 2006), as well as expression of the secreted protein CTGF (Omoto et al., 2004) and TGFβ3 with its signaling molecule Smad2 were observed (Blaney Davidson et al., 2006). PCNA and syndecan-3, the markers of early fetal chondrocyte differentiation, as well as annexin VI and alkaline phosphatase, which are involved in terminal stage of differentiation, all are upregulated near articular surface in human OA articular cartilage (Karpouzas & Terkeltaub, 1999; Pfander et al., 2001). At the same time annexin VIII and osteocalcin, which were never detected in normal articular cartilage, were observed in the mid- and deep zones in late OA cartilage (Pullig et al., 2000; White et al.,2002). An increase in BMP-2 expression (Blaney Davidson *et al.*, 2006) was associated with upregulation of tumor suppressor p53 expression (Yatsugi*et al.*, 2000) and cyclin-dependent kinase inhibitor p16INK4a upregulation in all the cartilage zones (Zhou *et al.*, 2004) indicating inhibition of proliferative potential in late OA chondrocytes. However, repression of anti-proliferative factor Tob1 has been also reported in the late stage knee OA cartilage (Gebauer *et al.*, 2005).

The most severely damaged rodent knee OA articular cartilage has shown significantly reduced expression of proliferation-related growth factors and their signaling molecules such as PTHrP, TGFβ3 and Smad2, TGFβ1 and its receptor II (Blaney Davidson *et al.*, 2006; Gomez-Barrena *et al.*, 2004). However, in human hip OA, both downregulation and upregulation of TGFβ1-3 isoform expression compared to healthy cartilage has been also reported (Verdier *et al.*, 2005; Pombo-Suarez *et al.*, 2009). Increased expression of Ihh was associated with the severity of OA evidenced by increased Mankin score, upregulation of chondrocyte hypertrophy markers: type X collagen and MMP-13, and larger chondocyte size in human OA cartilage (Wei *et al.*, 2012). However, one study failed to detect any upregulation of chondrocyte differentiation and hypertrophy markers associated with late OA (Brew *et al.*, 2010).

Antiangiogenic factor chondromodulin-1 downregulation concomitant to VEGF upregulation indicating increased vascular invasion into cartilage in advanced OA has been also observed (Pufe *et al.*, 2001). This was accompanied by upregulation of chondrocyte apoptosis, a marker of the final step of chondrocyte differentiation, which was more pronounced in OA cartilage compared to normal specimens (Yatsugi *et al.*, 2000). Overall degrading activity prevailed over synthesis; as serum levels of COL2A N-propeptide were lower than collagen degradation products in late OA patients compared to controls indicating the uncoupling of collagen synthesis and degradation in OA (Miosge *et al.*,2004). Moreover, serum increase in both COL2A N-propeptide and collagen degradation fragments was often indicative on the most aggressive disease progression (Sharif *et al.*, 2007).

Thus, the similarity in the gene expression profiles associated with matrix destruction in OA articular cartilage and in the hypertrophic zone of the growth plate observed in the majority of studies suggests an acquisition of fetal hypertrophic chondrocyte traits by OA articular chondrocytes.

7 Inhibition of Cartilage Degeneration is Accompanied by Downregulation of Articular Chondrocyte Hypertrophy

The similarity of ECM degradation in OA to that in the hypertrophic zone of primary growth plate involves upregulation of type II collagen cleavage by collagenase and expression of regulatory differentiation related growth factors and matrix proteins, which are associated with chondrocyte hypertrophy (Poole *et al.*, 2007; Tchetina *et al.*, 2005; von der Mark *et al.*, 1992; Kirsch *et al.*, 2000). Therefore, the above observation that hypertrophic changes in the growth plate chondrocytes are reversible (Szuts *et al.*, 1998) suggests a possibility for OA articular chondrocytes to regain healthier phenotype when they are treated by agents inhibiting fetal hypertrophy.

In fact, the same growth factors, namely, TGFβ2, FGF-2, and insulin, which were previously used indivi-dually or in combination to suppress hypertrophy in the growth plate chondrocytes (Szuts *et al.*, 1998), have been shown capable of arresting type II collagen cleavage, chondrocyte differentiation-related gene, and proinflammatory cytokine expression in human OA articular cartilage explants (Tchetina *et al.*, 2006). Furthermore, combination of TGFβ1 and IGF1 inhibited collagen degradation, a marker of extracellular matrix destruction, which was induced by oncostatin M and TNFα in bovine articular cartilage (Hui *et al.*, 2003). It has been also shown that TGFβ inhibition of chondrocyte differentiation is likely mediated by Smad2/3 pathway through modulation of Runx2 function (van der Kraan *et al.*, 2009).

In another study, a major proliferation-related growth factor PTHrP downregulated terminal differentia-tion–related genes in cultured mineralizing articular chondrocytes from the deep zone as well as in chondrogenic articular cartilage constructs (Jiang *et al.*, 2008). Overexpression of FGF-2 has been shown to enhance the survival and proliferation of human normal and OA chondrocytes, without stimulating the matrix synthetic processes (Cucchiarini *et al.*, 2009). However, these mitogenic properties of FGF-2 were associated with simultaneous co-overexpression of SOX9 and accompanied by an increase in the production of proteoglycans and type II collagen, and decreased expression of type X collagen, a marker of hypertrophy (Cucchiarini *et al.*, 2009). It is worth to note here that growth factors, which were capable of inhibiting collagen degradation in OA articular cartilage, are predominantly expressed in the proliferative zone of the growth plate and are required for chondrocyte proliferation in the development.

Similar effect on suppression of collagen cleavage in association with inhibition of chondrocyte hypertrophy-related genes and proinflammatory cytokines IL-1β and TNFα has been observed on treatment of OA cartilage explants with low concentrations of PGE2 (Tchetina *et al.*, 2007a). Although PGE2 is expressed in all the growth plate zones, it is primarily required for fetal chondrocyte proliferation (Brochhausen *et al.*, 2006) and is capable also of inhibiting their terminal differentiation (Li *et al.*, 2004b; Zhang *et al.*, 2004) and expression of proinflammatory mediators (Akaogi *et al.*, 2006). At the same, time PGE2 at higher concentrations has been shown to exert stimulating effects on cartilage degradation (Attur *et al.*, 2008).

Alternatively, downregulation of the genes, which are expressed in the hypertrophic zone of the growth plate and associated with chondrocyte terminal differentiation such as Hedgehog signaling, TGFβ1/BMP signaling, transforming growth factor –beta activated kinase (TAK) 1, cyclin-dependent kinase inhibitor p16INK4a, ADAMTS5, Runx2, and caspases, resulted in abrogation of matrix degeneration, less type X collagen production, and MMP-13 expression (Zhou *et al.*, 2004; D'Lima *et al.*, 2006; Scharstuhl *et al.*, 2003; Lin *et al.*, 2009; Araldi *et al.*, 2010; Glasson *et al.*, 2005; Kamekura *et al.*, 2006; Klatt *et al.*, 2006).

Although CTGF has been shown to be able of repairing cartilage defects in experimental OA in animal studies in vivo (Fu *et al.*, 2010; Nishida *et al.*,2004), downregulation of CTGF expression might ameliorate human knee OA condition as increased CTGF concentration in plasma and synovial fluid positively correlated with radiographic disease severity (Honsawek *et al.*, 2010).Therefore, upregulation of the genes associated with growth plate chondrocyte proliferation or downregulation of hypertrophy-related genes favors acquisition of healthier phenotype in OA articular chondrocytes (Figure 1).

However, while direct inhibition of cartilage degradation by the agents capable of regulating chondrocyte differentiation is an attractive means to counteract articular cartilage degeneration in OA, it has several limitations. Thus, following the inhibition of cartilage degradation by individual growth factors (GF) reparation of articular cartilage in OA in vivo may require a combination of GF (Attur *et al.*, 2011; Weisser *et al.*, 2001; Yamamoto *et al.*, 2004). For example, being the most efficient in suppressing OA articular cartilage destruction (Tchetina *et al.*, 2006), TGFβ2 alone may not be capable of restoring the anabolic functions in healthy articular cartilage since it has been reported to downregulate type II collagen and aggrecan synthesis (Bohme *et al.*, 1995; Elford *et al.*, 1992). In contrast, in responsive individuals insulin may facilitate tissue repair, as it is a principal anabolic agent in the articular cartilage (Trippel, 2004). FGF-2 can also promote cartilage repair (Yamamoto *et al.*, 2004) by itself or inducing local TGFβ or its own expression (Shida *et al.*, 2001). In addition, combinations of these and other growth factors

FETAL GROWTH PLATE

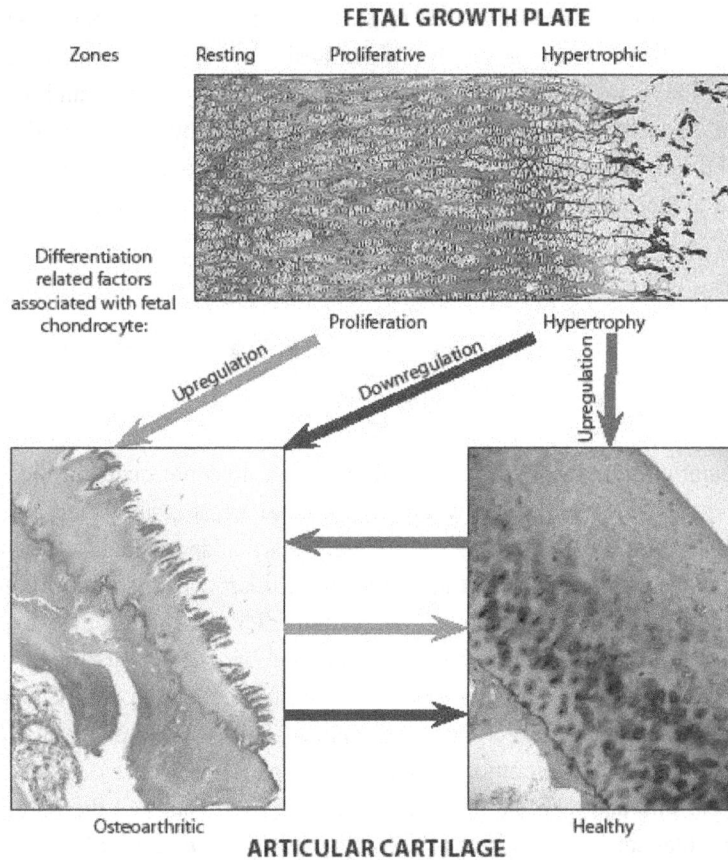

Figure 1: Mechanisms of articular cartilage destruction and recovery in osteoarthritis. Fetal growth plate is divided into zones: resting, proliferative, and hypertrophic. OA-related changes in healthy articular cartilage occur on upregulation of fetal chondrocyte hypertrophy-associated differentiation factors (red arrows). In contrast, upregulation of fetal chondrocyte proliferation-associated factors (green arrows) and/or downregulation of hypertrophy-associated differentiation factors (blue arrows) in OA articular cartilage result in suppression of OA-related traits producing healthier phenotype.

have been shown to produce synergistic effect in maintaining synthesis of matrix molecules in articular and growth plate chondrocytes (Bohme *et al.*, 1995; Yaeger *et al.*, 1997; Barbero *et al.*, 2004).

Another concern on GF application for therapy is related to their possible catabolic effects. Although no evidence has been obtained that TGFβ2 can act catabolically in human OA articular cartilage (Tchetina *et al.*, 2006) destructive potential of this growth factor at high concentration was observed in normal articular cartilge in vivo after its intraarticular injections, which produced joint swelling, fibroblastic proliferation of synovial membrane, and profound loss of articular cartilage proteoglycan in rabbit joints (Elford *et al.*, 1992).Therefore, the delivery of exact therapeutic amount of the growth factor to the site of articular cartilage destruction may be important. This has been demonstrated in a recent study, where deleterious effect of TGFβ1 capable of inducing synovial fibrosis and osteophyte formation has been counteracted by combined overexpression of TGFβ1 and its inhibitor Smad7 (Blaney Davidson *et al.*, 2006). This resulted both in prevention of proteoglycan (PG) loss and in increase in PG content in mouse OA cartilage.

Moreover, the response to TGFβ appeared to be age related as it has been shown that in the cartilage of young mice TGFβ stimulated proteoglycan synthesis, while in old mice reduced stimulation of aggrecan synthesis by TGFβ was associated with a loss in ALK5 expression, and an IL-1-mediated decrease of TGFβ type II receptor expression (Blaney Davidson et al., 2005; Pujol et al., 2008).

Therefore, TGFβ indeed maintains chondrocyte and cartilage homeostasis although changes in differentiation stage and associated alterations in receptor expression could modify the effect of TGFβ on chondrocyte function.

8   Induction of OA-related Changes in Healthy Articular Cartilage is Associated with Chondrocyte Hypertrophy

In healthy adult articular cartilage, chondrocyte differentiation does not occur in the non-calcified cartilage zone (Babarina et al., 2001). However, when maturational arrest is abolished, chondrocyte differentiation-related genes, which are barely expressed in healthy articular cartilage, become upregulated followed by hypertrophic changes in the cells and extracellular matrix. If this notion is true, stimulation of degradation in healthy articular cartilage should be accompanied by chondrocyte hypertrophy development. The relieve of transcriptional repression can be attained by cartilage treatment with azacytidine C (Aza-C), which replaces cytidine bases in genomic DNA during replication and disturbs methylation pattern of cytidines (CpG islands) in target gene promoters. This was associated with upregulation of PTHrP, governing chondrocyte proliferation in the growth plate, as well as chondrocyte hypertrophy-related type X collagen, Ihh, and alkaline phosphatase gene expression, and the increase in chondrocyte cell size in healthy articular cartilage (Cheung et al., 2001; Zuscik et al., 2004; Ho et al., 2006).

Functional disturbances in the regulatory genes involved in chondrocyte differentiation can also produce OA-related changes in healthy articular cartilage resembling chondrocyte maturation in the growth plate. Thus, deficiency in TGFβ signaling, which is essential for articular cartilage maintenance and had been induced either by over-expression of functionless TGFβ type II receptor (Serra et al., 1997) or by deletion of Smad3 signaling (Yang et al., 2001; Li et al., 2006) caused accelerated chondrocyte differentiation associated with type X collagen expression and OA-like changes in articular cartilage. It has been also shown that the absence of signaling through Fgfr (fibroblast growth factor receptor) 3 in the joints of Fgfr3(-/-) mice produced premature cartilage degeneration and early arthritis (Valverde-Franco et al., 2006). Similar maturation-dependent changes involving COL10A1 and ADAMTS5 upregulation, and downregulation of aggrecan expression were observed on inhibition of NAD+ dependent deacetylase, SIRT1 in human studies, or nuclear factor of activated T-cells (Nfat1) deficiency in mice (Fujita et al., 2011; Schroeppel et al., 2011).

In contrast, upregulation of specific regulatory molecules have been also shown to produce OA-like phenotypes in articular chondrocytes. For example, TGFα signaling suggests a catabolic potential of this growth factor as it has been shown to stimulate articular chondrocyte proliferation, formation of cell clusters followed by expression of matrix degrading enzymes MMP-13, cathepsin C and downregulation of Sox9, as well as collagen and aggrecan expression in rat articular osteochondral explants (Appleton et al., 2007b).Similar maturation dependent changes were observed in bovine immature articular cartilage explants after their treatment by FGF2 and TGFβ1 in combination (Khan et al.,2011). Treatment of cultured chondrocytes with BMP-2 resulted in increased β-catenin nuclear translocation and upregulation of a low-density-lipoprotein receptor-related protein 5 (LRP-5) mediated by Smad1/5/8 binding on LRP-5 promoter. This was accompanied by upregulation of type X collagen and MMPs expression (Schroeppel *et al.*, 2011; Papathanasiou *et al.*,2012). Treatment of normal chondrocytes with 1,25-dihydroxyvitamin D(3) (1a,25(OH)(2)D(3)), which has been shown to play an intracrine role of 1,25(OH)(2)D(3) in endochondral ossification and chondrocyte development in vivo (Naja *et al.*, 2009), or Pi resulted in significant upregulation of hypertrophy markers type X collagen, osteopontin, osteocalcin, as well as catabolic markers metalloproteinase-13, and the apoptotic marker caspase-9 (Naja *et al.*, 2009; Orfanidou *et al.*, 2012). Similar effects were observed during normal articular chondrocyte treatment by polyamines, lectin-like oxidized low-density lipoprotein (Ox-LDL) receptor 1 (LOX-1), or hypoxia-inducible factor-2alpha (Facchini *et al.*, 2012; Kishimoto *et al.*, 2010; Saito *et al.*, 2010).

On the other hand, alterations associated with chondrocyte hypertrophy in the growth plate are always ac-companied by overt extracellular matrix resorption producing its degradation fragments (Poole, 2005). Therefore, it is not surprising that collagen and/or fibronectin degrading peptides, which can be also released on mechanical destruction of articular cartilage caused by trauma or joint overload in case of anterior cruciate ligament transection, have been shown to be capable of inducing articular cartilage degradation by upregulation of collagenase and MMPs activity (Yasuda *et al.*, 2006; Yasuda & Poole, 2002; Homandberg, 2001). Besides, these peptides upregulated chondrocyte proliferation, production of type X collagen and apoptotic cells on the surface of articular cartilage explants (Homandberg, 2001; Tchetina *et al.*, 2007). Collagen fragments may also account for OA-like changes induced in healthy cartilage by over-expression of MMP-13, which were associated with chondocyte hypertrophy in mouse articular cartilage (Neuhold *et al.*, 2001). In addition, other matrix disturbances such as lack of matrilin-3 by a corresponding gene knockout produced premature chondrocyte maturation to hypertrophy and formed predisposition to develop severe OA in mice (van der Weyden *et al.*, 2006).

Being an important factor of OA articular cartilage pathology proinflammatory cytokines such as TNFα and IL-1β have been shown to mediate articular cartilage degradation by upregulation of matrix degrading MMPs (Goldring & Marcu, 2009). Several other cytokines including IL-6, IL-15, IL-17, IL-18, IL-21, leukemia inhibitory factor and IL-8 (a chemokine) have also been shown to be implicated in OA (Kapoor *et al.*, 2011). It has been observed recently that increased expression of proinflammatory agents such as TNFα, chemokine IL-8, growth-related oncogene (GRO)α, or the multiligand receptor for advanced glycation end products (RAGE) also induced chondrocyte hypertrophy evidenced by type X collagen expression (Cecil *et al.*, 2005; Merz *et al.*, 2003). This suggests a link between inflammation and altered differentiation in articular chondrocytes (Merz *et al.*, 2003). Interestingly, the impairment of TGFβ signaling by IL-1β was mediated by downregulation of TGFβRII (Baugé *et al.*, 2007). The loss of function of this receptor has been previously linked to chondrocyte hypertrophy induction and OA development in animal studies (Serra *et al.*, 1997).

In view of this it is worth to mention a dual role of nuclear factor kappa-light-chain-enhancer of activated B cells (NF-κB) transcription factor. Being induced by various inducers, including reactive oxygen species, TNFα, and IL-1β, NFkB positively regulates genes encoding cytokines, their receptors, and growth regulators (Marcu *et al.*, 2010). In human chondrocytes downregulation of NFkB induced by proinflammatory cytokines resulted both in repression of MMP-13 and induction of COL2A1 (Fan *et al.*, 2006), as well as produces upregulation of apoptotic activity mediated by downregulation of FGF2 and Bcl-2 (Kim *et al.*, 2012). This indicates that NFkB is required for cell survival but detrimental when it is deregulated.

Therefore, OA-like alterations in healthy articular cartilage induced by the mediators, which are upregulated in the hypertrophic zone during endochondral ossification, are accompanied by ECM degradation and associated with articular chondrocyte hypertrophy (Figure 1).

9   Implications to Future Therapies

The disability in OA is related to pain, reduced mobility and is thought to be primarily due to articular cartilage degeneration. However, inhibition of cartilage destruction by abrogation of local proteolysis of aggrecan and collagen by genetic manipulation in animal studies has only reduced experimental disease severity, subchondral bone thickness and pain while osteophyte development was not affected (Glasson, 2007; Little&Fosang, 2010; Botter et al., 2009). Moreover, clinical trials applying an inhibitor of proteinases or inflammatory cytokines have been also thus far unsuccessful (Botter et al., 2009; Bondeson, 2011; Chevalier et al., 2006). Therefore, identification of upstream factors that regulate the expression of catabolic molecules and/or chondrocyte hypertrophy in articular cartilage is important for a more sophisticated understanding of the regulatory mechanisms that control the function of articular chondrocytes (Schroeppel et al., 2011).

Previous studies have reported that the majority of the identified genes involved in OA encode signal-transduction proteins (Rousseau & Delmas, 2007; Wu et al., 2012). Signal transduction pathways are flexible and therefore potentially amenable to intervention and modification (Scanzello et al., 2008). Numerous signaling pathways have been shown to regulate chondrocyte activities. They involve Wnt/β-catenin pathway, the hypoxia-inducible factor (HIF)-1α/β pathway, the transforming growth factor (TGF) β/BMP pathway, the nuclear factor (NF)-kB cytokine pathway, the p38, JNK, and ERK MAP -kinase, the PI-3 kinase-Akt pathway, the Jak-STAT pathway, and Rho GTFase pathway, Toll-like receptor (TLR) pathway, and the thyroid pathway as well as apoptotic-related molecules (Wu et al., 2012; Scanzello et al., 2008; Marcu et al., 2010; Valdes&Spector, 2010).

Signaling molecules that regulate chondrocyte activities both in the growth plate and adult articular car-tilage during osteoarthritis could be of particular interest (Dreier, 2010). For example, the activation of ERK1/2 phosphorylation and suppression of p38 phosphorylation resulted in hypertrophic differentiation of articular cartilage chondrocytes (Prasadam et al., 2010; Li et al., 2010). However, targeting signaling pathways in osteoarthritis might be not easy due to their high variety and crosstalk (Berenbaum, 2004). For example, direct targeting of beta-catenin might be risky, because of its importance for the maintenance of articular chondrocyte phenotype stability and involvement in carcinogenesis (Blom, 2010).

With this regard, it is more convenient to track nutrient signaling pathways, which have been recently shown to be linked to 7 of the top 10 causes of sickness and death in North America including heart disease, obesity, several cancers, diabetes and others (Walker&Blackburn, 2004). Traditionally, nutrients such as amino acids, carbohydrates and lipids have been viewed as substrates for generation of high-energy molecules and as precursors for the biosynthesis of macromolecules. However at present it is apparent that nutrients can function as signaling molecules in nutrient sensing transduction pathways, which regulate various aspects of energy metabolism and control cell growth, proliferation, and survival (Marshall, 2006). In humans gene expression is regulated by nutrients interacting with signaling pathways involving primarily mammalian target of rapamycin (mTOR), hexosamine, and peroxisome proliferator activator proteins (PPARs) (Marshall, 2006; Maloney & Rees, 2005).

mTOR is considered a key regulator of cell growth and proliferation (Hay & Sonnenberg, 2004), which expression has been reported both in fetal chondrocytes in animal studies (Bohensky *et al.*, 2010; Kim *et al.*, 2009; Sanchez & He, 2009) and human articular chondrocytes (Cejka *et al.*, 2010). Nutrients, such as amino acids and glucose, acting through mTOR directly influence chondrocyte differentiation and long bone growth (Phornphutkul *et al.*, 2008). Moreover treatment of mice by mTOR inhibitors, ra-pamycin or its analogs, has been recently shown to reduce the severity of experimental osteoarthritis (Carames *et al.*, 2010, 2012) and inflammatory arthritis (Cejka *et al.*, 2010; Laragione & Gulko, 2010).

mTOR inhibition on cessation of growth is accompanied by activation of autophagy (Raught *et al.*, 2001), which was originally shown to affect fetal growth plate chondrocyte differentiation (Shapiro *et al.*, 2005) and was also observed in OA articular chondrocytes (Bohensky *et al.*, 2010; Carames *et al.*, 2010). This process occurs in lysosomes and favors cellular survival (Wei *et al.*, 2008; Lotz&Caramés, 2011).

Another important nutrient signaling pathway in OA development and progression might be a hexosamine signaling pathway. This pathway functions as a glucose sensor coupled to a transductional cascade that directly regulates intracellular energy metabolism. Uridine diphosphate- N-acetylglucosamine, which is generated through the conversion of fructose-6-phosphate through glucosa-mine-6-phosphate, serves as precursor for the formation of complex glycosylated proteins and lipids (Marshall, 2006). Glucosamine is an amino sugar that is widely used to relieve symptoms associated with OA. It has been shown to decrease both fetal and articular chondrocyte proliferation, differentiation, and mineralization (Nakatani *et al.*, 2007; Terry *et al.*, 2007). Glucosamine capacity to downregulate catabol-ic enzymes, such as MMPs and aggrecanases, and pro-inflammatory mediators, as well as to induce pro-anabolic hyaluronic acid was also observed in vitro (Piperno *et al.*,2000; Gouze *et al.*, 2006; Igarashi *et al.*, 2011). However, clinical trials show it equivocal efficacy. Some studies reported a decrease for pain and reduction of knee joint space loss (Pavelká *et al.*, 2002). These could be associated with induction of tissue TGFβ1 and CTGF expression, as well as reduction of a marker of degradation, cartilage oligomeric matrix protein (Petersen *et al.*, 2010; Ali *et al.*, 2011). However, the structure-modifying effect of glu-cosamine on OA joints remains controversial as the majority of clinical trials reported numerous non-responders or the absence of the effect compared to non-pharmacological means, such as exercise or weight loss (Durmus *et al.*, 2012; Henrotin *et al.*, 2012). Moreover, increased flux through the hex-osamine signaling pathway enhances glycosylation of transcrip-tion factors that regulate expression of proteins that are involved in controlling the insulin-responsive glucose transport system, namely induc-tion of insulin resistance often observed in OA patients (Marshall, 2006).

Lipids are sensed through binding to the peroxisome proliferator activator protein subfamily of nuclear hormone receptors (PRARs). These receptors modulate lipid and glucose metabolism by acting as transcriptional activators following fatty acid binding (Kota *et al.*, 2005). Activation of PPAR-gamma in growth plate chondrocytes inhibited terminal differentiation and promoted apoptosis (Shao *et al.*, 2005; Stanton *et al.*, 2010). PPARs expression was also observed in adult articular cartilage tissue and has been shown to counteract IL-1 effects in animal and human studies (Bordji *et al.*, 2000; Kobayashi *et al.*, 2005c; Clockaerts *et al.*, 2011).

Further understanding of the molecular mechanisms involved in nutrient signaling might open opportu-nities for identification of targets for therapeutic intervention, which hopefully will lead to safe and effective therapies that reduce the symptoms and slow the progression of OA.

10 Concluding Remarks

The data presented here shows a significant progress in our understanding of molecular mechanisms of articular cartilage degradation in OA. They involve at least in part similar machinery of extracellular matrix resorption in the hypertrophic zone of the growth plate and in OA articular cartilage in the course of its degeneration. The observation that profound cellular phenotypic changes in articular chondrocytes occur prior the overt cartilage matrix degradation monitored histologically suggests that articular chondrocyte phenotype modifications can be recognized very early in the disease at gene expression level favoring timely disease recognition, which could help its prevention. This implies also innovative opportunities in suppression of cartilage matrix degradation targeting inhibition of chondrocyte hypertrophy and suggests new targets for therapeutic intervention. For this purpose, further studies are required in search of new agents generating programmable articular chondrocyte phenotype modification.

List of Abbreviations

OA:	Osteoarthritis
ECM:	Extracellular matrix
MMP:	Metalloproteinases
IL:	Interleukin
ADAMTS:	A disintegrin and metalloprotease with thrombospondin motifs
PTHrP:	Parathyroid hormone related peptide
TNF:	Tumor necrosis factor
ALP:	Alkaline phosphatase
PCNA:	Proliferating cell nuclear antigen
SLRPs:	Small leucine-rich proteoglycans
BMP:	Bone morphogenetic protein
FGF:	Fibroblast growth factor
TGF:	Transforming growth factor
TGFR:	Transforming growth factor receptor
IGF:	Insulin growth factor
Bcl-2:	B-cell lymphoma 2
Sox9:	SRY-type high-mobility-group box transcription factor-9
GADD45beta:	Growth arrest and DNA damage-inducible 45beta
Bag1:	Bcl2-associated athanogen 1, a Bcl2 –binding protein capable ofenhancing Bcl2 activity
COL10A1:	Type X collagen
BMP:	Bone morphogenetic proteins
CTGF:	Connective tissue growth factor
VEGF:	Vascular endothelial growth factor
Ihh:	Indian hedgehog
RUNX2:	Runt-related transcription factor
COL2A1:	Type II collagen
Ank:	Ankylosis protein
PGE2:	Prostaglandin E2

Gas1:	Growth arrest specific protein1
Aza-C:	Azacytidine C
Fgfr3:	Fibroblast growth factor receptor 3
RAGE:	Multiligand receptor for advanced glycation end products
GRO:	Growth-related oncogene
PG:	Proteoglycan
TAK:	Transforming growth factor –beta activated kinase
GF:	Growth factor
mTOR:	Mammalian target of rapamycin
PPAR:	Peroxysome proliferator activator protein
HIF	Hypoxia inducible factor
LRP-5:	Low-density-lipoprotein receptor-related protein 5
NF-κB:	Nuclear factor kappa-light-chain-enhancer of activated B cells
ALK:	Activin receptor-like kinase
Smad:	Sma and Mad Related Family proteins

Acknowledgments

This chapter represents an updated and extended version of the review article by E.V. Tchetina "Developmental mechanisms in articular cartilage degradation in osteoarthritis" published in Arthritis 2011,2011:683970 (Hindawi Publishing Corporation). The study was supported by the Russian Foundation for Basic Research (projects no. 09-04-01158a and 12-04-00038a to EVT)

References

Abramson, S.B. &Attur, M. (2009).Developments in the scientificunderstanding of osteoarthritis.Arthritis Research & Therapy, 11, 227.

Aigner, T.&Gerwin, N.(2007). Growth plate cartilage as developmental model in osteoarthritis research-potentials and limitations. Current Drug Targets, 8, 377-385.

Aigner, T. & McKenna, L. (2002). Molecular pathology andpathobiology of osteoarthritic cartilage.Cellular & Molecular Life Sciences, 59, 5-18.

Aigner, T., Haag, J., Martin, J., &Buckwalter, J. (2007). Osteoarthritis: agingof matrix and cells- going to a remedy. Current Drug Targets, 8, 325-331.

Aigner, T., Hemmel, M., Neureiter, D., Gebhard, P.M., Zeiler, G., Kirchner,T., &McKenna, L. (2001). Apoptotic cell death is not a widespread phenomenon in normal aging and osteoarthritis human articular knee cartilage: a study of proliferation, programmed celldeath (apoptosis), and viability of chondrocytes in normal and osteoarthritic human knee-cartilage. Arthritis and Rheumatism, 44:1304-1312.

Aigner, T., Zien, A., Gehrsitz, A., Gebhard, P.M., &McKenna, I. (2001).Anabolic and catabolic geneexpression pattern analysis in normal versus osteoarthritic cartilage using complementary DNA-array technology. Arthritis&Rheumatism, 44, 2777-2789.

Aigner, T., Zien, A., Hanisch, D.,& Zimmer, R. (2003). Gene expression inchondrocytes assessed with useof microarrays.Journal of Bone &Joint Surgery American, 85-A Suppl 2,117-123.

Akaogi, J., Nozaki, T., Satoh, M., &Yamada, H. (2006). Role of PGE2 and EPreceptors in the pathogenesisof rheumatoid arthritis and as a novel therapeutic strategy.Endocrine, Metabolic & Immune Disorders Drug Targets, 6, 383-394.

Akiyama, H., Chaboissier, M.C., Martin, J.F., Schedl, A., &deCrombrugghe, B. (2002). The transcriptionfactor Sox9 has essential roles in successive steps of the chondrocyte differentiation pathway and is required for expression ofSox5 and Sox6. Genes&Development, 16, 2813-2828.

Ali, A.A., Lewis, S.M., Badgley, H.L., Allaben, W.T., &Leakey, J.E.(2011). Oral glucosamine increasesexpression of transforming growth factor β1 (TGFβ1) and connectivetissue growth factor (CTGF) mRNA in rat cartilage andkidney: implications for human efficacyand toxicity.Archives of Biochemistry & Biophysics, 510, 11-18.

Alvarez, J., Costales, L., Serra, R., Balbín, M., &López, J.M. (2005).Expression patterns of matrixmetalloproteinases and vascular endothelial growth factor during epiphyseal ossification.Journal of Bone & Mineral Research, 20, 1011-1021.

Amizuka, N., Warshawsky, H., Henderson, J.E., Goltzman, D., &Karaplis, A.C. (1994). Parathyroidhormone-related peptide-depleted mice show abnormal epiphysealcartilage development and altered endochondral boneformation. Journal of Cell Biology, 126,1611-1623.

Anderson, H.C., Hodges, P.T., Aguilera, X.M., Missana, L., &Moylan, P.E. (2000). Bone morphogeneticprotein (BMP) localization in developing human and rat growth plate, metaphysis, epiphysis, and articular cartilage. Journal ofHistochemistry & Cytochemistry, 48, 1493-1502.

Appleton, C.T., McErlain, D.D., Pitelka, V., Schwartz, N., Bernier, S.M., Henry, J.L., Holdsworth, D.W.& Beier, F. (2007). Forced mobilization accelerates pathogenesis: characterization of a preclinical surgical model of osteoarthritis.Arthritis Research and Therapy, 9, R13.

Appleton, C.T., Usmani, S.E., Bernier, S.M., Aigner, T., &Beier, F. (2007). Transforming growth factoralpha suppressionof articular chondrocyte phenotype and Sox9 expression in a rat model of osteoarthritis. Arthritis&Rheumatism, 56, 3693-3705.

Araldi, E., Shipani, E. (2010). MicroRNA-140 and silencing of osteoarthritis. Genes & Development,24,1075-1080.

Armstrong, A.L., Barrach, H.J., &Ehrlich, M.G. Identification of the metalloproteinase stromelysin inthe physis. Journal of Orthopedic Research, 20, 289-294.

Attur, M., Al-Mussawir, H.E., Patel, J., Kitay, A., Dave, M., Palmer, G., Pillinger, M.H., &Abramson, S.B. (2008). Prostaglandin E2 exerts catabolic effects in osteoarthritis cartilage: evidence for signaling via the EP4 receptor.Journalof Immunology, 181, 5082-5088.

Attur, M., Belitskaya-Lévy, I., Oh. C., Krasnokutsky, S., Greenberg, J., Samuels, J.,Smiles, S., Lee, S., Patel,J., Al-Mussawir, H., McDaniel, G., Kraus, V.B., &Abramson, S.B. (2011). Increased interleukin-1β gene expression in peri-pheral blood leukocytes is associated with increased pain and predicts risk for progression of symptomatic knee osteoarthritis.Arthritis & Rheumatism, 63, 1908-1917.

Babarina, A.V., Möllers, U., Bittner, K., Vischer, P., &Bruckner, P. (2001). Role of the subchondral vascular system in endochondral ossification: endothelial cell-derived proteinases derepress late cartilage differentiation in vitro. Matrix Biology, 20, 205-213.

Ballock, R.T., Heydemann, A., Wakefield. L.M., Flanders, K.C., Roberts, A.B., &Sporn, M.B. (1993). TGFbeta 1 prevents hypertrophy of epiphyseal chondrocytes: regulation of gene expression for cartilage matrix proteins and metalloproteases. Developmental Biology, 158, 414-429.

Barbero, A., Grogan, S., Schafer, D., Heberer, M., Mainil-Varlet, P., &Martin I. (2004). Age related changes in human articular chondrocyte yield, proliferation and post-expansion chondrogenic capacity. Osteoarthritis &Cartilage,12, 476-484.

Baugé, C., Legendre, F., Leclercq, S., Elissalde, J.M., Pujol, J.P., Galéra, P., &Boumédiene, K. (2007). Inter-leukin-1beta impairment of transforming growth factor beta1 signaling by down-regulation of transforming growth factor betareceptor type II and up-regulation of Smad7 in human articular chondrocytes. Arthritis & Rheumatism, 56, 3020-3032.

Bay-Jenson, A.C., Andersen, T.L., Charni-Ben Tabassi, N., Kristensen, P.W., Kjaersgaard-Andersen, P.,Sandell, L., Garnero, P., &deLaisse, J.M. (2008). Biochemical markers of type II collagen breakdown and synthesis are positionned at specific sites in human osteoarthritic knee cartilage. Osteoarthritis & Cartilage, 16, 615-623.

Beier, F., Ali, Z., Mok, D., Taylor, A.C., Leask, T., Albanese, C., Pestell, R.G., &LuValle, P. (2001).TGFbetaand PTHrP control chondrocyte proliferation by activating cyclin D1 expression. Molecular Biology of the Cell, 12, 3852-3863.

Berenbaum, F. (2004). Signalingtransduction: target in osteoarthritis.Current Opinion in Rheumatology, 16, 616-622.

Bi, W., Huang, W., Whitworth, D.J., Deng, J.M., Zhang, Z., Behringer, R.R., &de Crombrugghe, B. (2001).Haploinsufficiency of Sox9 results in defective cartilage primordia and premature skeletal mineralization. Proceedings of National Academy of Sciences of the United States of America, 98, 6698-6703.

Billinghurst, R.C., Dahlberg, L., Ionescu, M., Reiner, A., Bourne, R., Rorabeck, R., Mitchell, P., Hambor, J., Diekmann, O., Tschesche, H., Chen, J., van Wart, H., &Poole, A.R. (1997). Enhanced cleavage of type II collagen bycol-lagenases in osteoarthritic cartilage. Journal of Clinical Investigation, 99, 1534–1545.

Blanco, F.J., Guitian, R., Vazquez-Martul, E.,de Toro, F.J., &Galdo, F. (1998). Osteoarthritis chondrocytesdie by apoptosis: a possible pathway for osteoarthritis pathology. Arthritis &Rheumatism, 41, 284-289.

Blaney Davidson, E.N., Scharstuhl, A., Vitters, E.L., van der Kraan, P.M., &van den Berg, W.B.Reduced transforming growth factor-beta signaling in cartilage of old mice: role in impaired repair capacity. Arthritis Research& Therapy, 7, R1338-R1347.

Blaney Davidson, E.N., Vitters, E.L., van der Kraan, P.M., &van den Berg, W.B. (2006). Expression of transforming growth factor-beta (TGFbeta) and the TGFbeta signalling molecule SMAD-2P in spontaneous and instability-induced osteoarthritis: role in cartilage degradation, chondrogenesis and osteophyte formation. Annals of Rheumatic Diseases, 65, 1414-1421.

Blom, A.B., van Lent, P.L., van der Kraan, P.M., &van den Berg, W.B. (2010). To seek shelter from theWNT in osteoarthritis? WNT-signaling as a target for osteoarthritis therapy.Current Drug Targets, 11, 620-629.

Bohensky, J., Leshinsky, S., Srinivas, V., &Shapiro, I.M. (2010). Chondrocyte autophagy is stimulatedby HIF-1 dependent AMPK activation and mTOR suppression.Pediatric Nephrology,25, 633-642.

Bohme, K., Winterhalter, K.H., &Bruckner, P. (1995). Terminal differentiation of chondrocytes is a spontaneous process and is arrested by transforming growth factor-beta-2 and basic fibroblast growth factor in synergy. Experimental Cell Research, 216, 191-198.

Bondeson, J. (2011). Are we moving in the right direction with osteoarthritis drug discovery? Expert Opinionon Therapeutic Targets, 15, 1355-1368.

Borden, P., Solymar, D., Sucharczuk, A., Lindman, B., Cannon, P., &Heller, R.A. (1996). Cytokine controlof interstitial collagenase and collagenase 3 gene expression in human chondrocytes. Journal of Biological Chemistry, 271,23577-23581.

Bordji, K., Grillasca, J.P., Gouze, J.N., Magdalou, J., Schohn, H., Keller, J.M., Bianchi, A., Dauça, M.,Netter, P., &Terlain, B. (2000). Evidence for the presence of peroxisome proliferator-activated receptor (PPAR) alpha andgamma and retinoid Z receptor in cartilage. PPARgamma activation modulates the effects of interleukin-1beta on rat chondrocytes.Journal of Biological Chemistry, 275, 12243-12250.

Borzi, R.M., Olivotto, E., Pagani, S., Vitellozzi, R., Neri, S., Battistelli, M., Falcieri, E., Facchin, A., Flamigni,F.,Penzo, M., Platano, D., Santi, S., Facchini, A., &Marcu, K.B. (2010). MMP-13 loss associated with impaired ECM remodelling disrupts chondrocyte differentiation by concerted effects on multiple regulatory factors.Arthritis & Rheumatism, 62,2370-2381.

Bos, P.K., van Osch, J.V.M., Frenz, D.A., Verhaar, J.A.N., &Verwoerd-Verhoef, H.L. (2001). Growth factor expression in cartilage wound healing: temporal and spatial immunolocalization in a rabbit auricular cartilage wound model.Osteoarthritis & Cartilage, 9, 382-389.

Botter, S.M., Glasson, S.S., Hopkins, B., Clockaerts, S., Weinans, H., van Leeuwen, J.P., &van Osch, G.J.(2009). ADAMTS5-/- mice have less subchondral bone changes after induction of osteoarthritis through surgical instability:implications for a link between cartilage and subchondral bone changes. Osteoarthritis& Cartilage,17, 636-645.

Brew, C.J., Clegg, P.D., Boot-Handford, R.P., Andrew, J.G., &Hardingham, T. (2010). Gene expression inhuman chondrocytes in late osteoarthritis is changed in both fibrillated and intact cartilage without evidence of generalizedchondrocyte hypertrophy. Annals of Rheumatic Diseases, 69, 234-240.

Brochhausen, C., Neuland, P., Kirkpatrick, C.J., Nüsing, R.M., &Klaus, G. (2006). Cyclooxygenasesand prostaglandin E2 receptors in growth plate chondrocytes in vitro and in situ--prostaglandin E2 dependent proliferation of growth plate chondrocytes. Arthritis Research & Therapy, 8, R78.

Buckwalter, J.A., &Mankin. H.J. (1998). Articular cartilage repair and transplantation.Arthritisand Rheumatism, 41, 1331-1342.

Burton, D.W., Foster, M., Johnson, K.A., Hiramoto, M., Deftos, L.J., &Terkeltaub, R.(2005). Chondrocytealcium-sensing receptor expression is up-regulated in early guinea pig knee osteoarthritis and modulates PTHrP, MMP-13, and-TIMP-3 expression.Osteoarthritis & Cartilage,13, 395-404.

Cancedda, R. & Garofalo, S. (2003). Depletion of cartilage collagen fibrils in mice carrying a dominant negative Col2al transgene affects chondrocyte differentiation. American Journal of Physiology- Cell Physiology, 285,1504-1512.

Carames, B., Hasegawa, A., Taniguchi, N., Miyaki, S., Blanco, F.J.,& Lotz, M. (2012). Autophagy activetion by rapamycin reduces severity of experimental osteoarthritis. Annals ofthe Rheumatic Diseases, 71, 575-581.

Carames, B., Taniguchi, N., Otsuki, S., Blanco, F.J., &Lotz, M. (2010). Autophagy is a protective mechanism in normal cartilage, and its aging-related loss is linked with cell death and osteoarthritis. Arthritis and Rheumatism, 62, 791-801.

Cecil, D.L., Johnson, K., Rediske, J., Lotz, M., Schmidt, A.M., &Terkeltaub, R. (2005). Inflammation-induced chondrocyte hypertrophy is driven by receptor for advanced glycation end products. Journal of Immunology, 175, 8296302.

Cejka, D., Hayer, S., Niederreiter, B., Sieghart, W., Fuereder, T., Zwerina, J., &Schett, G. (2010). Mammalian target of rapamycin signaling is crucial for joint destruction in experimental arthritis and is activated in osteoclasts from patients with rheumatoid arthritis. Arthritis &Rheumatism,62, 2294-2302.

Chen, C.G., Thuillier, D., Chin, E.N., &Alliston, T.(2012). Chondrocyte-intrinsic Smad3 represses Runx2-inducible matrix metalloproteinase 13 expression to maintain articular cartilage and prevent osteoarthritis. Arthritis & Rheumatism, 64, 3278-3289.

Chen, Q., Johnson, D.M., Haudenschild, D.R., &Goetinck, P.F. (1995). Progression and recapitulation of thechondrocyte differentiation program: cartilage matrix protein is a marker for cartilage maturation.Developmental Biology, 172, 293-306.

Chen, X., Macica, C.M., Nasiri, A., &Broadus, A.E. (2008). Regulation of articular chondrocyte proliferationand differentiation by Indian hedgehog and parathyroid hormone-related protein in mice. Arthritis &Rheumatism, 58, 3788-3797.

Cheung, J.O.P., Hillarby, M.C., Ayad, S., Hoyland, J.A., Jones, C.J., Denton, J., Thomas, J.T.,Wallis, G.A.&Grant, M.E. (2001). A novel cell culture model of chondrocyte differentiation during mammalian endochondral ossification.Journal of Bone &Mineral Research, 16, 309–318.

Chevalier, X., Mugnier, B., &Bouvenot, G.(2006). Targeted anti-cytokine therapies for osteoarthritis.Bulletin de l Academie Nationale de Medecine, 190, 1411-1420.

Chlebova, K., Bryja, V., Dvorak, P., Kozubik, A., Wilcox, W.R., &Krejci, P.(2009). High molecular weight FGF2: the biology of a nuclear growth factor.Cellular & Molecular Life Science , 66, 225-235.

Clockaerts ,S., Bastiaansen-Jenniskens, Y.M., Feijt, C., Verhaar. J.A., Somville, J., De Clerck, L.S., &Van Osch, G.J.(2011). Peroxisome proliferator activated receptor alpha activation decreases inflammatory and destructive responses in osteoarthritic cartilage.Osteoarthritis & Cartilage, 19, 895-902.

Cucchiarini. M., Terwilliger, E.F., Kohn, D., &Madry, H. (2009). Remodelling of human osteoarthriticcartilage by FGF-2, alone or combined with Sox9 via rAAV gene transfer. Journal of Cellular & Molecular Medicine, 13,2476-2488.

Dahlberg, L., Billinghurst, R.C., Manner, P., Nelson, F., Webb, G., Ionescu, M., Reiner, A., Tanzer, M.,Zukor, D., Chen, J., van Wart, H.E., &Poole, A.R. (2000). Selective enhancement of collagenase-mediated cleavage of residenttype II collagen in cultured osteoarthritic cartilage and arrest with a synthetic inhibitor that's speres collagenase (matrix metalloproteinase).Arthritis &Rheumatism, 43, 673–682.

Damron, T.A., Mathur, S., Horton, J.A., Strauss, J., Margulies, B., Grant, W., Farnum, C.E., &Spadaro,J.A. (2004). Temporal changes in PTHrP, Bcl-2, Bax, caspase, TGF-beta, and FGF-2 expression following growth plate irradiation with or without radioprotectant. Journal of Histochemistry & Cytochemistry, 52, 157-167.

de Crombrugghe, B., Lefebvre, V., Behringer, R.R., Bi, W., Murakami, S., &Huang, W. (2000).Transcriptional mechanisms of chondrocyte differentiation.Matrix Biology, 19, 389-394.

de Jong, H., Berlo, S.E., Hombrink, P., Otten, H.G., van Eden, W., Lafeber, F.P., Heurkens, A.H., Bijlsma,J.W., Glant, T.T., &Prakken, B.J. (2010). Cartilage proteoglycan aggrecan epitopes induce proimflammatory autoreactive T-cell responses in rheumatoid arthritis and osteoarthritis.Annals of the Rheumatic Diseases, 69, 255-262.

de los Rios, P. &Hill, D.J. (1999). Cellular localization and expression of insulin-like growth factors (IGFs) and IGF binding proteins within the epiphyseal growth plate of the ovine fetus: possible functional implications. Canadian Journal of Physiology & Pharmacology, 77, 235-249.

D'Lima, D., Hermida, J., Hashimoto, S., Colwell, C., &Lotz, M. (2006). Caspase inhibitors reduce severity of cartilage lesions in experimental osteoarthritis.Arthritis & Rheumatism, 54,1814-1821.

Domowicz, M.S., Cortes, M., Henry, J.G., &Schwartz, N.B. (2009). Aggrecan modulation of growth plate morphogenesis. Developmental Biology, 329, 242-257.

Dong, Y.F., Soung do, Y., Schwarz, E.M., O'Keefe, R.J., &Drissi. H. (2006). Wnt induction of hypertrophy through the Runx2 transcription factor. Journal of Cellular Physiology, 208, 77-86.

Dreier, R. (2010). Hypertrophic differentiation of chondrocytes in osteoarthritis: the developmental aspect of degenerative joint disorders. Arthritis Research & Therapy, 12, 216.

Drissi, H., Zuscik. M., Rosier, R., &O'Keefe, R. (2005). Transcriptional regulation of chondrocyte maturation: potential involvement of transcription factors in OA pathogenesis. Molecular Aspects of Medicine, 26, 169-179.

Ducy, P., Zhang, R., Geoffroy, V., Ridall, A.L., &Karsenty, G. (1997). Osf2/Cbfa1: a transcriptional activator of osteoblast differentiation. Cell, 89, 747-754.

Dumond, H., Presle, N., Pottie, P., Pacquelet, S., Terlain, B., Netter, P., Gepstein, A., Livne, E., & Jouzeau J.Y. (2004). Site specific changes in gene expression and cartilage metabolism during early experimental osteoarthritis. Osteoarthritis & Cartilage, 12, 284-295.

Durmus, D., Alayli, G., Aliyazicioglu, Y., Buyukakıncak, O., &Canturk, F.(2012). Effects of glucosamine sulfate and exercise therapy on serum leptin levels in patients with knee osteoarthritis: preliminary results of randomized controlled clinical trial.Rheumatology International, Apr 3. [Epub ahead of print].

Elford, P.R., Graeber, M., Ohtsu, H., Aeberhard, M., Legendre, B., Wishart, W.L., &MacKenzie, A.(2008). Induction of swelling, synovial hyperplasia and cartilage proteoglycan loss upon intra-articular injection of transforming growth factor-β2 in the rabbit. Cytokine, 4, 232-238.

Ellman, M.B., An, H.S., Muddasani, P., &Im, H.J.(2008). Biological impact of the fibroblast growth factor family on articular cartilage and intervertebral disc homeostasis. Gene, 420, 82-89.

Eyre, D.R., Weis, M.A., &Wu, J.J.(2006). Articular cartilage collagen: an irreplaceable framework?European Cells& Materials, 12, 57-63.

Facchini, A., Borzì, R.M., Olivotto, E., Platano, D., Pagani, S., Cetrullo, S., &Flamigni, F. (2012). Role of polyamines in hypertrophy and terminal differentiation of osteoarthritic chondrocytes. Amino Acids, 42:667-78.

Fan, Z., Yang, H., Bau, B., Söder, S., &Aigner T.(2006). Role of mitogen-activated protein kinases and NFkappaB on IL-1beta-induced effects on collagen type II, MMP-1 and 13 mRNA expression in normal articular human chondrocytes.Rheumatology International, 26, 900-903.

Fergusson, C.M., Schwarz, E.M., Reynolds, P.R., Puzas, J.E., Rosier, R.N., &O'Keefe, R.J. (2000). Smad2 and 3 mediate treansforming growth factor eta1-induced inhibition of chondrocyte maturation. Endocrinology, 141, 4728-4735.

Fernandes, J.C., Martel-Pelletier, J., Lascau-Coman, V., Moldovan, F., Jovanovic, D., Raynauld, J.P.,& Pelletier, J.P. (1998). Collagenase-1 and collagenase-3 synthesis in normal and early experimental osteoarthritic canine cartilage: an immunohistochemical study. Journal of Rheumatology, 25, 1585-1594.

Findlay, D.M. (2007).Vascular pathology and osteoarthritis.Rheumatology (Oxford), 46, 1763-1768.

Fu, J.J., Chu, T.W., Zhou, Y., &Liu, Y.G. (2010). Expression and its significance of connective tissue growth factor in articular cartilage during repair after full-thickness cartilage injury in young rabbit model.Xi Bao Yu Fen Zi Mian Yi Xue Za Zhi, 26, 132-134.

Fujita, N., Matsushita, T., Ishida, K., Kubo, S., Matsumoto, T., Takayama, K., Kurosaka, M., &Kuroda, R.(2011). Potential involvement of SIRT1 in the pathogenesis of osteoarthritis through the modulation of chondrocyte gene expressions. Journal of Orthopaedic Research, 29, 511-515.

Fukunaga, T., Yamashiro, T., Oya, S., Takeshita, N., Takigawa, M., &Takano-Yamamoto, T. (2003).Connective tissue growth factor mRNA expression pattern in cartilages is associated with their type I collagen expression.Bone, 33, 911-918.

Garnero, P., Ayral, X., Rousseau, J.C., Christgau, S., Sandell, L.J., Dougados, M., &Delmas, P.D. (2002).Uncoupling of type II collagen synthesis and degradation predicts progression of joint damage in patients with knee osteoarthritis. Arthritis & Rheumatism, 46, 2613-2624.

Gebauer, M., Saas, J., Haag, J., Dietz, U., Takigawa, M., Bartnik, E., &Aigner, T. (2005). Repression of anti-proliferative factor Tob1 in osteoarthritic cartilage.Arthritis Research & Therapy, 7, R274-R284.

Ghayor, C., Chadjichristos, C., Herrouin, J.F., Ala-Kokko, L., Suske, G., Pujol, J.P., &Galera, P. (2001). Sp3 represses the Sp1-mediated transactivation of the human COL2A1 gene in primary and de-differentiated chondrocytes.Journal of Biological Chemistry, 276, 36881-36895.

Ghosh, P., &Cheras, P.A. (2001). Vascular mechanisms in osteoarthritis. Best Practice & Research:Clinical Rheumatology, 15, 693-709.

Gill, R.K., Turner, R.T., Wronski, T.J., &Bell, N.H. (1998). Orchiectomy markedly reduces the concentration of the three isoforms of transforming growth factor beta in rat bone, and reduction is prevented by testosterone. Endocrinology,139, 546-550.

Girkontaite, I., Frischholz, S., Lammi, P., Wagner, K., Swoboda, B., Aigner, T., & von der Mark, K.(1996). Immunolocalization of type X collagen in normal fetal and adult osteoarthritic cartilage with monoclonal antibodies.Matrix Biology, 15, 231-238.

Glasson ,S.S., Askew, R., Sheppard, B., Carito, B., Blanchet, T., Ma, H.L., Flannery, C.R., Peluso, D. Kanki, K., Yang, Z., Majumdar, M.K., &Morris, E.A. (2005). Deletion of active ADAMTS5 prevents cartilage degradation in amurine model of osteoarthritis. Nature, 434, 644-648.

Glasson, S.S. (2007). In vivo osteoarthritis target validation utilizing genetically-modified mice. CurrentDrug Targets, 8, 367-376.

Goldring, M.B. & Marcu, K.B. (2009). Cartilage homeostasis in health and rheumatic diseases.Arthritis Research & Therapy, 11, 224.

Gomez-Barrena, E., Sanchez-Pernaute, O., Largo, R., Calvo, E., Esbrit, P., &Herrero-Beaumont, G. (2004). Sequential changes of parathyroid hormone related protein (PTHrP) in articular cartilage during progression of inflammatory and degenerative arthritis. Annals of the Rheumatic Diseases, 63, 917-922.

Gouze, J.N., Gouze, E., Popp, M.P., Bush, M.L., Dacanay, E.A., Kay, J.D., Levings, P.P., Patel, K.R., Saran, J.P.,Watson, R.S., &Ghivizzani, S.C.(2006). Exogenous glucosamine globally protects chondrocytes from the arthritogenic effects of IL-1beta.Arthritis Research & Therapy, 8, R173.

Grimsrud, C.D., Romano, P.R., D'Souza, M., Pusas, J.E., Reynolds, P.R., Rosier. R.N., &O'Keefe, R.J. (1999). BMP-6 is an autocrine stimulator of chondrocyte differentiation. Journal of Bone& Mineral Research, 14, 475-482.

Haeusler, G., Walter, I., Helmreich, M., Egerbacher, M. (2005). Localization of matrix metalloproteinases, (MMPs) their tissue inhibitors, and vascular endothelial growth factor (VEGF) in growth plates of children and adolescents indicates a role for MMPs in human postnatal growth and skeletal maturation. Calcified Tissue International, 76, 326-335.

Ham, A.V. & Cormack, D.H. (1987). Ham's histology. Philadelphia:Lippincott.

Hardingham, T.E., Fosang, A.J., &Dudhia, J. (1992). Aggrecan, the chondroitin sulfate/keratan sulfateproteoglycan from cartilage. In: Kuettner K et al, editors. Articular Cartilage and Osteoarthritis, New York: Raven Press.

Hattori, T., Muller, C., Gebhard, S., Bauer, E., Pausch, F., Schlund, B., Bosl, M.R., Hess, A., Surmann-Schmidt, C., von der Mark, H., de Crombrugghe, B., &von der Mark, K. (2010). SOX9 is a major negative regulator of cartilage vascularization, bone marrow formation and endochondral ossification. Development, 137, 901-911.

Hay, N. & Sonnenberg, N. (2004). Upstream and downstream of mTOR. Genes & Development,8, 1926-1945.

Heinegård, D.(2009). Proteoglycans and more--from molecules to biology.International Journal of Experimental Pathology, 90, 575-586.

Henrotin, Y., Mobasheri, A., &Marty, M.(2012). Is there any scientific evidence for the use of glucosamine in the management of human osteoarthritis?Arthritis Research & Therapy,14, 201.

Henson, F.M., Davies, M.E., Skepper, J.N., &Jeffcott, L.B. (1995). Localization of alkaline phosphatase inequine growth cartilage. Journal of Anatomy, 187 (Pt 1), 151-159.

Hiraki, Y., Inoue, H., Iyama, K, Kamizono, A., Ochiai, M., Shukunami, C., Iijima, S., Suzuki, F., &Kondo, J. (1997). Identification of chondromodulin I as a novel endothelial cell growth inhibitor. Purification and its localization in theavascular zone of epiphyseal cartilage. Journal of Biological Chemistry, 272, 32419-32426.

Ho, M.-L., Chang, J.-K., Wu, S.-C., Chung, Y.-H., Chen, C.-H., Hung, S.-H., &Wang, G.-J. (2006). A novel terminal differentiation model of human articular chondrocytes in three-dimensional cultures mimicking chondrocytic changes inosteoarthritis. Cell Biology International, 30, 288–294.

Hollander, A.P., Pidoux, I., Reiner, A., Rorabeck, C., Bourne, R., Poole, A.R. (1995). Damage to type IIcollagen in aging and osteoarthritis starts at the articular surface, originates around chondrocytes, and extends into the cartilagewith progressive degeneration. Journal of Clinical Investigation, 96, 2859-2869.

Homandberg, G.A. (2001). Cartilage damage by matrix degradation products: fibronectin fragments.Clinical Orthopedics and Related Research, 391 (Suppl), S100-107.

Honsawek, S., Yuktanandana, P., Tanavalee, A., Chirathaworn, C., Anomasiri, W., Udomsinprasert, W., Saetan, N., Suantawee, T., &Tantavisut, S. (2012). Plasma and synovial fluid connective tissue growth factor levels are correlated with disease severity in patients with knee osteoarthritis. Biomarkers, 17, 303-308.

Horner, A., Kemp, P., Summers, C., Bord, S., Bishop, N.J., Kelsall, A.W., Coleman, N., &Compston, J.E.(1998). Expression and distribution of transforming growth factor-beta isoforms and their signaling receptors in growing humanbone. Bone, 23, 95-102.

Hui, W., Cawston, T., &Rowan, A.D. (2003). Transforming growth factor beta 1 and insulin-like growth factor 1 block collagen degradation induced by oncostatin M in combination with tumour necrosis factor alpha from bovine cartilage.Annals of the Rheumatic Diseases, 62, 172-174.

Hui, W., Rowan, A.D., &Cawston, T. (2001). Insulin-like growth factor 1 blocks collagen release and down regulates matrix metalloproteinase-1, -3, -8, and -13 mRNA expression in bovine nasal cartilage stimulated with oncostatin M in combination with interleukin 1alpha.Annals of the Rheumatic Diseases, 60, 254-261.

Hunter, D.J. & Felson, D.T. (2006). Osteoarthritis. BMJ, 332, 639-642.

Hutchison, M.R., Bassett, M.H., &White, P.C.(2007). Insulin-like growth factor-I and fibroblast growth factor, but not growth hormone, affect growth plate chondrocyte proliferation. Endocrinology, 148, 3122-3130.

Igarashi, M., Kaga, I., Takamori, Y., Sakamoto, K., Miyazawa, K., &Nagaoka, I.(2011). Effects of glucosemine derivatives and uronic acids on the production of glycosaminoglycans by human synovial cells and chondrocytes. International Journal of Molecular Medicine, 27, 821-827.

Ijiri, K., Zerbini LF, Peng H, Correa RG, Lu B, Walsh N, Zhao Y, Taniguchi N, Huang XL, Otu H, Wang H, Wang JF, Komiya S, Ducy. P., Rahman, M.U., Flavell, R.A., Gravallese, E.M., Oettgen, P., Libermann, T.A., & Goldring,M.B. (2005). A novel role for GADD45beta as a mediator of MMP-13 gene expression during chondrocyte terminal differentiation. Journal of Biological Chemistry, 280, 38544-38555.

Ijiri, K., Zerbini, L.F., Peng, H., Out, H.H., Tsuchimochi, K., Otero, M., Dragomir, C., Walsh, N., Bierbaum, B.E., Mattingly, D., van Flandern, G., Komiya, S., Aigner, T., Libermann, T.A., &Goldring, M.B. (2008). Differential expression of GADD45beta in normal and osteoarthritic cartilage: potential role in homeostasis of articular chondrocytes. Arthritis & Rheumatism, 58, 2075-2087.

Jiang, J., Leong, N.L., Mung, J.C., &Lu, H.H. (2008). Interaction between zonal populations of articular chondrocyte mineralization and this process is mediated by PTHrP. Osteoarthritis & Cartilage, 16, 70-82.

Jimenez, M.J.G., Balbin, M., Lopez, J.M., Alvarez, J., Komori, T., &Lopez-Otin, C. (1999). Collagenase 3 is a target of Cbfa1, a transcription factor of runt gene family involved in bone formation.Molecular & Cellular Biology, 19,4431-4442.

Johnson, K. & Terkeltaub, R. (2004). Upregulated ank expression in osteoarthritis can promote both chondrocyte MMP-13 expression and calcification via chondrocyte extracellular PPi excess. Osteoarthritis & Cartilage,12, 321-335.

Kamekura, S., Kawasaki, Y., Hoshi. K., Shimoaka, T., Chikuda, H., Maruyama, Z., Komori, T., Sato, S.,Takeda, S., Karsenty, G., Nakamura, K., Chung, U.I., &Kawaguchi, H. (2006). Contribution of Runt-related transcription factor 2 to the pathogenesis of osteoarthritis in mice after induction of knee joint osteoarthritis. Arthritis & Rheumatism, 54, 2462-2470.

Kapoor, M., Martel-Pelletier, J., Lajeunesse, D., Pelletier, J.P., &Fahmi, H.(2011). Role of proinflammatory cytokines in the pathophysiology of osteoarthritis.Nature Reviews. Rheumatology, 7, 33-42.

Karaplis, A.C., Luz, A., Glowacki, J., Bronson, R.T., Tybulewicz, V.L., Kronenberg, H.M., &Mulligan, R.C. (1994). Lethal skeletal dysplasia from targeted disruption of the parathyroid hormone-related peptide gene.Genes & Development, 8, 277-289.

Karpouzas, G.A. & Terkeltaub, R.A. (1999). New developments in the pathogenesis of articularcartilage calcification. Current Rheumatology Reports, 1, 121-127.

Kempson, G.E., Muir, H., Pollard, C., &Tuke, M. (1973). The tensile properties of the cartilage of human femoral condyles related to the content of collagen and glycosaminoglycans. Biochimica et Biophysica ACTA, 297, 456-472.

Khan, I.M., Evans, S.L., Young, R.D., Blain, E.J., Quantock, A.J., Avery, N., &Archer, C.W. (2011). Fibroblast growth factor 2 and transforming growth factor β1 induce precocious maturation of articular cartilage. Arthritis & Rheumatism, 63, 3417-3427.

Kiepe, D., Ciarmatori, S., Haarmann, A., &Tonshoff, B. (2006). Differential expression of IGF system components in proliferating vs. differentiating growth plate chondrocytes: the functional role of IGFBP-5. American Journal of Physiology, Endocrinology and Metabolism, 290, E363-371.

Kim, H.R., Heo, Y.M., Jeong, K.I., Kim, Y.M., Jang, H.L., Lee, K.Y., Yeo, C.Y., Kim, S.H., Lee, H.K., Kim, S.R., Kim, E.G., &Choi, J.K.(2012). FGF-2 inhibits TNF-α mediated apoptosis through upregulation of Bcl2-A1 and Bcl-xL in ATDC5 cells.BMB Reports, 45, 287-292.

Kim, M.S., Wu, K.Y., Auyeung, V., Chen, Q., Gruppuso, P.A., &Phornphutkul, C. (2009). Leucine restriction inhibits chondrocyte proliferation and differentiation through mechanisms both dependent and independent of mTOR signaling.American Journal of Physiology, Endocrinology and Metabolism,296, E1374-1382.

Kindblom, J.M., Nilsson, O., Hurme, T., Ohlsson, C., &Sävendahl, L. (2002). Expression and localization of Indian hedgehog (Ihh) and parathyroid hormone related protein (PTHrP) in the human growth plate during pubertal development. Journal of Endocrinology, 174, R1-6.

Kinkel, M.D., Yagi, R., McBurney. D., Nugent, A., &Horton, W.E. Jr. 92004). Age-related expression patterns of Bag-1 and Bcl-2 in growth plate and articular chondrocytes. The anatomical record. Part A, Discoveries in molecular,cellular, and evolutionary biology, 279, 720-728.

Kirsch, T., Swoboda, B., &Nah, H.(2000). Activation of annexin II and V expression, terminal differentiation, mineralization and apoptosis in human osteoarthritic cartilage. Osteoarthritis & Cartilage, 8, 294-302.

Kirsch, T. (2005). Annexins - their role in cartilage mineralization. Frontiers in Bioscience, 10, 576-581.

Kishimoto, H., Akagi, M., Zushi, S., Teramura., T., Onodera, Y., Sawamura, T., &Hamanishi, C. (2010). Induction of hypertrophic chondrocyte-like phenotypes by oxidized LDL in cultured bovine articular chondrocytes through increase in oxidative stress. Osteoarthritis & Cartilage, 18, 1284-1290.

Kitahara, H., Hayami, T., Tokunaga, K., Endo, N., Funak, H., Yoshida, Y., Yaoita, E., &Yamamoto, T.(2003). Chondromodulin-I expression in rat articular cartilage. Archives of Histology & Cytology, 66, 221-228.

Klatt, A.R., Klinger, G., Neumuller, O., Eidenmuller, B., Wagner, I., Achenbach, T., Aigner, T., &Bartnik, E. (2006). TAK1 downregulation reduces IL-1beta induced expression of MMP13, MMP1 and TNF-alpha. Biomedicine & Pharmacotherapy, 60, 55-61.

Kobayashi, M., Squires, G.R., Mousa, A., Tanzer, M., Zukor, D.J., Antoniou, J., Feige, U., &Poole, A.R. (2005). Role of interleukin-1 and tumor necrosis factor alpha in matrix degradation of human osteoarthritic cartilage.Arthritis & Rheumatism, 52, 128-135.

Kobayashi, T., Lyons, K.M., McMahon, A.P., &Kronenberg, H.M. (2005). BMP signaling stimulates cellular differentiation at multiple steps during cartilage development. Proceedings of National Academy of Sciences of the United States of America,, 102, 18023-18027.

Kobayashi, T., Notoya, K., Naito, T., Unno, S., Nakamura, A., Martel-Pelletier, J., &Pelletier, J.P.(2005). Pioglitazone, a peroxisome proliferator-activated receptor gamma agonist, reduces the progression of experimental osteoarthritis in guinea pigs.Arthritis & Rheumatism, 52, 479-487.

Komori, T. (2000). A fundamental transcription factor for bone and cartilage. Biochemical and Biophysical Research Communications, 276, 813–816.

Kota, B.P., Huang, T.H., &Roufogalis, B.D.(2005). An overview on biological mechanisms of PPARs. Pharmacological Research, 51, 85-94.

Krejci, P., Krakow, D., Mekikian, P.B., &Wilcox, W.R. (2007). Fibroblast growth factors 1, 2, 17, and 19 are the predominant FGF ligands expressed in human fetal growth plate cartilage. Pediatric Research, 61, 267-272.

Kronenberg, H.M. (2006). PTHrP and skeletal development. Annals of the New York Academy of Sciences, 1068, 1-13.

Kuhn, K., D'Lima, D.D., Hashimoto, S., &Lotz, M. (2004). Cell death in cartilage. Osteoarthritis & Cartilage, 12, 1-16.

Laragione ,T. & Gulko, P.S. (2010). mTOR regulates the invasive properties of synovial fibroblasts in rheumatoid arthritis. Molecular Medicine, 16, 352-358.

Laron, Z. (2001). Insulin growth factor 1 (IGF-1): a growth hormone. Molecular Pathology, 54, 311-316.

Lefebvre, V. & Smits, P. (2005). Transcriptional control of chondrocyte fate and differentiation.Birth Defects Research Part C: Embryo Today, 75, 200-212.

Li, C., Chen, L., Iwata, T., Kitagawa, M., Fu, X.Y., &Deng, C.X. (1999). A Lys644Glu substitution in fibroblast growth factor receptor 3 (FGFR3) causes dwarfism in mice by activation of STATs and ink4 cell cycle inhibitors. Human Molecular Genetics, 8, 35-44.

Li, T.F., Darowish, M., Zuscik, M.J., Chen, D., Schwarz, E.M., Rosier, R.N., Drissi, H., &O'Keefe, R.J. (2006). Smad3-deficient chondrocytes have enhanced BMP signaling and accelerated differentiation. Journal of Bone & Mineral Research, 21, 4-16.

Li, T.F., Dong, Y., Ionescu, A.M., Rosier, R.N., Zuscik, M.J., Schwarz, E.M., O'Keefe, R.J., &Drissi, H. (2004).Parathyroid hormone-related peptide (PTHrP) inhibits Runx2 expression through the PKA signaling pathway. Experimental Cell Research, 299, 128-136.

Li, T.F., Zuscik, M.J., Ionescu, A.M., Zhang, X., Rosier, R.N., Schwarz, E.M., Drissi, H., &O'Keefe, R.J. (2004). PGE2 inhibits chondrocyte differentiation through PKA and PKC signaling. Experimental Cell Research, 300:159-169.

Li, T.F., Gao, L., Sheu, T.J., Sampson, E.R., Flick, L.M., Konttinen, Y.T., Chen, D., Schwarz, E.M., Zuscik, M.J., Jonason, J.H., &O'Keefe, R.J.(2010). Aberrant hypertrophy in Smad3-deficient murine chondrocytes is rescued by restoringtransforming growth factor beta-activated kinase 1/activating transcription factor 2 signaling: a potential clinical implication for osteoarthritis.Arthritis & Rheumatism, 62, 2359-2369.

Lin, A.C., Seeto, B.L., Bartoszko, J.M., Khoury, M.A., Whetstone, H., Ho, L., Ali, S.A., &Alman, B.A. (2009).Modulating hedgehog signaling can attenuate the severity of osteoarthritis. Nature Medicine, 15, 1421-1425.

Lin, E.A. &Liu, C.J.(2010). The role of ADAMTSs in arthritis. Protein & Cell, 1, 33-47.

Little, C.B. & Forsang, A.J. (2010). Is cartilage matrix breakdown an appropriate therapeutic target inosteoarthritis- insights from studies of aggrecan and collagen proteolysis. Current Drug Targets, 11, 561-575.

Lorenz, H. & Richter, W. (2006). Osteoarthritis: cellular and molecular changes in degenerating cartilage. Progress in Histochemistry & Cytochemistry, 40, 135-163.

Lorenz, H., Wenz, W., Ivancic, M., Steck, E., &Richter, W. (2005). Early and stable upregulation of collagen type II, collagen type I and YKL40 expression levels in cartilage during early experimental osteoarthritis occurs independent of joint location and histological grading. Arthritis Research & Therapy, 7, R156-165.

Lotz, M.K. & Caramés, B. (2011). Autophagy and cartilage homeostasis mechanisms in joint health, aging and OA. Nature Reviews. Rheumatology, 7:579-587.

Ma, Q., Li, X., Vale-Cruz, D., Brown, M.L., Beier, F., &LuValle, P. (2007). Activating transcription factor 2 controls Bcl-2 promoter activity in growth plate chondrocytes. Journal of Cellular Biochemistry, 101, 477-487.

MacLean, H.E. &Kronenberg, H.M.(2005). Localization of Indian hedgehog and PTH/PTHrP receptor expression in relation to chondrocyte proliferation during mouse bone development. Development Growth and Differentiation, 47, 59-63.

Magee, C., Nurminskaya, M., Faverman, L., Galera, P., &Linsenmayer, T.F.(2005). SP3/SP1 transcriptionactivity regulates specific expression of collagen type X in hypertrophic chondrocytes.Journal of Biological Chemistry, 280, 25331-25338.

Mailhot, G., Yang, M., Mason-Savas, A., Mackay, C.A., Leav, I., &Odgren, P.R. (2008). BMP-5 expression increases during chondrocyte differentiation in vivo and in vitro and promotes proliferation and cartilage matrix synthesis in primary chondrocyte cultures. Journal of Cellular Physiology, 214, 56-64.

Maloney, C.A. &Rees, W.D. (2005). Gene-nutrient interactions during fetal development. Reproduction, 130:401-410.

Mankin, H.J., Dorfman, H., Lippiello, L., &Zarins, A.(1971). Biochemical and metabolic abnormalities inarticular cartilage from osteo-arthritic human hips. II. Correlation of morphology with biochemical and metabolic data. Journalof Bone & Joint Surgery American, 53, 523-537.

Marcu, K.B., Otero, M., Olivotto, E., Borzi, R.M., &Goldring, M.B.(2010). NF-kappaB signaling: multiple angles to target OA. Current Drug Targets, 11, 599-613.

Maroudas, A., Bayliss, M.T., & Venn, M.F. (1980). Further studies on the composition of human femoral head cartilage. Annals of the Rheumatic Diseases, 39, 514-523.

Marshall, S. (2006). Role of insulin, adipocyte hormones, and nutrient-sensing pathways in regulating fuel metabolism and energy homeostasis: a nutritional perspective of diabetes, obesity, and cancer. Sci STKE, 2006, re7.

Matsunaga, S., Yamamoto, T., &Fukumura, K. (1999). Temporal and spatial expressions of transforming growth factor-betas and their receptors in epiphyseal growth plate. International Journal of Oncology, 14, 1063-1067.

Matyas, J.R., Ehlers, P.F., Huang, D., &Adams, M.E. (1999). The early molecular natural history of experimental osteoarthritis. I. Progressive discoordinate expression of aggrecan and type II procollagen messenger RNA in the articular cartilage of adult animals. Arthritis & Rheumatism, 42, 993-1002.

Matyas, J.R., Huang, D., Chung, M., &Adam,s M.E. (2002). Regional quantification of cartilage type II collagen and aggrecan messenger RNA in joints with early experimental osteoarthritis. Arthritis & Rheumatism, 46,1536-1543.

Merz, D., Liu, R., Johnson, K., &Terkeltaub, R. (2003). IL-8/CXCL8 and growth-related oncogene α/CXCL1induce chondrocyte hypertrophic differentiation. Journal of Immunology, 171, 4406–4415.

Miosge, N., Hartmann, M., Maelicke, C., &Herken, R. (2004). Expression of collagen type I and type II inconsecutive stages of human osteoarthritis.Histochemistry &Cell Biology, 122, 229-236.

Moldovan, F., Pelletier, J.P., Jolicoeur, F.C., Cloutier, J.M., &Martel-Pelletier, J. (2000). Diacerhein and rhein reduce the ICE-induced IL-1beta and IL-18 activation in human osteoarthritic cartilage. Osteoarthritis & Cartilage, 8, 186-196.

Mwale, F., Billinghurst, C., Wu, W., Alini, M., Webber, C., Reiner, A., Ionescu, M., Poole, J., &Poole, A.R. (2000). Selective assembly and remodelling of collagens II and IX associated with expression of the chondrocyte hypertrophicphenotype. Developmental Dynamics, 218, 648-662.

Mwale, F., Tchetina, E., Wu, C.W., &Poole, A.R. (2002). The assembly and remodeling of the extracellular matrix in the growth plate in relationship to mineral deposition and cellular hypertrophy: an in situ study of collagens II and IX and proteoglycan. Journal of Bone & Mineral Research, 17, 275-283.

Nagai, H. &Aoki, M. (2002). Inhibition of growth plate angiogenesis and endochondral ossification with diminished expression of MMP-13 in hypertrophic chondrocytes in FGF-2-treated rats. Journal of Bone & Mineral Metabolism, 20, 142-147.

Naja, R.P., Dardenne, O., Arabian, A., &St Arnaud, R.(2009). Chondrocyte-specific modulation of Cyp27b1 expression supports a role for local synthesis of 1,25-dihydroxyvitamin D3 in growth plate development. Endocrinology, 150, 4024-4032.

Nakatani, S., Mano, H., Im, R., Shimizu, J., &Wada, M.(2007). Glucosamine regulates differentiation of a chondrogenic cell line, ATDC5.Biological & Pharmaceutical Bulletin, 30, 433-438.

Neuhold, L.A., Killar, L., Zhao, W., Sung, M.L., Warner, L., Kulik, J., Turner, J., Wu, W., Billinghurst, C., Meijers, T., Poole, A.R., Babij, P., &DeGennaro, L.J. (2001). Postnatal expression in hyaline cartilage of constitutively active human collagenase-3 (MMP-13) induces osteoarthritis in mice. Journal of Clinical Investigation, 107, 35-44.

Ng, L.J., Wheatley, S., Muscat, G.E.O., Conway-Campbell, J., Bowles, J., Wright, E., Bell, D.M., Tam, P.P.I.,Cheah, K.S.E., &Koopman, P. (1997). Sox9 binds DNA, activates transcription, and coexpresses with type II collagen during-chondrogenesis in the mouse. Developmental Biology, 183, 108–121.

Nilsson, O., Parker, E.A., Heghe, A., Chan, M., &Baron, J. (2007). Gradients in bone morphogenetic protein-related gene expression across the growth plate. Journal of Endocrinology, 193, 75-84.

Nishida, T., Kubota, S., Kojima, S., Kuboki, T., Nakao, K., Kushibiki, T., Tabata, Y., &Takigawa, M. (2004).Regeneration of defects in articular cartilage in rat knee joints by CCN2 (connective tissue growth factor.Journal of Bone & Mineral Research, 19, 1308-1319.

Olney, R.C., Wang, J., Sylvester, J.E., &Mougey, E.B. (2004). Growth factor regulation of human growthplate chondrocyte proliferation in vitro. Biochemical and Biophysical Research Communications, 317, 1171-1182.

Omoto, S., Nishida, K., Yamaai, Y., Shibahara, M., Nishida, T., Doi, T., Asahara, H., Nakanishi, T., Inoue, H.,&Takigawa, M. (2004). Expression and localization of connective tissue growth factor (CTGF/Hcs24/CCN2) in osteoarthritic cartilage. Osteoarthritis & Cartilage, 12, 771-778.

Orfanidou, T., Malizos, K.N., Varitimidis, S., &Tsezou, A.(2012). 1,25-Dihydroxyvitamin D(3) and extracellular inorganic phosphate activate mitogen-activated protein kinase pathway through fibroblast growth factor 23 contributing to hypertrophy and mineralization in osteoarthritic chondrocytes.Experimental Biology & Medicine, 237, 241-253.

Pacifici, M., Shimo, T., Gentili, C., Kirsch, T., Freeman, T.A., Enomoto-Iwamoto, M., Iwamoto, M.,& Koyama, E. (2005). Syndecan-3: a cell-surface heparan sulfateproteoglycan important for chondrocyte proliferation and function during limb skeletogenesis.Journal of Bone & Mineral Metabolism, 23, 191-199.

Papathanasiou, I., Malizos, K.N., &Tsezou, A.(2012). Bone morphogenetic protein-2-induced Wnt/β-catenin signaling pathway activation through enhanced low-density-lipoprotein receptor-related protein 5 catabolic activity contributes to hypertrophy in osteoarthritic chondrocytes.Arthritis Research & Therapy, 14, R82.

Pateder, D.B., Rosier, R.N., Schwartz, E.M., Reynolds, P.R., Puzas, J.E., D'Souza, M., &O'Keefe, R.J. (2000). PTHrP expression in chondrocytes, regulation by TGF-β, and interaction between epiphyseal and growth plate chondrocytes. Experimental Cell Research, 256, 555–562.

Pavelká, K., Gatterová, J., Olejarová, M., Machacek, S., Giacovelli, G., &Rovati, L.C.(2002). Glucosamine sulfate use and delay of progression of knee osteoarthritis: a 3-year, randomized, placebo-controlled, double-blind study.Archives of Internal Medicine, 162, 2113-2123.

Petersen, S.G., Saxne, T., Heinegard, D., Hansen, M., Holm, L., Koskinen, S., Stordal, C., Christensen, H.,Aagaard, P., &Kjaer, M.(2010). Glucosamine but not ibuprofen alters cartilage turnover in osteoarthritis patients in response to physical training.Osteoarthritis & Cartilage, 18, 34-40.

Pfander, D., Cramer, T., Schipani, E., &Johnson, R.S. (2003). HIF-1alpha controls extracellular matrix synthesis by epiphyseal chondrocytes. Journal of Cell Science, 116(Pt 9), 1819-1826.

Pfander, D., Rahmanzadeh, R., &Scheller, E.E. (1999). Presence and distribution of collagen II, collagen I, fibronectin, and tenascin in rabbit normal and osteoarthritic cartilage. Journal of Rheumatology, 26, 386-394.

Pfander, D., Swoboda, B., &Kirsch. T. (2001). Expression of early and late differentiation markers (prolife-rating cell nuclear antigen, syndecan-3, annexin VI, and alkaline phosphatase) by human osteoarthritic chondrocytes.AmericanJournal of Pathology, 159, 1777-1783.

Phornphutkul, C., Wu, K.Y., Auyeung, V., Chen, Q., &Gruppuso, P.A. (2008). mTOR signaling contributes to chondrocyte differentiation. Developmental Dynamics, 237, 702-712.

Piperno, M., Reboul, P., Hellio Le Graverand, M.P., Peschard, M.J., Annefeld, M., Richard, M., & Vignon,E. (2000). Glucosamine sulfate modulates dysregulated activities of human osteoarthritic chondrocytes in vitro.Osteoarthritis& Cartilage, 8, 207-212.

Pogue, R. & Lyons, K. (2006). BMP signaling in the cartilage growth plate.Current Topics in Developmental Biology, 76, 1-48.

Pombo-Suarez, M., Castaño-Oreja, M.T., Calaza, M., Gomez-Reino, J., &Gonzalez, A. (2009). Differential upregulation of the three transforming growth factor beta isoforms in human osteoarthritic cartilage. Annals of the Rheumatic Diseases, 68, 568-571.

Poole, A.R., Alini, M., &Hollander, A.P.(1995).Cellular biology of cartilage degradation, In: Mechanisms and Models in Rheumatoid arthritis(pp. 163-203).

Poole, A.R., Guilak, F., &Abramson, S.B.(2007). Etiopathogenesis of osteoarthritis. In: Osteoarthritis: Diagnosis and Medical/Surgical Management. 4th ed. Edited by Moskowitz RW, Altman RD Hochberg MC, Buckwalter JA, Goldberg VM. Williams &Wilkins, Pa, USA (pp.27-49).

Poole, A.R., Kobayashi, M., Yasuda, T., Laverty, S., Mwale, F., Kojima, T., Sakai, T., Wahl, C., El-Maadawy, S., Webb, G., Tchetina, E., &Wu, W. (2002). Type II collagen degradation and its regulation in articular cartilage in osteoarthritis. Annals of the Rheumatic Diseases, 61 Suppl 2, ii78-81.

Poole, A.R., Nelson, F., Dahlberg, L., Tchetina, E., Kobayashi, M., Yasuda, T., Laverty, S., Squires, G., Kojima, T., Wu, W., &Billinghurst, R.C. (2003). Proteolysis of the collagen fibril in osteoarthritis. Biochemical SocietySymposia, 70, 115-123.

Poole, A.R., Rosenberg, L.C., Reiner, A., Ionescu, M., Bogoch, E., &Roughley, P.J. (1996). Contents and distribution of the proteoglycans decorin and biglycan in normal and osteoarthritic human articular cartilage. Journal of Orthopaedic Research, 14, 681-689.

Poole, A.R. (2003). What type of cartilage repair are we attempting to attain? Journal of Bone & Joint Surgery, 85A(Suppl 2), 40-44.

Poole, A.R. (2005). Cartilage in health and disease. In: Arthritis and Allied Conditions: a Textbook of Rheumatology. 15th ed. Edited by Koopman W. Philadelphia, Lippincott, Williams &Wilkins, Pa, USA(pp.223-269).

Porte, D., Tuckermann, J., Becker, M., Baumann, B., Teurich, S., Higgins, T., Owen, M.J., Schorpp-Kistner, M., &Angel, P. (1999). Both AP-1 and Cbfa1-like factors are required for the induction of interstitial collagenase by parathyroid hormone. Oncogene, 18, 667-678.

Prasadam, I., van Gennip, S., Friis, T., Shi, W., Crawford, R., &Xiao, Y.(2010). ERK-1/2 and p38 in the regulation of hypertrophic changes of normal articular cartilage chondrocytes induced by osteoarthritic subchondral osteoblasts.Arthritis & Rheumatism, 62, 1349-1360.

Pufe, T., Petersen, W., Tillmann, B., &Mentlein. R. (2001). The spice variants VEGF121 and VEGF 189 of theangiogenic peptide vascular endothelial growth factor are expressed in osteoarthritic cartilage.Arthritis & Rheumatism, 44, 1082-1088.

Pujol, J.P., Chadjichristos, C., Legendre, F., Bauge, C., Beauchef, G., Andriamanalijaona, R., Galera, P.,&Boumediene. K.(2008). Interleukin-1 and transforming growth factor-beta 1 as crucial factors in osteoarthritic cartilage metabolism. Connective Tissue Research, 49, 293-297.

Pullig, O., Weseloh, G., Ronneberger, D., Käkönen, S., &Swoboda, B. (2000). Chondrocyte differentiation inhuman osteoarthritis: expression of osteocalcin in normal and osteoarthritic cartilage and bone. Calcified Tissue International, 67, 230-240.

Pucci, B., Adams, C.S., Fertala, J., Snyder, B.C., Mansfield, K.D., Tafani, M., Freeman, T., &Shapiro, I.M. (2007). Development of the terminally differentiated state sensitizes epiphyseal chondrocytes to apoptosis through caspase-3activation. Journal of Cellular Physiology, 210, 609-615.

Quintavalla, J., Kumar, C., Daouti, S., Slosberg, E., &Uziel-Fust, S. (2005). Chondrocyte cluster formation in agarose cultures as a functional assay to identify genes expressed in osteoarthritis. Journal of Cellular Physiology, 204, 560-566.

Raught, B., Gingras, A.C., &Sonenberg, N. (2001). The target of rapamycin (TOR) proteins. Proceedings of National Academy of Sciences of the United States of America,98, 7037-7044.

Reppe, S., Rian, E., Jemtland, R., Olstad, O.K., Gautvik, V.T., &Gautvik, K.M. (2000).Sox-4 messenger RNA is expressed in the embryonic growth plate and regulated via the parathyroid hormone/parathyroid hormone-related protein receptor in osteoblast-like cells. Journal of Bone & Mineral Research, 15, 2402-2412.

Roach, H.I., Mehta, G., Oreffo, R.O., Clarke, N.M., &Cooper, C. (2003). Temporal analysis of rat growth plates: cessation of growth with age despite presence of a physis. Journal of Histochemistry & Cytochemistry, 51, 373-383.

Roberts, A.B. & Sporn, M.B. (1993). Physiological actions and clinical applications of transforminggrowth factor-β (TGFβ). Growth Factors, 8, 1-9.

Robertson, C.M., Pennock, A.T., Harwood, F.L., Pomerleau, A.C., Allen, R.T., &Amiel, D. (2006). Characterization of proapoptotic and matrix-degradative gene expression following induction of osteoarthritis in mature and aged rabbits. Osteoarthritis & Cartilage, 14, 471-476.

Rolauffs, B., Williams, J.M., Aurich, M., Grodzinsky, A.J., Kuettner, K.E., &Cole, A.A.(2010). Proliferative remodeling of the spatial organization of human superficial chondrocytes distant from focal early osteoarthritis. Arthritis &Rheumatism, 62, 489-498.

Rousseau, J.C. &Delmas, P.D. (2007). Biological markers in osteoarthritis. Nature Clinical PracticeRheumatology, 3, 346-356.

Saito, T., Fukai, A., Mabuchi, A., Ikeda, T., Yano, F., Ohba, S., Nishida, N., Akune, T., Yoshimura, N., Nakagawa, T.,Nakamura, K., Tokunaga, K., Chung, U.I., &Kawaguchi, H. (2010). Transcriptional regulation of endochondral ossification by HIF-2alpha during skeletal growth and osteoarthritis development. Nature Medicine, 16, 678-686.

Sakkas, L.I. & Platsoucas, C.D. (2007). The role of T cells in the pathogenesis of osteoarthritis. Arthritis & Rheumatism, 56, 409-424.

Sakou, T., Onishi, T., Yamamoto, T., Nagamine, T., Sampath, T., &Ten Dijke, P. (1999). Localization of Smads, the TGF-beta family intracellular signaling components during endochondral ossification. Journal of Bone & MineralResearch, 14, 1145-1152.

Sanchez, C.P. & He, Y-Z. (2009). Bone growth during rapamycin therapy in young rats. BMC Pediatrics, 9, 3.

Scanzello, C.R., Plaas, A., &Crow, M.K. (2008). Innate immune system activation in osteoarthritis: is osteoarthritis a chronic wound? Current Opinion in Rheumatology, 20, 565-572.

Scharstuhl, A., Glansbeek, H.L., van Beuningen, H.M., Vitters, E.L., van der Kraan, P.M., &van den Berg, W.B. (2002). Inhibition of endogenous TGF-β during experimental osteoarthritis prevents osteophyte formation and impairs cartilage repair. Journal of Immunology, 169, 507-514.

Scharstuhl, A., Vitters, E.L., van der Kraan, P.M., &van den Berg, W.B. (2003). Reduction of osteophyte formation and synovial thickening by adenoviral overexpression of transforming growth factor beta/bone morphogenetic protein inhibitors during experimental osteoarthritis. Arthritis & Rheumatism, 48, 3442-3451.

Schroeppel, J.P., Crist, J.D., Anderson, H.C., &Wang, J. (2011). Molecular regulation of articular chondrocyte function and its significance in osteoarthritis. Histology & Histopathology, 26, 377-3.

Schwarz, Z., Gilley, R.M., Sylvia, V.L., Dean, D.D., &Boyan, B.D. (1998). The effect of prostaglandin E2on costochondral chondrocyte differentiation is mediated by cyclic adenosine 3', 5' – monophosphate and protein kinase C. Endocrinology, 139:1825-1834.

Semevolos, S.A., Strassheim, M.L., Haupt, J.L., &Noxin, A.J. (2005). Expression patterns of hedgehog signaling peptides in naturally acqired equine osteochondrosis. Journal of Orthopaedic Research, 23, 1152-1159.

Serra, R., Johnson, M., Filvaroff, E.H., LaBorde, J., Sheehan, D.M., Derynck, R., &Moses, H.L. (1997). Expression of a truncated, kinase-defective TGF-beta type II receptor in mouse skeletal tissue promotes terminal chondrocyte differentiation and osteoarthritis. Journal of Cell Biology, 139, 541-552.

Serra, R., Karaplis, A., &Sohn, P. (1999). Parathyroid hormone-related peptide (PTHrP)-dependent and –independent effects of transforming growth factor beta (TGF-beta) on endochondral bone formation. Journal of Cell Biology, 145, 783-794.

Shao, Y.Y., Wang, L., Hicks, D.G., Tarr, S., &Ballock, R.T.(2005). Expression and activation of peroxisome proliferator-activated receptors in growth plate chondrocytes.Journal of Orthopaedic Research, 23, 1139-1145.

Shapiro, I.M., Adams, C.S., Freeman, T., & Srinivas, V. (2005). Fate of the hypertrophic chondrocyte; microenvironmental perspectives on apoptosis and survival in the epiphyseal growth plate. Birth Defects Research Part C: Embryo Today, 75, 330-339.

Sharif, M., Kirwan, J., Charni, N., Sandell, L.J., Whittles, C., &Ganero, P. (2007). A 5-year longitudinal studyof type IIA collagen synthesis and total type II collagen degradation in patients with knee osteoarthritis--association with disease progression. Rheumatology (Oxford), 46, 938-943.

Shida, J.-I., Jingushi, S., Izumi, T., Ikenoue, T., &Iwamoto, Y. (2001). Basic fibroblast growth factor regulates expression of growth factors in rat epiphyseal chondrocytes. Journal of Orthopaedic Research, 19, 259-264.

Shinar, D.M., Endo, N., Halperin, D., Rodan, G.A., &Weinreb, M. (1993). Differential expression of insulinlike growth factor-I (IGF-I) and IGF-II messenger ribonucleic acid in growing rat bone. Endocrinology, 132, 1158-1167.

Solomon, L.A., Bérubé, N.G., &Beier. F. (2008). Transcriptional regulators of chondrocyte hypertrophy.Birth Defects Research Part C: Embryo Today, 84, 123-130.

Soung do, Y., Dong, Y., Wang, Y., Zuscik, M.J., Schwarz, E.M., O'Keefe, R.J., &Drissi, H. (2007). Runx3/AML2/Cbfa3 regulates early and late chondrocyte differentiation.Journal of Bone & Mineral Research, 22, 1260-1270.

Stanton, L.A., Li, J.R., &Beier, F.(2010). PPARgamma2 expression in growth plate chondrocytes is regulated by p38 and GSK-3. Journal of Cellular & Molecular Medicine, 14, 242-256.

Stewart, M.C., Kadlcek, R.M., Robbins, P.D., MacLeod, J.N., &Ballock, R.T. (2004). Expression and activity of the CDK inhibitor p57Kip2 in chondrocytes undergoing hypertrophic differentiation. Journal of Bone & Mineral Research, 19, 123-132.

St-Jacques, B., Hammerschmidt, M., &McMahon, A.P. (1999). Indian hedgehog signaling regulates proliferation and differentiation of chondrocytes and is essential for bone formation. Genes & Development, 13, 2072-2086.

Studer, D., Millan, C., Öztürk, E., Maniura-Weber, K., &Zenobi-Wong, M.(2012). Molecular and biophysical mechanisms regulating hypertrophic differentiation in chondrocytes and mesenchymal stem cells.European Cells& Materials, 24, 118-135.

Szuts, V., Mollers, U., Bittner, K., Schurmann, G., Muratoglu, S., Deak, F., Kiss, I., &Bruckner, P.(1998). Terminal differentiation of chondrocytes is arrested at distinct stages identified by their expression repertoire of marker genes.Matrix Biology,17, 435-448.

Takahashi, T., Morris, E.A., &Trippel, S.B. (2007). Bone morphogenetic protein-2 and -9 regulate the interaction of insulin-like growth factor-1 with rowth plate chondrocytes. International Journal of Molecular Medicine, 20, 53-57.

Takeda, S., Bonnamy, J.-P., Owen, M.J., Ducy, P., &Karsenty, G. (2001). Continuous expression of Cbfa1in nonhypertrophic chondrocytes uncovers its ability to induce hypertrophyc chondrocyte differentiation and partially rescuesCbfa1-deficient mice. Genes & Development, 15, 467-481.

Tchetina, E., Mwale, F., &Poole, A.R. (2003). Distinct phases of coordinated early and late gene expression in growth plate chondrocytes in relationship to cell proliferation, matrix assembly, remodeling, and cell differentiation. Journal of Bone & Mineral Research, 18, 844-851.

Tchetina, E.V., Antoniou, J., Tanzer, M., Zukor, D.J., &Poole, A.R. (2006). Transforming growth factor-beta2 suppresses collagen cleavage in cultured human osteoarthritic cartilage, reduces expression of genes associated with chondrocyte hypertrophy and degradation, and increases prostaglandin E(2) production.American Journal of Pathology, 168, 131-140.

Tchetina, E.V., Di Battista, J.A., Zukor, D.J., Antoniou, J., &Poole, A.R. (2007). Prostaglandin PGE2 at very low concentrations suppresses collagen cleavage in cultured human osteoarthritic articular cartilage: this involves a decrease in expression of proinflammatory genes, collagenases, and COL10A1, a gene linked to chondrocyte hypertrophy. Arthritis Research & Therapy, 9, R75.

Tchetina, E.V., Kobayashi, M., Yasuda, T., Meijers, T., Pidoux, I., &Poole, A.R. (2007). Chondrocyte hypertrophy can be induced by a cryptic sequence of type II collagen and is accompanied by the induction of MMP-13 and collagenase activity: implications for development and arthritis. Matrix Biology, 26, 247-258.

Tchetina, E.V., Squires, G., &Poole, A.R. (2005). Increased type II collagen degradation and very early focal cartilage degeneration is associated with upregulation of chondrocyte differentiation related genes in early human articular cartilage lesions.Journal of Rheumatology, 32, 876-886.

Terkeltaub, R., Lotz, M., Johnson, K., Deng, D., Hashimoto, S., Goldring, M.B., Burton, D., &Deftos,L.J. (1998). Parathyroid hormone-related protein is abundant in osteoarthriticcartilage and the parathyroid hormone-relatedprotein 1-173 isoform is selectively induced by transforming growth factor β in articular chondrocytes and suppresses generation of extracellularinorganic pyrophosphate. Arthritis & Rheumatism, 41, 2152-2164.

Terkeltaub, R.A., Johnson, K., Rohnow, D., Goomer, R., Burton, D., &Deftos, L.J. (1998). Bone morphogenetic proteins and bFGF exert opposing regulatory effects on PTHrP expression and inorganic pyrophosphate elaborationin immortalized murine endochondral hypertrophic chondrocytes (MCT cells). Journal of Bone & Mineral Research, 13, 931-941.

Terry, D.E., Rees-Milton, K., Pruss, C., Hopwood, J., Carran, J., &Anastassiades, T.P. (2007). Modulation ofarticular chondrocyte proliferation and anionic glycoconjugate synthesis by glucosamine (GlcN), N-acetyl GlcN (Glc-NAc)GlcN sulfate salt (GlcN.S) and covalent glucosamine sulfates (GlcN-SO4). Osteoarthritis & Cartilage, 15, 946-956.

Tetlow, L.C., Adlam, D.J., &Woolley, D.E. (2001). Matrix metalloproteinase and proinflammatory cytokineproduction by chondrocytes of human osteoarthritic cartilage: associations with degenerative changes. Arthritis & Rheumatism, 44, 585-594.

Trippel, S.B. (2004). Growth factor inhibition. Potential role in the etiopathogenesis of osteoarthritis. Clinical Orthopedics & Related Research, 427, S47–S52.

Troeberg, L.&Nagase, H.(2012). Proteases involved in cartilage matrix degradation in osteoarthritis.Biochimica et Biophysica ACTA, 1824, 133-145.

Tsuchimochi, K., Otero, M., Dragomir, C.L., Plumb, D.A., Zerbini, L.F., Libermann, T.A., Marcu, K.B., Komija, S., Ijiri, K., &Goldring, M.B. (2010). GADD45beta enhances Col10a1 transcription via the MTK/MKK3/6/p38 axis and activation of C/EBPbeta-TAD4 in terminally differentiating chondrocytes. Journal of Biological Chemistry, 285, 8395-8407.

Tuckermann, J.P., Pittois, K., Partridge, N.C., Merregaert, J., &Angel, P. (2000). Collagenase-3 (MMP-13) and integral membrane protein 2a (Itm2a) are marker genes of chondrogenic/osteoblastic cells in bone formation:sequential temporal, and spatial expression of Itm2a, alkaline phosphatase, MMP-13, and osteocalcin in the mouse. Journal of Bone & Mineral Research, 15, 1257-1265.

Ueta, C., Iwamoto, M., Kanatani, N., Yoshida, C., Liu, Y., Enomoto-Iwamoto, M., Ohmori, T., Enomoto, H., Nakata, K., Takada, K., Kurisu, K., &Komori, T. (2001). Skeletal malformations caused by overexpression of Cbfa1 or its dominant negative form in chondrocytes. Journal of Cell Biology, 153, 87-100.

Uria, J.A., Balbin, M., Lopez, J.M., Alvarez, J., Vizoso, F., Takigawa, M., &Lopez-Otin, C. (1998). Collagenase-3 (MMP-13) expression in chondrosarcoma cells and its regulation by basic fibroblast growth factor. American Journal of Pathology, 153, 91-101.

Valdes, A.M. &Spector, T.D. (2010). The clinical relevance of genetic susceptibility to osteoarthritis.Best Practice & Research: Clinical Rheumatology, 24, 3-14.

Valverde-Franco, G., Binette, J.S., Li, W., Wang, H., Chai, S., Laflamme, F., Tran-Khanh, N., Quenneville, E., Meijers, T., Poole, A.R., Mort, J.S., Buschmann, M.D., &Henderson, J.E. (2006). Defects in articular cartilage metabolism and early arthritis in fibroblast growth factor receptor 3 deficient mice. Human Molecular Genetics, 15, 1783-1792.

van den Berg, W.B. (1995). Growth factors in experimental osteoarthritis: Transforming growth factor βpathogenic? Journal of Rheumatology, 22(Suppl 43), 143-145.

van der Kraan, P.M.&van den Berg, W.B.(2012). Chondrocyte hypertrophy and osteoarthritis: role in initiation and progression of cartilage degeneration?Osteoarthritis & Cartilage, 20, 223-232.

van der Kraan, P.M., Blaney Davidson, E.N., Blom, A., &van den Berg, W.B. (2009). TGF-beta signaling in chondrocyte terminal differentiation and osteoarthritis: modulation and integration of signaling pathways through receptor-Smads. Osteoarthritis & Cartilage, 17, 1539-1545.

van der Kraan, P.M., Blaney Davidson, E.N., &van den Berg, W.B. (2010). A role for age-related changes in TGFbeta signaling in aberrant chondrocyte differentiation and osteoarthritis. Arthritis Research & Therapy, 12, 201-214.

van der Weyden, L., Wei, L., Luo, J., Yang, X., Birk, D.E., Adams, D.J., Bradley, A., &Chen, Q. (2006).Functional knockout of the matrilin-3 gene causes premature chondrocyte maturation to hypertrophy and increases bone mineral density and osteoarthritis.American Journal of Pathology, 169, 515-527.

Veje, K., Hyllested-Winge, J.L., &Ostergaard, K. (2003). Topographic and zonal distribution of tenascin in human articular cartilage from femoral heads: normal versus mild and severe osteoarthritis. Osteoarthritis & Cartilage, 11, 217-227.

Verdier,M.P., Seité, S., Guntzer, K., Pujol, J.P., &Boumédiène, K. (2005). Immunohistochemical analysis of transforming growth factor beta isoforms and their receptors in human cartilage from normal and osteoarthritic femoralheads. Rheumatology International, 25, 118-124.

von der Mark, K., Kirsch, T., Nerlich, A., Kuss, A., Weseloh, G., Gluckert, K., &Stoss, H.(1992). Type X collagen synthesis in human osteoarthritic cartilage – indication of chondrocyte hypertrophy. Arthritis & Rheumatism, 35, 806-811.

Vortkamp, A., Lee, K., Lanske, B., Segre, G.V., Kronenberg, H.M., &Tabin, C.J. (1996). Regulation of rate of cartilage differentiation by Indian hedgehog and PTH-related protein. Science, 273, 613-622.

Walker, G.D., Fischer, M., Gannon, J., Thompson, R.C., &Oegema, T.R. (1995). Expression of type X collagen in osteoarthritis. Journal of Orthopaedic Research, 3, 4-12.

Walker, W.A. &Blackburn, G. (2004). Symposium introduction: nutrition and gene regulation. Journal of Nutrition, 134, 2434S-2436S.

Wang, W., Xu, J., Du, B., &Kirsch, T. (2005). Role of the progressive ankylosis gene (ank) in cartilage mineralization. Molecular & Cellular Biology, 25, 312-323.

Wang, W., Xu, J., &Kirsch, T. (2005). Annexin V and terminal differentiation of growth plate chondrocytes. Experimental Cell Research, 305, 156-165.

Wang, Q., Green, R.P., Zhao, G., &Ornitz, D.M. (2001). Differential regulation of endochondral bone growth and joint development by FGFR1 and FGFR3 tyrosine kinase domains. Development, 128, 3867–3876.

Wang, Q., Wei, X., Zhu, T., Zhang, M., Shen, R., Xing, L., O'Keefe, R.J., &Chen, D. (2007). Bone morphogenetic protein 2 activates Smad6 gene transcription through bone-specific transcription factor Runx2. Journal of Biological Chemistry, 282, 10742-10748.

Wang, W.&Kirsch, T.(2006). Annexin V/beta5 integrin interactions regulate apoptosis of growth plate chondrocytes. Journal of Biological Chemistry, 281, 30848-30856.

Wang, W., Xu, J., &Kirsch, T. (2003). Annexin-mediated Ca^{2+} influx regulates growth plate chondrocyte maturation and apoptosis. Journal of Biological Chemistry, 278, 3762-3769.

Wang, Y., Middleton, F., Horton, J.A., Reichel, L., Farnum, C.E., &Damron, T.A. (2004). Microarray analysis of proliferative and hypertrophic growth plate zones identifies differentiation markers and signal pathways. Bone, 35, 1273-1293.

Wang, Y., Nishida, S., Sakata, T., Elalieh, H.Z., Chang, W., Halloran, B.P., Doty, S.B., &Bikle, D.D. (2006). Insulin-like growth factor-I is essential for embryonic bone development. Endocrinology, 147, 4753-4761.

Wei, F., Zhou, J., Wei, X., Zhang, J., Fleming, B.C., Terek, R., Pei, M., Chen, Q., Liu, T., &Wei, L.(2012). Activation of Indian hedgehog promotes chondrocyte hypertrophy and upregulation of MMP-13 in human osteoarthritic cartilage. Osteoarthritis & Cartilage, 20, 755-763.

Wei, L., Kanbe, K., Lee, M., Wei, X., Pei, M., Sun, X., Terek, R., &Chen, Q. (2010). Stimulation of chondrocyte hypertrophy by chemokine stromal cell-derived factor 1 in the chondro-osseous junctionduring endochondral bone formation. Developmental Biology, 241, 236-245.

Wei, Y., Sinha, S., &Levine, B. (2008). Dual role of JNK1-mediated phosphorylation of Bcl-2 in autophagyand apoptosis regulation. Autophagy, 4, 949-951.

Weir, E.C., Philbrick, W.M., Amling, M., Neff, L.A., Baron, R., &Broadus, A.E. (1996).Targeted overexpression of parathyroid hormone-related peptide in chondrocytes causes chondrodysplasia and delayed endochondral bone formation. Proceedings of National Academy of Sciences of the United States of America, 93, 10240-10245.

Weisser, J., Rahforth, B., Timmermann, A., Aigner, T., Brauer, R., & von der Mark, K.(2001). Role ofgrowth factors in rabbit articular cartilage repair by chondrocytes in agarose. Osteoarthritis & Cartilage, 9, S48-S54.

Wezeman, F.H. &Bollnow, M.R. (1997). Immunohistochemical localization of fibroblast growthfactor-2 in normal and brachymorphic mouse tibial growth plate and articular cartilage. Histochemical Journal, 29, 505-514.

White, A.H., Watson, R.L., Newman, B., Freemont, A.J., &Wallis, G.A. (2002). Annexin VIII is differentially expressed by chondrocytes in the mammalian growth plate during endochondral ossification and in osteoarthritic cartilage. Journal of Bone & Mineral Research, 17, 1851-1858.

Wu, C.W., Tchetina, E.V., Mwale, F., Hasty, K., Pidoux, I., Reiner, A., Chen, J., Van Wart, H.E., &Poole, A.R. (2002). Proteolysis involving matrix metalloproteinase 13 (collagenase-3) is required for chondrocyte differentiation that is associated with matrix mineralization. Journal of Bone & Mineral Research, 17, 639-651.

Wu, W., Billinghurst, R.C., Pidoux, I., Antoniou, J., Zukor, D., Tanzer, M., &Poole, A.R. (2002). Sites of collagenase cleavage and denaturation of type II collagen in aging and osteoarthritic articular cartilage and their relationship to thedistribution of matrix metalloproteinase 1 and matrix metalloproteinase 13. Arthritis & Rheumatism, 46, 2087-2094.

Wu, L., Huang, X., Li, L., Huang, H., Xu, R., &Luyten, W. (2012). Insights on Biology and Pathology of HIF1α/-2α, TGFβ/BMP, Wnt/β-Catenin, and NF-κB Pathways in Osteoarthritis. Current Pharmaceutical Design, 18, 3293-3312.

Wuelling, M. &Vortkamp, A. (2010). Transcriptional networks controlling chondrocyte proliferation and differentiation during endochondral ossification. Pediatric Nephrology, 25, 625-631.

Yaeger, P.C., Masi, T.L., Buck de Ortiz, J.L., Binette, F., Tubo, R., &McPherson, M.(1997). Synergistic action of transforming growth factor-β and insulin-like growth factor-I induces expression of type II collagen and aggrecan genesin adult human articular chondrocytes. Experimental Cell Research, 237, 318-325.

Yagi, R., McBurney, D., Laverty, D., Weiner, S., &Horton, W.E.Jr. (2005). Intrajoint comparison of gene expression patterns in human osteoarthritis suggest a change in chondrocyte phenotype. Journal of Orthopaedic Research, 23,1128-1138.

Yamamoto, T., Wakitani, S., Imoto, K., &Hattori, T. (2004). Fibroblast growth factor-2 promotes the repair of partial thickness defects of articular cartilage in immature rabbits but not in mature rabbits. Osteoarthritis & Cartilage, 12, 636-641.

Yamane, S., Cheng, E., You, Z., &Reddi, A.H. (2007). Gene expression profiling of mouse articular andgrowth plate cartilage. Tissue Engineering, 13, 2163-2173.

Yamashita, F., Sakakida, K., Kusuzaki, K., Takeshita, H., &Kuzuhara, A. (1989). Immunohistochemicallocalization of interleukin 1 in human growth cartilage. Nippon Seikeigka Gakkai Zasshi, 63, 562-568.

Yang, X., Chen, L., Xu, X., Li, C., Huang, C., &Deng, C.X. (2001). TGFbeta-Smad3 signals repress chondrocyte hypertrophic differentiation and are required for maintaining articular cartilage. Journal of Cell Biology, 153, 35–46.

Yasuda, T., &Poole, A.R. (2002). A fibronectin fragment induces type II collagen degradation by collagenase through an interleukin-1-mediated pathway. Arthritis & Rheumatism, 46, 138-148.

Yasuda, T., Tchetina, E., Ohsawa, K., Roughley, P.J., Wu, W., Mousa, A., Ionescu, M., Pidoux, I., &Poole, A.R. (2006). Peptides of type II collagen can induce the cleavage of type II collagen and aggrecan in articular cartilage.MatrixBiology, 25, 419-429.

Yatsugi, N., Tsukazaki, T., Osaki, M., Koji, T., Yamashita, S., &Shindo, H. (2000). Apoptosis of articular chondrocytes in rheumatoid arthritis and osteoarthritis: correlation of apoptosis with degree of cartilage destruction and expression of apoptosis-related proteins of p53 and c-myc. Journal of Orthopaedic Science, 5, 150-156.

Yoon, B.S., Pogue, R., Ovchinnikov, D.A., Yoshii, I., Mishina, Y., Behringer, P.R., &Lyons, K.M. (2006).BMPs regulate multiple aspects of growth plate chonderogenesis through opposing actions on FGF pathways. Development,133, 4667-4678.

Yoshida, E., Noshiro, M., Kawamoto, T., Tsutsumi, S., Kuruta, Y., &Kato, Y. (2001). Direct inhibition of Indian hedgehog expression by parathyroid hormone (PTH)/PTH-related peptide and upregulation by retinoic acid in growthplate chondrocyte cultures. Experimental Cell Research, 265, 64-72.

Zhang, D., Schwarz, E.M., Rosier, R.N., Zuscik, M.J., Puzas, J.E., &O'Keefe, R.J. (2003). ALK2 functionsas a BMP type I receptor and induces Indian hedgehog in chondrocytes during skeletal development. Journal of Bone & Mineral Research, 18, 1593-1604.

Zhang, X., Ziran, N., Goater, J.J., Schwarz, E.M., Puzas, J.E., Rosier, R.N., Zuscik, M., Drissi, H., &O'Keefe, R.J. (2004). *Primary murine limb bud mesenchimal cells in long-term culture complete chondrocyte differentiation:TGF-β delays hypertrophy and PGE2 inhibits terminal differentiation. Bone, 34, 809-817.*

Zhao, Q., Eberspaecher, H., Lefebvre, V., &De Crombrugghe, B. (1997). *Parallel expression of Sox9 andCol2a1 in cells undergoing chondrogenesis. Developmental Dynamics, 209, 377-386.*

Zhou, H.W., Lou, S.Q., &Zhang, K. (2004). *Recovery of function in osteoarthritic chondrocytes induced by p16INK4a-specific siRNA in vitro. Rheumatology (Oxford), 43, 555-568.*

Zuscik, M.J., Baden, J.F., Wu, Q., Sheu, T.J., Schwarz, E.M., Drissi, H., O'Keefe, R.J., Pusas, J.E., &Rosier,R.N. (2004). *5-azacytidine alters TGF-β and BMP signaling and induces maturation in articular chondrocytes. Journal of Cellular Biochemistry, 92, 316–331.*

Effect of Flotillin-1 and cCbl-Associated Protein on the Cellular Localization of Fibroblast Growth Factor Receptor Substrate 2

Ana Tomasovic
Institute of Biochemistry
University of Giessen, Germany

Melanie Meister
Institute of Biochemistry
University of Giessen, Germany

Ritva Tikkanen
Institute of Biochemistry
University of Giessen, Germany

1   Introduction

The regulation of receptor tyrosine kinases (RTK) is accomplished by a complex network of multiple participants. One malfunctioning factor within this network may already result in an aberrant signaling leading to, e.g. cancerogenesis. These networks are based on proteins with enzymatic activities, such as kinases and phosphatases, but also on scaffolding proteins which can serve as adaptors that interact with multiple partners at the same time, recruit novel partners for further signal transduction or modulate the interactor's intracellular translocation. This chapter will shed light on how three protein families, namely flotillins, sorbin homology (SoHo) adaptor proteins and the fibroblast growth factor receptor substrate (FRS) family cooperate in scaffolding processes during RTK signaling.

1.1   Flotillin Protein Family

Liquid-ordered state microdomains, also known as membrane rafts, are structures that are capable of facilitating protein interactions and endocytosis as well as regulating signaling pathways. They are enriched in cholesterol and sphingolipids and float in low density fractions of detergent-resistant membrane preparations (Lingwood & Simons 2010; Simons & Gerl 2010; Simons & Ikonen 1997; Simons & Sampaio 2011). Members of the flotillin protein family were discovered and named after this property (Bickel *et al.* 1997). In the same year, another group described them as 'reggies' as they were upregulated during the regeneration of axons after a lesion of goldfish optic nerve (Schulte *et al.* 1997). Unfortunately, the numbering is inversed, with flotillin-1 (flot-1) being the same as reggie-2 and flotillin-2 (flot-2) corresponding to reggie-1.

The propensity of flotillins to associate with membrane rafts and to form higher-order oligomers was found to be due to post-translational modifications and their structural domain organization (Babuke *et al.* 2009; Morrow *et al.* 2002; Neumann-Giesen *et al.* 2004; Solis *et al.* 2007). The N-terminal globular SPFH (stomatin/prohibitin/flotillin/HflK/C) domain, also known as PHB (prohibitin homology) domain (Tavernarakis *et al.* 1999), promotes the association with membrane rafts (Morrow & Parton 2005; Morrow *et al.* 2002; Neumann-Giesen *et al.* 2004). Flot-1 exhibits a palmitoyl modification on cysteine 34 (Morrow *et al.* 2002), and flot-2 is palmitoylated on cysteines 4, 19 and 20 by DHHC5, a member of the Asp-His-His-Cys palmitoyltransferase family (Li *et al.* 2012; Neumann-Giesen *et al.* 2004). In addition, the membrane association of flot-2 is dependent on the myristoylation, and a point mutation Gly2Ala renders flot-2 soluble (Neumann-Giesen *et al.* 2004). The C-terminal domain is called 'flotillin-domain' (Babuke & Tikkanen 2007) since it contains several EA repeats (Glu–Ala) and promotes the homo- as well as hetero-oligomerization of flotillins by coiled-coil structures (Babuke *et al.* 2009; Frick *et al.* 2007; Solis *et al.* 2007). Besides post-translational modifications with fatty acids, flotillins contain several putative phosphorylation sites with functional relevance (Neumann-Giesen *et al.* 2007).

The subcellular localization of flotillins is highly dynamic and seems to depend on several factors, such as cell type, differentiation and stimuli. Flotillins have been detected in several subcellular compartments, e.g. the plasma membrane, late endosomes, lysosomes, phagosomes, exosomes, the Golgi network and the nucleus (Dermine *et al.* 2001; Glebov *et al.* 2006; Langhorst *et al.* 2006; Neumann-Giesen *et al.* 2007; Santamaria *et al.* 2005; Stuermer *et al.* 2001). Flot-1 levels increase during cellular differentiation processes in skeletal myoblasts, osteoclasts and 3T3 fibroblasts (Bickel *et al.* 1997; Ha *et al.* 2003; Volonte *et al.* 1999). Especially for the cell line 3T3-L1, a translocation of flot-1 from endosomal compartments towards the plasma membrane has been observed upon differentiation (Liu *et al.* 2005). Several stimuli can induce a change in the cellular localization of flotillins. For example, a translocation to uropods was observed during cell migration in hematopoietic cells, and during T-cell activation flotillins move to the immunological synapse (Affentranger *et al.* 2011; Rajendran *et al.* 2009; Rajendran *et al.* 2003). Furthermore, growth factors can influence the intracellular trafficking of flotillins. Our group has shown that upon treatment with epidermal growth factor (EGF), flot-2 is Tyr phosphorylated by Src kinases and endocytosed together with flot-1 from the plasma membrane to late endosomes (Babuke *et al.* 2009). This is dependent on the proper hetero-oligomerization with flot-1 and on Tyr163, since a point mutation of this Tyr into Phe (Y163F) will constitutively localize flot-2 to the plasma membrane (Babuke *et al.* 2009; Neumann-Giesen *et al.* 2007). Nichols and coworkers showed similar results for the corresponding Y160 in flot-1 (Riento *et al.* 2009).

Flotillins, which are constitutive residents of membrane microdomains, were shown to display a functional impact on endocytic processes, cellular adhesion and RTK signaling pathways. Nichols and colleagues described a novel membrane raft mediated endocytosis pathway that depends on flot-1 but seems to be independent of the classical endocytosis components, such as clathrin (Frick *et al.* 2007; Glebov *et al.* 2006). Cargo proteins of this endocytosis pathway are the GPI-anchored protein CD59, the ganglioside GM1 and the Nodal coreceptor cripto (Ait-Slimane *et al.* 2009; Blanchet *et al.* 2008; Frick *et al.* 2007; Glebov *et al.* 2006). Additionally, while flot-2 has been shown to be involved in the endocytosis of the amyloid precursor protein (APP) and its subsequent amyloidogenic processing (Schneider *et al.* 2008), flot-1 was shown to colocalize with Aß42 to membrane rafts and to interact with the intracellular domain of APP (Chen *et al.* 2006; Kokubo *et al.* 2005). Another role for flotillins in cellular uptake processes was supported by the observation that flotillins might bind cholesterol and are involved in cholesterol uptake into cells (Ge *et al.* 2011; Strauss *et al.* 2010 and our unpublished data). Furthermore, the protein kinase C driven phosphorylation of Ser315 of flot-1 is indispensable for the endocytosis of the dopamine transporter DAT (Cremona *et al.* 2011). Recently, our group established that flot-1 is important for the activation of receptor tyrosine kinases, such as epidermal growth factor receptor (EGFR) and fibroblast growth factor receptor (FGFR), as well as for downstream mitogen activated protein kinase (MAPK) signaling resulting in the activation of ERK and Akt. Especially flot-1 seems to be a central scaffolding factor during MAPK signaling, and it was found to bind to another adaptor protein of the same cascade, FRS2 (Amaddii *et al.* 2012; Tomasovic *et al.* 2012). Another signaling pathway in which flot-1 seems to be involved is the PI3K independent insulin signaling pathway. In this context, flot-1 was shown to interact with one of the regulators of this pathway, c-Cbl associated protein (CAP) and to mediate the translocation of the glucose transporter GLUT4 to the plasma membrane (Baumann *et al.* 2000; Fecchi *et al.* 2006; Kimura *et al.* 2001; Liu *et al.* 2005; Zhang *et al.* 2003).

1.2   Fibroblast Growth Factor Receptor Substrate 2

The first described mammalian substrate of fibroblast growth factor receptor kinase (FGFR) was phospholipase C-γ (PLCγ) (Gotoh 2008; Mohammadi *et al.* 1991). Later on, other substrates were discovered, among them the two members of the fibroblast growth factor receptor substrate 2 family – FRS2α alias FRS2 and FRS2β alias FRS3 (Gotoh *et al.* 2004b). FRS2, also known as suc1-associated neurotrophic factor target (SNT), was described as a protein that becomes Tyr phosphorylated upon nerve growth factor (NGF) and fibroblast growth factor (FGF) treatment of PC12 and NIH3T3 cells (Kouhara *et al.* 1997; Meakin *et al.* 1999; Rabin *et al.* 1993). FRS3 was discovered later and found to be highly homologous to FRS2 (Gotoh *et al.* 2004b; McDougall *et al.* 2001; Xu *et al.* 1998; Zhou *et al.* 2003).

Both FRS2 family proteins show a similar organization of their functional domains. A myristoylation consensus sequence at the N-terminus mediates the constitutive association with the plasma membrane (Kouhara *et al.* 1997), whereas the phosphotyrosine-binding (PTB) domain is important for the binding to RTKs as well as to signaling partners (Ong *et al.* 2000). While the PTB domain of FRS2 binds FGFR irrespective of its activation state, the binding to the neurotrophin receptors TrkA and B is dependent on receptor activation (Dhalluin *et al.* 2000; Easton *et al.* 2006; Ong *et al.* 2000; Xu *et al.* 1998). FRS3 is important for the inhibition of EGFR kinase activity and for the negative feedback regulation in that it forms a ternary complex with the cytoplasmic domain of the EGFR and the MAPK ERK (Huang *et al.* 2004; Huang *et al.* 2006).

In their C-terminus, the FRS2 proteins harbor several Tyr phosphorylation sites – for FRS2 6 Tyr and for FRS3 5 Tyr have been reported (Hadari *et al.* 1998; Kouhara *et al.* 1997). FRS2 and -3 are Tyr phosphorylated upon activation of the respective RTKs with NGF, FGF or BDNF (Dixon *et al.* 2006; Hadari *et al.* 1998; Kurokawa *et al.* 2001; Melillo *et al.* 2001). Upon Tyr phosphorylation, both FRS2 and 3 recruit the SH2-containing protein Grb2 and the Tyr phosphatase Shp2 (Hadari *et al.* 1998; Kouhara *et al.* 1997). While the recruitment of Grb2 to the YXNX motifs in FRS2 results in a strong activation of the PI3K signaling pathway and only a moderate activation of ERK, the recruitment of Shp2 results in a strong activation of ERK (Gotoh *et al.* 2004a; Hadari *et al.* 2001; Kouhara *et al.* 1997; Ong *et al.* 2001). Furthermore, during a negative feedback mechanism, FRS2 is Thr phosphorylated by ERK, which inhibits further Tyr phosphorylation of FRS2 (Lax *et al.* 2002; Wu *et al.* 2003) Besides FGF, NGF, BDNF and PDGF, insulin stimulation also results in Tyr phosphorylation of FRS2. However, the functional implications of this observation are still unknown (Delahaye *et al.* 2000).

1.3   CAP

CAP, a member of the sorbin homology (SoHo) adaptor protein family, is a well characterized adaptor protein that is involved in cellular signaling processes and organization of the cytoskeleton. The SoHo adaptor protein family consists of 3 members, namely CAP/sorbin/SH3P12, the Arg-binding protein 2 (ArgBP2) and vinexin-α. Due to alternative splicing, various isoforms for the members of this family exist. Structurally, the main hallmarks of this family are the N-terminal SoHo domain and three Src homology 3 (SH3) domains at the C-terminus (Kioka *et al.* 2002; Roignot & Soubeyran 2009).

Regulation of cell-cell as well as cell-matrix adhesion, organization of the actin cytoskeleton and growth factor receptor downstream signaling are functions that have been assigned to SoHo protein family members (Cestra *et al.* 2005; Kioka *et al.* 2002; Roignot & Soubeyran 2009). Accordingly, ArgBP2 is involved in regulatory processes during cytoskeletal dynamics (Cestra *et al.* 2005), while vinexin-α is a modulator of the EGFR/MAPK signaling pathway (Matsuyama *et al.* 2005; Mitsushima *et al.* 2006; Mitsushima *et al.* 2007; Suwa *et al.* 2002) and participates in remodeling processes of the actin cytoskeleton (Kioka *et al.* 2010; Kioka *et al.* 1999; Mizutani *et al.* 2007).

The adapter functions of CAP have been suggested to play a role during signaling events in integrin-mediated cellular adhesion and focal adhesion turnover (Fernow *et al.* 2009; Ribon *et al.* 1998b). Focal adhesions and cellular motility often are controlled by focal adhesion kinase (FAK) (Chacon & Fazzari 2011). The third SH3 domain of CAP interacts with FAK, and overexpression of CAP was shown to result in a reduced phosphorylation of FAK (Ribon *et al.* 1998a). CAP localizes to stress fibers and is recruited to focal adhesions by vinculin (Fernow *et al.* 2009; Mandai *et al.* 1999; Zhang *et al.* 2006). Furthermore, CAP was shown to be phosphorylated by c-Abl and Src kinases (Fernow *et al.* 2009). Other interactors that assist CAP in cellular adhesion and cytoskeletal regulation are 1-afadin (Mandai *et al.* 1999; Takai *et al.* 2008), paxillin (Gehmlich *et al.* 2007; Zhang *et al.* 2006; Zhang *et al.* 2007), filamin C (Zhang *et al.* 2007), dynamin-1 and -2 (Tosoni & Cestra 2009) and SHIP2 (Vandenbroere *et al.* 2003). A myogenic program remodels cell-matrix contacts that are mediated by focal adhesions into so-called costameres during muscle differentiation (Le Grand & Rudnicki 2007). During this program, cellular CAP protein levels rise and CAP changes its localization from focal adhesions to costameres (Gehmlich et al. 2007; Mandai et al. 1999). This implies a role for CAP in modulation or turnover of focal adhesions and the connected actin cytoskeleton.

Scaffolding roles have been defined for CAP in RTK signaling downstream of both the neurotrophin receptor TrkA and the insulin receptor. Upon NGF stimulation, CAP associates with TrkA and, together with flot-1, facilitates its translocation to membrane rafts (Huang & Reichardt 2003; Limpert et al. 2007). CAP was also shown to be a central component of the PI3K-independent arm of the insulin signaling pathway (Baumann et al. 2000; Kimura et al. 2001). Once the insulin receptor is activated by ligand binding, CAP-c-Cbl complex becomes associated with the receptor (Ahn et al. 2004; Ribon et al. 1998a) which phosphorylates c-Cbl, inducing a translocation of the c-Cbl-CAP complex to membrane rafts to facilitate proper downstream signaling (Mastick et al. 1998; Ribon & Saltiel 1997). Again, this translocation depends on the interaction of CAP and flot-1 (Liu et al. 2005).

1.4   Interplay of Flotillin-1, FRS2 and CAP

As putative scaffolding proteins, flot-1, FRS2 and CAP serve as crucial regulators of many different signaling pathways. A direct interaction has been described between each of these three proteins (Baumann et al. 2000; Tomasovic et al. 2012), and the interacting domains are overlapping (Tomasovic et al. 2012). The pathways in which these proteins have been shown to be involved include insulin signaling (Baumann et al. 2000; Delahaye et al. 2000) and TrkA signaling (Limpert et al. 2007). Generally, FRS2 tethers signaling components to RTKs that use FRS2 as a docking molecule (Dhalluin et al. 2000; Hadari et al. 2001; Kurokawa et al. 2001; Melillo et al. 2001; Ong et al. 2000; Xu et al. 1998). Furthermore, FRS2 is a coordinator of negative feedback signals and helps to attenuate the pathway (Lax et al. 2002; Wong et al. 2002; Wu et al. 2003). Similary to FRS2, flot-1 recruits signaling proteins to membrane rafts, which is the "meeting point" for many components of the respective pathway (Baumann et al. 2000; Haglund et al. 2004; Limpert et al. 2007). By binding to several kinases of MAPK cascade, flot-1 propagates the transmission of the signal more downstream and possibly insulates correct signaling complexes from competing proteins (Amaddii et al. 2012). On the other hand, CAP serves as a shuttling protein. It binds RTKs (TrkA and insulin receptor) indirectly (Ahn et al. 2004; Limpert et al. 2007) and helps recruiting the TrkA receptor or the downstream components (Cbl) to membrane rafts by means of a direct interaction with flot-1 (Baumann et al. 2000; Limpert et al. 2007). Thus, it is likely that these three proteins, by their virtue of interacting with each other, form a signaling network that regulates RTK signaling.

2   Results

Apart from signaling sequences and posttranslational modifications, protein interactors are the third important determinant of the protein localization. Myristoylation was suggested to assist FRS2 in the attachment to cellular membranes (Kouhara et al. 1997). However, myristoylation alone was shown to be insufficient in providing a strong membrane anchor, and some further modification, such as palmitoylation, should be present to assist the protein in membrane binding (Shahinian & Silvius 1995). FRS2 does not exhibit such modifications, but several of its interaction partners were demonstrated to preferentially localize at cellular membranes, e.g. FGFR and flot-1 (Ong *et al.* 2000; Tomasovic *et al.* 2012; Xu *et al.* 1998). Indeed, interaction with flot-1 was found to represent "the secondary signal" for membrane localization of FRS2 (Tomasovic *et al.* 2012). Furthermore, studies by us and others have shown that membrane association of flot-1 is mediated by palmitoylation, oligomerization and association with flot-2 (Babuke *et al.,* 2009; Morrow *et al.,* 2002; Neumann-Giesen *et al.,* 2004; Solis *et al.,* 2007). Previously, we could demonstrate by means of immunofluorescence that in Hep3B cells depleted of flot-1, FRS2 showed a prominent localization in the cytosol and was almost absent from the plasma membrane, whereas in control cells it exhibited a plasma membrane localization (Tomasovic *et al.,* 2012). To rule out the possibility of nonspecific immunofluorescence staining of FRS2 antibody, membrane fractionation experiments were performed, using the same stable clones in which flot-2 or flot-1 were knocked down (Tomasovic *et al.,* 2012). The cells were homogenized without a detergent and then fractionated with high-speed centrifugation to cytosolic (C) and membrane-bound (M) fractions (Figure 1). For FRS2, we observed several bands in the Western Blots which could be due to posttranslational modifications. The results from three independent experiments were quantified (Figure 1B and D). Quantification of the FRS2 distribution between C and M fractions showed that about 60-70% of FRS2 was membrane associated in the control cells. On the other hand, in flot-2 (Figure 1B) and in flot-1 (Figure 1D) knockdown cells, about an equal distribution (50% each) of FRS2 between those two fractions was detected. However, due to variation between the experiments, these data were not significant. The effect of flot-2 knockdown on the membrane localization of FRS2 is probably caused by the lack of flot-1 in these cells, since flot-1 is also downregulated upon depletion of flot-2 (Babuke *et al.,* 2009). These data suggest that FRS2 membrane localization may be facilitated by the presence of flotillins.

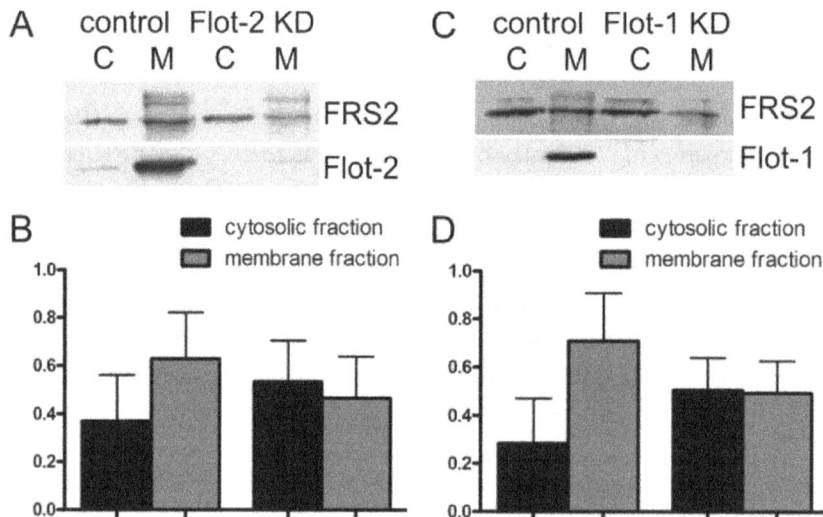

Figure 1. Membrane localization of FRS2 is reduced in cells depleted of flot-2 or flot-1. Hep3B cells were homogenized without detergent and fractionated into membrane bound (M) and cytoplasmic fractions (C) by means of centrifugation. In flot-2 (A) and flot-1 (C) knockdown cells, more FRS2 was found in the cytoplasmic fraction in comparison to the control cells. (B) and (D): densitometric quantification of the soluble and membrane bound FRS2 in flot-2 (B) and flot-1 (D) knockdown cells. Bars represent mean ±SD of three individual experiments.

To check whether the observed effect is specific for the Hep3B cell line, HeLa cells were also tested (Figure 2). Cells transiently knocked down of flot-1 and overexpressing FRS2-GFP were grown on coverslips under steady-state conditions, fixed and stained for the endogenous flot-1. Whereas FRS2-GFP was detected at the plasma membrane in control cells, it became more soluble and did not localize at the plasma membrane in flot-1 knockdown cells, verifying the data obtained with Hep3B cells (Tomasovic *et al.*, 2012).

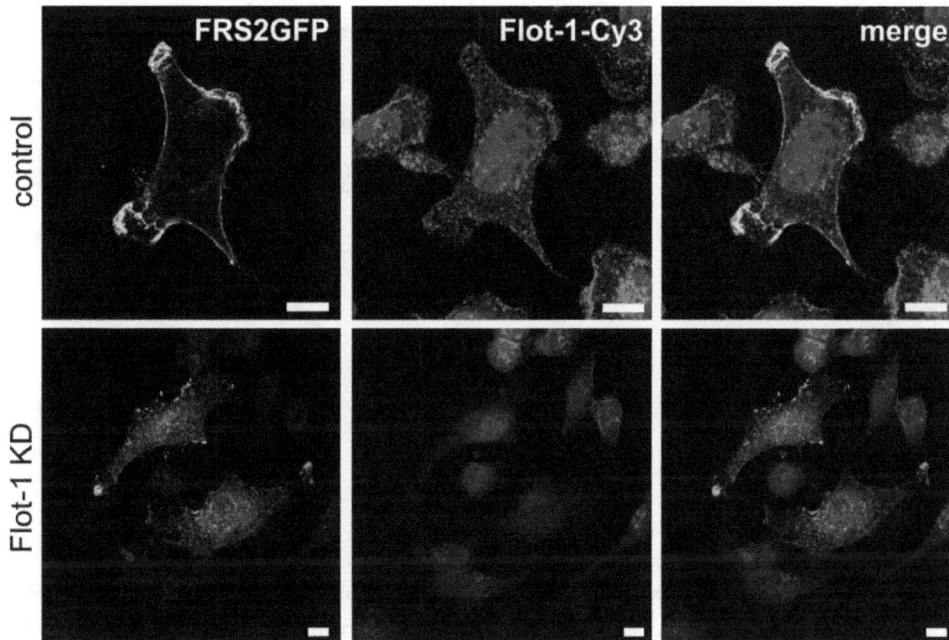

Figure 2: FRS2-GFP is mislocalized in HeLa cells after transient knockdown of flotillin-1. Cells were transfected with FRS2-GFP, grown in serum containing medium, fixed with methanol and stained with antibodies against flot-1 (middle panel). In control cells (upper row), FRS2 was localized at plasma membrane, whereas in flot-1 knockdown cells (lower row), it was found mainly in the cytosol and cytoplasmic inclusions. Scale bars 10 μm.

Flotillins have been shown to be constitutive residents of membrane rafts. FRS2 was also published to be constitutively associated with membrane rafts in PC12 cells (Limpert *et al.*, 2007), and we could show that it becomes recruited to rafts upon pervanadate stimulation of Hep3B cells (Tomasovic *et al.*, 2012). To test if FRS2 raft association is dependent on flot-1 in SHSY5Y cells, which express high amounts of both FRS2 and flot-1, rafts were extracted at 4°C with the non-ionic detergent Triton X-100 from SHSY5Y control cells and stable clones depleted of flot-1. Western blot of the fractions with Cholera toxin-B subunit, which specifically binds to the lipid raft ganglioside GM1, was used to determine the lipid raft-enriched fractions (Figure 3). Rafts were found in fractions 1-4, starting from the top of the gradient. To detect the heavy non-raft fractions, an antibody against transferrin receptor was used. This receptor has been shown to be absent from membrane rafts (Chamberlain & Gould 2002; Limpert *et al.*, 2007), and was detected in fractions 7-9. Flot-1 was mainly found to be localized in the light fractions (fractions 2-5) (Figure 3A), which is in agreement with its constitutive association with membrane rafts. Similarly, a portion of FRS2 was found to be present in the same light fractions (fractions 2 and 3) in both control (Figure 3A) and flot-1 knockdown cells (Figure 3B and C), demonstrating that a fraction of FRS2 is constitutively associated with rafts in SHSY5Y cells, as it was already shown for FRS2 in PC12 cells, and this localization is not dependent on flot-1.

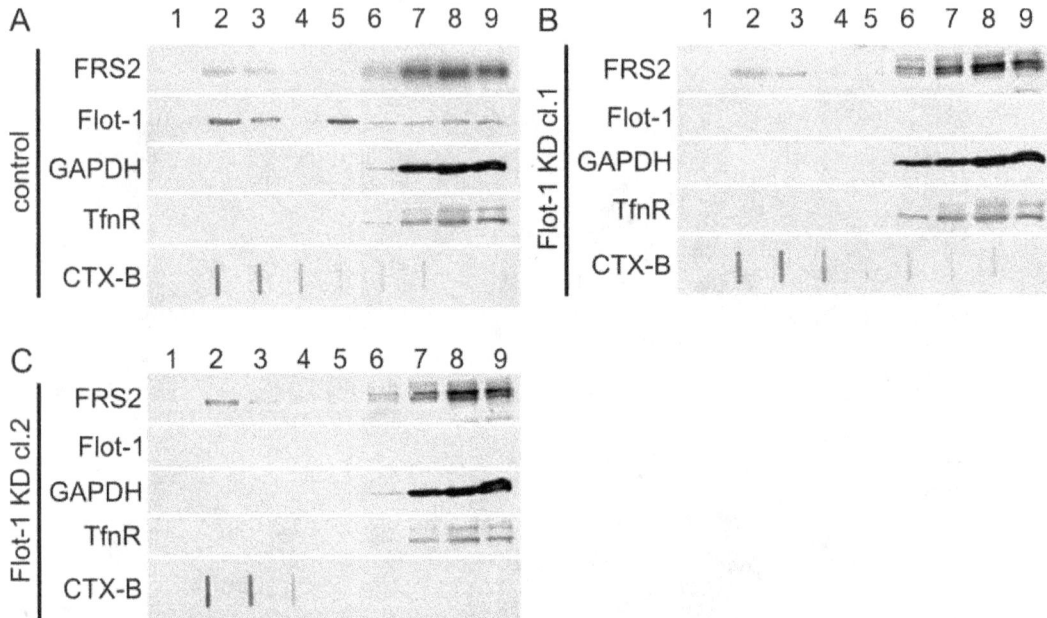

Figure 3: FRS2 localizes to membrane rafts independently of flot-1 in SHSY5Y cells. SHSY5Y cells depleted of flot-1 (B and C) and control cells (A) were grown in serum containing media and rafts were isolated from the cells. Fractions were collected from the top (fraction 1 = the lightest fraction), run on SDS-PAGE and analyzed by Western blot. FRS2 was present in the raft fractions (fractions 2 and 3) in both control and flot-1 knockdown cells. Transferrin receptor (TfnR) was used as a marker for heavy fractions and GAPDH for the cytoplasmic fraction. The raft marker GM1 was detected with HRP-coupled cholera toxin B.

Stimulation of cells with growth factors often results in a change in protein localization. To be able to visualize the cellular localization of FRS2 induced by the stimulation, immunofluorescence stainings of the endogenous FRS2 was done in Hep3B cells (Figure 4). Control cells (Figure 4A) and stable clones depleted of flot-1 (Figure 4B) were either serum starved or stimulated with insulin or pervanadate. Pervanadate is a very potent protein tyrosine phosphatase inhibitor and was described as insulin-mimicking agent which keeps proteins in their hyperphosphorylated state (Shisheva & Shechter, 1993; Tsiani *et al.*, 1997). Surprisingly, in control cells, insulin and pervanadate stimulation led to a translocation of FRS2 into the nucleus, whereas flot-1 remained mainly associated with endosomal structures. As already shown with the serum-grown cells (Figure 1), in starved flot-1 knockdown cells, FRS2 was more soluble when compared to starved control cells. However, upon treatment with insulin or pervanadate, FRS2 was recruited to the nucleus also in flot-1 knockdown cells, indicating that the expression of flot-1 is not necessary for the nuclear transport of FRS2.

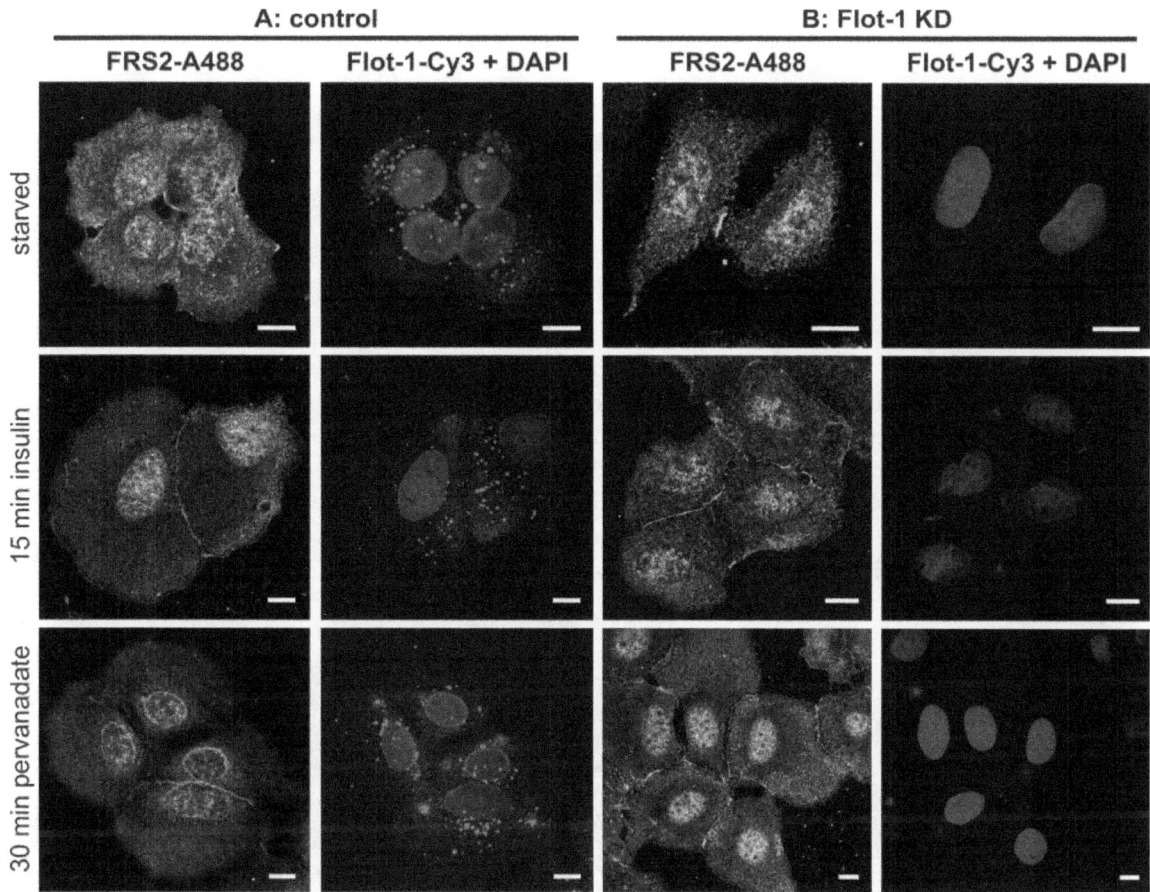

Figure 4: FRS2 is transported to the nucleus upon insulin or pervanadate stimulation independently of flot-1 expression. Hep3B cells depleted of flot-1 (B) and control cells (A) were starved and then treated with insulin or pervanadate. They were fixed with methanol and stained with antibodies against FRS2 and flot-1. FRS2 was translocated to the nucleus upon insulin or pervanadate treatment in both control and flot-1 knockdown cells. Scale bars 10 μm.

To confirm the immunofluorescence data and to exclude possible experimental artefacts due to antibody crossreactivity, biochemical analysis of FRS2 localization was done. Cells were either serum-starved or stimulated with pervanadate and then fractionated to obtain nuclear (N) and non-nuclear (C) fractions (Figure 5). Indeed, after pervanadate stimulation a higher fraction of FRS2 was detected in the nuclear fraction of both control and flot-1 knockdown cells. Pervanadate treatment resulted in the shift of the mobility of FRS2 on the gel, resulting in several bands in the 75–100 kDa range. The uppermost band appeared in the nuclear fraction, pointing to a possible role of post-translational modifications in the nuclear transport of FRS2.

To verify the nuclear localization of FRS2 in other cell lines, immunofluorescence staining of endogenous FRS2 was done using mouse embryonic fibroblasts (MEFs) (Figure 6A). Cells were grown under steady-state conditions, fixed with methanol and stained with antibodies against FRS2 and flot-1. While flot-1 was localized at the plasma membrane and in vesicular structures, FRS2 showed a prominent nuclear localization together with staining residing at the plasma membrane (Figure 6A). The immune

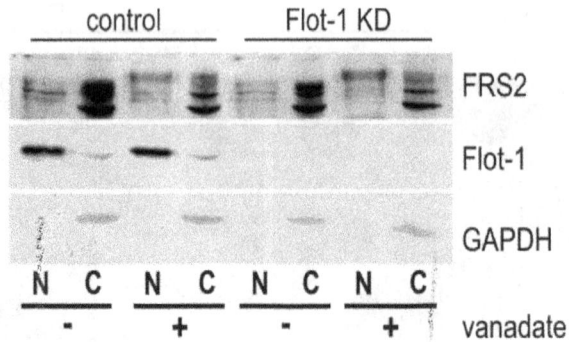

Figure 5: FRS2 nuclear localization upon pervanadate stimulation is independent of flot-1.
Hep3B cells depleted of flot-1 (right) and control cells (left) were starved, treated with pervanadate for 30 min, and the nuclei were isolated. FRS2 was found to be present in the nuclear fraction (N) upon pervanadate stimulation in both control and flot-1 knockdown cells. The amount of the nuclear fraction loaded onto the gel corresponds to a five times higher percentage than that of the cytosolic fraction. GAPDH, a cytoplasmic protein, was used to control the purity of the nuclear fraction.

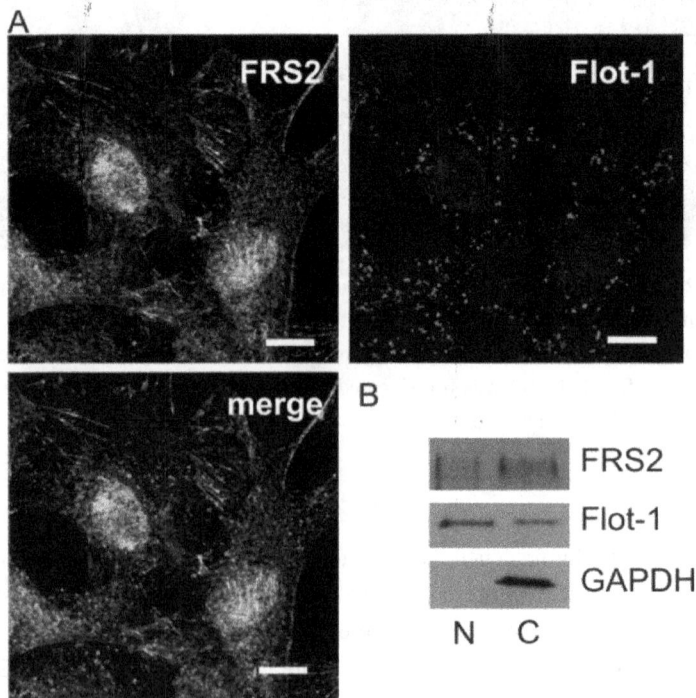

Figure 6: FRS2 is localized in the nucleus of mouse embryonic fibroblasts. A: Cells were grown in serum containing medium, fixed with methanol and stained with antibodies against FRS2 and flot-1. FRS2 was localized in the nucleus, whereas flot-1 was found mainly in cytosolic vesicles. Scale bars 10 µm. B: Nuclear fractionation: FRS2 and flot-1 were present in the nuclear as well as in the cytosolic fraction of MEFs.

fluorescence staining was verified by nuclear fractionation experiments (Figure 6B). The results clearly show that FRS2 is transported to the nucleus despite the lack of a nuclear localization sequence. The nuclear transport is independent of flot-1, which also may localize in the nucleus, as shown here and previously (Gomez *et al.*, 2010; Santamaria *et al.*, 2005).

We were able to show that FRS2 directly interacts with CAP *in vitro* (Tomasovic *et al.*, 2012). Together with flot-1, CAP was found to be one of the major players of the PI3K independent insulin signaling and TrkA signaling pathway (Baumann *et al.*, 2000; Limpert *et al.*, 2007). To test whether the interaction between FRS2 and CAP is dependent on flot-1, coimmunoprecipitation studies were done using Hep3B cells (Figure 7). Immunoprecipitation of FRS2 was done from control cells or stable clones depleted of flotillins, which were grown under steady-state conditions. A CAP isoform of the size around 100 kDa coprecipitated with FRS2 from Hep3B cells, showing that the interaction indeed exists *in vivo*. A similar degree of coprecipitation was detected in control and flot-1 or flot-2 knockdown cells, although the coprecipitation may even be slightly increased in flot-1 knockdown cells. These results imply that the interaction between FRS2 and CAP is independent of flot-1.

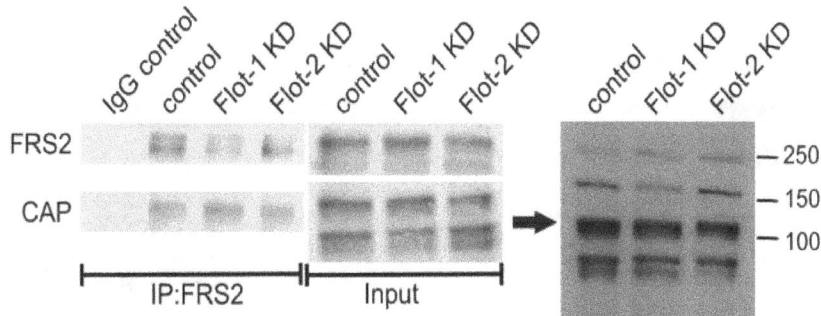

Figure 7: CAP coimmunoprecipitates with FRS2 from Hep3B cells. FRS2 was immuno-precipitated from Hep3B cells. The amount of coprecipitated CAP was slightly increased in flot-1 and flot-2 knockdown cells as compared to the control. No CAP was detected with an isotype-matched control antibody. The right panel shows different CAP isoforms expressed in Hep3B cells.

Since flot-1 has been shown to translocate to the nucleus and the same was shown here for FRS2, the possibility that CAP1 would do the same was also tested. For one of the murine CAP isoforms, CAP2, and its human homologue, R85, it was shown previously that they localize in the nucleus, owing to the presence of a bipartite nuclear localization signal (Lebre *et al.*, 2001; Nunes *et al.*, 2005). Even though this sequence was not found to be present in the CAP1 isoform used in this study, the possibility that some other protein would facilitate its nuclear import remained. To check if CAP1 is able to localize in the nucleus, HeLa cells exogenously expressing CAP1-GFP were subjected to the process of nuclear fractionation (Figure 8A). The nuclear (N) and the cytosolic (C) fractions were then analysed for the presence of CAP1-GFP by means of Western blot. The data show that both the endogenous FRS2 as well as CAP1-GFP can be detected in both fractions. However, when comparing the nuclear level of FRS2 in CAP1-GFP expressing cells with that in GFP expressing control cells, one can see that the forced expression of CAP1 does not recruit more FRS2 protein to the nucleus. The cytosolic marker, GAPDH, was present only in the cytosol, and its absence from the nuclear fraction was used as a measure of the purity of this fraction. Since HeLa cells do not express any detectable levels of endogenous CAP, MEFs were used for further experiments to confirm that the endogenous CAP is able to localize in the nucleus (Figure 8B and C). One has to keep in mind, though, that when checking the endogenous CAP using antibodies against this protein, all CAP isoforms containing the antigen peptide will be detected. Nuclear localization was first checked by immunofluorescence (Figure 8B). For this purpose, MEFs were grown on coverslips under steady-state conditions and stained with antibodies against endogenous CAP which showed a prominent localization in the nucleus, together with a distinct staining of the focal adhesions. Next, to exclude the antibody crossreactivity in staining, biochemical analysis of the CAP localization was done (Figure 8C). MEFs were fractionated to obtain nuclear and non-nuclear fractions, which were then tested for the presence of CAP. Both fractions were positive for several CAP isoforms. GAPDH was exclusively present in the non-nuclear fraction. Thus, biochemical analysis verified immunofluorescence data showing the nuclear localization of endogenous CAP, whose localization in the nucleus seems not to facilitate the nuclear import of FRS2. It still remains to be elucidated whether CAP nuclear localization is dependent on flot-1.

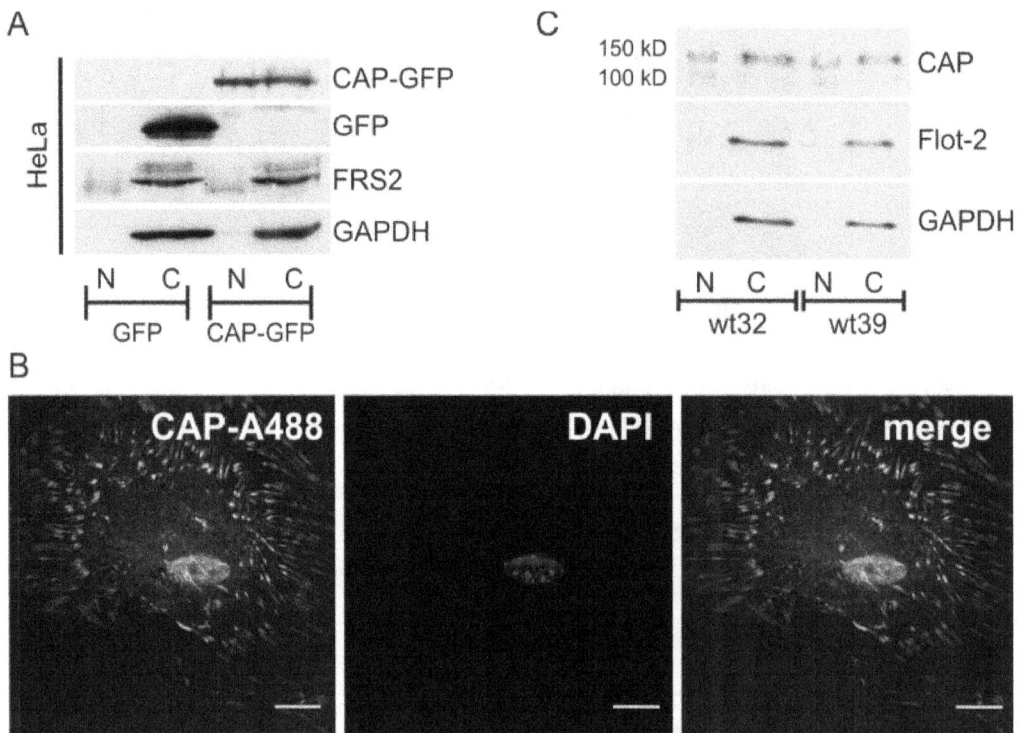

Figure 8: Localization of CAP in mouse embryonic fibroblasts. A: After nuclear fractionation of Hela cells, overexpressed CAP1-GFP (detected with an anti-GFP antibody) was found localized in the nuclear (N) as well as in the cytosolic fraction (C). **B:** Immunofluorescence staining of the endogenous CAP in MEFs. DAPI was used to visualize the nucleus. CAP localized in the nucleus and in focal adhesions. Scale bars 10 μm. **C:** Nuclear fractionation of serum grown MEFs was performed to check the localization of endogenous CAP which localized in the nuclear (N) and cytosolic fractions (C). GAPDH was used as a cytosolic marker to control the purity of the nuclear fraction.

3   Materials and Methods

Plasmid constructs and Antibodies. Full-length FRS2α (GenBank NM_006654) cDNA was amplified from HeLa cDNA by standard PCR and cloned into pEGFP-N1 vector (Clontech) at Eco RI and Bam HI sites. GFP fusion construct of CAP (murine isoform 1, GenBank U58883) was as described previously (Fernow *et al.* 2009; Tomasovic *et al.* 2012). The primary antibodies were as follows: FRS2: Santa Cruz, CAP: Upstate Biotech, flotillins: BD Biosciences, GAPDH: Abcam, GFP: Roche. HRP-coupled Cholera Toxin subunit B (Invitrogen) was used to detect GM1.

Culture of eukaryotic cell lines and transfection of plasmid DNA. HeLa cells were cultured at 8% CO_2 and 37°C in Dulbecco's modified Eagle's medium (DMEM), supplemented with 10% fetal calf serum, 100 U/ml Penicillin and 100 μg/ml Streptomycin. Hep3B and SHSY5Y cells were maintained in DMEM with supplements but at 5% CO_2. Mouse embryonic fibroblasts were cultured at 8% CO_2 and 37°C in DMEM supplemented with 10% fetal calf serum, 100 U/ml Penicillin, 100 μg/ml Streptomycin, 1% sodium pyruvate and 1% non-essential amino acids. For transient transfection with plasmids, Hela cells on 6 well plates were transfected with 1 μg plasmid DNA using Lipofectamine 2000. Hep3B flotillin knockdown cells were generated as described previously (Tomasovic *et al.* 2012). Transient knockdown of flotillin-1 using siRNA oligos was obtained as described previously (Amaddii *et al.* 2012; Tomasovic *et al.* 2012).

Growth factor treatment. Hep3B cells were serum starved for 18 h prior to treatment with 100 nM insulin (Sigma-Aldrich) for indicated times or with 100 μM sodium pervanadate for 30 min.

Immunofluorescence. Hep3B cells were grown on coverslips, starved and then treated with insulin or pervanadate for the indicated time. Cells were fixed with methanol, blocked with 1% BSA in PBS, labeled with primary antibodies for 1 h and then stained with Cy3 and Alexa Fluor 488 conjugated secondary antibodies for 45 min at room temperature. The cells were embedded in Gelmount (Biomeda) supplemented with 1,4-diazadicyclo(2,2,2)octane (DABCO). Images were taken with a confocal laser-scanning microscope (Zeiss LSM510 Meta) with constant imaging settings between the knockdown and control cells.

Coimmunoprecipitation and membrane fractionation. Coimmunoprecipitation assay was peformed as already described (Tomasovic et al, 2012). Membrane fractionation was done as follows: the cells were washed once with homogenization buffer (10 mM Hepes pH 7.2, 1 mM EGTA, 0.25 M sucrose), scraped in the same buffer, supplemented with Protease Inhibitor Cocktail, and homogenized on ice by 20 strokes with a glass homogenizer. The homogenate was centrifuged at 2,000 g for 5 min. This procedure was repeated with the pellet. Both supernatants were then collected and subjected to ultracentrifugation at 100,000 g for 1 h. The resulting supernatant with cytosolic proteins was kept, and the pellet, which represents the membrane fraction, was lysed in membrane fractionation lysis buffer (10 mM Tris pH 8.0, 1 mM EDTA, 0.5% Triton X-100, 60 mM n-Octyl-β-D-glucopyranoside). Proteins of both fractions were enriched by acetone precipitation, solubilized in 4x SDS sample buffer containing 100 mM dithiothreitol by boiling for 5 min at 94°C, separated by SDS-PAGE and subjected to immunoblotting with specific antibodies.

Preparation of membrane rafts using Triton X-100. Cells were grown in 15 cm dishes until reaching 100% confluency. Membrane rafts were prepared as described (Tomasovic *et al.* 2012).

Nuclear fractionation. Cells were grown under steady state or starved conditions, followed by pervana-date treatment for 30 min. They were washed once and scraped in hypotonic buffer (20 mM Hepes pH 7.9, 10 mM KCl, 1 mM EDTA, 10% Glycerol, 0.2% NP-40, 10 mM β-mercaptoethanol). After 5 min of hypotonic shock, the membrane was disrupted by pipetting cells up and down 10 times. Separation of nuclei from the cytosol was achieved by centrifugation at 18,900 g for 10 s. Nuclear pellet was washed twice, dissolved in 250 µl of hypotonic buffer, overlaid on 1 ml of 50 % sucrose cushion and centrifugated for 10 min at 17,200 g. The resulting nuclear pellet was solubilized in 2x SDS sample buffer containing 10% β-mercaptoethanol.

4   Discussion & Conclusions

Our earlier findings have shown that flotillins, FRS2 and CAP are involved in RTK signaling, and all three proteins can interact in a pairwise manner (Amaddii *et al.* 2012; Tomasovic *et al.* 2012). However, since the interaction domains of FRS2 and CAP with flot-1 are overlapping, it is plausible that they compete for the binding to flot-1, rather than forming trimeric complexes (Tomasovic *et al.* 2012). Flot-1, FRS2 and CAP are likely to be involved in the signaling of at least EGF and FGF receptors (Amaddii *et al.* 2012; Tomasovic *et al.* 2012) and the neurotrophin receptor Trk A (Limpert *et al.* 2007) . Furthermore, insulin receptor is another candidate since all three proteins have been shown to be connected with insulin signaling (Baumann *et al.* 2000; Delahaye *et al.* 2000).

Previously, it has been shown that upon NGF stimulation of PC12 cells, flot-1, FRS2 and CAP all localize to membrane rafts (Limpert *et al.* 2007) . Although it is known that FRS2 is a key docking protein for TrkA and necessary for the signal propagation elicited by NGF, no direct evidence exist of a detailed molecular mechanism of the receptor recruitment to membrane rafts. Following the activation and phosphorylation of TrkA receptor, a constitutive complex formed between CAP and Cbl was reported to be recruited to TrkA. Limpert *et al.* drew a parallel with the insulin signaling pathway and speculated that the possible link between this complex and the receptor is mediated by adapter protein with Pleckstrin homology and Src homology domain (APS) (Limpert *et al.* 2007). However, there are no data supporting this assumption. We recently shed new light on the possible sequence of events following the activation of TrkA and insulin receptor (Tomasovic *et al.* 2012). Since FRS2 is capable of interacting with both TrkA (Dhalluin *et al.* 2000; Ong *et al.* 2000) and CAP (Tomasovic *et al.* 2012), it is plausible that CAP/Cbl complex is recruited to the receptor via FRS2. Another possibility would be that CAP, by being a shuttle for TrkA trafficking and by the ability to directly bind to FRS2, might bring TrkA in the close proximity with its substrate, FRS2, which is enriched in membrane rafts in PC12 cells. With the help of flot-1, downstream kinases of MAPK pathway are clustered together (Amaddii *et al.* 2012) and this enables the propagation of the signal. However, so far the direct connection between flot-1, FRS2 and CAP has only been established by our findings (Tomasovic *et al.* 2012). Thus, the details how the interactions modulate the downstream signaling of the said receptors still remains to be clarified.

In this study, we have extended our previous findings concerning the flot-1-FRS2-CAP interaction to see how the binding partners influence the cellular localization of each other. Our earlier findings showed that the PTB and carboxy terminal (CT) domains of FRS2 interact with the CT half of flot-1 (Tomasovic *et al.* 2012). Although flot-1 and flot-2 are relatively homologous, we were not able to detect a direct interaction of flot-2 with FRS2 *in vitro*. However, in the cells, flot-1 and flot-2 are mostly engaged as hetero-oligomers, and an indirect association with flot-2 may also influence the function of

FRS2. Importantly, depletion of flot-2 results in destabilization and degradation of flot-1, so that an effect of flot-2 on FRS2 localization and function may be observed.

Previously, FRS2 was shown to be myristoylated, and this lipid modification facilitates its membrane association (Kouhara *et al.* 1997). However, myristoylation alone has been shown to be insufficient for a stable membrane anchorage of a protein (Resh 1994; Resh 1999). Therefore, it was speculated that constitutive interaction between PTB domain of FRS2 and the juxtamembrane domain of FGFR would contribute to the membrane localization of FRS2 (Kouhara *et al.* 1997). Since the interaction with flot-1 is also constitutive and mainly mediated by the PTB domain (Tomasovic *et al.* 2012), it might further contribute to the binding of FRS2 to cellular membranes. This was supported by our data showing that in the absence of flot-1, FRS2 becomes slightly more soluble. In the cells depleted of flot-2, which also lack flot-1, the membrane association of FRS2 is reduced in a similar fashion. The reduced membrane localization of FRS2 could also be observed by immunofluorescence staining. It has to be noted, however, that FRS2 was not completely solubilized upon flotillin depletion, implicating that further binding partners, such as FGFR, may support its membrane association.

FRS2 has been shown to be constitutively associated with membrane rafts in some cell types. In Hep3B cells, however, FRS2 becomes rafts associated upon a stimulus such as insulin or pervanadate (Tomasovic *et al.* 2012). This signal induced association of FRS2 with rafts requires the expression of flot-1, since in flot-1 depleted cells, FRS2 was not able to translocate into rafts (Tomasovic *et al.* 2012). On the contrary, we here show that the constitutive raft localization of FRS2 in SHSY5Y neuroblastoma cells does not require flotillins. These findings suggest that the signal independent, constitutive raft localization of FRS2 is also independent of flotillins, and may rely on an interaction with some other partner. However, in the cell types in which FRS2 is recruited into rafts only after a signal that activates RTKs or prolongs signaling by inhibition of dephosphorylation, flotillins are essential for the recruitment of FRS2 into detergent insoluble domains. In these cell types, it is possible that the interaction between flot-1 and FRS2 is not constitutive but modulated by the signaling.

Another interesting outcome of our study was the nuclear localization of FRS2, which was detected in several cell lines. When FRS2 was originally discovered as Suc-1, it was shown to localize in the nucleus (Rabin *et al.* 1993), but the nuclear transport of FRS2 has not been studied further. In this study, the nuclear localization of FRS2 was demonstrated by means of immunofluorescence staining and nuclear fractionation. Contamination of nuclear fractions with rafts is a known problem (Say & Hooper 2007). However, several facts speak against the possibility that raft associated FRS2 is actually detected in the nuclear fractions: 1) nuclear localization was shown by two different methods (immunofluorescence and biochemical fractionation), 2) nuclear localization was demonstrated in two different cell lines (Hep3B and MEF), and 3) insulin or pervanadate treatment of Hep3B cells stimulated the nuclear import of FRS2.

Previously, flot-1 has been shown to localize in the nucleus where it exerts a mitogenic effect together with a protein phosphatase PTOV1 (Santamaria *et al.* 2005). Nuclear flot-1 is also important for the regulation of the kinase activity of the mitotic kinase Aurora B (Gomez *et al.* 2010). Since FRS2 does not exhibit a nuclear localization signal, its interaction partner could provide the signal for the nuclear import of FRS2. However, the nuclear localization of FRS2 is independent of flot-1. A mobility shift of the nuclear FRS2 was observed on the gel, running slower than the non-nuclear FRS2. This might implicate that the phosphorylation of FRS2 regulates the nuclear import of the protein. Therefore, phosphorylation and association with some other shuttling protein, which is not flot-1, might mediate its nuclear translocation. One obvious candidate is CAP, which we here show to be partly nuclear in several cell lines. However, ectopic expression of CAP-GFP was unable to increase the nuclear localization of FRS2, implicating that yet another protein may be responsible for their nuclear import. Several growth factor receptors, such as EGFR, insulin receptor and FGFR, have been reported to undergo nuclear translocation after ligand stimulation (Gletsu *et al.* 1999; Jans & Hassan 1998; Lin *et al.* 2001). FGFR, which forms a constitutive complex with FRS2, undergoes importin beta mediated nuclear import upon FGF stimulation (Reilly & Maher 2001). Localization of FGFR in the nucleus has been shown to affect signaling and cell proliferation and to be part of a specific signaling module that is required to coordinate the transcriptional responses of growth factors (Stachowiak *et al.* 1997; Stachowiak *et al.* 2003). Hence, FRFR might even serve as a nuclear "FRS2-carrier". However, the exact molecular mechanism of nuclear import and the biological function which FRS2 and its binding partners flot-1 and CAP exhibit in the nucleus still remain to be clarified in the future.

Acknowledgements

This study has been supported by the German Research Council (DFG) personal grant Ti291/6-2 to RT. We thank Nina Kurrle for the critical reading of the manuscript.

References

Affentranger S, Martinelli S, Hahn J, Rossy J, Niggli V (2011) Dynamic reorganization of flotillins in chemokine-stimulated human T-lymphocytes. BMC Cell Biol 12: 28.

Ahn MY, Katsanakis KD, Bheda F, Pillay TS (2004) Primary and essential role of the adaptor protein APS for recruitment of both c-Cbl and its associated protein CAP in insulin signaling. J Biol Chem 279: 21526-21532.

Ait-Slimane T, Galmes R, Trugnan G, Maurice M (2009) Basolateral internalization of GPI-anchored proteins occurs via a clathrin-independent flotillin-dependent pathway in polarized hepatic cells. Mol Biol Cell 20: 3792-3800.

Amaddii M, Meister M, Banning A, Tomasovic A, Mooz J, Rajalingam K, Tikkanen R (2012) Flotillin-1/reggie-2 protein plays dual role in activation of receptor-tyrosine kinase/mitogen-activated protein kinase signaling. J Biol Chem 287: 7265-7278.

Babuke T, Ruonala M, Meister M, Amaddii M, Genzler C, Esposito A, Tikkanen R (2009) Hetero-oligomerization of reggie-1/flotillin-2 and reggie-2/flotillin-1 is required for their endocytosis. Cell Signal 21: 1287-1297.

Babuke T, Tikkanen R (2007) Dissecting the molecular function of reggie/flotillin proteins. Eur J Cell Biol 86: 525-532.

Baumann CA, Ribon V, Kanzaki M, Thurmond DC, Mora S, Shigematsu S, Bickel PE, Pessin JE, Saltiel AR (2000) CAP defines a second signalling pathway required for insulin-stimulated glucose transport. Nature 407: 202-207.

Bickel PE, Scherer PE, Schnitzer JE, Oh P, Lisanti MP, Lodish HF (1997) Flotillin and epidermal surface antigen define a new family of caveolae-associated integral membrane proteins. J Biol Chem 272: 13793-13802.

Blanchet MH, Le Good JA, Mesnard D, Oorschot V, Baflast S, Minchiotti G, Klumperman J, Constam DB (2008) Cripto recruits Furin and PACE4 and controls Nodal trafficking during proteolytic maturation. EMBO J 27: 2580-2591.

Cestra G, Toomre D, Chang S, De Camilli P (2005) The Abl/Arg substrate ArgBP2/nArgBP2 coordinates the function of multiple regulatory mechanisms converging on the actin cytoskeleton. Proc Natl Acad Sci U S A 102: 1731-1736.

Chacon MR, Fazzari P (2011) FAK: dynamic integration of guidance signals at the growth cone. Cell Adh Migr 5: 52-55.

Chamberlain LH, Gould GW (2002) The vesicle- and target-SNARE proteins that mediate Glut4 vesicle fusion are localized in detergent-insoluble lipid rafts present on distinct intracellular membranes. J Biol Chem 277: 49750-49754.

Chen TY, Liu PH, Ruan CT, Chiu L, Kung FL (2006) The intracellular domain of amyloid precursor protein interacts with flotillin-1, a lipid raft protein. Biochem Biophys Res Commun *342:* 266-272.

Cremona ML, Matthies HJ, Pau K, Bowton E, Speed N, Lute BJ, Anderson M, Sen N, Robertson SD, Vaughan RA, Rothman JE, Galli A, Javitch JA, Yamamoto A (2011) Flotillin-1 is essential for PKC-triggered endocytosis and membrane microdomain localization of DAT. Nature neuroscience *14:* 469-477.

Delahaye L, Rocchi S, Van Obberghen E (2000) Potential involvement of FRS2 in insulin signaling. Endocrinology *141:* 621-628.

Dermine JF, Duclos S, Garin J, St-Louis F, Rea S, Parton RG, Desjardins M (2001) Flotillin-1-enriched lipid raft domains accumulate on maturing phagosomes. J Biol Chem *276:* 18507-18512.

Dhalluin C, Yan KS, Plotnikova O, Lee KW, Zeng L, Kuti M, Mujtaba S, Goldfarb MP, Zhou MM (2000) Structural basis of SNT PTB domain interactions with distinct neurotrophic receptors. Mol Cell *6:* 921-929.

Dixon SJ, MacDonald JI, Robinson KN, Kubu CJ, Meakin SO (2006) Trk receptor binding and neurotrophin/fibroblast growth factor (FGF)-dependent activation of the FGF receptor substrate (FRS)-3. Biochim Biophys Acta *1763:* 366-380.

Easton JB, Royer AR, Middlemas DS (2006) The protein tyrosine phosphatase, Shp2, is required for the complete activation of the RAS/MAPK pathway by brain-derived neurotrophic factor. J Neurochem *97:* 834-845.

Fecchi K, Volonte D, Hezel MP, Schmeck K, Galbiati F (2006) Spatial and temporal regulation of GLUT4 translocation by flotillin-1 and caveolin-3 in skeletal muscle cells. FASEB J *20:* 705-707.

Fernow I, Tomasovic A, Siehoff-Icking A, Tikkanen R (2009) Cbl-associated protein is tyrosine phosphorylated by c-Abl and c-Src kinases. BMC Cell Biol *10:* 80.

Frick M, Bright NA, Riento K, Bray A, Merrified C, Nichols BJ (2007) Coassembly of flotillins induces formation of membrane microdomains, membrane curvature, and vesicle budding. Curr Biol *17:* 1151-1156.

Ge L, Qi W, Wang LJ, Miao HH, Qu YX, Li BL, Song BL (2011) Flotillins play an essential role in Niemann-Pick C1-like 1-mediated cholesterol uptake. Proc Natl Acad Sci U S A *108:* 551-556.

Gehmlich K, Pinotsis N, Hayess K, van der Ven PF, Milting H, El Banayosy A, Korfer R, Wilmanns M, Ehler E, Furst DO (2007) Paxillin and ponsin interact in nascent costameres of muscle cells. J Mol Biol *369:* 665-682.

Glebov OO, Bright NA, Nichols BJ (2006) Flotillin-1 defines a clathrin-independent endocytic pathway in mammalian cells. Nat Cell Biol *8:* 46-54.

Gletsu N, Dixon W, Clandinin MT (1999) Insulin receptor at the mouse hepatocyte nucleus after a glucose meal induces dephosphorylation of a 30-kDa transcription factor and a concomitant increase in malic enzyme gene expression. J Nutr *129:* 2154-2161.

Gomez V, Sese M, Santamaria A, Martinez JD, Castellanos E, Soler M, Thomson TM, Paciucci R (2010) Regulation of aurora B kinase by the lipid raft protein flotillin-1. J Biol Chem *285:* 20683-20690.

Gotoh N (2008) Regulation of growth factor signaling by FRS2 family docking/scaffold adaptor proteins. Cancer Sci *99:* 1319-1325.

Gotoh N, Ito M, Yamamoto S, Yoshino I, Song N, Wang Y, Lax I, Schlessinger J, Shibuya M, Lang RA (2004a) Tyrosine phosphorylation sites on FRS2alpha responsible for Shp2 recruitment are critical for induction of lens and retina. Proc Natl Acad Sci U S A *101:* 17144-17149.

Gotoh N, Laks S, Nakashima M, Lax I, Schlessinger J (2004b) FRS2 family docking proteins with overlapping roles in activation of MAP kinase have distinct spatial-temporal patterns of expression of their transcripts. FEBS Lett *564:* 14-18.

Ha H, Kwak HB, Lee SK, Na DS, Rudd CE, Lee ZH, Kim HH (2003) Membrane rafts play a crucial role in receptor activator of nuclear factor kappaB signaling and osteoclast function. J Biol Chem *278:* 18573-18580.

*Hadari YR, Gotoh N, Kouhara H, Lax I, Schlessinger J (2001) Critical role for the docking-protein FRS2 alpha in FGF receptor-mediated signal transduction pathways. Proc Natl Acad Sci U S A **98**: 8578-8583.*

*Hadari YR, Kouhara H, Lax I, Schlessinger J (1998) Binding of Shp2 tyrosine phosphatase to FRS2 is essential for fibroblast growth factor-induced PC12 cell differentiation. Mol Cell Biol **18**: 3966-3973.*

*Haglund K, Ivankovic-Dikic I, Shimokawa N, Kruh GD, Dikic I (2004) Recruitment of Pyk2 and Cbl to lipid rafts mediates signals important for actin reorganization in growing neurites. J Cell Sci **117**: 2557-2568.*

*Huang EJ, Reichardt LF (2003) Trk receptors: roles in neuronal signal transduction. Annu Rev Biochem **72**: 609-642.*

*Huang L, Gotoh N, Zhang S, Shibuya M, Yamamoto T, Tsuchida N (2004) SNT-2 interacts with ERK2 and negatively regulates ERK2 signaling in response to EGF stimulation. Biochem Biophys Res Commun **324**: 1011-1017.*

*Huang L, Watanabe M, Chikamori M, Kido Y, Yamamoto T, Shibuya M, Gotoh N, Tsuchida N (2006) Unique role of SNT-2/FRS2beta/FRS3 docking/adaptor protein for negative regulation in EGF receptor tyrosine kinase signaling pathways. Oncogene **25**: 6457-6466.*

*Jans DA, Hassan G (1998) Nuclear targeting by growth factors, cytokines, and their receptors: a role in signaling? Bioessays **20**: 400-411.*

*Kimura A, Baumann CA, Chiang SH, Saltiel AR (2001) The sorbin homology domain: a motif for the targeting of proteins to lipid rafts. Proc Natl Acad Sci U S A **98**: 9098-9103.*

*Kioka N, Ito T, Yamashita H, Uekawa N, Umemoto T, Motoyoshi S, Imai H, Takahashi K, Watanabe H, Yamada M, Ueda K (2010) Crucial role of vinexin for keratinocyte migration in vitro and epidermal wound healing in vivo. Exp Cell Res **316**: 1728-1738.*

*Kioka N, Sakata S, Kawauchi T, Amachi T, Akiyama SK, Okazaki K, Yaen C, Yamada KM, Aota S (1999) Vinexin: a novel vinculin-binding protein with multiple SH3 domains enhances actin cytoskeletal organization. J Cell Biol **144**: 59-69.*

*Kioka N, Ueda K, Amachi T (2002) Vinexin, CAP/ponsin, ArgBP2: a novel adaptor protein family regulating cytoskeletal organization and signal transduction. Cell Struct Funct **27**: 1-7.*

*Kokubo H, Kayed R, Glabe CG, Saido TC, Iwata N, Helms JB, Yamaguchi H (2005) Oligomeric proteins ultrastructurally localize to cell processes, especially to axon terminals with higher density, but not to lipid rafts in Tg2576 mouse brain. Brain Res **1045**: 224-228.*

*Kouhara H, Hadari YR, Spivak-Kroizman T, Schilling J, Bar-Sagi D, Lax I, Schlessinger J (1997) A lipid-anchored Grb2-binding protein that links FGF-receptor activation to the Ras/MAPK signaling pathway. Cell **89**: 693-702.*

*Kurokawa K, Iwashita T, Murakami H, Hayashi H, Kawai K, Takahashi M (2001) Identification of SNT/FRS2 docking site on RET receptor tyrosine kinase and its role for signal transduction. Oncogene **20**: 1929-1938.*

*Langhorst MF, Reuter A, Luxenhofer G, Boneberg EM, Legler DF, Plattner H, Stuermer CA (2006) Preformed reggie/flotillin caps: stable priming platforms for macrodomain assembly in T cells. FASEB J **20**: 711-713.*

*Lax I, Wong A, Lamothe B, Lee A, Frost A, Hawes J, Schlessinger J (2002) The docking protein FRS2alpha controls a MAP kinase-mediated negative feedback mechanism for signaling by FGF receptors. Mol Cell **10**: 709-719.*

*Le Grand F, Rudnicki MA (2007) Skeletal muscle satellite cells and adult myogenesis. Curr Opin Cell Biol **19**: 628-633.*

*Lebre AS, Jamot L, Takahashi J, Spassky N, Leprince C, Ravise N, Zander C, Fujigasaki H, Kussel-Andermann P, Duyckaerts C, Camonis JH, Brice A (2001) Ataxin-7 interacts with a Cbl-associated protein that it recruits into neuronal intranuclear inclusions. Hum Mol Genet **10**: 1201-1213.*

*Li Y, Martin BR, Cravatt BF, Hofmann SL (2012) DHHC5 protein palmitoylates flotillin-2 and is rapidly degraded on induction of neuronal differentiation in cultured cells. J Biol Chem **287**: 523-530.*

*Limpert AS, Karlo JC, Landreth GE (2007) Nerve growth factor stimulates the concentration of TrkA within lipid rafts and extracellular signal-regulated kinase activation through c-Cbl-associated protein. Mol Cell Biol **27**: 5686-5698.*

Lin SY, Makino K, Xia W, Matin A, Wen Y, Kwong KY, Bourguignon L, Hung MC (2001) Nuclear localization of EGF receptor and its potential new role as a transcription factor. Nat Cell Biol **3:** 802-808.

Lingwood D, Simons K (2010) Lipid rafts as a membrane-organizing principle. Science **327:** 46-50.

Liu J, Deyoung SM, Zhang M, Dold LH, Saltiel AR (2005) The stomatin/prohibitin/flotillin/HflK/C domain of flotillin-1 contains distinct sequences that direct plasma membrane localization and protein interactions in 3T3-L1 adipocytes. J Biol Chem **280:** 16125-16134.

Mandai K, Nakanishi H, Satoh A, Takahashi K, Satoh K, Nishioka H, Mizoguchi A, Takai Y (1999) Ponsin/SH3P12: an l-afadin- and vinculin-binding protein localized at cell-cell and cell-matrix adherens junctions. J Cell Biol **144:** 1001-1017.

Mastick CC, Brady MJ, Printen JA, Ribon V, Saltiel AR (1998) Spatial determinants of specificity in insulin action. Mol Cell Biochem **182:** 65-71.

Matsuyama M, Mizusaki H, Shimono A, Mukai T, Okumura K, Abe K, Shimada K, Morohashi K (2005) A novel isoform of Vinexin, Vinexin gamma, regulates Sox9 gene expression through activation of MAPK cascade in mouse fetal gonad. Genes Cells **10:** 421-434.

McDougall K, Kubu C, Verdi JM, Meakin SO (2001) Developmental expression patterns of the signaling adapters FRS-2 and FRS-3 during early embryogenesis. Mech Dev **103:** 145-148.

Meakin SO, MacDonald JI, Gryz EA, Kubu CJ, Verdi JM (1999) The signaling adapter FRS-2 competes with Shc for binding to the nerve growth factor receptor TrkA. A model for discriminating proliferation and differentiation. J Biol Chem **274:** 9861-9870.

Melillo RM, Santoro M, Ong SH, Billaud M, Fusco A, Hadari YR, Schlessinger J, Lax I (2001) Docking protein FRS2 links the protein tyrosine kinase RET and its oncogenic forms with the mitogen-activated protein kinase signaling cascade. Mol Cell Biol **21:** 4177-4187.

Mitsushima M, Ueda K, Kioka N (2006) Vinexin beta regulates the phosphorylation of epidermal growth factor receptor on the cell surface. Genes Cells **11:** 971-982.

Mitsushima M, Ueda K, Kioka N (2007) Involvement of phosphatases in the anchorage-dependent regulation of ERK2 activation. Exp Cell Res **313:** 1830-1838.

Mizutani K, Ito H, Iwamoto I, Morishita R, Deguchi T, Nozawa Y, Asano T, Nagata KI (2007) Essential roles of ERK-mediated phosphorylation of vinexin in cell spreading, migration and anchorage-independent growth. Oncogene **26:** 7122-7131.

Mohammadi M, Honegger AM, Rotin D, Fischer R, Bellot F, Li W, Dionne CA, Jaye M, Rubinstein M, Schlessinger J (1991) A tyrosine-phosphorylated carboxy-terminal peptide of the fibroblast growth factor receptor (Flg) is a binding site for the SH2 domain of phospholipase C-gamma 1. Mol Cell Biol **11:** 5068-5078.

Morrow IC, Parton RG (2005) Flotillins and the PHB domain protein family: rafts, worms and anaesthetics. Traffic **6:** 725-740.

Morrow IC, Rea S, Martin S, Prior IA, Prohaska R, Hancock JF, James DE, Parton RG (2002) Flotillin-1/reggie-2 traffics to surface raft domains via a novel golgi-independent pathway. Identification of a novel membrane targeting domain and a role for palmitoylation. J Biol Chem **277:** 48834-48841.

Neumann-Giesen C, Falkenbach B, Beicht P, Claasen S, Luers G, Stuermer CA, Herzog V, Tikkanen R (2004) Membrane and raft association of reggie-1/flotillin-2: role of myristoylation, palmitoylation and oligomerization and induction of filopodia by overexpression. Biochem J **378:** 509-518.

Neumann-Giesen C, Fernow I, Amaddii M, Tikkanen R (2007) Role of EGF-induced tyrosine phosphorylation of reggie-1/flotillin-2 in cell spreading and signaling to the actin cytoskeleton. J Cell Sci **120:** 395-406.

Nunes SM, Ferralli J, Choi K, Brown-Luedi M, Minet AD, Chiquet-Ehrismann R (2005) The intracellular domain of teneurin-1 interacts with MBD1 and CAP/ponsin resulting in subcellular codistribution and translocation to the nuclear matrix. Exp Cell Res **305:** 122-132.

Ong SH, Guy GR, Hadari YR, Laks S, Gotoh N, Schlessinger J, Lax I (2000) FRS2 proteins recruit intracellular signaling pathways by binding to diverse targets on fibroblast growth factor and nerve growth factor receptors. Mol Cell Biol 20: 979-989.

Ong SH, Hadari YR, Gotoh N, Guy GR, Schlessinger J, Lax I (2001) Stimulation of phosphatidylinositol 3-kinase by fibroblast growth factor receptors is mediated by coordinated recruitment of multiple docking proteins. Proc Natl Acad Sci U S A 98: 6074-6079.

Rabin SJ, Cleghon V, Kaplan DR (1993) SNT, a differentiation-specific target of neurotrophic factor-induced tyrosine kinase activity in neurons and PC12 cells. Mol Cell Biol 13: 2203-2213.

Rajendran L, Beckmann J, Magenau A, Boneberg EM, Gaus K, Viola A, Giebel B, Illges H (2009) Flotillins are involved in the polarization of primitive and mature hematopoietic cells. PLoS One 4: e8290.

Rajendran L, Masilamani M, Solomon S, Tikkanen R, Stuermer CA, Plattner H, Illges H (2003) Asymmetric localization of flotillins/reggies in preassembled platforms confers inherent polarity to hematopoietic cells. Proc Natl Acad Sci U S A 100: 8241-8246.

Reilly JF, Maher PA (2001) Importin beta-mediated nuclear import of fibroblast growth factor receptor: role in cell proliferation. J Cell Biol 152: 1307-1312.

Resh MD (1994) Myristylation and palmitylation of Src family members: the fats of the matter. Cell 76: 411-413.

Resh MD (1999) Fatty acylation of proteins: new insights into membrane targeting of myristoylated and palmitoylated proteins. Biochim Biophys Acta 1451: 1-16.

Ribon V, Herrera R, Kay BK, Saltiel AR (1998a) A role for CAP, a novel, multifunctional Src homology 3 domain-containing protein in formation of actin stress fibers and focal adhesions. J Biol Chem 273: 4073-4080.

Ribon V, Printen JA, Hoffman NG, Kay BK, Saltiel AR (1998b) A novel, multifuntional c-Cbl binding protein in insulin receptor signaling in 3T3-L1 adipocytes. Mol Cell Biol 18: 872-879.

Ribon V, Saltiel AR (1997) Insulin stimulates tyrosine phosphorylation of the proto-oncogene product of c-Cbl in 3T3-L1 adipocytes. Biochem J 324 (Pt 3): 839-845.

Riento K, Frick M, Schafer I, Nichols BJ (2009) Endocytosis of flotillin-1 and flotillin-2 is regulated by Fyn kinase. J Cell Sci 122: 912-918.

Roignot J, Soubeyran P (2009) ArgBP2 and the SoHo family of adapter proteins in oncogenic diseases. Cell Adh Migr 3: 167-170.

Santamaria A, Castellanos E, Gomez V, Benedit P, Renau-Piqueras J, Morote J, Reventos J, Thomson TM, Paciucci R (2005) PTOV1 enables the nuclear translocation and mitogenic activity of flotillin-1, a major protein of lipid rafts. Mol Cell Biol 25: 1900-1911.

Say YH, Hooper NM (2007) Contamination of nuclear fractions with plasma membrane lipid rafts. Proteomics 7: 1059-1064.

Schneider A, Rajendran L, Honsho M, Gralle M, Donnert G, Wouters F, Hell SW, Simons M (2008) Flotillin-dependent clustering of the amyloid precursor protein regulates its endocytosis and amyloidogenic processing in neurons. J Neurosci 28: 2874-2882.

Schulte T, Paschke KA, Laessing U, Lottspeich F, Stuermer CA (1997) Reggie-1 and reggie-2, two cell surface proteins expressed by retinal ganglion cells during axon regeneration. Development 124: 577-587.

Shahinian S, Silvius JR (1995) Doubly-lipid-modified protein sequence motifs exhibit long-lived anchorage to lipid bilayer membranes. Biochemistry 34: 3813-3822.

Shisheva A, Shechter Y (1993) Mechanism of pervanadate stimulation and potentiation of insulin-activated glucose transport in rat adipocytes: dissociation from vanadate effect. Endocrinology 133: 1562-1568.

Simons K, Gerl MJ (2010) Revitalizing membrane rafts: new tools and insights. Nat Rev Mol Cell Biol 11: 688-699.

Simons K, Ikonen E (1997) Functional rafts in cell membranes. Nature 387: 569-572.

Simons K, Sampaio JL (2011) Membrane organization and lipid rafts. Cold Spring Harbor perspectives in biology 3: a004697.

Solis GP, Hoegg M, Munderloh C, Schrock Y, Malaga-Trillo E, Rivera-Milla E, Stuermer CA (2007) Reggie/flotillin proteins are organized into stable tetramers in membrane microdomains. Biochem J 403: 313-322.

Stachowiak EK, Maher PA, Tucholski J, Mordechai E, Joy A, Moffett J, Coons S, Stachowiak MK (1997) Nuclear accumulation of fibroblast growth factor receptors in human glial cells--association with cell proliferation. Oncogene 14: 2201-2211.

Stachowiak MK, Fang X, Myers JM, Dunham SM, Berezney R, Maher PA, Stachowiak EK (2003) Integrative nuclear FGFR1 signaling (INFS) as a part of a universal "feed-forward-and-gate" signaling module that controls cell growth and differentiation. J Cell Biochem 90: 662-691.

Strauss K, Goebel C, Runz H, Mobius W, Weiss S, Feussner I, Simons M, Schneider A (2010) Exosome secretion ameliorates lysosomal storage of cholesterol in Niemann-Pick type C disease. J Biol Chem 285: 26279-26288.

Stuermer CA, Lang DM, Kirsch F, Wiechers M, Deininger SO, Plattner H (2001) Glycosylphosphatidyl inositol-anchored proteins and fyn kinase assemble in noncaveolar plasma membrane microdomains defined by reggie-1 and -2. Mol Biol Cell 12: 3031-3045.

Suwa A, Mitsushima M, Ito T, Akamatsu M, Ueda K, Amachi T, Kioka N (2002) Vinexin beta regulates the anchorage dependence of ERK2 activation stimulated by epidermal growth factor. J Biol Chem 277: 13053-13058.

Takai Y, Ikeda W, Ogita H, Rikitake Y (2008) The immunoglobulin-like cell adhesion molecule nectin and its associated protein afadin. Annu Rev Cell Dev Biol 24: 309-342.

Tavernarakis N, Driscoll M, Kyrpides NC (1999) The SPFH domain: implicated in regulating targeted protein turnover in stomatins and other membrane-associated proteins. Trends Biochem Sci 24: 425-427.

Tomasovic A, Traub S, Tikkanen R (2012) Molecular Networks in FGF Signaling: Flotillin-1 and Cbl-Associated Protein Compete for the Binding to Fibroblast Growth Factor Receptor Substrate 2. PLoS ONE 7(1): e29739. doi:10.1371.

Tosoni D, Cestra G (2009) CAP (Cbl associated protein) regulates receptor-mediated endocytosis. FEBS Lett 583: 293-300.

Tsiani E, Abdullah N, Fantus IG (1997) Insulin-mimetic agents vanadate and pervanadate stimulate glucose but inhibit amino acid uptake. Am J Physiol 272: C156-162.

Vandenbroere I, Paternotte N, Dumont JE, Erneux C, Pirson I (2003) The c-Cbl-associated protein and c-Cbl are two new partners of the SH2-containing inositol polyphosphate 5-phosphatase SHIP2. Biochem Biophys Res Commun 300: 494-500.

Volonte D, Galbiati F, Li S, Nishiyama K, Okamoto T, Lisanti MP (1999) Flotillins/cavatellins are differentially expressed in cells and tissues and form a hetero-oligomeric complex with caveolins in vivo. Characterization and epitope-mapping of a novel flotillin-1 monoclonal antibody probe. J Biol Chem 274: 12702-12709.

Wong A, Lamothe B, Lee A, Schlessinger J, Lax I (2002) FRS2 alpha attenuates FGF receptor signaling by Grb2-mediated recruitment of the ubiquitin ligase Cbl. Proc Natl Acad Sci U S A 99: 6684-6689.

Wu Y, Chen Z, Ullrich A (2003) EGFR and FGFR signaling through FRS2 is subject to negative feedback control by ERK1/2. Biol Chem 384: 1215-1226.

Xu H, Lee KW, Goldfarb M (1998) Novel recognition motif on fibroblast growth factor receptor mediates direct association and activation of SNT adapter proteins. J Biol Chem 273: 17987-17990.

Zhang M, Kimura A, Saltiel AR (2003) Cloning and characterization of Cbl-associated protein splicing isoforms. Mol Med 9: 18-25.

Zhang M, Liu J, Cheng A, Deyoung SM, Chen X, Dold LH, Saltiel AR (2006) CAP interacts with cytoskeletal proteins and regulates adhesion-mediated ERK activation and motility. EMBO J 25: 5284-5293.

*Zhang M, Liu J, Cheng A, Deyoung SM, Saltiel AR (2007) Identification of CAP as a costameric protein that interacts with filamin C. Mol Biol Cell **18:** 4731-4740.*

*Zhou L, McDougall K, Kubu CJ, Verdi JM, Meakin SO (2003) Genomic organization and comparative sequence analysis of the mouse and human FRS2, FRS3 genes. Mol Biol Rep **30:** 15-25.*

Analyses of Mouse Liver Microsomal Proteome

Xianquan Zhan, Zhuchu Chen, Fang Peng, Maoyu Li
Key Laboratory of Cancer Proteomics of Chinese Ministry of Health
Hunan Engineering Laboratory for Structural Biology and Drug Design
Xiangya Hospital, Central South University, China

1   Introduction

A major role is played by the liver in metabolism, biosynthesis, and chemical neutralizing in the processes of extensive physiological functions (Tananova *et al.*, 2012, Wong & Adeli, 2009). Liver diseases including viral hepatitis and liver cancer pose a worldwide public health challenge (He, 2005). With the rapid development of proteomics in the era of post-genomics, it brings the promise for the discovery of biomarkers to fight against liver diseases. However, no single analysis strategy can sufficiently address all components of a proteome due to the complexity of proteome. Analysis of the subcellular proteome would be a short-cut for insight into the functions of a given tissue or cell because subcellular proteomics reduces the complexity of a proteome (Jung *et al.*, 2000, Taylor *et al.*, 2003), detects some low-abundance proteins, and offers more detailed information (Arnold *et al.*, 2004), for the understanding of the function of the entire proteome.

Microsomes are primarily closed sacs of membrane that are derived mostly from endoplasmic reticulum (ER). As for liver, in addition to components of the protein secretary pathways, microsomes contain many proteins that are involved in the processes of lipid/lipoprotein biosynthesis and drug metabolism. The liver microsome is the ideal target to analyze compound metabolism, membrane-bound enzyme functions, lipid-protein interactions, and drug-drug interactions (Heinemann & Ozols, 1998, Wong & Adeli, 2009). Isolating and mapping the liver microsomal proteome in combination with bioinformatics annotation would reveal more and unknown essential information regarding the liver molecular functions.

Integration of gel-method with mass spectrometry (MS) is an effective approach to isolate and map the components of a proteome. Two-dimensional gel electrophoresis (2DE) is one of the most common techniques to array soluble proteins, and visualizes isoforms and post-translational modifications in a proteome (Okuzawa *et al.*, 1994, Chen *et al.*, 2007). However, membrane proteins are less amenable to solubilization in protein extraction buffers and are also susceptible to precipitation due to the pH environment that is around its isoelectric point (pI) or acidic pH during isoelectric focusing (IEF). The analytical capability of one-dimensional gel electrophoresis (1DE) in the separation of ER membrane proteins is incomparably greater than that of 2DE (Galeva & Altermann, 2002, Lisitsa *et al.*, 2009, Santoni *et al.*, 2000). The approach that combined 1DE and 2DE was suggested by some studies (Chen *et al.*, 2007, Kanaeva *et al.*, 2005) to analyze the proteome of a subcellular organelle such as microsome that contains a considerable number of highly hydrophobic membrane proteins. Also, the high efficiency of the carbonate procedure in separating membrane proteins was further confirmed (Friso *et al.*, 2004, Fujiki *et al.*, 1982). The Na$_2$CO$_3$ wash followed by sodium dodecyl sulfate polyacrylamide gel electrophoresis (SDS-PAGE) prior to in-gel tryptic digestion and liquid chromatography-tandem mass spectrometry (LC-MS/MS) is effective for detection of microsomal membrane proteins (Peng *et al.*, 2011). 2D liquid phase fraction (PF2D)-MS/MS is another effective system for the analysis of membrane proteins (Lee *et al.*, 2008). Furthermore, bioinformatics is a rapid and direct method to annotate those characterized protein component in a microsomal proteome and assists in the understanding of its biological functions.

In this chapter, we mainly review our own work (Peng *et al.*, 2012) in the analysis of mouse liver microsomal proteome, and compare our work with other researchers' work (Zgoda *et al.*, 2006 and 2009, Gilchrist *et al.*, 2006) in analysis of microsomal proteome so that an overall systems procedure will be present for global identification and functional annotation of the protein components of the liver microsomes to provide insight into the biological functions of the liver. In our work, mouse liver microsomes were isolated and enriched with differential centrifugation and sucrose gradient centrifugation, and microsomal membrane proteins were further extracted from isolated microsomal fractions by the carbonate method. The enriched microsomal proteins were arrayed with 2DE and carbonate-extraction microsomal membrane proteins with 1DE. A total of 183 2DE-arrayed proteins and 99 1DE-separated proteins were characterized with MS/MS. A total of 260 nonredundant microsomal proteins were obtained and represent the proteomic profile of mouse liver microsomes, including 62 definite microsomal membrane proteins. The comprehensive bioinformatics analyses annotated the functional categories of those microsomal proteins and provided clues into biological functions of the liver. Our gained data and established method (Peng *et al.*, 2012) complemented the published data and methods (Zgoda *et al.*, 2006 and 2009, Gilchrist *et al.*, 2006). A proposed method that combined 2D/3D LC-MS/MS (Gilchrist *et al.*, 2006) with carbonate extraction (Peng *et al.*, 2012) plus Triton X-114 extraction (Mathias *et al.*, 2011) of isolated microsomes would be effective in significant improvement of the coverage of microsomal membrane proteome.

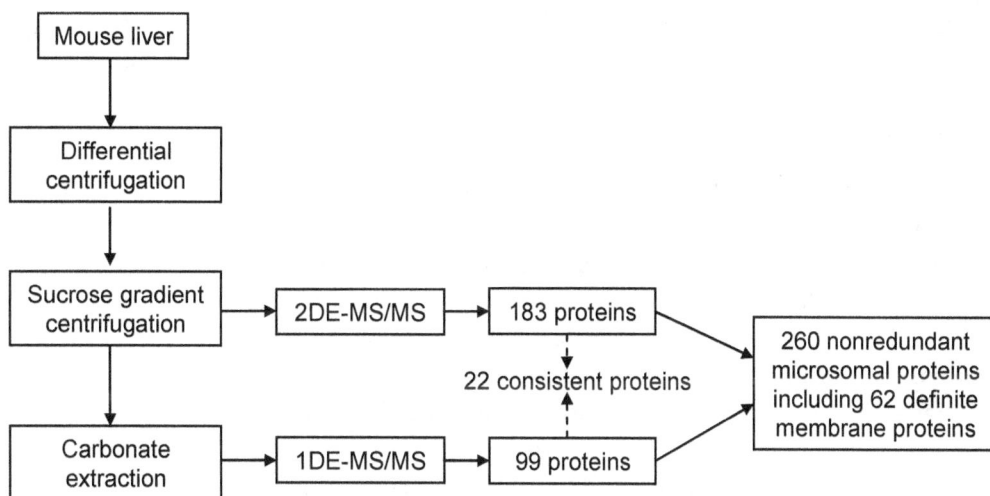

Scheme: Experimental flow-chart of identification of mouse liver microsomal proteins.

2 Preparation of Liver Microsomes

2.1 Preparation of Microsomes

The differential centrifugation and sucrose gradient centrifugation as described (Fleischer & Kervina, 1974) were used to prepare microsome apparatus-rich fractions from mice livers (male C57 mice, 9 weeks old, purchased from the Experimental Animal Center of Central South University). Mice livers (approximately 10 g each) were drained of blood, minced thoroughly with scalpels, and transferred to 50 mL of chilled homogenization solution that contained 0.25 M sucrose (pH 7.4, 5–10 min, occasional stirring). The liquid was decanted and replaced with fresh homogenization solution (50 ml) and then homogenized (30–60 sec.) on a TAMATO homogenizer (1,000 rpm× 3 and 1,500 rpm × 3). The homogenate was squeezed through a single layer of microcloth and centrifuged (1,000 g, 10 min; HITACHI centrifuge). The supernatant was centrifuged (3,000 g, 30 min,), and sequentially centrifuged (8,000 g, 30 min) after discarding the sediment. The remainder supernatant was centrifuged (34,000 g, 30 min), carefully decanted, and centrifuged again (130,000 g, 1 h; Beckman Instruments, Palo Alto, CA) to get the pellets as the crude smooth microsomes. The pink sediment was gently resuspended with a glass homogenizer in ~7 mL of 52 % sucrose-0.1 M H_3PO_4 buffer (pH 7.1), and the density of sucrose was adjusted to 43.7 %. The fraction was placed in one type-70i rotor centrifuge tube; overlayered sequentially with 7 mL, 5 mL, 5 mL, and 6 mL of 38.7 %, 36.0 %, 33.0 %, and 29.0 % sucrose, respectively, and centrifuged (80,000 g, 1 h). The upper four layers of the sucrose gradient were discarded by aspiration, and the bottom layer (43.7 %) was diluted with two volumes of cold distilled water and centrifuged (130,000 g, 1 h) in a type- 70i rotor to get the pellets as the crude rough microsomes. The crude smooth and rough microsome pellets were suspended in 3 mL of 0.25 M sucrose (pH 7.0) and combined. The mixture was diluted to a volume (14 mL) with 0.25 M sucrose containing CsCl with its final concentration of 0.015 M. The suspension was layered into an equal volume of 1.3 M sucrose/0.015 M CsCl and then centrifuged (240,000 g, 1 h) in an SW 55Ti rotor. The rough microsomes were in the pink sediment, and the smooth microsomes at the interface were collected carefully and diluted with an equal volume of 0.25 M sucrose (pH 7.0) and centrifuged (140,000 g, 1 h) in an SW55i rotor to get the pellets as the smooth microsomes. The smooth and rough microsomes were combined as the prepared microsome sample for futher analyses.

2.2   Validation of the Purity of Microsomes

A highly pure fraction was essential to conduct proteomic characterization of microsomes. The purity of prepared microsomes was assessed by electron microscopy (EM) and Western blot (WB). For electron microscope analysis, the prepared microsomes were fixed with 2.5% glutaraldehyde (24 h) and 2 % OsO_4 (2 h), dehydrated with alcohol (50 %, 70 %, 90 %, and 100 % in turn), and processed into epoxy resin. Thin sections (500 Å) were prepared and stained with uranyl acetate and lead citrate and then examined with a transmission electron microscope (H-600-1, Hitachi, Japan). For Western blotting analysis, the microsome fractions were lysed (4 °C; 30 min) in lysis buffer [50 mM Tris-HCl, 150 mM NaCl, 1 mM ethylene diamine tetraacetic acid (EDTA), 1% Triton-X100, and 0.1 % SDS]. The protein samples (50 µg) were subjected to electrophoresis on SDS-PAGE with 12 % gel and transferred to polyvinylidene fluoride (PVDF) membrane (Millipore). The protein on the PVDF membranes were immunoblotted with antibodies to endoplasmin (ER marker), OxPhos complex IV subunit I (mitochondrial marker), catalase (peroxisomal marker), and cadherin (cytoplasmic marker), respectively.

The EM analyses showed that a large number of nearly spherical membrane vesicles were visualized with EM without other contaminated organelles (Figure 1A). The WB analyses showed that, with the standard immunoblotting protocol, the ER marker endoplasmin was enriched in the isolated microsome fractions without the contamination marker (mitochondrial marker OxPhos Complex IV subunit I, peroxisomal marker catalase, and cytoplasmic marker cadherin) being detected (Figure 1B). The results demonstrated an optimized preparation of microsomes.

3   Separation and Identification of Microsome Proteins with the 2DE-MS/MS strategy

3.1   Separation of Microsome Proteins with 2DE

2DE was carried out according to the manufacturer (Amersham Biosciences). Protein samples (400 µg) from the prepared microsome sample were diluted to a volume (450 µL) with rehydration solution [7 mol/L urea, 2 mol/L thiourea, 0.2 % dithiothreitol (DTT), 0.5 % (v/v) pH3–10 non-linear (NL) immobi-

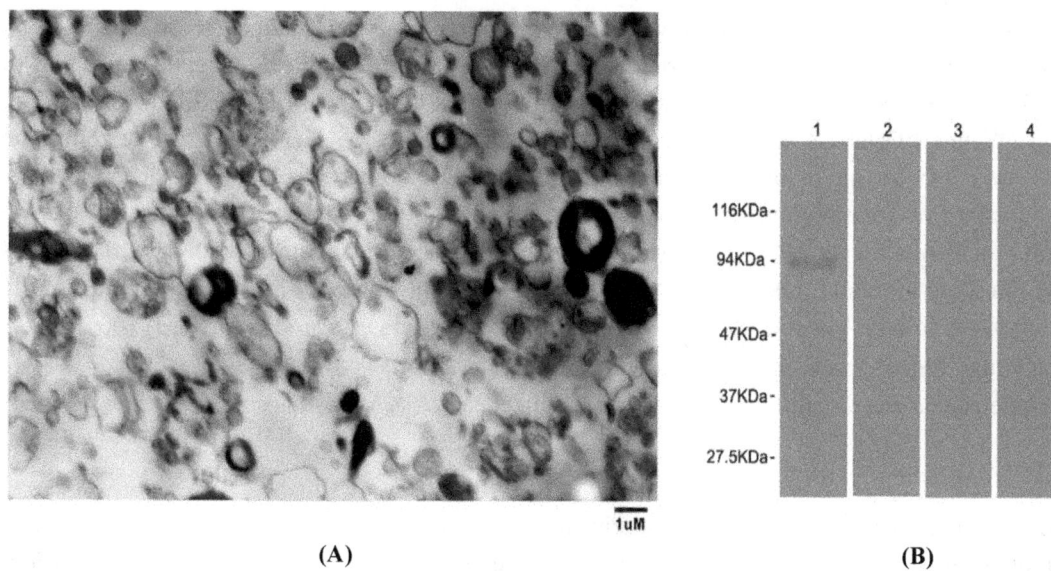

Figure 1: Validation of the purity of isolated microsomes. A. Electron microscope image shows a representative area of ER vesicles. B. Western blotting image. A amount (50 μg) of proteins were loaded at each lane, and lanes 1, 2, 3 and 4 were sequentially detected with anti-endoplasmin (92.5 kDa; ER marker), anti-OxPhos Complex IV subunit I (56.9 kDa; mitochondrial marker), anti-Catalase (59.8 kDa; peroxisomal marker), and anti-cadherin (98.3 kDa; cytoplasmic marker), respectively. Reproduced from Peng et al. (Peng *et al.*, 2012), with permission from Hindawi publisher open accession journal; copyright remains with authors.

lized pH gradient (IPG) buffer, and trace bromophenol blue], applied to IPG strips (pH 3–10 NL; 24 cm) for rehydration (14 h; 30 V), and then were focused (1 h at 500 V, 1 h at 1,000 V, and 8.5 h at 8,000 V) to achieve a total of 68 kVh on an IPGphor. After equilibration in a solution containing 65 mM DTT (15 min) and in another solution containing 135 mM iodacetamide (15 min), SDS-PAGE was performed with 12% gel on Ettan DALT II system. Then, the blue silver staining method was used to visualize the protein spots on the 2DE gels (Candiano *et al.*, 2004).

3.2   In-Gel Digestion with Trypsin

The proteins in the 2D gel spots were subjected to in-gel digestion with trypsin (Sigma-Aldrich). Gel spots were excised and destained in a solution of 100 mM NH_4HCO_3 with 50 % acetonitrile (ACN) at room temperature. The proteins were reduced (10 mM DTT and 100 mM NH_4HCO_3; 56 °C; 30 min) and alkylated (50 mM iodoacetamide and 100 mM NH_4HCO_3; dark, room temperature, 30 min). The gel pieces that contained proteins were dried and then incubated in the digestion solution (40 mM NH_4HCO_3, 9 % ACN, and 20 μg/mL Sigma-Aldrich trypsin; 18 h, 37 °C). The tryptic peptides were extracted with 50 % ACN/2.5 % trifluoroacetic Acid (TFA) and then dried using a Speed-Vac.

3.3   Protein Identification with MS/MS

The tryptic peptide mixture was fractionated with reverse-phase high-performance liquid chromatography (RP-HPLC) in a Dionex Ultimate nano-HPLC system. Peptide samples were purified with a C18-PepMap precolumn and then separated on an analytical C18-PepMap column (75 μm ID × 150 mm, 100 Å pore size, 3-mm particle size) at a column flow rate (300 nL/min). The ACN gradient (solution A: 0.1 % formic acid, 2 % ACN; solution B: 0.1% formic acid, 80% ACN) started at 5% B and ended at 70% B in 45 min. MS and MS/MS data were acquired using a Micromass quadrupole time-of-flight (Q-TOF) spectrometer (Waters). Database searches were carried out with the MASCOT server by the concatenated forward-reverse mouse international protein index (IPI) database (version 3.07). A mass tolerance (0.3 Da) for both parent (MS) and fragmented (MS/MS) ions, allowance for up to one trypsin miscleavage, variable amino acid modifications (methionine oxidation and cysteine carbamidomethylation) were used. MS/MS ion score threshold was determined to produce a false-positive rate less than 5% for a significant hit (P < 0.05). The false-positive rate was calculated with 2* reverse/(reverse + forward)/100. In the current study, the MS/MS ion score threshold was 23 and a false-positive rate was approximately 3.1%. For all the proteins that were identified with only one peptide, each MS/MS spectrum was checked manually.

3.4   2DE mapping of Microsome Proteins

The 2DE reference maps display 514±83 protein spots (n = 10 gels). A representative 2DE map of microsome proteins was shown (Figure 2). A total of 183 proteins were characterized with electrospray ionization (ESI)-Q-TOF MS/MS from 204 excised gel spots. Those proteins are summarized (Table 1), including 2D gel-spot number, protein name, predicted transmembrane domain (TMD), and subcellular location. The microsomal marker proteins such as endoplasmin (Spot 2) and UDP glucuronosyltransferase (Spots 6 and 7) were identified. Those proteins were located in different subcellular locations (Table 1) including ER, mitochondrial membrane, cytoplasmic, ribosome, microbody, microsome membrane, nuclear, vesicular membrane, sarcolemma, extracellular space, cilium, ER-Golgi intermediate compartment, and secreted proteins. Those non-ER proteins would be derived from the complexity of liver microsomes because it contained not only components of the protein secretary pathways but also many proteins that are involved in the processes of lipid/lipoprotein biosynthesis and drug metabolism. The possible reasons regarding the non-ER proteins was explained in the last paragraph of section 5. Figure 3 shows the percentage of each group of proteins, according to their subcellular locations, derived from the annotations in the Swiss-Prot database and Gene Ontology (GO): 22% of proteins (n = 41) from ER and Golgi, 11% of proteins (n = 20) from mitochondria and other membranes, 50% of proteins (n = 91) from cytosolic and other soluble proteins, 8% of secreted proteins (n = 15), 9% of proteins without unambiguous location (n = 16).

4   Fractionation and Identification of Microsomal Membrane Proteins with the Na_2CO_3-1DE-MS/MS strategy

4.1 Na_2CO_3-Extraction and 1DE Analysis of Microsomal Membrane Proteins

Microsomal membrane proteins were further extracted by the carbonate method from the prepared microsomal samples (Fujiki et al., 1982). Microsomal fractions were diluted 50- to 1,000-fold with 100 mM sodium carbonate (pH 11.5; final protein concentration to 0.02 to 1 mg/mL), and incubated [0 °C; 30 min; slow stirring; and bath sonication (15 sec; 3-4 W) at 0 min, 15 min, and 30 min]. The suspensions were centrifuged and decanted, and the membrane pellets were gently rinsed (ice-cold distilled water; 3x). These pellets were diluted with denaturing sample buffer that contained 5 % mercapto ethanol, 2 % SDS, 0.06 M Tris-HCl, pH 6.8, and 10 % glycerol, heated (95 °C; 5 min), and then subjected to 1D SDS-PAGE

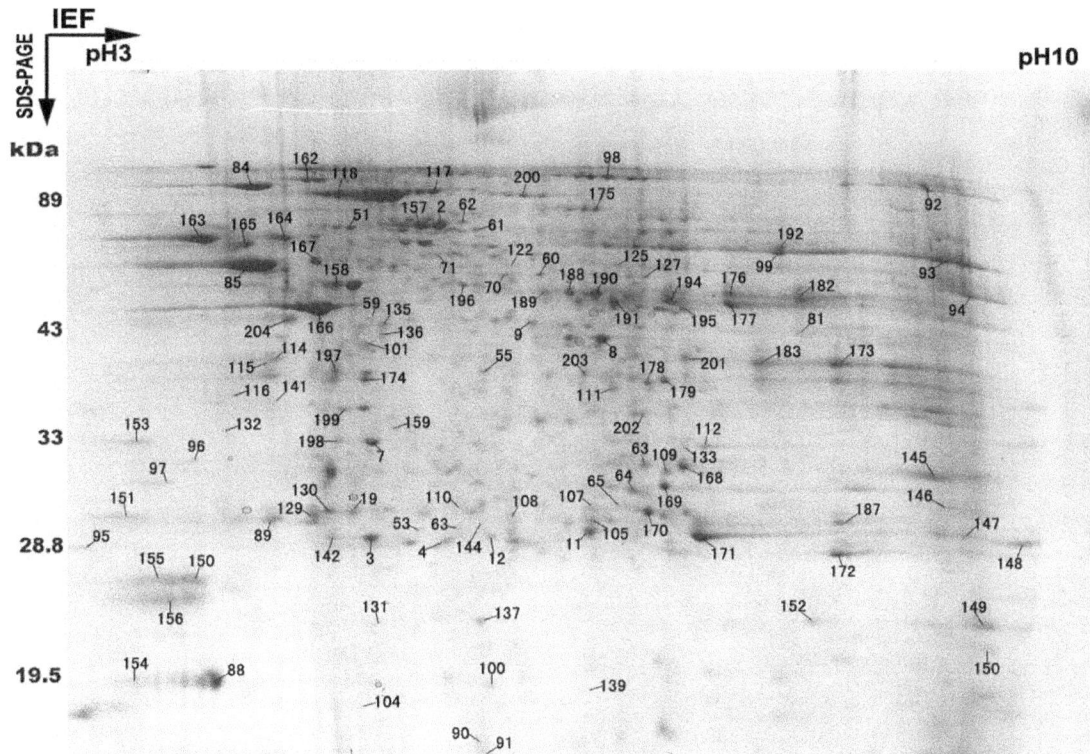

Figure 2: 2DE map of mouse liver microsome. Microsomal proteins (400 µg) were arrayed by 2DE with IPG strip (pH 3–10 NL; 24 cm) and SDS-PAGE with 12% gel, and visualized with blue silver staining method. Reproduced from Peng *et al.* (Peng *et al.*, 2012), with permission from Hindawi publisher open accession journal; copyright remains with authors.

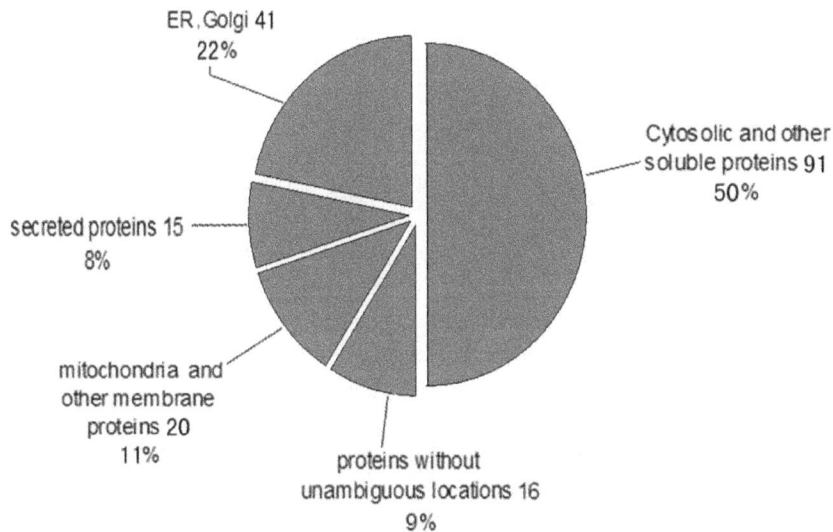

Figure 3: Distribution of subcellular locations of 2DE-derived proteins. The subcellular locations were derived from Swiss-Prot database and the Gene Ontology. Reproduced from Peng *et al.* (Peng *et al.*, 2012), with permission from Hindawi publisher open accession journal; copyright remains with authors.

Spot No. / Band No.	Protein Name	Predicted TMD	Location	Methods
156	Left-right dynein	0	Cilium	2DE-MS/MS
153	Splice Isoform 1 of Tropomyosin 1 alpha	0	Cytoplasm	2DE-MS/MS
116	Senescence marker protein-30	0	Cytoplasm	2DE-MS/MS
89,129,130,151,152	Heme-binding protein	0	Cytoplasm	2DE-MS/MS
88	Tubulin beta-4 chain	0	Cytoplasmic	2DE-MS/MS
105,138	Tubulin alpha-1 chain	0	Cytoplasmic	2DE-MS/MS
90	Fatty acid-binding protein, epidermal	0	Cytoplasmic	2DE-MS/MS
145	T-complex protein 1, delta subunit	0	Cytoplasmic	2DE-MS/MS
144	DJ-1 protein	0	Cytoplasmic	2DE-MS/MS
137,138,164	Tubulin alpha-4 chain	0	Cytoplasmic	2DE-MS/MS
141,153,165,132	Tubulin beta-5 chain	0	Cytoplasmic	2DE-MS/MS
152	21 kDa protein	0	Cytoplasmic	2DE-MS/MS
107,108,139,143,182	Argininosuccinate synthase	0	Cytoplasmic	2DE-MS/MS
191	Glutamine synthetase	0	Cytoplasmic	2DE-MS/MS
176,182,194	Betaine--homocysteine S-methyltransferase	0	Cytoplasmic	2DE-MS/MS
99	UDP-glucose pyrophosphorylase 2	0	Cytoplasmic	2DE-MS/MS
204	Gamma actin-like protein	0	Cytoplasmic	2DE-MS/MS
101,132	Tubulin beta-2C Chain	0	Cytoplasmic	2DE-MS/MS
202,133	Alcohol dehydrogenase A chain	0	Cytoplasmic	2DE-MS/MS
89	Actin, cytoplasmic type 5 homolog	0	Cytoplasmic	2DE-MS/MS
168	Carbonic anhydrase III	0	Cytoplasmic	2DE-MS/MS
202,133	Guanine nucleotide-binding protein beta subunit 2-like 1	0	cytoplasmic	2DE-MS/MS
159	T-complex protein 1, eta subunit	0	Cytoplasmic	2DE-MS/MS
154	Tubulin, beta 2	0	Cytoplasmic	2DE-MS/MS
141	Similar to tubulin Mbeta 1	0	Cytoplasmic	2DE-MS/MS
136	Microtubule-associated protein	0	Cytoplasmic	2DE-MS/MS
153	Tropomyosin alpha 4 chain	0	Cytoplasmic	2DE-MS/MS
194,195	Similar to Argininosuccinate synthase	0	Cytoplasmic	2DE-MS/MS
60	2-phospho-D-glycerate hydro-lyase	0	Cytoplasmic	2DE-MS/MS
178	Glycine N-methyltransferase	0	Cytoplasmic	2DE-MS/MS
63,109	Triosephosphate isomerase	0	Cytoplasmic	2DE-MS/MS
153	Alpha-tubulin 2	0	Cytoplasmic	2DE-MS/MS
162	Ubiquitin-activating enzyme E1 1	0	Cytoplasmic and nuclear	2DE-MS/MS
64	Proteasome subunit,alpha type 2	0	Cytoplasmic and nuclear	2DE-MS/MS
145	Oxidoreductase HTATIP2	0	Cytoplasmic and nuclear envelope	2DE-MS/MS
145	Oxidoreductase HTATIP2	0	Cytoplasmic and nuclear envelope	2DE-MS/MS
90,91	Glyceraldehyde-3-phosphate dehydro-Genase, spermatoGenic	0	ER	2DE-MS/MS
6	UDP-glucuronosyltransferase 1-2 precur-	1	ER	2DE-MS/MS

	sor, microsomal			
145	Acetyl-Coenzyme A acyltransferase 1	0	ER	2DE-MS/MS
102	Transitional Endoplasmic Reticulum ATPase	0	ER	2DE-MS/MS
6,61,194	Prolyl 4-hydroxylase, beta polypeptide	0	ER	2DE-MS/MS
17	Similar to GAPDH,37 kDa protein	0	ER	2DE-MS/MS
134,135	Hypoxia up-regulated 1	1	ER	2DE-MS/MS
139	Nucleoside diphosphate kinase A	0	ER	2DE-MS/MS
179	Splice Isoform 1 of Monoglyceride lipase	0	ER	2DE-MS/MS
49	Thioredoxin domain containing protein 4	0	ER	2DE-MS/MS
108,145,65	Similar to GAPDH isoform 1	0	ER	2DE-MS/MS
147,148,149	Mus musculus adult male kidney cDNA	1	ER	2DE-MS/MS
174,178,179,183	Similar to GAPDH	0	ER	2DE-MS/MS
49,50	Thioredoxin domain containing protein 5	0	ER	2DE-MS/MS
137	Thioredoxin	0	ER	2DE-MS/MS
148	ADAM4	1	ER	2DE-MS/MS
148	Similar to GAPDH	0	ER	2DE-MS/MS
146,147,149,150,153	GAPDH	0	ER	2DE-MS/MS
187	Glutathione S-transferase P 1	0	ER	2DE-MS/MS
144	Glutathione peroxidase	0	ER	2DE-MS/MS
153	Elongation factor 1-beta	0	ER	2DE-MS/MS
118	Heat shock cognate 71 kDa protein	0	ER	2DE-MS/MS
173	Similar to GAPDH	0	ER	2DE-MS/MS
145,201	Similar to GAPDH	0	ER	2DE-MS/MS
127	Alpha-2-macroglobulin receptor-associated protein precursor	0	ER	2DE-MS/MS
143,152,203	2700050F09Rik protein	0	ER	2DE-MS/MS
162	Leucine-rich repeat-containing protein 7	0	ER (integral to membrane)	2DE-MS/MS
149,150	Flavin containing monooxygenase 5	1	ER (integral to membrane)	2DE-MS/MS
131	GTP-binding protein SAR1b	0	ER (Peripheral membrane protein)	2DE-MS/MS
107	Stromal cell-derived factor 2-like protein 1	0	ER lumen	2DE-MS/MS
145	Expressed sequence AA959742	1	ER membrane	2DE-MS/MS
152	Multiple coagulation factor deficiency protein 2 homolog precursor	0	ER-Golgi intermediate compartment	2DE-MS/MS
170	RAS-RELATED PROTEIN RAB-7	0	Golgi, Endosomes, lysosomes	2DE-MS/MS
101,139	Keratin Kb40	0	Intermediate filament	2DE-MS/MS
101	Branched chain ketoacid dehydrogenase E1, beta	0	Membrane	2DE-MS/MS
197	G-protein G(I)/G(S)/G(T) beta subunit 1	0	Membrane	2DE-MS/MS
21,137	cytochrome c oxidase, subunit va	0	Membrane	2DE-MS/MS

129	Catechol O-methyltransferase	1	Membrane	2DE-MS/MS
174	G-protein G(I)/G(S)/G(T) beta subunit 2	0	Membrane	2DE-MS/MS
88,154	Cytochrome b5	1	Membrane	2DE-MS/MS
199,200	Annexin A4	0	Membrane	2DE-MS/MS
19	NADH-ubiquinone oxidoreductase 24 kDa subunit	0	Mitchondrial inner membrane	2DE-MS/MS
158	Ubiquinol-cytochrome-c reductase complex core protein I, mitochondrial	0	Mitchondrial inner membrane	2DE-MS/MS
175	Electron transfer flavoprotein-ubiquinone oxidoreductase, mitochondrial	0	Mitchondrial inner membrane	2DE-MS/MS
196	NADH-ubiquinone oxidoreductase 49 kDa subunit, mitochondrial	0	Mitchondrial inner membrane	2DE-MS/MS
145	Endonuclease G, mitochondrial	0	Mitochondrial	2DE-MS/MS
70	2-oxoisovalerate dehydrogenase alpha subunit, mitochondrial	0	Mitochondrial	2DE-MS/MS
94,95	Trifunctional enzyme beta subunit, mitochondrial	0	Mitochondrial	2DE-MS/MS
145	NipSnap1 protein	0	Mitochondrial	2DE-MS/MS
22	Cytochrome c oxidase, subunit vb	0	Mitochondrial	2DE-MS/MS
15,146,147,148 ,149,100	ATP synthase oligomycin sensitivity conferral protein, mitochondrial	0	Mitochondrial	2DE-MS/MS
127	Ubiquinol-cytochrome-c reductase complex core protein 2, mitochondrial	0	Mitochondrial	2DE-MS/MS
147,148	NADH-ubiquinone oxidoreductase 19 kDa subunit	0	Mitochondrial	2DE-MS/MS
137	Ubiquinol-cytochrome c reductase complex 11 kDa protein, mitochondrial	0	Mitochondrial	2DE-MS/MS
93,99,100,192, 203	ATP synthase alpha chain, mitochondrial	0	Mitochondrial	2DE-MS/MS
149,150	Tetratricopeptide repeat protein 11	1	Mitochondrial	2DE-MS/MS
150,151	NADH-ubiquinone oxidoreductase B15	1	Mitochondrial	2DE-MS/MS
101,132,137,14 1,153	NADH-ubiquinone oxidoreductase 23 kDa subunit, mitochondrial	0	Mitochondrial	2DE-MS/MS
92,93,94,95,96	Hydroxyacyl-Coenzyme A dehydrogenase/3-ketoacyl-Coenzyme A	0	Mitochondrial	2DE-MS/MS
142,143,152	ATP synthase D chain, mitochondrial	0	Mitochondrial	2DE-MS/MS
162	NADH-ubiquinone oxidoreductase 75 kDa subunit, mitochondrial precursor	0	mitochondrial	2DE-MS/MS
149	13KDA differentiation-associated protein	0	Mitochondrial	2DE-MS/MS
145,146	Hydroxymethylglutaryl-CoA synthase, mitochondrial	0	Mitochondrial	2DE-MS/MS
51	60 kDa heat shock protein, mitochondrial	0	Mitochondrial	2DE-MS/MS
153	Similar to adenine nucleotide translocase	3	Mitochondrial	2DE-MS/MS
85,165,167,203	ATP synthase beta chain, mitochondrial	0	mitochondrial	2DE-MS/MS
147	Phospholipid hydroperoxide glutathione peroxidase, mitochondrial	0	Mitochondrial and cytoplasmic	2DE-MS/MS
169	Ubiquinol-cytochrome c reductase iron-sulfur subunit, mitochondrial	0	Mitochondrial inner membrane	2DE-MS/MS
200,201	Succinate dehydrogenase [ubiquinone] flavoprotein subunit, mitochondrial	0	Mitochondrial inner membrane	2DE-MS/MS

174	Pyruvate dehydrogenase E1 component beta subunit, mitochondrial	0	Mitochondrial matrix	2DE-MS/MS
145,146	Succinate dehydrogenase [ubiquinone] iron-sulfur protein, mitochondrial	0	Mitochondrion	2DE-MS/MS
147	Splice Isoform 2 of Transcription factor BTF3	0	Nuclear	2DE-MS/MS
149	Nucleolin	0	Nuclear	2DE-MS/MS
53	UMP-CMP kinase	0	Nuclear	2DE-MS/MS
150	SIMILAR TO ZNF91L ISOFORM 1	0	Nuclear	2DE-MS/MS
6	E1A binding protein p300	0	Nuclear	2DE-MS/MS
55	RIKEN cDNA 4931406C07, PTD012 homolog	0	Nuclear	2DE-MS/MS
150,151	40S ribosomal protein S19	0	Ribosome	2DE-MS/MS
104	similar to 40s ribosomal protein S12	0	Ribosome	2DE-MS/MS
147	60S ribosomal protein L12	0	Ribosome	2DE-MS/MS
81,127,145	26S protease regulatory subunit S10B	0	Ribosome	2DE-MS/MS
199	40S ribosomal protein SA	0	Ribosome	2DE-MS/MS
125	26S protease regulatory subunit 8	0	Ribosome	2DE-MS/MS
149,150,151	60S ribosomal protein L23	0	Ribosome	2DE-MS/MS
149,150	60S ribosomal protein L22	0	Ribosome	2DE-MS/MS
145	60S acidic ribosomal protein P0	0	Ribosome	2DE-MS/MS
149	40S ribosomal protein S14	0	Ribosome	2DE-MS/MS
146	40S ribosomal protein S4, X isoform	0	Ribosome	2DE-MS/MS
149,150	60S ribosomal protein L11	0	Ribosome	2DE-MS/MS
188	Similar to ribosomal protein	0	Ribosome	2DE-MS/MS
148	60S ribosomal protein L12	0	Ribosome	2DE-MS/MS
149	40S ribosomal protein S17	0	Ribosome	2DE-MS/MS
199	40S ribosomal protein SA	0	Ribosome	2DE-MS/MS
4,11	Apolipoprotein A-I precursor	0	Secreted	2DE-MS/MS
149	Ribonuclease 4 precursor	1	Secreted	2DE-MS/MS
12	Plasma retinol-binding protein precursor	0	Secreted	2DE-MS/MS
163	Alpha-1-antitrypsin 1-3 precursor	0	Secreted	2DE-MS/MS
163	Alpha-1-antitrypsin 1-4 precursor	0	Secreted	2DE-MS/MS
163	Alpha-1-antitrypsin 1-5 precursor	0	Secreted	2DE-MS/MS
162	Hemopexin precursor	1	Secreted	2DE-MS/MS
3,117,118	Serum albumin precursor	0	Secreted	2DE-MS/MS
98	Serotransferrin precursor	0	Secreted	2DE-MS/MS
199	Apolipoprotein E precursor	0	Secreted	2DE-MS/MS
135,136	Apolipoprotein A-IV precursor	0	Secreted	2DE-MS/MS
163	Alpha-1-antitrypsin 1-1 precursor	0	Secreted	2DE-MS/MS
100,155,156	21 kDa protein	0	Secreted	2DE-MS/MS
156	Major urinary protein 1 precursor	0	Secreted	2DE-MS/MS
122	Tripeptidyl-peptidase I precursor	0	Secreted (Lyso-somal.)	2DE-MS/MS
110	Neighbor of COX4	0	Unknown	2DE-MS/MS
143	Hypothetical S-Adenosyl-L-Methioninedependent Metjyltransferases Structure Containing Protein	0	Unknown	2DE-MS/MS
144,108	RIKEN cDNA 6330409N04，CLLL6	0	Unknown	2DE-MS/MS

	protein homolog			
101	Eukaryotic translation initiation factor 3 subunit 2	0	Unknown	2DE-MS/MS
149,150	51 kDa protein	0	Unknown	2DE-MS/MS
203	Sid6061p	0	Unknown	2DE-MS/MS
105	Similar to GAPDH	0	Unknown	2DE-MS/MS
189,190,194	Glutamine synthetase	0	Unknown	2DE-MS/MS
50	86 kDa protein	0	Unknown	2DE-MS/MS
51	45 kDa protein	0	Unknown	2DE-MS/MS
133	77 kDa protein	0	Unknown	2DE-MS/MS
144	Probable ubiquitin-conjugating enzyme E2 FLJ25076 homolog	0	Unknown	2DE-MS/MS
146,147,150,173	44 kDa protein	0	Unknown	2DE-MS/MS
156	Major urinary protein 26	0	Unknown	2DE-MS/MS
59	169 kDa protein	0	Unknown	2DE-MS/MS
100,155,156	21 kDa protein	0	Unknown	2DE-MS/MS
149	Splice Isoform 1 of SNARE-associated protein Snapin	0	Vesicular membrane	2DE-MS/MS
9	Arginase 1	0	Cytoplasmic	2DE-MS/MS; Na_2CO_3-1DE-MS/MS
6	tubulin beta-4 chain homolog	0	Cytoplasmic	2DE-MS/MS; Na_2CO_3-1DE-MS/MS
8	Actin, alpha skeletal muscle	0	Cytoplasmic	2DE-MS/MS; Na_2CO_3-1DE-MS/MS
10,11	Actin, cytoplasmic 1	0	Cytoplasmic	2DE-MS/MS; Na_2CO_3-1DE-MS/MS
7	Carbamoyl-phosphate synthase	0	Cytoplasmic	2DE-MS/MS; Na_2CO_3-1DE-MS/MS
13	Tubulin alpha-2 chain	0	Cytoplasmic	2DE-MS/MS; Na_2CO_3-1DE-MS/MS
9	Argininosuccinate synthase	0	Cytoplasmic	2DE-MS/MS; Na_2CO_3-1DE-MS/MS
9	UDP-glucuronosyltransferase 2B5	1	ER	2DE-MS/MS; Na_2CO_3-1DE-MS/MS
9	Endoplasmin precursor	0	ER	2DE-MS/MS; Na_2CO_3-1DE-MS/MS
	Similar to 40S ribosomal protein S6	0	ER	2DE-MS/MS; Na_2CO_3-1DE-MS/MS
8	Glucose regulated protein	0	ER	2DE-MS/MS; Na_2CO_3-1DE-MS/MS
9	78 kDa glucose-regulated protein	0	ER	2DE-MS/MS; Na_2CO_3-1DE-MS/MS
9	Protein disulfide-isomerase A6	1	ER	2DE-MS/MS; Na_2CO_3-1DE-MS/MS
15	Microsomal glutathione S-transferase 1	3	ER and mitochondrial outer membrane	2DE-MS/MS; Na_2CO_3-1DE-MS/MS
5	Protein disulfide-isomerase precursor	0	ER.	2DE-MS/MS; Na_2CO_3-1DE-MS/MS

13	Membrane associated progesterone receptor component 1	1	ER; membrane-bound	2DE-MS/MS; Na$_2$CO$_3$-1DE-MS/MS
10	Polyposis locus protein 1-like 1	3	Integral to membrane	2DE-MS/MS; Na$_2$CO$_3$-1DE-MS/MS
8	Ras-related protein Rap-1A	0	Membrane	2DE-MS/MS; Na$_2$CO$_3$-1DE-MS/MS
9,10	Peroxiredoxin 1	0	Microbody	2DE-MS/MS; Na$_2$CO$_3$-1DE-MS/MS
17	Cytochrome c oxidase subunit IV isoform 1, mitochondrial	1	Mitochondrial inner membrane	2DE-MS/MS; Na$_2$CO$_3$-1DE-MS/MS
17	Cytochrome b5 outer mitochondrial membrane isoform	1	Mitochondrial outer membrane	2DE-MS/MS; Na$_2$CO$_3$-1DE-MS/MS
8	Voltage-dependent anion-selective channel protein 2	0	Outer mitochondrial Membrane	2DE-MS/MS; Na$_2$CO$_3$-1DE-MS/MS
9	Keratin, type II cytoskeletal 6B	0	Sarcolemma	2DE-MS/MS; Na$_2$CO$_3$-1DE-MS/MS
17	Protein ERGIC-53	1	ER-Golgi intermediate compartment (ER-GIC).Type I membrane protein	Na$_2$CO$_3$-1DE-MS/MS
9	Carcinoembryonic antigen-related cell adhesion molecule 1	1	Type I membrane protein.	Na$_2$CO$_3$-1DE-MS/MS
15,16	Fatty acid-binding protein, liver	0	Cytoplasmic	Na$_2$CO$_3$-1DE-MS/MS
13	Similar to tubulin, alpha 3c isoform 1	0	Cytoplasmic	Na$_2$CO$_3$-1DE-MS/MS
13	Betaine--homocysteine S-methyltransferase	0	Cytoplasmic	Na$_2$CO$_3$-1DE-MS/MS
7	UDP glucuronosyltransferase 2 family, polypeptide B36	1	ER	Na$_2$CO$_3$-1DE-MS/MS
8	UDP glycosyltransferase 1 family polypeptide A5	1	ER	Na$_2$CO$_3$-1DE-MS/MS
9	Cytochrome P450, family 2, subfamily d, polypeptide 9	2	ER	Na$_2$CO$_3$-1DE-MS/MS
5,6	40S ribosomal protein S6	0	ER	Na$_2$CO$_3$-1DE-MS/MS
1,10,12,14,15	Short-chain dehydrogenase CRAD2	0	ER	Na$_2$CO$_3$-1DE-MS/MS
8	Similar to GDH/6PGL endoplasmic bi-functional protein	0	ER	Na$_2$CO$_3$-1DE-MS/MS
8,17	Paraoxonase 1	0	ER	Na$_2$CO$_3$-1DE-MS/MS
10	NADH-cytochrome b5 reductase 3	0	ER ,membrane bound	Na$_2$CO$_3$-1DE-MS/MS
10,12,14	Cytochrome P450 2A5	1	ER ,Membrane bound.	Na$_2$CO$_3$-1DE-MS/MS
1,2,3	Cytochrome P450 2C38	0	ER ,Membrane-bound.	Na$_2$CO$_3$-1DE-MS/MS
1,8,9,13	Cis-retinol androgen dehydrogenase 1	0	ER lumen.	Na$_2$CO$_3$-1DE-MS/MS
9,10,11,12,13	UDP-glucuronosyltransferase 1-1 precursor, microsomal	2	ER, integral to plasma membrane	Na$_2$CO$_3$-1DE-MS/MS
17	Cytochrome P450 1A2	1	ER, Membrane-bound	Na$_2$CO$_3$-1DE-MS/MS
9	Cytochrome P450 2D11	2	ER, Membrane-	Na$_2$CO$_3$-1DE-MS/MS

			bound.	
1-11,13,17	Cytochrome P450 2F2	1	ER, Membrane-bound.	Na_2CO_3-1DE-MS/MS
1,4,6,10,11,14, 15	Cytochrome P450 2D10	2	ER, Membrane-bound.	Na_2CO_3-1DE-MS/MS
3,4	Long-chain-fatty-acid--CoA ligase 1	1	ER,Type III membrane protein.	Na_2CO_3-1DE-MS/MS
17	Cytochrome P450 2D9	0	ER. Membrane-bound	Na_2CO_3-1DE-MS/MS
9	Calnexin precursor	1	ER. Type I membrane protein	Na_2CO_3-1DE-MS/MS
14,15	Scavenger receptor class B member 1	2	Integral membrane protein	Na_2CO_3-1DE-MS/MS
1	Splice Isoform 1 of Solute carrier organic anion transporter family, member 1B2	12	Integral membrane protein	Na_2CO_3-1DE-MS/MS
1	Integrin associated protein precursor	5	Integral membrane protein	Na_2CO_3-1DE-MS/MS
1	Cytochrome c oxidase subunit 2	2	Integral membrane protein	Na_2CO_3-1DE-MS/MS
6	Secretedretory carrier-associated membrane protein 3	4	Integral membrane protein	Na_2CO_3-1DE-MS/MS
2	Solute carrier organic anion transporter family, member 1A1	11	Integral membrane protein	Na_2CO_3-1DE-MS/MS
10	Platelet glycoprotein IV	2	Integral membrane protein	Na_2CO_3-1DE-MS/MS
1,12,16,17	Sodium/potassium-transporting ATPase alpha-1	10	Integral membrane protein	Na_2CO_3-1DE-MS/MS
17	Prolow-density lipoprotein receptor-related protein 1	1	Integral to membrane	Na_2CO_3-1DE-MS/MS
5,8	Asialoglycoprotein receptor major subunit	1	Integral to membrane	Na_2CO_3-1DE-MS/MS
10,11,12	Camello-like protein 1	1	Integral to membrane	Na_2CO_3-1DE-MS/MS
9	Keratin, type II cytoskeletal 1	0	Intermediate filament	Na_2CO_3-1DE-MS/MS
15	Cell cycle control protein 50A	2	Membrane	Na_2CO_3-1DE-MS/MS
6	Splice Isoform 2 of Cell division control protein 42	0	Membrane	Na_2CO_3-1DE-MS/MS
1	Splice Isoform Pl-VDAC1 of Voltage-dependent anion-selective channel protein 1	0	Membrane	Na_2CO_3-1DE-MS/MS
9	Ras-related C3 botulinum substrate 1	0	Membrane	Na_2CO_3-1DE-MS/MS
15	MRNA	1	MHC class I protein complex	Na_2CO_3-1DE-MS/MS
17	Pyruvate carboxylase, mitochondrial	0	Mitochondrial	Na_2CO_3-1DE-MS/MS
16,17	Hemoglobin subunit beta-1	0	Mitochondrial	Na_2CO_3-1DE-MS/MS
8	Dihydrolipoyllysine-residue succinyl-transferase component of 2- oxoglutarate dehydroge complex	0	Mitochondrial	Na_2CO_3-1DE-MS/MS

15	prohibitin-2	0	Mitochondri-al,cytoplasmic, nuclear	Na$_2$CO$_3$-1DE-MS/MS
13	Histone H2A type 1	0	Nuclear	Na$_2$CO$_3$-1DE-MS/MS
15	Histone H2B F	0	Nuclear	Na$_2$CO$_3$-1DE-MS/MS
8	Keratin, type II cytoskeletal 8	0	Sarcolemma	Na$_2$CO$_3$-1DE-MS/MS
10	Similar to VH Coding Regio oding region	0	Secreted	Na$_2$CO$_3$-1DE-MS/MS
4	Cation-dependent mannose-6-phosphate receptor precursor	1	Type I membrane protein	Na$_2$CO$_3$-1DE-MS/MS
3,4	H-2 class I histocompatibility antigen, D-B alpha	1	Type I membrane protein	Na$_2$CO$_3$-1DE-MS/MS
2	Integrin alpha-V	1	Type I membrane protein	Na$_2$CO$_3$-1DE-MS/MS
5	Epidermal growth factor receptor	2	Type I membrane protein	Na$_2$CO$_3$-1DE-MS/MS
13	Macrophage mannose receptor 1	1	Type I membrane protein	Na$_2$CO$_3$-1DE-MS/MS
3	Splice Isoform LAMP-2A of Lysosome-associated membrane glycoprotein 2	1	Type I membrane protein	Na$_2$CO$_3$-1DE-MS/MS
4	Low-density lipoprotein receptor	1	Type I membrane protein	Na$_2$CO$_3$-1DE-MS/MS
5	Transmembrane emp24 domain-containing protein 10	2	Type I membrane protein	Na$_2$CO$_3$-1DE-MS/MS
16	Malectin	1	Type I membrane protein	Na$_2$CO$_3$-1DE-MS/MS
2,3	Polymeric-immunoglobulin receptor	1	Type I membrane protein. Also secreted	Na$_2$CO$_3$-1DE-MS/MS
10	Sodium/potassium-transporting ATPase beta-1 chain	1	Type II membrane protein	Na$_2$CO$_3$-1DE-MS/MS
3	Glutamyl aminopeptidase	1	Type II membrane protein	Na$_2$CO$_3$-1DE-MS/MS
3	ADP-ribosyl cyclase 1	1	Type II membrane protein	Na$_2$CO$_3$-1DE-MS/MS
9	Aminopeptidase N	1	Type II membrane protein	Na$_2$CO$_3$-1DE-MS/MS
7	Ectonucleotide pyrophospha-tase/phosphodiesterase 3	1	Unknown	Na$_2$CO$_3$-1DE-MS/MS
9	CD1D1 protein	1	Unknown	Na$_2$CO$_3$-1DE-MS/MS
1	NADPH--cytochrome P450 reductase	1	Unknown	Na$_2$CO$_3$-1DE-MS/MS
16	Cytochrome P450 2D26	2	Unknown	Na$_2$CO$_3$-1DE-MS/MS
8	Hydroxysteroid 17-beta dehydrogenase 6	0	Unknown	Na$_2$CO$_3$-1DE-MS/MS
16	Hypothetical krab box containing protein	0	Unknown	Na$_2$CO$_3$-1DE-MS/MS
17	Hypothetical Peptidase Family M20/M25/M40 Containning Protein	0	Unknown	Na$_2$CO$_3$-1DE-MS/MS
15	Ferritin light chain 2	0	Unknown	Na$_2$CO$_3$-1DE-MS/MS
3	17 kDa protein	0	Unknown	Na$_2$CO$_3$-1DE-MS/MS
2	Similar to ferrintin light chain 2	0	Unknown	Na$_2$CO$_3$-1DE-MS/MS
11	Plexin B2	0	Unknown	Na$_2$CO$_3$-1DE-MS/MS
15	Structure-specific endonuclease subunit	0	Unknown	Na$_2$CO$_3$-1DE-MS/MS

	SLX4			
10	Hypothetical protein LOC72792 isoform 1	0	Unknown	Na$_2$CO$_3$-1DE-MS/MS
10	Similar to Ferritin light chain 1	0	Unknown	Na$_2$CO$_3$-1DE-MS/MS

Table 1: Proteins identified from mouse liver microsomal preparations with 2DE-based strategy and from Na$_2$CO$_3$-extracted mouse liver microsomal membrane preparations with 1DE-based strategy. Modified from Peng *et al.* (Peng *et al.*, 2012), with permission from Hindawi publisher open accession journal; copyright remains with authors.

with a 12 % gel. Electrophoresis was performed (80 V, 20 min; 100 V, 2 h). The proteins in gels were visualized with Coomassie Brilliant Blue G (Candiano *et al.*, 2004).

4.2   In-Gel Digestion with trypsin

The proteins contained in 1D gel bands were subjected to in-gel digestion with trypsin. The detailed procedure was the same as described in the section 3.2.

4.3   Protein Identification with MS/MS

The tryptic peptide mixture was analyzed with LC-MS/MS. The detailed procedure was the same as described in the section 3.3.

4.4   1DE mapping of Microsomal Membrane Proteins

The carbonate-extracted microsomal membrane proteins were fractioned by SDS-PAGE gels and visualized by Coomassie brilliant blue staining (Figure 4A). A total of 99 proteins (Table 1) was characterized with MS/MS from 17 gel bands (Figure 4A). Those proteins were derived from the ER, type I/II membrane proteins, integral membrane proteins, major histocompatibility complex class I protein, ER-Golgi intermediate compartment, mitochondrial membrane, nuclear, cytoplasm, microbody, sarcolemma, and secreted and unknown proteins (Table 1). Those membrane proteins were classified into three categories (Figure 4B): (a) proteins with known membrane associations (55%; n = 54) that had the predicted trasmembrane regions and/or the reported annotaton, (b) putative membrane proteins (5%; n = 5) that had the reported annotation, and (c) other proteins (40%; n = 40) that had neither the predicted transmembrane regions nor the reported annotations. Those categorized criteria were from the reported annotation in the UniProt database (http://www.uniprot.org/) and predictions for transmembrane regions (http://www.cbs.dtu.dk/services/TMHMM/). Of the 99 proteins, 59 (60%) were described as "membrane-associated" proteins (category (a) and (b)), including ER characteristic proteins (cytochromes P-450 and b5, calnexin, integral membrane enzymes such as NADPH-cytochrome c reductase, and microsomal glutathione S-transferase 1). The possible reasons regarding the non-ER proteins was explained in the last paragraph of section 5.

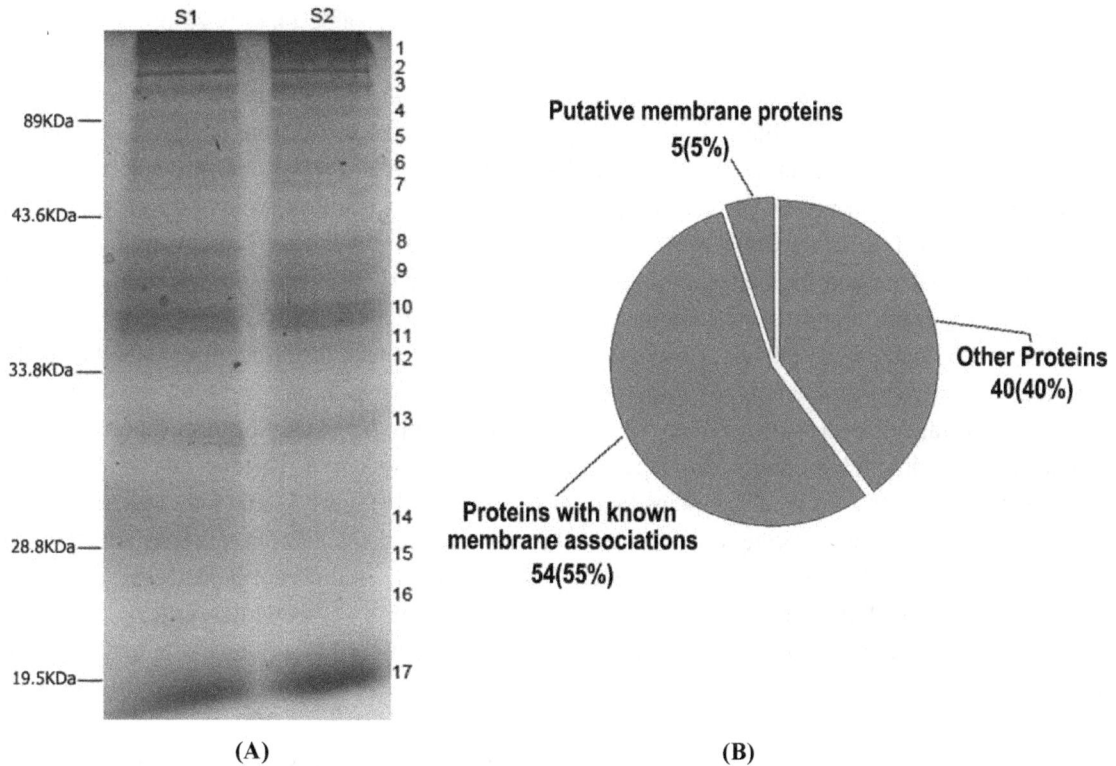

Figure 4: 1DE pattern and membrane-associated characteristic classification of Na$_2$CO$_3$-extracted microsomal membrane proteins. **A.** 1DE pattern. Molecular weight markers are shown on the left and 17 gel-bands excised for MS analysis are indicated on the right. Lanes S1 and S2 were loaded with the same protein samples (50 μg per lane). **B.** Classification based on membrane-associated characteristic. Reproduced from Peng *et al.* (Peng *et al.*, 2012), with permission from Hindawi publisher open accession journal; copyright remains with authors.

5 Overlay analysis of two Datasets from the 2DE-MS/MS and Na$_2$CO$_3$-1DE-MS/MS Strategies in analysis of mouse liver microsomal proteins

The main reasons why proteome analysis of the cell membrane-bound microsomes is a daunting task are (a) isolation of membrane that is free from nonconstituents and (b) solubilization of membrane proteins in a manner amenable to IEF (Santoni *et al.*, 2000). 2DE is one of the most common tool to survey biological complexity and provides a systematic and comprehensive study of the proteins. However, because of the pI value range limited by the IPG strip and the high dependence on sample preparation, some problems remain for the available 2DE protocols to resolve membrane-associated proteins (Santoni *et al.*, 2000, Adessi *et al.*, 1997). The analytical capability of 1DE in the separation of ER membrane proteins is greater than that of 2DE (Galeva & Altermann, 2002, Lisitsa *et al.*, 2009). Therefore, in our work, the whole microsome lysate from the prepared microsome samples was arrayed with 2DE, and the membrane fraction of microsomes purified by the carbonate procedure was separated with 1DE. Among the 2DE dataset (n = 183 proteins; Table 1) and 1DE dataset (n = 99 proteins; Table 1), only 22 proteins (Table 1) were found in both 2DE and 1DE datasets (12% of 2DE dataset, and 22% of 1DE dataset). A total of 260 nonredundant proteins (n = 183 + 99 − 22) were characterized in the microsome through the strategy of combining 2DE with 1DE technologies followed by LC-MS/MS. The microsome consisted of a complex network of continuous membranes including ER, ER-Golgi intermediate complex—also referred to as the vesiculotubular clusters or pre-Golgi intermediates—and the Golgi apparatus. Among those characterized proteins, 62 located in ER and Golgi were definitely classified as microsomal proteins by annotation in the Swiss-Prot database and the Gene Ontology. The complementary 2DE and 1DE approaches provided a much wider coverage of microsome proteome.

Hydrophobicity and relatively low abundance are the bottle neck for proteomic method to analyze membrane proteins. Hydrophobicity, an important characteristic of a membrane protein, can be evaluated by the grand average of hydropathy (GRAVY) scores (> −0.4) (http://us.expasy.org/tools/ protparam.html) that indicates a hydrophobic protein and suggests a membrane association (Kyte & Doolittle, 1982). In the 1DE dataset, 69 (70%) of the 99 proteins had a GRAVY > −0.4 (Figure 5) that indicates the probability for membrane association (Kyte & Doolittle, 1982). Moreover, some alkaline proteins with pI values close to or greater than 10 were separated by 1DE (Figure 6), but they could not be detected in a conventional 2DE map. Only 22 proteins were found in both 2DE and 1DE datasets with 6 proteins classified as membrane proteins (Table 1). All these results further indicate that 1DE is a potent supplement to 2DE, and the combination of the two approaches is necessary in protein profiling of microsomes (Peng *et al.*, 2012, Kanaeva *et al.*, 2004).

Microsome-sealed sacs could be converted into flat membrane sheets with cisternal contents in the treatment solution (100 mM Na$_2$CO$_3$; 0 °C) that is as effective as the low detergent procedure in selectively releasing microsomal content. In our work, the fact that some characterized proteins from carbonate-extracted fraction were classified as membrane association is mainly based on published reports even though their predicted TMDs did not suggest a membrane origin. Thus points out the fact that structure alone might not be the deciding factor, as far as the association of proteins with integral membrane is concerned. (1) Some proteins might be bound to the membrane simply to perform their functional obligations. As a result, they would become part of complexes involving membrane proteins, and would not depart from them easily under the sample preparation. Many enzymes were the example to be identified in the extracted membrane fraction. For instance, Cis-retinol androgen dehydrogenase 1 is anchored to the ER membrane facing the cytoplasm by an N-terminal signaling sequence of 22 residues and takes part in the membrane-associated retinoid metabolism (Zhang *et al.*, 2004), so it is fatty acid-binding protein that is involved in the palmitic acid or retinylester metabolism that is incorporated in microsomal membranes (Zanetti & Catala, 1990) and the free fatty acid that is transferred to the membrane. (2) Some truly cytosolic proteins may simply integrate with membrane sacs during the sonication process and become difficult to be removed by the extraction procedure (Friso & Wikström, 1990). Study (Wong & Adeli, 2009) has demonstrated that hepatic microsomes are derived from the ER and other cell organelles. The ER represents a membrane tubular network that crosses the cytoplasm from the nucleus membrane to the plasma membrane. (3) Some proteins perform their functions between cytoplasm and ER, such as fatty-acid-binding proteins (Stan *et al.*, 2005). From those points of view, 60%–70% of the characterized proteins can be regarded as microsome proteins in our work. A part (~15%) of the characterized proteins did not have unambiguous locations in published reports or annotations in the genome database.

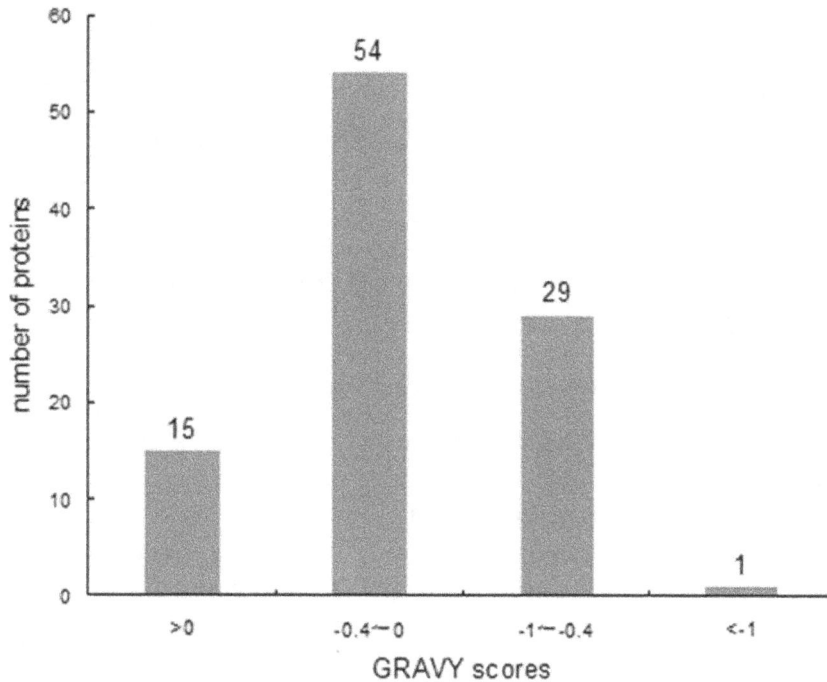

Figure 5: Distribution of 1DE-derived proteins over the GRAVY scores. The value (-0.4) is the mean GRAVY score for cytosolic proteins; it is the borderline between cytosolic proteins and membrane proteins. A score >-0.4 indicates probability for membrane association (the higher the score is, the greater the probability is). Reproduced from Peng *et al.* (Peng *et al.*, 2012), with permission from Hindawi publisher open accession journal; copyright remains with authors.

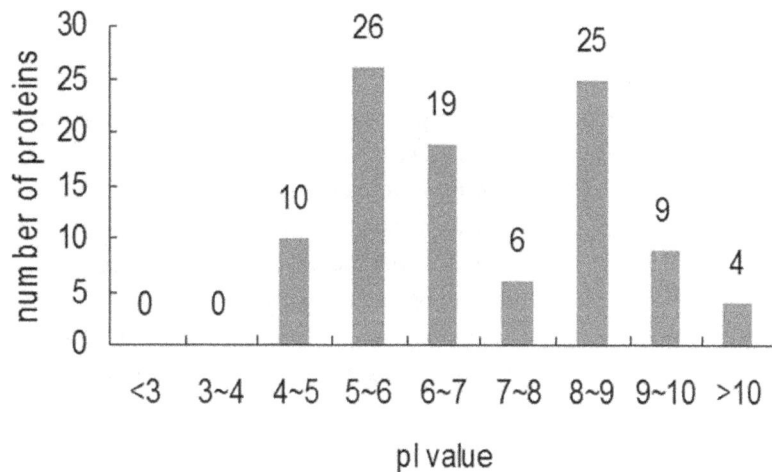

Figure 6: Distribution of 1DE-derived proteins over the pI values. Reproduced from Peng *et al.* (Peng *et al.*, 2012), with permission from Hindawi publisher open accession journal; copyright remains with authors.

6   Bioinformatics Analysis of Identified Microsomal Proteins

6.1   Tools and software

Protein annotations were obtained primarily from UniProt 7.0 including accession, entry name, comments such as function, catalytic activity, subcellular location, and similarity. The Cytoscape plugin, Biological Networks Gene Ontology (BiNGO), was used to find statistically overrepresented GO categories of the protein dataset. An online tool, WebGestalt (http://bioinfo.vanderbilt.edu/webgestalt/), was used to map target proteins to Kyoto Encyclopedia of Genes and Genomes (KEGG) pathways. The pathway visualization was based on the pathway mapping service provided in KEGG.

6.2   Significantly Enriched GO Terms for Mouse Liver Microsomal Proteins

BiNGO (Maere *et al.*, 2005) and Cytoscape (Shannon *et al.*, 2003) plugins that find statistically overrepresented GO categories were used for the enrichment analysis of our protein datasets. The microsomal protein dataset (n = 260, from 1DE and 2DE datasets) was compared to a reference set of complete mouse proteome (IPI mouse) that was provided by BiNGO. The analysis was done with a hypergeometric test for association of categories and genes that computes hypergeometric p-values over- and under-representation of each term in the specified category among the specified gene test, and all significant (p < 0.01) GO terms were selected after correcting for a multiple term testing with a Benjamini and Hochberg false discovery rate (FDR) that was used to increase the power of statistical tests. The analysis was performed for molecular function, cellular component, and biological process categories, separately, and x-fold enrichment for every overrepresented term in three GO categories was calculated (Figure 7). The results showed that the terms were related to mostly catalytic activity in terms of molecular function, including metabolism-related oxidoreductase, hydrolase, and dehydrogenase. Similarly, terms belonging to the cellular component namespace include mitochondrion, ER, and ribosome. Finally, terms from the biological process namespace included metabolic process, localization, transport, and translation. All of the information suggested the main functions and compositions of liver microsomes.

6.3   Significant Enrichment of KEGG Pathway for Mouse Liver Microsomal Proteins

The KEGG pathway database-based biological pathways analysis was carried out with an analysis toolkit—WebGestalt (http://bioinfo.vanderbilt.edu/webgestalt/) (Zhang *et al.*, 2005). This toolkit allowed the functional annotation of gene/protein sets into the well-characterized functional signaling pathways (KEGG: http://www.genome.jp/kegg/). An enrichment score was obtained of the frequency of occurrence of a specific protein (or gene) within any given experimental subset with respect to a species-specific background set. Thus, an enrichment factor [the observed frequency in input set (microsome protein list; Figure 7)/the expected frequency in background set (reference protein list that represents all proteins in the KEGG database; Figure 7)] was created with a statistical value that indicated that the protein (or gene) was specifically overrepresented in the input dataset. In our work, all the proteins except 81 (n = 260 − 81 = 179) were linked to a total of 99 biological pathways in the KEGG database, including metabolic pathway, glycolysis/gluconeogenesis, metabolism of xenobiotics by cytochrome P450, and peroxisome proliferator activated receptor (PPAR) signaling pathway. Among those pathways, 34 significantly (p < 0.01) enriched biological processes analyzed by WebGestalt were obtained (Figure 8). Those biological processes were involved in cell metabolism, benzoate degradation, metabolism of xenobiotics, ribosome, biosynthesis, signaling pathway, and oxidative stress. These results are known to be related to microsome (Peng, *et al.*, 2012).

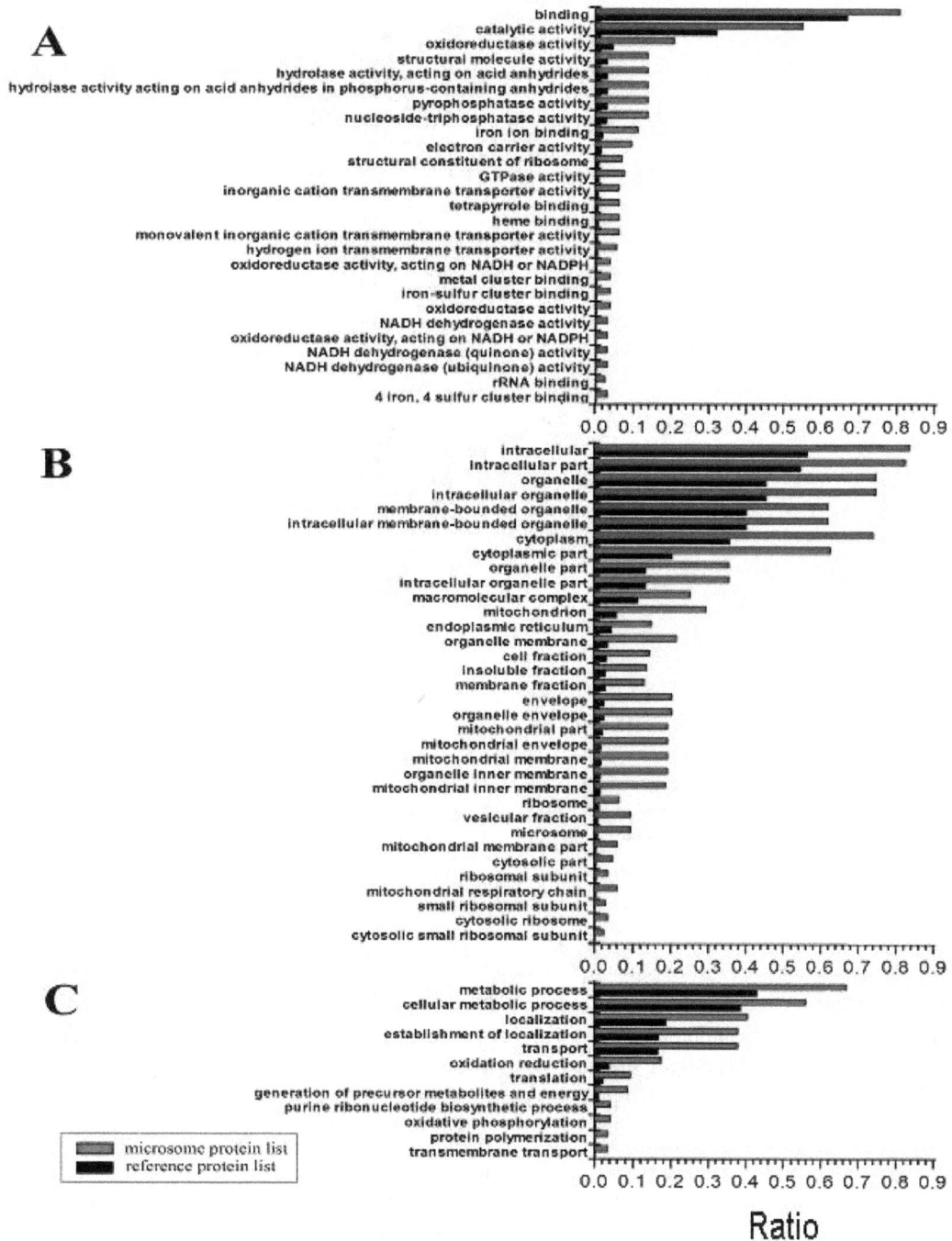

Figure 7: Significant enrichment of GO terms for mouse liver microsomal proteins (n = 260) that were derived from the 2DE-MS/MS and Na$_2$CO$_3$-1DE-MS/MS strategies. The set of identified microsomal proteins was compared with the reference list of IPI entries (provided by BiNGO), and significantly over-represented GO terms (P < 0.01) are shown. The ratio shown is the number of microsome and reference IPI proteins annotated to each GO term divided by the number of microsome and reference IPI proteins linked to at least one annotation term within the indicated GO molecular function (A), cellular component (B), and biological process categories(C). Reproduced from Peng *et al.* (Peng *et al.*, 2012), with permission from Hindawi publisher open accession journal; copyright remains with authors.

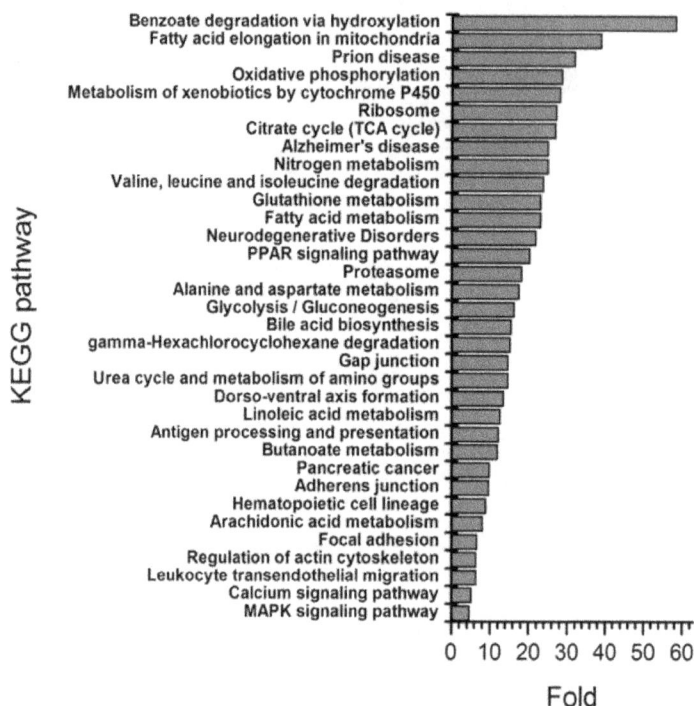

Figure 8: Significantly enriched KEGG pathways for mouse liver microsomal proteins (n = 260) that were derived from the 2DE-MS/MS and Na$_2$CO$_3$-1DE-MS/MS strategies. KEGG pathway enrichment analysis was performed using WebGestalt. The pathways having enrichment (P < 0.01) are presented. For each KEGG pathway, the bar shows the x-fold enrichment of the pathway in our dataset, and x-fold = the ratio in the microsome protein dataset/the ratio in the reference protein dataset. Reproduced from Peng *et al*. (Peng *et al*., 2012), with permission from Hindawi publisher open accession journal; copyright remains with authors.

The KEGG search service was used to map our dataset on the KEGG pathways in order to ascertain the coverage of our dataset with the enriched pathways or biological processes. Two enriched KEGG pathways (metabolism of xenobiotics and ribosome) were related to the well-known function and composition of the microsome. Enzyme Commission numbers (EC., e.g, 1.14.14.1) are used to represent enzymes in the process of metabolism. All enzymes (n = 9) that were involved in every pathway of metabolism of xenobiotics were found in our dataset (Table 2). Also, 13 proteins from large and small subunits of ribosome were found in our dataset (Table 2), and they interact physically with each other and form a large protein complex—the ribosome. All the characterized proteins that were involved in those two pathways are summarized in Table 2, including their KEGG pathway, protein ID, and protein name.

7   Comparison between Different Research Groups in Analysis of Liver Microsome Proteomes

Several research groups have studied the mammalian liver microsome proteomes (Zgoda *et al*., 2006, Zgoda *et al*., 2009, Gilchrist *et al*., 2006). A comparison was performed of our work with the literature

KEGG Pathway		Protein ID	Protein Name	MS-identified proteins
A. Metabolism of Xexnobiotics	EC:1.14.14.1	IPI00128287	Cytochrome P450 1A2	+
		IPI00123964	Cytochrome P450 2A5	+
		IPI00116572	Cytochrome P450 2D9	+
		IPI00323908	Cytochrome P450 2D10	+
		IPI00321644	Cytochrome P450 2D26	+
		IPI00114779	Cytochrome P450 2C38	+
		IPI00308328	Cytochrome P450 2F2	+
	EC:2.5.1.18	IPI00331322	Microsomal glutathione S-transferase 1	+
	EC:1.1.1.1	IPI00221400	Alcohol dehydrogenase A chain	+
B. Ribosome	Small subunit	IPI00135640	26S protease regulatory subunit 8	+
		IPI00125971	26S protease regulatory subunit S10B	+
		IPI00331092	40S ribosomal protein S4, X isoform	+
		IPI00116908	Similar to 40s ribosomal protein S12	+
		IPI00322562	40S ribosomal protein S14	+
		IPI00465880	40S ribosomal protein S17	+
		IPI00113241	40S ribosomal protein S19	+
		IPI00123604	40S ribosomal protein SA	+
		IPI00314950	60S acidic ribosomal protein P0	+
	Large subunit	IPI00331461	60S ribosomal protein L11	+
		IPI00849793	60S ribosomal protein L12	+
		IPI00222546	60S ribosomal protein L22	+
		IPI00139780	60S ribosomal protein L23	+

Table 2: Proteins involved in KEGG pathways. A. Metabolism of exnobiotics (cytochrome P450 pathway). B. Ribosome. Reproduced from Peng *et al.* (Peng *et al.*, 2012), with permission from Hindawi publisher open accession journal; copyright remains with authors.

data (Zgoda *et al.*, 2006, Zgoda *et al.*, 2009, Gilchrist *et al.*, 2006) and summarized in Tables 3. Zgoda group (Zgoda *et al.*, 2006) used differential ultracentrifugation to separate mouse liver microsome proteome; 2DE and silver stain yielded 1,100 protein spots, and 138 proteins contained in 2D gel spots were characterized with peptide mass fingerprint (PMF). The differential ultracentrifugation was also used by Zgoda group (Zgoda *et al.*, 2009) to separate mouse liver microsome proteome with 1DE and MS/MS; 519 proteins were characterized including 138 (138/519 = 27%) predicted membrane proteins that have at least one transmembrane domain in a protein. Gilchrist group (Gilchrist *et al.*, 2006) used differential ultracentrifugation and density gradient centrifugation to separate rat ER and Golgi followed by 1DE and MS/MS analyses; 832 ER proteins were identified including 183 (183/832 = 22%) membrane proteins

	Our work (Peng et al., 2012)	Zgoda et al., 2009	Zgoda et al., 2006	Gilchrist et al., 2006
Comparison regarding method and results				
Species	Mouse	Mouse	Mouse	Rat
Sample	Liver microsome	Liver microsome	Liver microsome	ER,Golgi
Pretreatment	None	Phenobarbital	Phenobarbital or 3-methylcholantrene	None
Sample preparation	Subfractionated by differential ultra-centrifugation + sucrose gradient centrifugation + Na$_2$CO$_3$	Subfractionated by differential ultra-centrifugation	Differential ultra-centrifugation	Subfractionated by differential ultra-centrifugation + Density Gradient Centrifugation
Protein separation	2DE, 1DE	1DE	2DE	1DE
1D/2D-Gel Stain	Coomassie brilliant blue (2DE; 1DE)	-	Silver Stain	-
Protein identification	MS/MS	MS/MS	MS	MS/MS
Protein spots on 2D-Gel	514	-	1100	-
Proteins identified in 2D-Gel	183	-	139	-
Proteins identified in 1DE	99	519	-	832(ER)
Proteins identified in 2-D LC	-	1410	-	-
Proteins identified in 3-D LC	-	3703	-	-
Total identified proteins	260	4142	Unspecified	832(ER)
Membrane proteins	2DE: 41 (41/183 = 22%) 1DE: 54 (54/99 = 55%) Total: 62 (62/260 = 24%)	1DE: 138 (138/519 = 27%) 2-D LC: 259 (259/1410 = 21%) 3-D LC: 659 (659/3703 = 18%)	Unspecified	183 (183/832 = 22%)
Protein superfamily				
P450 family members	10	29	2	11
Ribosomal proteins	13	16	Unspecified	45
UDP-glycosyltransferases, UGTs	6	8	Unspecified	3
Tubulins	11	5	Unspecified	2
Short-chain Dehydrogenase/ reductase	32	9	Unspecified	56
Protein disulfide isomerase	2	4	Unspecified	1
Comparison of selected proteins				
P450 family members	2D9, 2A5, 2C38, 1A2, 2D11, 2F2, 2D10, 2D26		2C37	17A1, 20A1, 2B2, 2J3, 4A1, 4A8, 4F1, 4F4, 4V3, 8B1, NA2

GRP-170	Hypoxia up-regulated protein 1		170 kDa glucose regulated protein	-
Endoplasmin	Endoplasmin		Tumor rejection antigen gp96	
Serotransferrin	Serotransferrin		Transferrin	-
78 kDa glucose-regulated protein	78 kDa glucose-regulated protein		78 kDa glucose-regulated protein	-
Stress-induced phosphoprotein 1	-		Stress-induced phosphoprotein 1	-
Calreticulin family	Calnexin		Calreticulin	-
Protein disulfide-isomerase	Protein disulfide-isomerase precursor (PDI)		Protein disulfide-isomerase precursor (PDI)	SIMILAR TO DISULFIDE ISOMERASE
Glucose regulated protein similar to ER-60 protease	-		Glucose regulated protein similar to ER-60 protease	-
Erp58	-		Erp58	-
Vitamin D-binding protein	-		Vitamin D-binding protein	-
Tubulins	Tubulin beta-4, alpha-1, alpha-2, alpha-4, beta-5, beta-2C, beta 2		Tubulin alpha	Tubulin alpha 6
Fibrinogen	-		Fibrinogen, gamma polypeptide	-
Serine protease inhibitor	-		Similar to serine protease inhibitor 1–4	-
Argininosuccinate synthetase 1	Argininosuccinate synthetase 1		Argininosuccinate synthetase 1	-
Interferon-inducible GTPase	-		Interferon-inducible GTPase	
Progesterone receptor membrane component	Progesterone receptor membrane component		Progesterone receptor membrane component	-
Major urinary protein 2	Major urinary protein 2		Major urinary protein 2	-
Superoxide dismutase I	-		Superoxide dismutase I	-

| ribosomal proteins | 26S protease regulatory subunit 8, S10B; 40S ribosomal protein S17, SA, S6, S19, S12, SA, S14, S4 X isoform; 60S ribosomal protein L11, L12, L23, L22, P0 | | Unspecified | 40S Ribosomal Protein S10, S12, S18, S20, S21, S23, S24, S25, S26, S27, S29, S30, S6, S9 60S Ribosomal protein L12, L15, L18A, L19, L21, L22, L23, L23A, L24, L26, L27, L27A, L28, L3, L32, L34, L35, L35A, L36, L37, L37A, L39, L4, L40, L44, L6, L7A |
| UDP-glycosyltransferases, UGTs | UDP-glucuronosyltransferase 2B5, 2B36, 1A5 UDP-glucuronosyltransferase 1-1 precursor UDP-glucuronosyltransferase 1-2 precursor | | Unspecified | UDP-glucuronosyltrans-ferase 1A7 UDP-glucuronosyltrans-ferase GTNA2 |

Table 3: Comparison of our work (Peng *et al.*, 2012) with the literature data (Zgoda *et al.*, 2006 and 2009, Gilchrist *et al.*, 2006). Note: No protein list was obtained from the publication (Zgoda *et al.*, 2009). – means "not included". Modified from Peng *et al.* (Peng *et al.*, 2012), with permission from Hindawi publisher open accession journal; copyright remains with authors.

that have at least one transmembrane domain in a protein. Our study (Peng, *et al.*, 2012) combined differential ultracentrifugation and sucrose gradient centrifugation to prepare mouse liver microsomes; 2DE and Coomassie brilliant blue stain yielded 514 protein spots, and 183 proteins were characterized with MS/MS from 204 excised gel spots, including 41 (41/183 = 22%) membrane proteins. Carbonate method was used to further purify membrane proteins from isolated microsome fraction; 1DE and Coomassie brilliant blue stain yield 17 protein bands, and 99 proteins were characterized with MS/MS, including 54 (54/99 = 55%) membrane proteins. A total of 260 nonredundant proteins were characterized including 62 (62/260 = 24%) membrane proteins. Compared to the literature data (Zgoda *et al.*, 2006, Zgoda *et al.*, 2009, Gilchrist *et al.*, 2006), the advantages of our work (Peng, *et al.*, 2012) were (1) that the carbonate method significantly increased the identification rate of microsomal membrane proteins, (2) that some proteins and functional annotations from our work had not been identified in other literature, which expanded and enriched the literature data, and (3) that the established analysis system and data would benefit the discovery of liver disease-related microsomal membrane proteins. Meanwhile, we also noted that our study (Peng, et al., 2012) had a relatively low coverage (n = 260 proteins) of mouse liver microsome proteome relative to other literature data (n = 519 proteins (Zgoda *et al.*, 2009) and 832 proteins (Gilchrist *et al.*, 2006)), which might be derived from several factors: (i) inconsistent protein extraction procedures and protein-staining methods were used, (ii) only part of 2D gel spots were excised to identify proteins, (iii) only visualized 1D gel bands (not the entire 1D gel lane) were used for protein identification, (iv) MS/MS (not PMF) was used to identify 2D gel proteins, (v) mass spectrometers with different sensitivities were used, (vi) different parameters were used to search protein database. The use of 2D/3D LC-MS/MS (Gilchrist *et al.*, 2006) and carbonate extraction of isolated microsomes (Peng, *et al.*, 2012) would significantly improve the coverage of microsomal membrane proteome.

8   Conclusion

Microsome is an ideal target for analyzing membrane-bound enzyme functions, compound metabolism, lipid-protein interactions, and drug-drug interactions. This chapter presents an overall systems procedure to analyze mouse liver microsomal proteome. Mouse liver microsomes were effectively isolated and enriched with differential centrifugation and sucrose gradient centrifugation, and the prepared microsomal proteins were arrayed by 2DE and characterized by LC-MS/MS. The microsomal membrane proteins were further maximally extracted from isolated microsomal fractions by the carbonate method, fractioned by 1DE, and characterized by LC-MS/MS. The 2DE-MS/MS and Na_2CO_3-1DE-MS/MS strategies demonstrated their complementary ability to analyze the intracellular microsomes that contain considerable numbers of highly hydrophobic membrane proteins. An integrated bioinformatics analysis of all of the microsome proteins can provide a relatively complete understanding of the protein composition and cellular function of the target microsome organelles. Furthermore, the Triton X-114 extraction is able to significantly maximally enrich microsomal membrane proteins from carbonate extraction (Mathias *et al.*, 2011). A facile system that couples formic acid assisted solubilization and online immobilized pepsin digestion with strong cation exchange and microflow reversed-phase liquid chromatography with electrospray ionization MS/MS (SCX-μRPLC-ESI-MS/MS) was developed to analyze integral membrane proteome such as microsome (Ma *et al.*, 2010). We recommend that the use of 2D/3D LC-MS/MS (Gilchrist *et al.*, 2006) and carbonate extraction (Peng *et al.*, 2012) plus Triton X-114 extraction (Mathias *et al.*, 2011) of isolated microsomes should significantly improve the coverage of microsomal membrane proteome. Also, the present methods will easily translate to the development of a quantitative proteomics to analyze liver disease-related microsome proteins for biomarker discovery and mechanism clarification of a liver disease.

Abbreviations

ACN: acetonitrile

BiNGO: Biological Networks Gene Ontology

DTT: dithiothreitol

ER: endoplasmic reticulum

ESI: electrospray ionization

EDTA: ethylene diamine tetraacetic acid

FDR: false discovery rate

GO: gene ontology

GRAVY: grand average of hydropathy

HPLC: high-performance liquid chromatography

IEF: isoelectric focusing

IPG: immobilized pH gradient

IPI: international protein index

KEGG: Kyoto Encyclopedia of Genes and Genomes

LC: liquid chromatography

MS: mass spectrometry

MS/MS: tandem mass spectrometry

NL: non-linear

pI: isoelectric point

PF2D: two-dimensional liquid phase fraction

PMF: peptide mass fingerprint

PPAR: peroxisome proliferator activated receptor

PVDF: polyvinylidene fluoride

Q-TOF: quadrupole time-of-flight

RP: reverse phase

SCX: strong cation exchange

SDS-PAGE: sodium dodecyl sulfate polyacrylamide gel electrophoresis

2DE: two-dimensional electrophoresis

2D/3D: two- or three-dimensional

TFA: trifluoroacetic Acid

TMD: transmembrane domains

1DE: one-dimensional electrophoresis

Acknowledgments

This work was supported by the National Human Liver Proteome Project of China (Grant no. 2004 BA711A18), the National Basic Research Program of China (Grant No. 2011CB910704), the National Natural Science Foundation of China (Grant No. 81272798), and the Xiangya Hospital Funds for Talent Introduction (X.Z.).

References

Adessi, C., Miege, C., Albrieux, C., Rabilloud, T. (1997). Two-dimensional electrophoresis of membrane proteins: a current challenge for immobilized pH gradients. Electrophoresis, 18 (1), 127–135.

Arnold, R. J., Hrncirova, P., Annaiah, K., Novotny, M. V. (2004). Fast proteolytic digestion coupled with organelle enrichment for proteomic analysis of rat liver. J. Proteome Res., 3 (3), 653-657.

Candiano, G., Bruschi, M., Musante, L., et al. (2004). Blue silver: a very sensitive colloidal Coomassie G-250 staining for proteome analysis. Electrophoresis, 25 (9), 1327–1333.

Chen, P., Zhang, L., Li, X., et al. (2007). Evaluation of strategy for analyzing mouse liver plasma membrane proteome. Science in China Series C, 50(6), 731–738.

Fleischer, S., Kervina, M. (1974). Subcellular fractionation of rat liver. Methods in Enzymology, 31, 6–41.

Friso, G., Giacomelli, L., Ytterberg, A. J., et al. (2004). In-depth analysis of the thylakoid membrane proteome of Arabidopsis thaliana chloroplasts: new proteins, new functions, and a plastid proteome database. Plant Cell, 16 (2), 478–499.

Friso, G., Wikström, L. (1999). Analysis of proteins from membrane-enriched cerebellar preparations by two-dimensional gel electrophoresis and mass spectrometry. Electrophoresis, 20 (4-5), 917–927.

Fujiki, Y., Hubbard, A. L., Fowler, S., Lazarow, P. B. (1982). Isolation of intracellular membranes by means of sodium carbonate treatment: application to endoplasmic reticulum. Journal of Cell Biology, 93 (1), 97–102.

Galeva, N., Altermann, M. (2002). Comparison of one-dimensional and two-dimensional gel electrophoresis as a separation tool for proteomic analysis of rat liver microsomes: cytochromes P450 and other membrane proteins. Proteomics, 2(6), 713–722.

Gilchrist, A., Au, C. E., Hiding, J., et al. (2006). Quantitative proteomics analysis of the secretory pathway. Cell, 127 (6), 1265–1281.

He, F. (2005). Human liver proteome project: plan, progress, and perspectives. Molecular and Cellular Proteomics, 4(12), 1841–1848.

Heinemann, F. S., Ozols, J. (1998). Isolation and structural analysis of microsomal membrane proteins. Frontiers in Bioscience, 3, 483–493.

Jung, E., Heller, M., Sanchez, J. C., Hochstrasser, D. F. (2000). Proteomics meets cell biology: the establishment of subcellular proteomes. Electrophoresis, 21 (16), 3369–3377.

Kanaeva, I. P., Petushkova, N. A., Lisitsa, A. V., et al. (2005). Proteomic and biochemical analysis of the mouse liver microsomes. Toxicology In Vitro, 19 (6), 805–812.

Kanaeva, I. P., Petushkova, N. A., Lokhov, P. G., Zgoda, V. G., Karuzina, I. I., Lisitsa, A. V., Archakov, A. I. (2004). Study of the mouse liver microsomes by the methods of proteome analysis. Biomed. Khim., 50 (4), 367-375.

Kyte, J., Doolittle, R. F. (1982). A simple method for displaying the hydropathic character of a protein. Journal of Molecular Biology, 157 (1), 105–132.

Lee, H. J., Kwon, M. S., Lee, E. Y., Cho, S. Y., Paik, Y. K. (2008). Establishment of a PF2D-MS/MS platform for rapid profiling and semiquantitative analysis of membrane protein biomarkers. Proteomics, 8 (11), 2168-2177.

Lisitsa, A. V., Petushkova, N. A., Nikitin, I. P., Zgoda, V. G., Karuzina, I. I., Moshkovskii, S. A., Larina, O. V., Skipenko, O. G., Polyschuk, L. O., Thiele, H., Archakov, A. I. (2009). One-dimensional proteomic mapping of human liver cytochromes p450. Biochemistry (Mosc), 74 (2), 153-161.

Ma, J., Hou, C., Sun, L., Tao, D., Zhang, Y., Shan, Y., Liang, Z., Zhang, L., Yang, L., Zhang, Y. (2010).Coupling formic acid assisted solubilisation and online immobilized pepsin digestion with strong cation exchange and microflow reversed-phase liquid chromatography with electrospray ionization tandem mass spectrometry for integral membrane proteome analysis. Anal Chem., 82 (23), 9622-9625.

Maere, S., Heymans, K., Kuiper, M. (2005). BiNGO: a cytoscape plugin to assess overrepresentation of Gene Ontology categories in Biological Networks. Bioinformatics, 21 (16), 3448–3449.

Mathias, R. A., Chen, Y. S., Kapp, E. A., Greening, D. W., Mathivanan, S., Simpson, R. J. (2011). Triton X-114 phase separation in the isolation and purification of mouse liver microsomal membrane proteins. Methods, 54 (4), 396-406.

Okuzawa, K. Franzen, B., Lindholm, J., et al. (1994). Characterization of gene expression in clinical lung cancer materials by two-dimensional polyacrylamide gel electrophoresis. Electrophoresis, 15 (3-4), 382–390.

Peng, F., Zhan, X., Li, M. Y., et al. (2012). Proteomic and bioinformatics analyses of mouse liver microsomes. International Journal of Proteomics, doi: 10.1155/2012/832569.

Peng, L., Kapp, E. A., McLauchlan, D., Jordan, T. W. (2011). Characterization of the Asia Oceania Human Proteome Organisation Membrane Proteomics Initiative Standard using SDS-PAGE shotgun proteomics. Proteomics, 11 (22), 4376-4384.

Santoni, V., Molloy, M., Rabilloud, T. (2000). Membrane proteins and proteomics: un amour impossible? Electrophoresis, 21 (6), 1054–1070.

Shannon, P., Markiel, A., Ozier, O., et al. (2003). Cytoscape: a software environment for integrated models of biomolecular interaction networks. Genome Research, 13 (11), 2498–2504.

Stan, S., Lambert, M., Delvin, E., et al. (2005). Intestinal fatty acid binding protein and microsomal triglyceride transfer protein polymorphisms in French-Canadian youth. Journal of Lipid Research, 46 (2), 320–327.

Tananova, O. N., Arianova, E. A., Gmoshinskii, I. V., Aksenov, I. V., Zgoda, V. G., Khotimchenko, S. A. (2012). Effect of titanium dioxide nanoparticles on protein expression profiles in rat liver microsomes. Vopr Pitan. 81 (2), 18-22.

Taylor, S. W., Fahy, E., Ghosh, S. S. (2003). Global organellar proteomics. Trends in Biotechnology, 21 (2), 82–88.

Wong, D. M., Adeli, K. (2009). Microsomal proteomics. Methods in Molecular Biology, 519, 273–289.

Zanetti, R., Catala, A. (1990). Interaction of fatty acid binding protein with microsomes: removal of palmitic acid and retinyl esters. Archives Internationales de Physiologie et de Biochimie, 98 (4), 173–177.

Zhang, M., Hu, P., Napoli, J. L. (2004). Elements in the Nterminal signaling sequence that determine cytosolic topology of short-chain dehydrogenases/reductases: studies with retinol dehydrogenase type 1 and cis-retinol/androgen dehydrogenase type 1. Journal of Biological Chemistry, 279 (49), 51482–51489.

Zhang, B., Kirov, S., Snoddy, J. (2005). WebGestalt: an integrated system for exploring gene sets in various biological contexts. Nucleic Acids Research, 33 (2), W741–W748.

Zgoda, V. G., Moshkovskii, S. A., Ponomarenko, E. A., et al. (2009). Proteomics of mouse liver microsomes: performance of different protein separation workflows for LC-MS/MS. Proteomics, 9 (16), 4102–4105.

Zgoda, V. G., Tikhonova, O., Viglinskaya, A., Serebriakova, M., Lisitsa, A., Archakov, A. (2006). Proteomic profiles of induced hepatotoxicity at the subcellular level. Proteomics, 6 (16), 4662–4670.

Methylation Level of Genes and MiRNA-Mediated Methylation Modification Mechanism In Glioma

Minghua Wu, Zuping Zhang, Xiaoping Liu, Hailin Tang
Cancer Research Institute
Central South University, China

1   Introduction

Aberrant DNA methylation patterns are common in the genesis and progression of tumors (Jones & Baylin, 2007). In cancer cells, a general decline in the methylated cytosine levels (genomic hypomethylation) is accompanied by local locus-specific hypermethylation (Baylin *et al.*, 2001; Laird, 2005). Genomic hypomethylation may lead to genome instability and the hypomethylation of protooncogenes, which leads to their stronger expression (Ehrlich, 2002). On the other hand, local promoter hypermethylation induces the functional silencing of tumor-associated genes (Herman & Baylin, 2003). Therefore, cancer cells undergo massive alterations to their DNA methylation that result in aberrant gene expression and malignant phenotypes.

Glioma is the most frequent and devastating primary brain tumor affecting adults. Aberrant DNA methylation contributes to glioma development and progression (Kim *et al.*, 2006). Promoter hypermethylation and the epigenetic silencing of the O6-methylguanine-DNA methyltransferase（MGMT）gene has been widely described in glioma (Komine *et al.*, 2003; Yin *et al.*,2003; Hegi *et al.*, 2004). The silencing of several other genes involved in key cellular functions, such as the cell cycle (Ohta *et al.*, 2006), tumor suppression (Amatya *et al.*, 2005; Hesson *et al.*, 2004; Horiguchi *et al.*, 2003; Wiencke *et al.*, 2007; Zhang *et al.*, 2008), DNA repair(Fukushima *et al.*, 2005; Nakamura *et al.*,2001), tumor invasion (Waha *et al.*, 2005) and apoptosis (Stone *et al.*, 2004), are also associated with promoter hypermethylation in malignant glioma. Despite these important findings, the aberrant DNA methylation in glioma on a genome-wide scale is not fully understood.

Methylation changes to the genome are controlled by DNA methyltransferases (DNMTs). Currently, three catalytically active DNMTs, DNMT1, DNMT3A and DNMT3B, have been identified (Jeltsch, 2002). Whereas DNMT1 preferentially replicates already existing methylation patterns, DNMT3A and DNMT3B are responsible for establishing de novo methylation. Although the mechanisms leading to aberrant DNA methylation are not fully elucidated, the increased expression of DNMT1 and DNMT3B and the decreased expression of DNMT3A have been observed in glioblastoma (Foltz *et al.*, 2009; Fanelli *et al.*, 2008), suggesting that the abnormal expression of DNMTs contributes to aberrant DNA methylation and in turn to gliomagenesis.

MicroRNAs (miRNAs) are ~20–22-nucleotide non-coding RNA molecules that tend to negatively regulate genes by binding to the 3' untranslated region of the target mRNA via the RNA-induced silencing complex, causing mRNA destabilization and/or translational inhibition (Bartel, 2004; He&Hannon, 2004). Growing evidence supports a role for miRNAs as both targets and effectors in aberrant mechanisms of DNA methylation (Saito *et al.*, 2006; Fabbri *et al.*, 2007). The miRNA silencing by promoter DNA hypermethylation is involved in various cancers (Lujambio *et al.*, 2008; Datta *et al.*, 2008; Toyota *et al.*, 2008). Meanwhile, miRNAs are also involved in the control of DNA methylation by targeting the DNA methylation machinery (Benetti *et al.*, 2008; Wu et al., *2010*).

In this study, we used the MeDIP-chip to investigate the whole-genome differential methylation patterns of glioma and normal brain samples. The MeDIP-chip is a novel high-throughput array-based method that uses a monoclonal antibody raised against 5-methylcytidine to enrich the methylated DNA fragments and to hybridize to the promoter and CpG island microarrays that cover the entire human genome (Jacinto *et al.*, 2008). To confirm the results of the microarray, the promoter methylation status of fourteen candidate genes, including 8 hypermethylated genes and 6 hypomethylated genes were verified, and the possible mechanisms of the epigenetic regulation of expression were examined. Our study demonstrated that miR-185 targets DNMT1 directly, leading to the reduction of global DNA methylation

(GDM) and the reexpression of the promoter-hypermethylated genes described. The miR-101 regulates the histone-mediated methylation of hypomethylated genes by targeting EZH2, EED and DNMT3A.

2 Materials and Methods

2.1 Cell lines and Tissue Samples

Human glioblastoma-derived cell lines U251, U87, SF126 and SF767 were obtained from the Cell Research Institute of Peking Union Medical College (Peking, China). U251 and U87 were maintained in DMEM supplemented with 10% fetal calf serum (FCS) and standard antibiotics; SF126 and SF767 were cultured in minimal essential medium. All cells were cultured in a $37^\circ C$ humidified incubator supplied with 5% CO_2.

Primary tumor samples were obtained from randomly selected cancer patients at Xiangya Hospital (Hunan, People's Republic of China). Tumors were graded according to the revised classification of the World Health Organization (2007) (Louis *et al.*, 2007). For comparison, normal human brain white matters from person without cancer were obtained at the time of autopsy. Informed consent was obtained from all patients and controls. The glioma samples for methylation analysis include astrocytoma (gradeI(1), gradeII(18), gradeIII(11)), glioblastoma multiforme(gradeIV(6)), oligoastrocytoma(gradeII(3), gradeIII(1)). All specimens were utilized in accordance with an Institutional Review Board-approved protocol.

2.2 MeDIP and Microarray Hybridization

6 cases glioma tissues (T1, T2, T3, T4, T5, T6) and 4 cases normal brain tissues (N1, N2, N3, N5) with matched age and sex were selected to perform methylated DNA immunoprecipitation and microarray hybridization by Nimblegen MeDIP-chip protocol. Briefly, 11μg genomic DNA was sheared by sonication on ice to generate random fragments of 100–500 bp. Heat-denatured DNA was incubated with 5 μg of mouse anti-5-methylcytidine monoclonal antibody (Eurogenetec, San Diego, CA, USA) in 1×IP buffer (0.5% NP40, 1.1% Triton X-100, 1.5mM EDTA, 50mM Tris-HCl and 150mM NaCl) with rotating at 4°C overnight. Sheep anti-mouse IgG-conjugated magnetic beads (Bangs laboratories. Inc) were added to the IP buffer and incubated for an additional rotation for 2h at 4°C. The beads were washed five times with 500 μl wash buffer and then resuspended in 250 μl digestion buffer (50mM Tris, pH 8.0, 10mM EDTA, 0.5% SDS). The antibodies were digested with 80 μg of proteinase-K for 3 h at 50°C. DNA was extracted with phenol–chloroform and precipitated with ethanol. Precipitated DNA was resuspended in 20μl of 10mM Tris-HCl pH 8.0 and used for real-time quantitative PCR (qPCR) (for validation of IP efficiency) or for microarray hybridization. Immunoprecipitated methylated DNA was labled with Cy5 fluorophere and the input genomic DNA was labeled with Cy3 fluorophere. Labeled DNA from enriched and input pools were combined and hybridized to HG18 CpG promoter microarray 385K (Nimblegen). Arrays were washed and scanned on GenePix 4000B scanner (Nimblegen). Data were extracted and exported to excel using GenePix Pro6.0.

2.3 Microarray Data Analysis

Raw excel data files obtained from tiling array experiments were analyzed using NimbleScan[TM]2.3 software. The ratio between Cy5 and Cy3 signals were caculated for all high-quality hybridization dots. Then ratios were normalized and transformed to Log_2Ratio. One-side Kolmogorov-Smirnov (KS) test was conducted to obtain *p value* and P Value (-Log10 *p value*) of each probe according to Log_2Ratio of ambient probes within 750bp sliding window width. Peak score was generated by interval anaylsis with P Value cutoff at 2, maximum gap at 500bp and a minimum run at least two consecutive probes. The regions with Peak score were defined as methylated and level of methylation was positive correlation with Peak score. GFF files of Log_2Ratio, P Value, Peak score and HG18 CpG Promoter Annotation data were exported to Signalmap 1.0 software for visual analysis and review.

2.4 MassARRAY Measurements for DNA Methylation Analysis

The Sequenom MassARRAY platform (CapitalBio, Beijing, China) was used to perform the quantitative methylation analysis. Genomic DNA was isolated by means of standard procedures from cell lines and tissue samples obtained for diagnostic reasons from patients with glioma or nonmalignant diseases for control purposes. The target regions were amplified using bisulfite-modified DNA. The PCR reactions were carried out in a total volume of 5 μL using 5ηg/μL DNA, 1 pmol of each primer, 40 μM dNTP, 0.1 unit of Hot Star Taq DNA polymerase (Qiagen), 1.5 mM MgCl2, and buffer supplied with the enzyme (final concentration 1×). The reaction mix was preactivated for 15 minutes at 94°C. The reactions were amplified in 45 cycles of 94°C for 20 seconds, 62°C for 30 seconds, and 72°C for 1 minutes followed by 72°C for 3 minutes. Unincorporated dNTPs were dephosphorylated by adding 1.7 μL H_2O and 0.3 units of shrimp alkaline phosphatase (SAP; Sequenom, San Diego, CA). The reaction was incubated at 37°C for 20 minutes, and SAP was then heat inactivated for 10 minutes at 85°C.

Two microliters of the PCR reaction were directly used as template in a 7 μL transcription reaction. Twenty units of T7 DNA polymerase (Epicentre, Madison,WI) were used to incorporate either dCTP or dTTP in the transcripts. Ribonucleotides were used at 1 mM and the dNTP substrate at 2.5 mM; other components in the reaction were as recommended by the supplier. In the same step, RNase A (Sequenom) was added to cleave the in vitro transcript. The mixture was then further diluted with H_2O to a final volume of 27 μL. Conditioning of the phosphate backbone prior to matrix-assisted laser desorption / ionization time-of-flight mass spectrometry (MALDI-TOF MS) was achieved by the addition of 6 mg CLEAN Resin (Sequenom). Further experimental analysis for DNA methylation determination has been described previously (Ehrich *et al.*, 2005).

2.5 Bisulfite Sequencing PCR (BSP) and Methylation Specific PCR (MSP)

BSP and MSP were conducted as described previously (Reed K), commencing with the amplification of the bisulfite-treated gene promoter containing CpG sites. For PCR, 2.5 U of Taq mix (Takara, Dalian, Liaoning, China), 0.5 μl 1 μM forward and reverse primers were used in a 50 μl total reaction volume. Here 100 ng of bisulfite-treated DNA was used as the template of the PCR. The PCR products were purified by gel extraction from a 1% agarose gel and ligated into the pGEM-T vector (Promega, Madison, WI, USA) in a 3:1 vector/PCR product ratio. The ligation products were used to transform competent Escherichia coli cells (strain JM109) using standard procedures, and blue/white screening was used to select a minimum of 5 bacterial transformants (clones). The gene promoter of positive clones was sequenced by the Genscript Company (Nanjing, China) and Invitrogen. The methylation decrease for each sample was calculated as the percentage of unmethylated CpG dinucleotides from the total number of CpG dinucleotides analyzed. For MSP, 2.5 U of Taq mix (Takara, Dalian, Liaoning, China), 0.5 μl 1 μM forward and reverse primers, were used in a 25 μl total reaction volume. Here 50 ng of bisulfite-treated

DNA was used as the template of the PCR. PCR products were separated on 1% agarose gels and analyzed by ethidium bromide staining.

2.6   5-aza-2'-deoxycytidine Treatment of Cell Lines

To study the effect of epigenetic modulation, glioma cell lines were culutured in media supplement with 5 µmol/L of 5-aza-2'-deoxycytidine (Sigma, Aldrich) for 4 days. Fresh drug was added every 24h. Mock-treated cells were cultured similarly.

2.7   Chromatin Immunoprecipitations

The chromatin immunoprecipitations were performed according to the protocol of EZ ChIP[TM] Chromatin Immunoprecipitation Kit (Upstate,USA).Briefly, cells were crosslinked with 1% formaldehyde for 10 minutes. After washing with ice-cold PBS, the cell pellets were resuspended in SDS lysis buffer and sonicated for 70 seconds at 50% amplitude. The lysates were incubated either with 5 µg anti-K4 trimethylated histone H3 antibody, anti-K9 trimethylated histone H3 antibody or antiacetylated histone H3 antibody (Upstate Biotechnology) at 4°C overnight. Isotype control IgG antibody was used as a negative control. Protein A/G plus agarose beads were added for 1 hour at 4°C. After washing, the immunoprecipitates were eluted by incubating with elution buffer. Samples were treated with RNaseA and incubated overnight at 65°C to reverse the crosslinks. Proteins were removed by treatment with EDTA, 1 M Tris Cl (pH 6.5), and proteinase K for 1 hour at 42°C. DNA was extracted using a DNA purification kit and eluted in 50 µL Elution Reagent C.

2.8   Quantitative Real-time PCR

RNA was isolated from harvested cells with Trizol (Invitrogen) reagent and then treated with DNase (Roche) to eliminate contaminated DNA. Reverse transcription of the RNA was performed according to the instructions of Promega. The SYBR green-based real-time PCR was performed in Bio-Rad IQ5 Real-Time PCR System and the level of gene expression was normalised by β-actin. For real-time quantification of miR-185 or miR-101, total RNAs were extracted and cDNA was synthesized from 1 µg of total RNA using miRNA specific primers with SYBR-green-based PCR kit (GenePharma) and normalized by U6 snRNA.

2.9   Western Blotting

Western blot was performed as previously described (Wu *et al.*, 2006). Protein extracts (30 µg) were resolved on 10 % SDS-polyacrylamide gels. The proteins were transferred onto PVDF membranes, incubated with 5% skim milk at room temperature in TTBS (20 mM Tris-HCl, pH 7.5, 500 mM NaCl, 0.1% Tween-20), and then incubated at 4°C for 12 h with primary antibody. After washed with TTBS, the membranes were incubated at 37°C for 1 h with secondary antibodies. The membranes were developed using the chemiluminescent substrate ECL detection system (Amersham) and bands were visualized on X-ray film (Kodak).

2.10   Luciferase Assays

The 3'-untranslated regions (UTRs) of the gene were synthesized and annealed, then inserted into the pMIR-REPORT(TM) Luciferase vector (Ambion), using the Hind III (aagctt) and Spe I(actagt) site downstream from the stop codon of luciferase. We also generated an insert with deletions of 4 bp from the site of perfect complementarity of the gene. U251 cells were cotransfected using Lipofectamine 2000 (Invitrogen) according to the manufacturer's protocol using 0.8 μg of the firefly luciferase report vector and 0.2 μg of the Psv-β-galactosidase control vector (Promega) in 12-well plates. Firefly luciferase activities were measured consecutively using the Luciferase Assays System (Promega) 48 hours after transfection. β-galactosidase activity was measured using β-galactosidase Enzyme Assay System (promega).

2.11   GDM Analysis

Genomic DNA was isolated from cells, according to the manufacturer's instructions (TaKaRa). A High performance liquid chromatography / Diode array detectors (HPLC-DAD) method was used for determination of GDM. The HPLC-DAD was performed as previously described (Liu et al., 2007). Briefly, 1 mg of genomic DNA was first denatured by heating at 100°C for 3 min and then chilling on ice. After adding a 1/10 volume of 0.1M ammonium acetate (pH 5.3) and two units of nuclease P1, the mixture was incubated at 45°C for 2 h. One-tenth volume of 1M ammonium bicarbonate and 0.002 unit of venom phosphodiesterase I were added, and the mixture was incubated at 37°C for 1 h. Next, 0.5 unit of alkaline phosphatase was added, and the mixture was incubated at 37°C for 1 h.The separation was performed on a Phenomenex C18 column (250mm×4.6mm, 5 μm) with ammonium formate–methanol (3:7) as mobile phase at the flow rate of 1 mL/min, The column temperature was at 20°C, UV detection wavelength was at 260 nm.

2.12   Statistical Analysis

To analyze methylation levels of genes in glioma samples or controls, the mean level of methylation for each sample and each gene was caculated according to percentage of methylation for every CpG site of target promoter regions. Statistical analyses were done with SPSS 10.0. One-way ANOA was used to compare differences in methylation levels. To assess correlation between gene expression and methylation levels, we used Pearson correlation and linear regression analysis. All reported $p < 0.05$ was taken as statistically significant.

3   Results

3.1   Identification of Differential Methylation Regions in Primary Glioma on a Genome-wide based Platform

To better understand the global change in DNA methylation in primary gliomas, the genome-wide methylation analyses were performed in six cases of primary glioma and four cases of normal brain white matter, which were matched for age and sex. The methylated DNA fragments in the genome of each sample were enriched using MeDIP, followed by a whole-genome investigation by hybridization to the HG18 CpG promoter microarrays (Nimblegen, 385K) that cover 28, 226 CpG islands and 17,000 reference gene promoter regions in the entire human genome.

To highlight the aberrant methylated regions and to allow downstream processing and analyses, the methylated regions in at least four cases of primary gliomas and no more than one case of normal brain white matter were defined as hypermethylation differential regions. In contrast, the regions that were methylated in at least three of the cases of normal brain white matter and no more than two of the cases of primary glioma were defined as hypomethylation differential regions in glioma. We identified

524 hypermethylated and 104 hypomethylated differential regions in the primary gliomas. Intriguingly, a number of the human genome differential methylation regions (DMRs), 199 hypermethylation and 30 hypomethylated differential regions, were mapped to genomic regions without gene annotation (Figure 1A). Only 325 hypermethylation and 74 hypomethylation differential regions were mapped to the annotated gene regions, including promoter, intragenic and downstream regions of the genes. A high percentage of the DMRs, 63.0% (216) of the hypermethylated and 79.0% (60) of the hypomethylated, mapped to the promoter regions of known genes (Figure 1B), and 53 of the hypermethylated and 27 of the hypomethylated differential regions mapped to the promoters of known genes and CpG islands (Figure 1C). Therefore, many novel DMRs residing in promoters, intragenic regions, downstream of known genes and in unannotated genomic regions were identified in the primary gliomas.

Because the change in promoter methylation status may be closely related to gene expression and involved in tumor development, we focused on the investigation of glioma DMRs that mapped to gene promoter regions. The 216 promoter hypermethylated genes and 60 promoter hypomethylated genes identified using the MeDIP-chip were analyzed according to their chromosomal location, and the physical distribution of the loci was analyzed further (Figure 1D, Figure 2[1]). With the exception of the intensive promoter hypermethylated genes found in chromosomes 1, 2, 3, 17 and the X chromosome, the promoter hypermethylated genes were distributed evenly throughout the other chromosomes. However, the majority of the promoter hypomethylated genes were distributed mainly in chromosomes 1, 11, 16, 19, 20 and 22.

We performed function and pathway analyses of the promoter methylated differential genes using the DAVID bioinformatics tools (Tables 1 and 2). The majority of the promoter methylated differential genes clustered into several networks, which are involved in a wide variety of biological functions including cell communication, neurological system processes, the negative regulation of biological processes, homeostatic processes, brain development, cell adhesion, ion transport, cytoskeletal protein binding, the regulation of transcription, and apoptosis. Meanwhile several of these genes were also involved in a number of pathways that are important in the development of cancer, such as the MAPK signaling pathway, Wnt signaling pathway and Jak-STAT signaling pathway. In addition, several of the promoter hypermethylated genes identified using the MeDIP-chip in this study were reported in the literature to undergo promoter hypermethylation and gene silencing in various human cancers, including the GIPC2, DIRAS3, TYSPL6, EDNRB, FYN, GDNF, RASSF1 and RASSF2 genes (Kuang *et al.*, 2008; Riemenschneider *et al.*, 2008; Yates *et al.*, 2007; Wu *et al.*, 2010; Huang *et al.*, 2009; Huang *et al.*, 2009). These data validate the techniques used in this study.

3.2   Validation of 8 Candidate Promoter Hypermethylation Genes in Glioma

To confirm the results of the microarray experiments, 8 candidate promoter hypermethylation genes identified using the MeDIP-chip were selected randomly (Figure 2) and detected using Sequenom's MassAR

---

[1] In 2A: Each chromosome is numbered at the top. The number below the chromosome number represents the number of promoter hypermethylated genes identified in each chromosome. Gene names are indicated beside each hypermethylated locus. In 2B: Chromosomal localization of 60 promoter hypomethylated genes identified by MeDIP-chip. Each chromosome is numbered at the top. The number below the chromosome number represents the number of promoter hypomethylated genes identified in each chromosome. Gene names are indicated beside each hypomethylated locus.

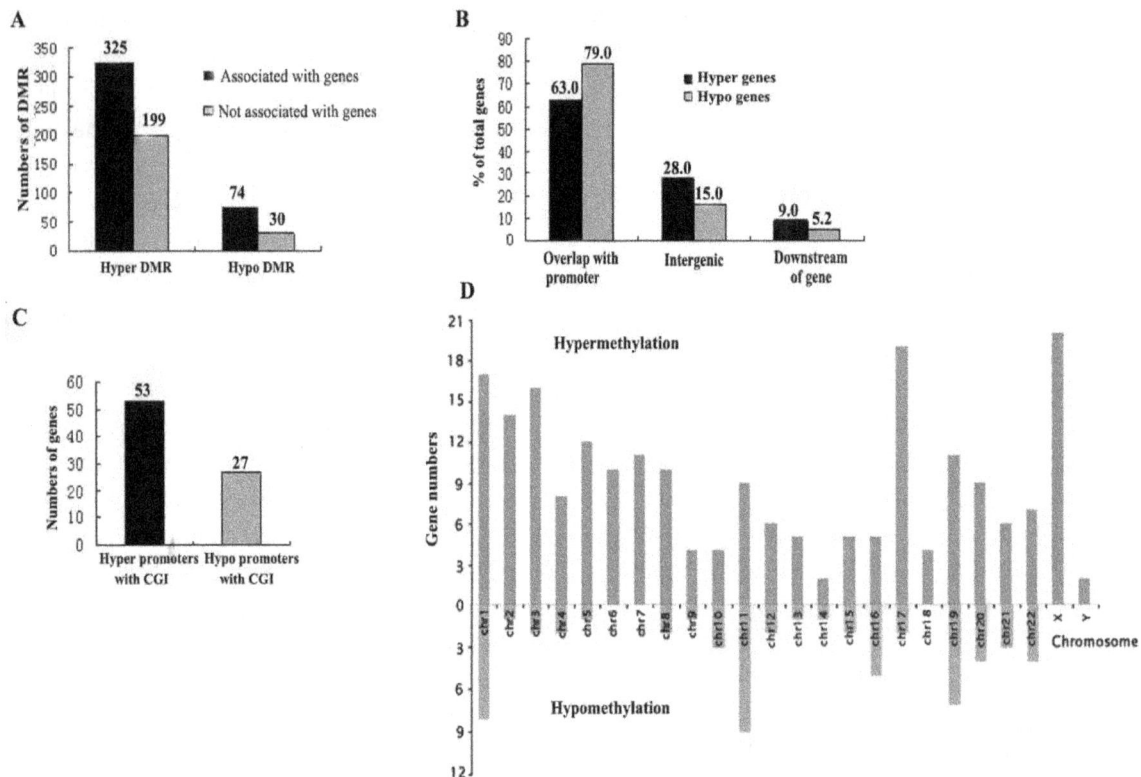

Figure 1: Genome-wide analysis of DMRs in primary glioma. (A) Number of differentially methylated regions that are associated with or without genes. (B) Distribution of diifferentially methylated regions associated with genes. Most of the identified DMRs associated with genes were mapped to gene promoters. (C) Number of DMRs which were both gene promoters and CpG islands. (D) Chromosomal distribution of 216 promoter hypermethylated genes and 60 promoter hypomethylated genes.

RAY System in samples screened by the microarray. For the tested genes, significant hypermethylation in the promoter regions was observed in the glioma samples compared with the normal controls (Figure 4A[2]). The degree of methylation, determined by the MassARRAY, correlated with the results obtained using the MeDIP-chip.

To determine whether the 8 promoter hypermethylated genes were hypermethylated in other primary glioma samples and cell lines, we evaluated the methylation status of the 8 genes in 4 glioma cell lines, in 40 samples from patients with primary glioma and in 11 normal brain white matter samples using

---

[2] Promoter methylation levels of hypermethylation genes identified from MeDIP-chip. MassARRAY assay were performed using gDNA from samples screened by microarray. Circles mark the position of CpG dinucleotides within the sequence (straight line), with different color of the circle indicating the methylation level. Gray circles represents CpG sites that could not be analysed.The ruler on top of each gene sequence indicate the base pair position within in the sequence on top and CpG sites number at the bottom. For all tested genes, significant hypermethylation in promoter regions were observed in glioma samples compared with normal controls. T1,T2,T3,T4,T5 and T6 represent glioma samples; N1,N2,N3 and N5 represent normal brain white matter samples. Glioma samples and normal control samples were ages and sexes matched.

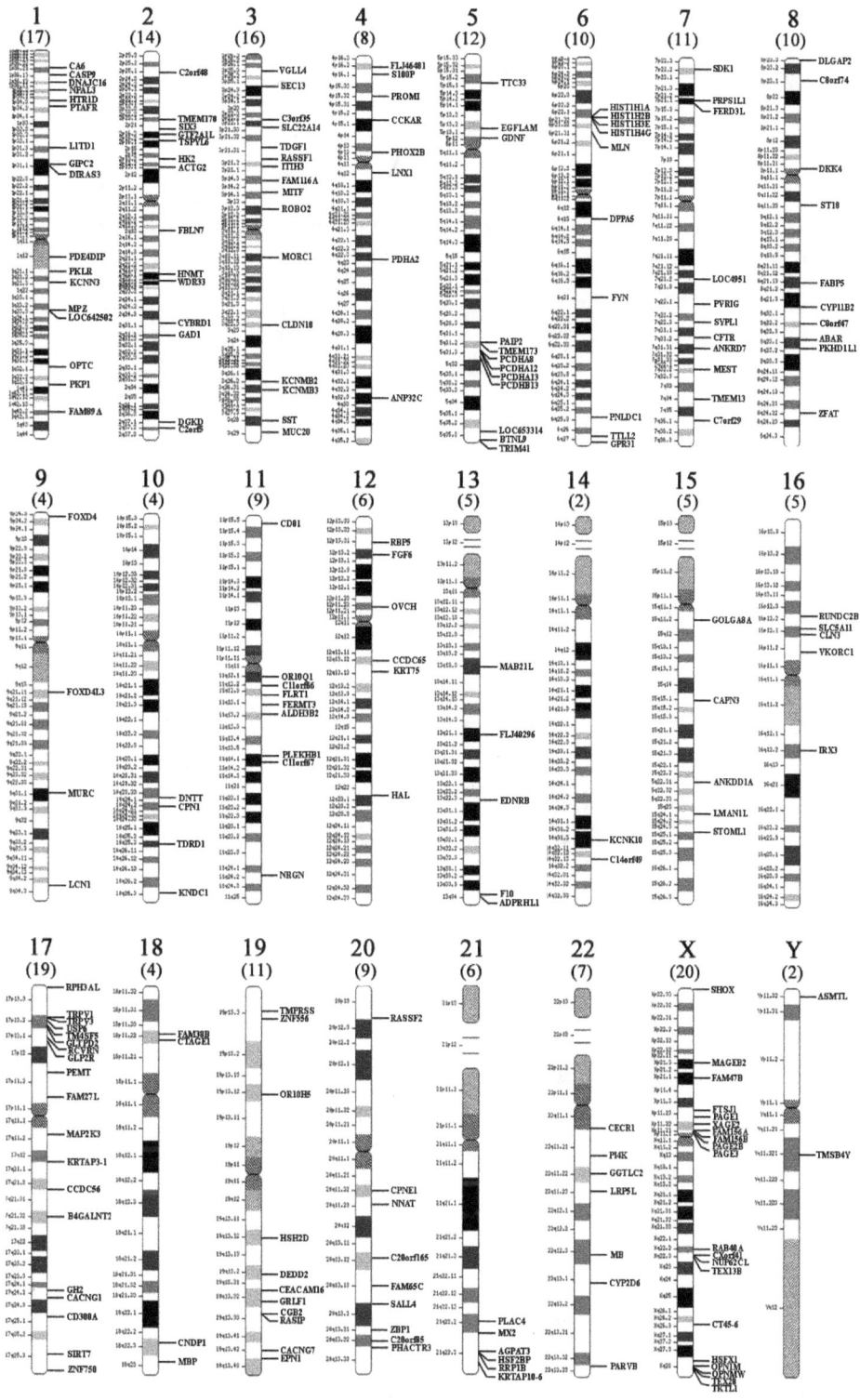

(continued on next page)

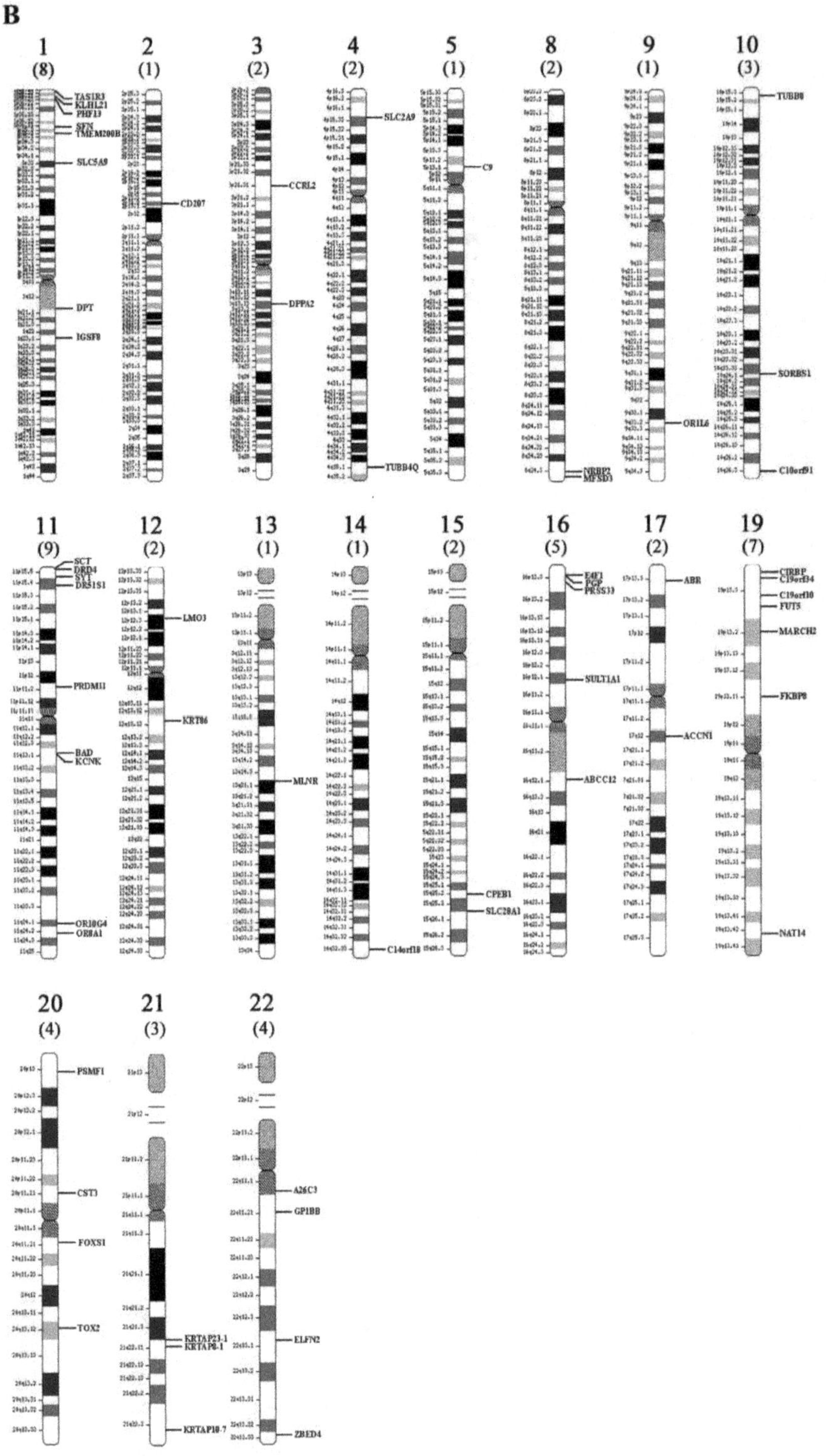

Figure 2: Chromosomal localization of hyper/hypo-methylated genes identified by MeDIP-chip. **A:** Chromosomal localization of 216 promoter hypermethylated genes identified by MeDIP-chip. **B**: Chromosomal localization of 60 promoter hypomethylated genes identified by MeDIP-chip.

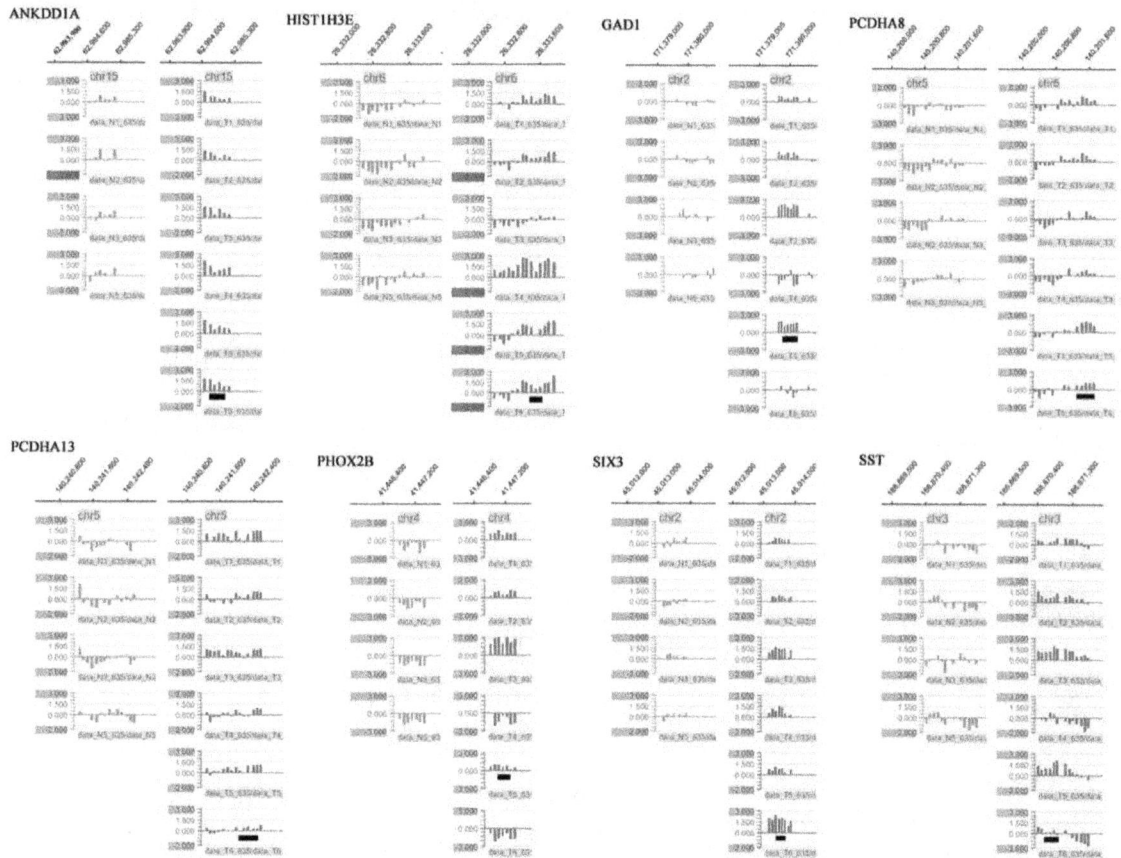

Figure 3: Examples of 8 promoter hypermethylated genes methylation array profiles. The green represent normal brain white matter samples (N1, N2, N3 and N5). The red represent the glioma primary samples (T1, T2, T3, T4, T5 and T6). The black bars indicate the regions analyzed by MassARRAY assay.

Term	Promoter Hypermethylation Genes
Go Term	
cell communication , intracellular signaling cascade, signal transduction	23 genes: SST, DIRAS3, PTAFR, KCNN3, OR10Q1, CD81, ABRA,CASP9, FYN, MBP, OR10H5, RCVRN, GPR31, KCNMB2, TDGF1, ANKDD1A, OPN1MW, PKP1, PCDHB13, PI4KA, HSH2D,KNDC1, KCNMB3
neurological system process, system process, synaptic transmission , transmission of nerve impulse	21 genes: KCNMB3,CLN3,MPZ,S100P,TRPV1,DLGAP2, SIX3, PI4KA,RCVRN,PCDHB13,OR10H5,MBP,KCNMB2,PROM1, FYN, SYPL1,KCNN3,OR10Q1,HTR1D,SST,GAD1
negative regulation of biological process, negative regulation of metabolic process, negative regulation of cellular process, negative regulation of transcription, transcription repressor activity	16 genes: SST, ST18, B4GALNT2, DEDD2, GRLF1, SALL4, RASSF2, PAIP2, TDGF1, RASSF1, CLN3, GDNF, SIX3, DKK4, TMSB4Y, CFTR
homeostatic process, chemical homeostasis, ion homeostasis, regulation of pH, regulation of biological quality	13 genes: KCNMB3,CCKAR,CLN3,MPZ,TRPV1,CYP11B2, RPH3AL, KCNMB2,MBP,EDNRB,DNAJC16,DEDD2,MB
brain development, generation of neurons, neuron migration	8 genes: FYN,NNAT, CCKAR, ROBO2, SIX3, CFTR, GRLF1, GDNF
cell adhesion, biological adhesion, homophilic cell adhesion, Cadherin	14 genes: FGF6,FLRT1,CLDN18,PKP1,CD300A,FERMT3, SDK1, FBLN7,PCDHB13,ROBO2,PCDHA12,PARVB,PCDHA8, PCDHA13
ion transport,Calcium channel, cation channel activity, gated channel activity, ion transmembrane transporter activity, transmembrane transporter activity	10 genes: KCNMB3,TRPV1,FYN,CACNG7,KCNN3,TRPV3, CACNG1, SLC5A11,KCNK10,KCNMB2
cell migration, cell motility, localization of cell, cellular morphogenesis during differentiation, cellular structure morphogenesis	9 genes: SST, GDNF, ROBO2, S100P, FYN, CCKAR, TDGF1, EDNRB, CFTR
cytoskeletal protein binding, actin binding	7 genes: PARVB, ABRA, C14orf49, RPH3AL, TMSB4Y, PDE4DIP, FYN, PHACTR3
induction of apoptosis by extracellular signals	2 genes: SST, DEDD2
KEGG_PATHWAY	
Neuroactive ligand-receptor interaction	7 genes: TRPV1, EDNRB, SST, PTAFR, GH2, CCKAR, HTR1D
MAPK signaling pathway	4 genes: CACNG7, MAP2K3, CACNG1, FGF6
Wnt signaling pathway	1 genes: DKK4
Jak-STAT signaling pathway	1 genes: GH2

Table 1: Function and pathway analysis of promoter hypermethylated genes identified by MeDIP-chip

Term	Promoter Hypomethylation Genes
Go Term	
signal transduction, cell communication	14 genes:OR10G4, BAD, C9, OR51S1, CCRL2, OR8A1, SFN, ABR, OR1L6, FKBP8, DRD4, SORBS1, GP1BB, MLNR
protein metabolic process, cellular metabolic process, biopolymer metabolic process	11 genes: CPEB1, C9, NRBP2, PSMF1, OR51S1, KLHL21, FKBP8, TUBB4Q, PRSS33, FUT5, TUBB8
transport, ion channel activity, metal ion transport, cation transport	10 genes:ACCN1, ABCC12, MFSD3, SLC28A1, SLC5A9, SLC2A9, KCNK4, TUBB4Q, TUBB8, SORBS1
hydrolase activity, serine hydrolase activity	5 genes:ABCC12, OR51S1, TUBB4Q, PRSS33, TUBB8
regulation of gene expression,regulation of transcription,DNA binding,transcription factor activity	5 genes: CPEB1,TOX2, LMO3, PHF13, NAT14
nervous system development, system development, organ development	3 genes: IGSF8, ACCN1, ABR
apoptotic program, induction of apoptosis ,cell death	3 genes: BAD, SFN, C9
KEGG_PATHWAY	
Neuroactive ligand-receptor interaction	3 genes: SCT, MLNR, DRD4
Insulin signaling pathway	2 genes: BAD, SORBS1

Table 2: Function and pathway analysis of promoter hypomethylated genes identified by MeDIP-chip.

MassARRAY (Figure 4B[3]). In 7 genes (ANKDD1A, GAD1, SIX3, SST, PHOX2B, PCDHA8 and HIST1H3E), the promoter methylation levels in the glioma patients and cell lines were significantly higher than in the normal controls (p<0.01). The PCDHA13 promoter methylation levels in the glioma primary samples were also significantly higher than in the normal controls (p < 0.01); however, in the glioma cell lines, the methylation levels did not differ from the normal controls. Based on these data, we conclude that in gliomas, the ANKDD1A, GAD1, SIX3, SST, PHOX2B, PCDHA8, HIST1H3E and PCDHA13 genes contain hypermethylated promoters. Meanwhile, the accuracy of the microarray results was verified.

To clarify whether the promoter methylation status of the 8 genes in the glioma samples correlated with the clinicopathological features of the glioma patients, Chi-square analyses were performed. Promoter methylation in the 8 genes was defined as methylation levels that were above the mean methylation levels in the controls plus 2 times the standard deviation of the controls. As shown in Table 3, the promoter methylation of the ANKDD1A and PHOX2B genes correlated with the age of the glioma patients and the differentiation status of the glioma. The two genes were more likely to be methylated in the younger age group and in the low-grade glioma samples.

---

[3] Merhylation levels of 8 selected genes identified by MeDIP-chip in normal controls, primary glioma patients and glioma cell lines. DNA methylation was analyzed using MassARRAY assay. The name of each gene is shown in the upper of each graph. N represents the number of cases studied for each gene and each group. Each graph represents the results of an individual gene indicated in the upper of each graph.

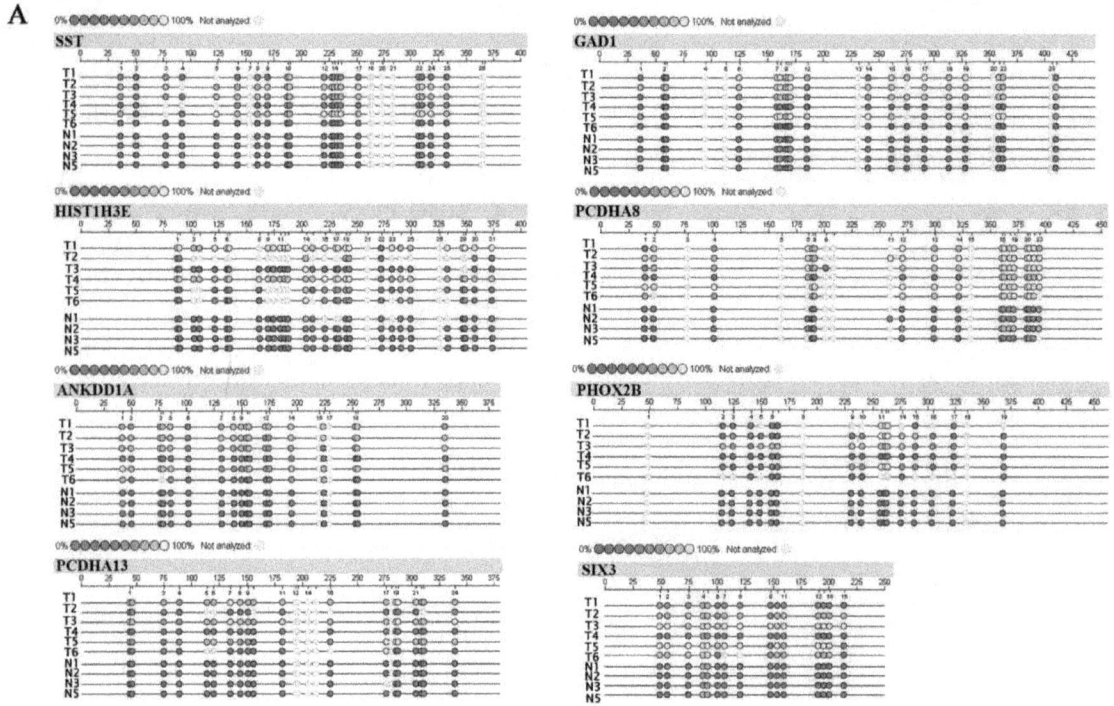

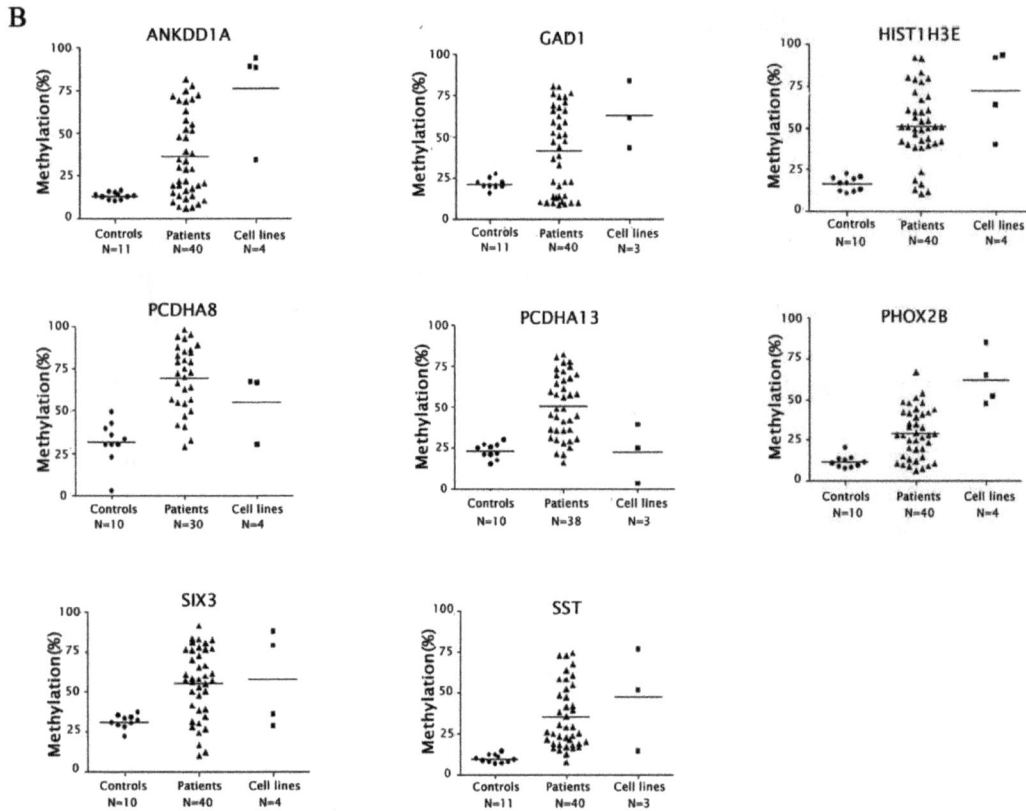

Figure 4: MassARRAY methylation analysis for primary gliomas.

Variable	Methylation n (%)							
	ANKD D1A	GAD1	HIST1H3 E	PCDHA 8	PCDHA1 3	PHOX2 B	SIX3	SST
Sex								
Male	18 (64.3)	15 (53.6)	25 (89.3)	13 (65.0)	20 (76.9)	19 (67.9)	19 (67.9)	27 (96.4)
Female	11 (91.7)	9 (75.0)	9 (75.0)	7 (70.0)	9 (75.0)	10 (83.3)	10 (83.3)	11 (91.7)
p-vablue	0.076	0.205	0.246	0.784	0.897	0.315	0.315	0.527
Age								
<45y	18 (90.0)	13 (65.0)	17 (85.0)	12 (60.0)	17 (85.0)	18 (90.0)	14 (70.0)	19 (95.00)
≥45y	11 (55.0)	11 (55.0)	17 (85.0)	8 (40.0)	12 (60.0)	11 (55.0)	15 (75.0)	19 (95.0)
p-vablue	0.013 *	0.519	1.000	0.121	0.077	0.013 *	0.723	1.000
Differentiation								
Grade I - II	20 (90.9)	16 (72.7)	19 (86.4)	14 (63.6)	18 (81.8)	19 (86.4)	18 (81.8)	22 (100.0)
Grade III - IV	9 (50.0)	8 (44.4)	15 (83.3)	6 (54.5)	11 (68.8)	10 (55.6)	11 (68.8)	16 (88.9)
p-vablue	0.004 **	0.069	0.789	0.425	0.350	0.030 *	0.145	0.109
Tumor type								
A	22 (73.3)	18 (60.0)	27 (90.0)	15 (68.2)	22 (73.3)	23 (76.7)	20 (66.7)	29 (96.7)
GBM	3 (50.0)	3 (50.0)	4 (66.7)	2 (50.0)	4 (100.0)	3 (50.0)	5 (83.3)	5 (83.3)
OA	4 (100.0)	3 (75.0)	3 (75.0)	3 (75.0)	3 (75.0)	3 (75.0)	4 (100.0)	4 (100.0)
p-value	0.217	0.732	0.289	0.723	0.498	0.407	0.304	0.349

Table 3: Genes promoter methylation and glioma patients clinical characteristics p-values from Chi-square test, *p-value < 0.05, ** p-value < 0.005. A, Astrocytoma; GBM, Glioblastoma multiforme; OA, Oligoastrocytoma

3.3   Epigenetic Regulation of Promoter Hypermethylated Gene Expression

To examine the role of the promoter methylation in the control of gene expression, the eight genes validated in this study were investigated. The expression of the hypermethylated genes was detected using real-time PCR in the primary glioma and normal brain white matter samples. The results indicated that the expression of these genes in the primary glioma samples were significantly lower than in the normal brain white matter samples (p < 0.05) (Figure 5A[4]). To determine whether the promoter methylation was responsible for the down-regulation of these genes, we examined the in vitro effects of treatment with the demethylating agent 5-aza-2'-deoxycytidine in the U251, SF767 and SF126 cell lines using real-time PCR. In the methylated glioma cell lines, the 8 genes exhibited the restoration or upregulation of gene

---

[4] Promoter hypermethylated genes expression were dected by real-time PCR in primary glioma and normal brain tissue samples. Each graph represents the results of an individual gene indicated in the upper of each graph. Each plot represents a sample.

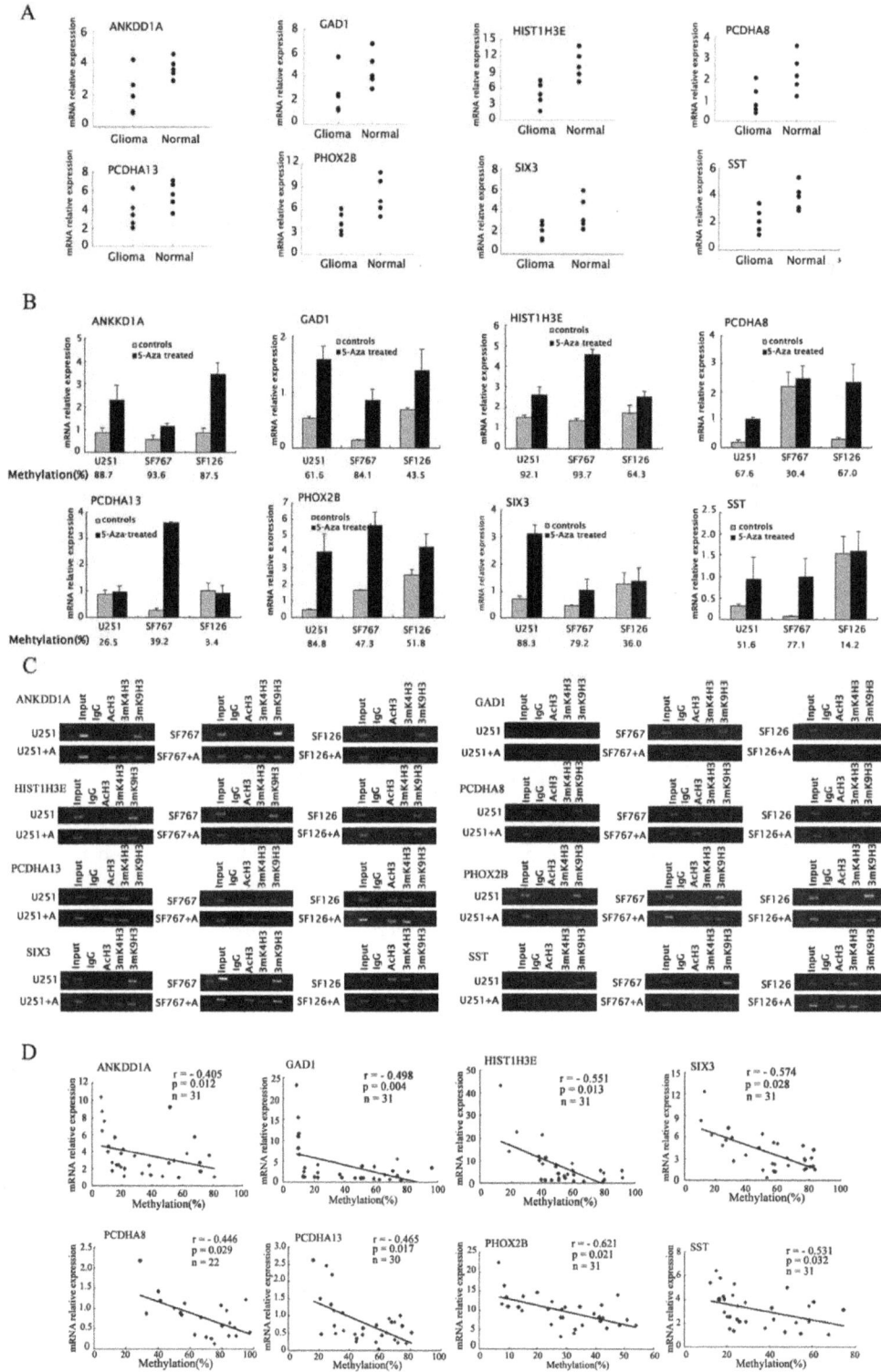

Figure 5: Promoter hypermethylated genes expression was regulated epigenetically in glioma.

expression following the demethylation treatment (p < 0.05). In contrast, in the unmethylated cell lines, similar expression levels were observed before and after the treatment, e.g., in the SST and SIX3 genes in the SF126 cell lines, the PCDHA13 gene in the U251 and SF126 cell lines, and the PCDHA8 gene in the SF767 cell line (Figure 5B[5]). A relationship was also observed between methylation and gene expression in the primary glioma samples, which were detected by MassARRAY, supporting the role of DNA methylation in the control of gene expression. In general, we observed an inverse relationship between promoter methylation levels and mRNA expression in the genes investigated (Figure 5D[6]).

Because there is crosstalk between DNA methylation and histone modification in the regulation of gene expression, the CHIP analysis of the histone markers AcH3 (histone H3 acetylation), 3mK4H3 (trimethyl-histone H3 lys4) and 3mK9H3 (trimethyl-histone H3 lys9) was performed for the promoters of the genes in the U251, SF767 and SF126 cell lines. The 8 promoter hypermethylated genes exhibited high levels of the 3mK9H3 markers in the methylated glioma cell lines. However, after treatment of the methylated or unmethylated cell lines with 5-aza-2'-deoxycytidine, we observed a decrease in the 3mK9H3 and an increase in AcH3 and 3mK4H3 markers, which are associated with an open chromatin structure (Figure 5C[7]).

The data suggested that the promoter methylation and histone modification of the genes were associated with the gene expression.

3.4   DNTM1 is the Target of miR-185

The available miRNA target prediction programs indicated that DNMT1 is a putative target of miR-185 (Lewis et al., 2003) (Figure 6F[8]). We confirmed this finding in glioma cells using luciferase reporter assays. The DNMT1 complementary sites were cloned downstream of the firefly luciferase gene. A mutated construct in which 4 nucleotides (UNCUT) were deleted from the miR-185 predicted sites was also cloned. The wild type or mutated constructs were transfected with miR-185 or with a scrambled oligonucleotide into U251 cells. The luciferase activity was measured 24 hours after transfection. As shown in Figure 6C[9], the deletion of the miR-185 interaction sites abrogated the miR-185/DNMT1 interaction,

[5] Derepression of promoter hypermethylated genes by 5-aza-2'-deoxycytidine. Gene expression was analyzed with real-time PCR in glioma cell lines U251, SF126 and SF767. The figure below each cell line indicates the percent of methylation. The name of each gene is shown in the left upper of each graph.

[6] Correlation of geme promoter methylation levels with its mRNA expression. Gene expression was analyzed with real-time PCR in primary glioma samples. Promoter methylation level was dertermined by MassARRAY. There were inverse relationship between promoter methylation levels and mRNA expression in the interrogated genes. r represents regression coefficient; p represnts statistical ananlysis p value; n represents the number of samples analyzed. The straight line indicates the regression line. Each graph represents the results of an individual gene indicated in the left upper of each graph.

[7] CHIP-PCR analysis for histone marks AcH3 (histone H3 acetylation), 3mK4H3 (trimethyl-histone H3 lys4) and 3mK9H3 (trimethyl-histone H3 lys9) in hypermethylated genes promoter. U251+A, SF767+A and SF126+A represent cell lines were treated by demethylating agent 5-aza-2'-deoxycytidine. Input represents amplification from 1% chromatin before immunoprecipitating. IgG represents negative control, immunoprecipitated by normal rabbit serum. AcH3, immunoprecipitated by rabbit anti-acytyl-H3; 3mK4H3, immunoprecipitated by rabbit anti-trimethyl-H3(lys4); 3mK9H3, immunoprecipitated by rabbit anti-trimethyl-H3(lys9).

[8] Schema of the firefly luciferase reporter constructs for DNMT1, indicating the interaction sites between miR-185 and the 3'-UTRs of the DNMT1.

[9] Luciferase assay of U251cells cotransfected with firefly luciferase constructs containing the DNMT1 wild-type or mutated 3-UTRs and miR-185 or scrambled oligonucleotides as indicated.The firefly luciferase activity was normalized to β-galactosidase activity. The data are shown as relative luciferase activity of miR-185 transfected cells with respect to the control (scrambled oligonucleotide) from 3 independent transfections. Bars represent SD.

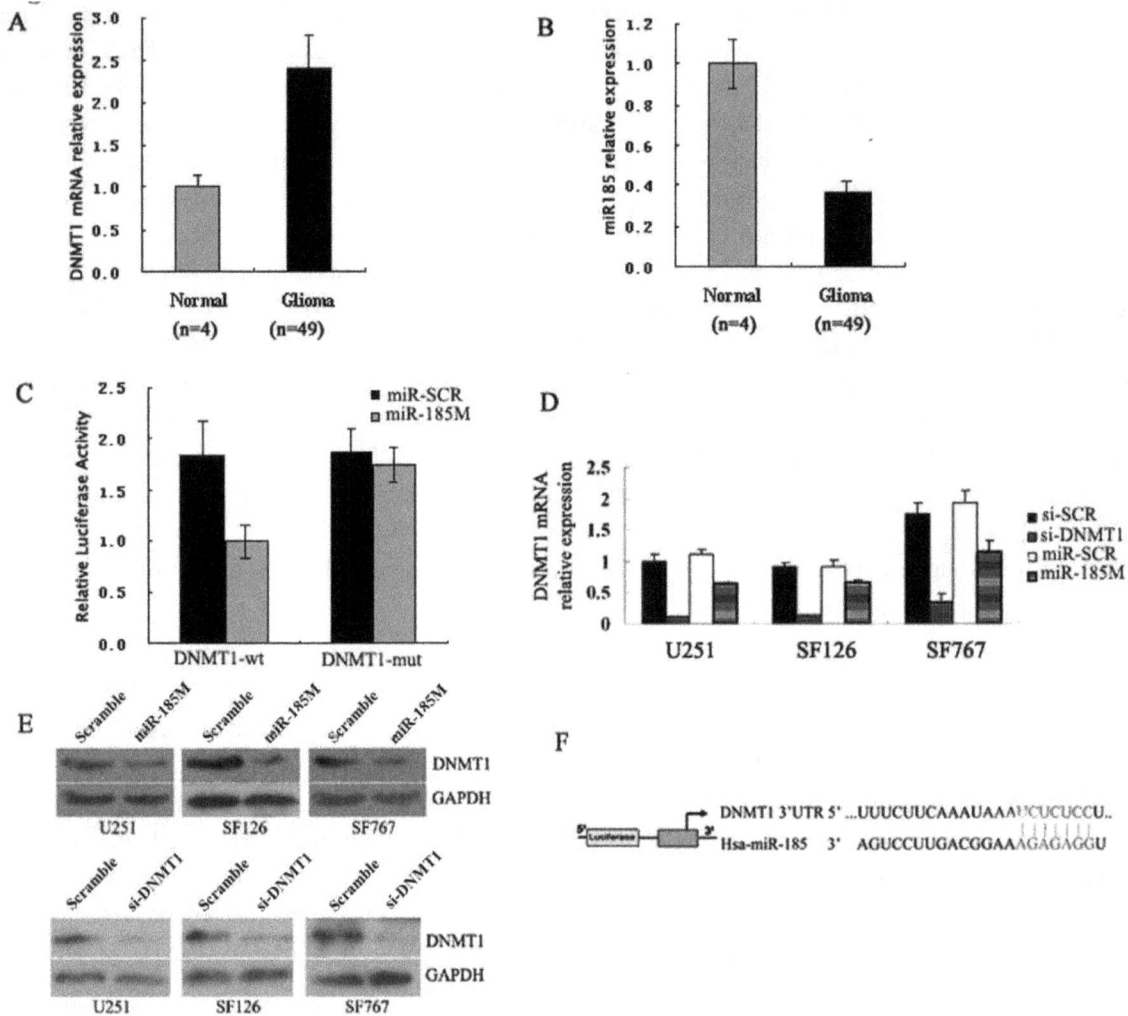

Figure 6: miR-185 targets DNMT1 mRNA at 3'-UTR.

demonstrated by the absence of changes in the normalized luciferase activity. The cells transfected with miR-185 exhibited approximately 40% reduction in the DNMT1 mRNA expression compared with the cells transfected with the scrambled oligonucleotide (Figure 6D[10]). The western blotting indicated that the DNMT1 protein expression also decreased in the glioma cells transfected with miR-185 compared with the scrambled oligonucleotide (Figure 6E[11]). In addition, si-DNMT1 transfected into glioma cells was used as a control to demonstrate the DNMT1 mRNA and protein expression. Furthermore, the expression of DNMT1 and miR-185 were determined using real-time PCR in normal brain tissue and primary glioma samples. We determined that miR-185 and DNMT1 were inversely expressed in these samples (Fig-

---

[10] Glioma cells were transfected with miR-185 or interfered by si-DNMT1 for 48h. Expression of DNMT1 was evaluated by real-time PCR quantification of mRNAs. Results are presented as mean±S.D. from three independent experiments.

[11] Western blot indicating that DNMT1 is markedly diminished in glioma cells transfected by miR-185 or interfered by si-DNMT1 versus transfected by the corresponding scrambled sequence.

ure 6A[12], 6B[13]). The results indicate that the effect of miR-185 on DNMT1 is direct and is mediated by specific 3'-UTR target sites.

3.5   Overexpression of miR-185 Reduces Global DNA Methylation and Induces Re-expression of Promoter Hypermethylation Genes

Because miR-185 targeted DNMT1, which maintained an established DNA methylation pattern, we investigated whether the enforced expression of miR-185 functionally caused DNA hypomethylation. The GDM was measured using the HPLC-DAD method in the U251, SF126 and SF767 cell lines 48 hours after transfection with miR-185M or scrambled oligonucleotides. Meanwhile, an si-DNMT1 sequence was also transfected into the glioma cells as the positive control. We observed a 20%-30% reduction in the GDM in the glioma cell lines transfected with miR-185M compared with the negative controls (Figure 7A). The miR-185M-induced reduction in GDM in the glioma cells was slightly less than that achieved following the si-DNMT1 treatment at the same time point (Figure 7A).

To assess whether the overexpression of miR-185 leads to promoter demethylation and reexpression of the hypermethylated genes, we measured the mRNA levels of the 8 hypermethylated genes under investigation using quantitative real-time PCR and detected the promoter methylation level changes using the MassARRAY System in the glioma cell lines after transfection with miR-185M or a scrambled oligonucleotide. In the expression experiment, the si-DNMT1 sequence was transfected into the glioma cell lines as a positive control. At 48 hours after transfection with the miR-185M or the si-DNMT1 sequence, significant expression of the PCDHA8, PCDHA13, ANKDD1A, GAD1, HIST1H3E, PHOX2B, SIX3 and SST genes was induced in the methylated glioma cell lines compared with the controls (Figure 7B). Furthermore, after the transfection with miR-185M, the reexpression of these hypermethylated genes coincided with a significant reduction in their promoter DNA methylation levels compared with scrambled oligonucleotides, which was also seen in the methylated glioma cell lines (Figure 7C).

3.6   The promoter hypomethylation gene was overexpressed and correlated with a poor outcome in glioma

To validate further the MeDIP-chip results, we designed and validated BSP and MSP to investigate the promoter methylation status of promoter hypo methylation genes. In this study, the CPEB1 gene, which contains 17 CpGs or 10 CpGs (Figure. 8A), was selected to further verify the promoter methylation status and expression of this promoter hypomethylation gene. The methylation status of the CPEB1 promoter was determined in four glioma cell lines using MSP and in 50 glioma samples and 10 normal brain tissue samples using BSP. The tumor cell lines were significantly hypomethylated (Figure. 8B). The CpG dinucleotides were heavily methylated in the normal brain samples, and the methylation decrease varied from 9.6 to 25.7% with a mean of 20.1% and a median of 18.4%. In contrast, the methylation decrease observed in the glioma samples ranged from 28.6 to 89.0%, with a mean of 71.8% and a median of 77.0% ($P<0.001$) (Figure. 8C). The decrease in methylation levels of >45.3% were considered hypomethylation. CPEB1 was hypomethylated in 43 (86.0%) out of the 50 tumors. A statistically significant correlation between the sex, age, histological grade, and CPEB1 hypomethylation was not observed (Table 4). In addition, the increased expression of the CPEB1 protein in the glioma cell lines and in 25 of the 50 glioma tissue samples was demonstrated by the real-time PCR (Figure 8D) and immunohistochemical anal-

---

[12] DNMT1 mRNA expression in normal brain tissue and primary gliomas. n represents the number of samples detected.

[13] miR-185 expression in normal brian tissue and primay gliomas. n represents the number of samples detected.

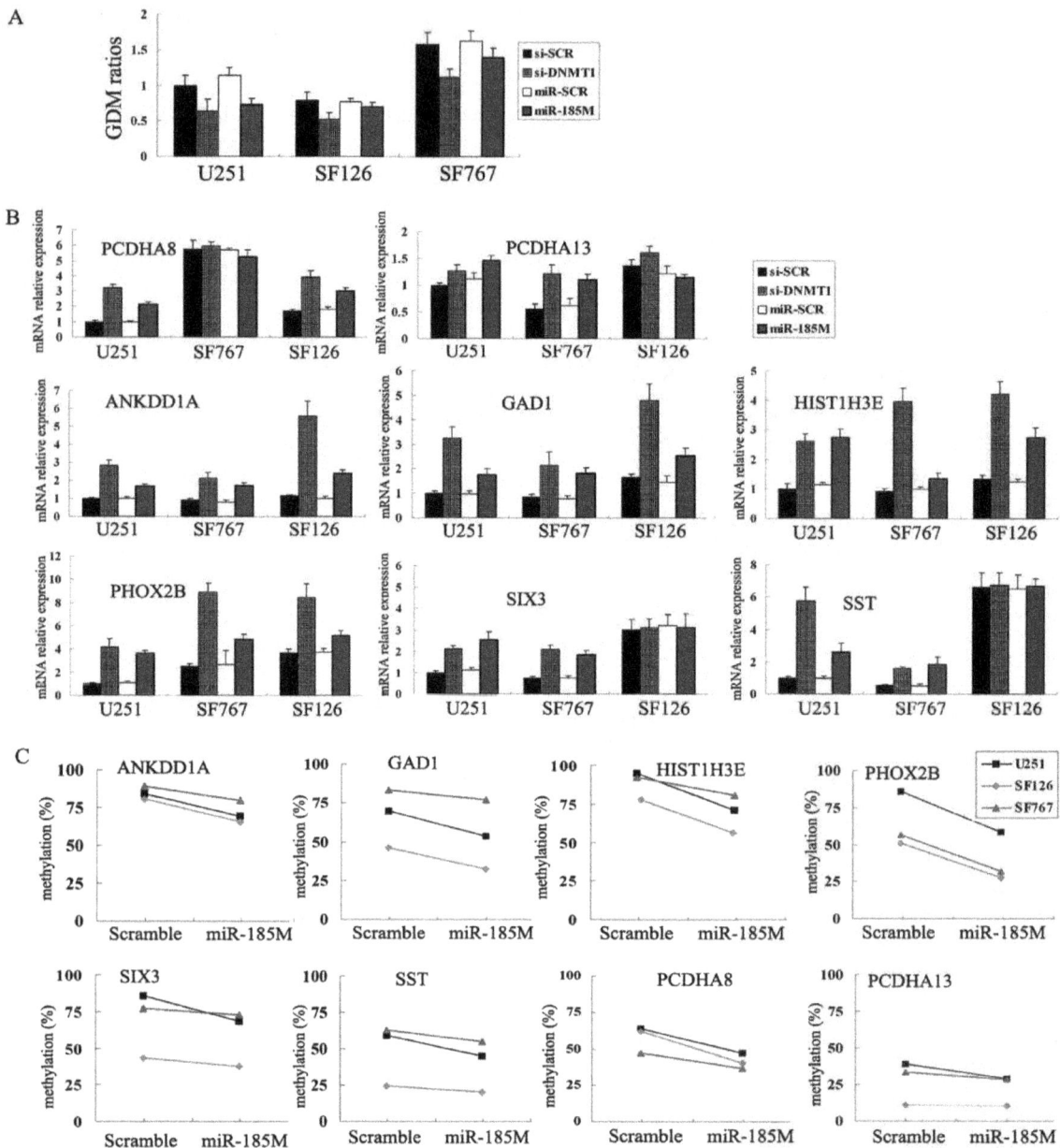

Figure 7: miR-185 reduces GDM and restores hypermethylated genes expression in the glioma cell lines. (A) Overexpression of miR-185M in glioma cell lines reduces GDM. U251, SF126 and SF767 cell lines were transfeted with miR-185M or interfered by si-DNMT1 after 48 hours to observe the global DNA methylation levels by HPLC-DAD. The data are shown as relative GDM. Bar represent range of 3 independent experiments. (B) Real-time PCR for hypermethylated genes in glioma cell lines transfeted with miR-185M or interfered by si-DNMT1 after 48 hours. Results are presented as mean±S.D. from three independent experiments. Each graph represents the results of an individual gene indicated in the upper of each graph. (C)The mean promoter methylation levels of hypermethylated genes in glioma cell lines after transfected with miR-185M or a scrambled oligonucleotide obtained using the MassArray System. The lines connecting the dots indicate the corresponding cell lines. Each graph represents the results of an individual gene indicated in the upper of each graph.

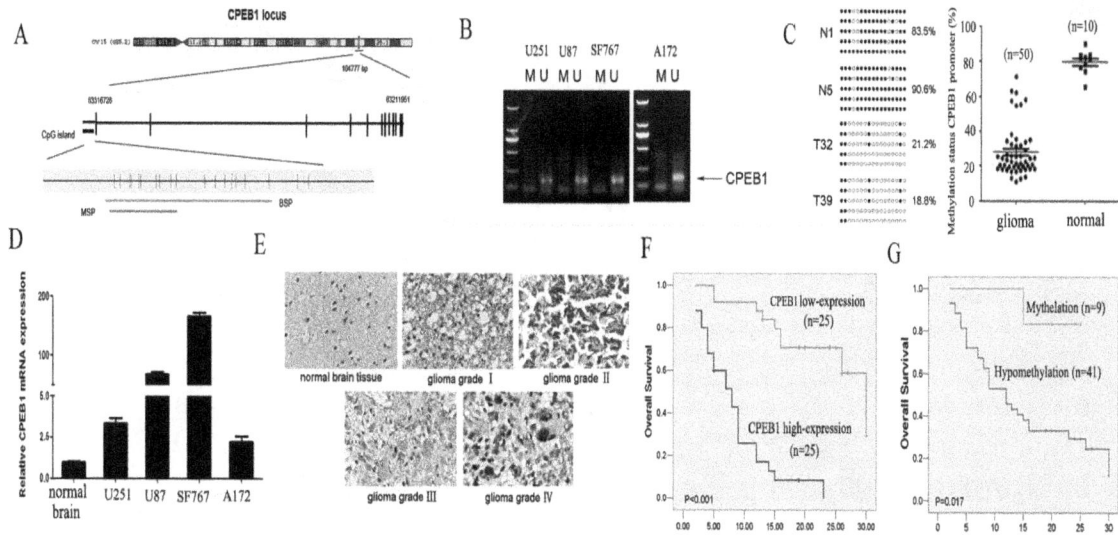

Figure 8: CPEB1 is overexpressed by promoter hypomethylation, correlated with poor outcome in glioma. (A) Schematic diagram of CpG dinucleotides within the CPEB1 promoter. Nucleotide number is relative to the transcription start site of CPEB1. The red line indicates the region tested in BSP, the blue line indicates the region detected in MSP. (B) The methylation status of CPEB1 in glioma cell lines is detected by MSP. U: unmethylated primer, M: methylated primer. (C) BSP of the upstream regulatory region of CPEB1 is performed for representative tissues (N normal brain tissue, T glioma sample). For each sample, at least five separate clones are sequenced and the results are shown here. Unmethylated CpG sites are shown as open circles whereas methylated CpG sites are indicated by closed circles. For each row of circles sequence results for an individual clone of the bisulfite-PCR product are given. The number of methylated CpGs divided by the total number of true CpGs analyzed is given as a percentage on the right of each bisulfite result. (D) Real-time PCR detects the expression of CPEB1 in normal brain tissue and four glioma cell lines. (E) ISH tests the expression of CPEB1 in normal brain tissue and glioma tissues. (F) Correlation between CPEB1 protein expression in the tumor and OS of glioma patients. (G) Correlation between CPEB1 methylation in tumor and OS of glioma patients.

yses (Figure 8E), respectively. A statistically significant correlation between the sex, age, histological grade, and CPEB1 expression was not observed (Table 5).

The comparison of the methylation data and the immunohistochemistry findings revealed that the 25 tumors with a high-level of CPEB1 protein expression harbored CPEB1 hypomethylation. In comparison, methylated CPEB1 was observed in 18/25 (52.9%) of the tumors exhibiting a reduced or loss of CPEB1 expression (Table 5). A significant relationship was observed between the CPEB1 promoter hypomethylation and protein overexpression ($P=0.001$; Table 4). The Kaplan–Meier survival analysis was performed to determine the prognostic potential of CPEB1 expression and the methylation status. The correlation between the CPEB1 expression, methylation status and OS was statistically significant. A markedly decreased OS was observed in the glioma patients exhibiting CPEB1 over-expression compared with the patients exhibiting low expression of the gene (Figure 8F). Nevertheless, the glioma patients with CPEB1 hypomethylation suffered a worse outcome than those with CPEB1 methylation (Figure 8G). The results suggest that CPEB1 overexpression and hypomethylation is involved in glioma carcinogenesis.

Variable	CPEB1		P
	<8	≥8	
Total (N=50)	25	25	
Sex			1.000
Male(34)	17	17	
Female(16)	8	8	
Age(years)[a]			0.145
<42(23)	14	9	
≧42(27)	11	16	
Grade			0.868
low grade (I + II)(26)	14	12	
high grade (III+IV)(24)	11	13	

Table 4: Relationship of CPEB1 expression to clinical parameters of glioma patients

Variable	CPEB1		P
	hypomethylation	methylation	
Total (N=50)	43	7	
Expression			0.004
<8(25)	18	7	
≥8(25)	25	0	
Sex			1.000
Male(34)	29	5	
Female(16)	14	2	
Age(years)[a]			0.145
<42(23)	18	5	
≧42(27)	25	2	
Grade			0.697
low grade (I + II)(26)	23	3	
high grade (III+IV)(24)	20	4	

Table 5: Correlation between CPEB1 methylation status, protein expression and clinical parameters of glioma patients

3.7   CPEB1 is a Direct and Epigenetic Target of miR-101

Having established a role for CPEB1 in glioma cell senescence, we next investigated the mechanism of regulation. The roles of microRNAs (miRNAs) in gene regulation and phenotype determination are established. The CPEB gene family members CPEB2, CPEB3 and CPEB4 are downregulated by miR-92 and miR-26 (Morgan et al., 2010). Currently, only one study has demonstrated the repression of CPEB1 by miR-122 (Burns et al., 2011). To elucidate the roles of miRNAs in CPEB1 regulation, we performed an online TargetScan 5.1 to predict the potential miRNA binding sites in the 3'-UTR sequence of CPEB1. CPEB1 was predicted as a target of miR-101. Recent data have demonstrated the suppressor role of miR-101 in tumors (Semaan et al., 2011; Saito et al., 2012; Ma &Tao, 2012). To demonstrate the direct inter-action of miR-101 with CPEB1 in glioma cells, the 3'-UTR of CPEB1 (with the predicted binding sites for the miR-101 included) was cloned downstream of the firefly luciferase gene in the pMIR-REPORT vector (Figure 9A). The miR-101 was co-transfected with pMIR-CPEB1-3'-UTR-WT and produced a significant reduction in luciferase activity compared with the cells transfected with the negative control (Figure 9B). The mutation of the seed region for miR-101 binding in the pMIR-CPEB1-3'-UTR-MUT vector abrogated the regulatory activity (Figure 9B), confirming that miR-101 directly interacted with the 3'-UTR of CPEB1 in the glioma cells. Next, we determined the relationship between the expression of CPEB1 and miR-101 in the glioma cells. It was gratifying to observe that the miR-101 inhibited the expression of CPEB1 (Figure 9C), supporting the concept of CPEB1 regulation by miR-101 in glioma. Therefore, CPEB1 can be considered a new target for miR-101 in glioma.

EZH2 and EED are the core subunits of the polycomb repressive complex 2 (PRC2) and are tar-gets of miR-101(Varambally et al., 2008; Chiang et al., 2010). The polycomb group proteins (PcGs) form macromolecular complexes that function as epigenetic gene silencers (Sessa et al., 2007). Many studies have demonstrated that PcGs accumulate at specific DNA regions that are associated with regulatory genes and direct the post-translational modification of histones (Gieni& Hendzel, 2009) . The signature activity of PRC2 is to methylate histone H3 lysine 27 (H3K27), adding up to three methyl groups to this target Lys residue. Trimethylated H3K27 (H3K27me3) is thought to be the main form of H3K27 that functions in PRC2 silencing. Although H3K27 trimethylation is viewed as crucial, recent studies also emphasize PRC2 functions beyond this enzymatic activity (Simon&Kingston, 2009). DNA methylation is correlated to histone modification. In general, permissive regions exhibit an open chromatin structure marked by the hyperacetylation of histones H3 and H4 and the di- and tri-methylation of histone H3 at lysine 4 (H3K4me2/3). In contrast, repressed regions exhibit a compact chromatin structure that is en-riched in the "repressive" modifications, the di-and tri-methylation of H3K9 (H3K9me2/3), H3K27me3, and the trimethylation of H4K20 (H4K20me3) (Jenuwein &Allis, 2001; McCabe et al.,2009). Although the code is not fully deciphered, it is apparent that DNA methylation influences and is influenced by his-tone modifications. We hypothesized that miR-101 regulates the promoter methylation status of CPEB1 by targeting EZH2 and EED. To support our findings, we determined the expression level of CPEB1 in EZH2 siRNA- and EED siRNA-transfected glioma cells. To confirm that miR-101 regulates the methyla-tion status of CPEB1, BSP was performed. The BSP demonstrated the miR-101-mediated reduction in the methylation level of CPEB1 in U251 and U87 cells (Figure 9D). Therefore, in these experiments, miR-101 epigenetically downregulated the expression of CPEB1 by inhibiting EZH2 and EED. Next, we in-vestigated how miR-101 reverses the promoter methylation status of CPEB1. Because EZH2 and EED are considered the specific histone methyltransferases of the repressed gene expression marker H3K27 and are associated with the active gene expression marker H3K4 and the repressed gene expression markers H3K9 and H4K20 (Hong&Bain, 2012; Shumaker *et al.*, 2006; Murata *et al.*, 2012), we hypothe-sized that the miR-101-mediated histone modifications contribute to the DNA methylation recovery of the CPEB1 promoter. To determine whether miR-101 regulates the histone modification of the CPEB1 promoter, we identified the core promoter of CPEB1. The luciferase activity driven by the CPEB1 pro-moter constructs was measured 48 h following transfection. The results demonstrated that four fragments

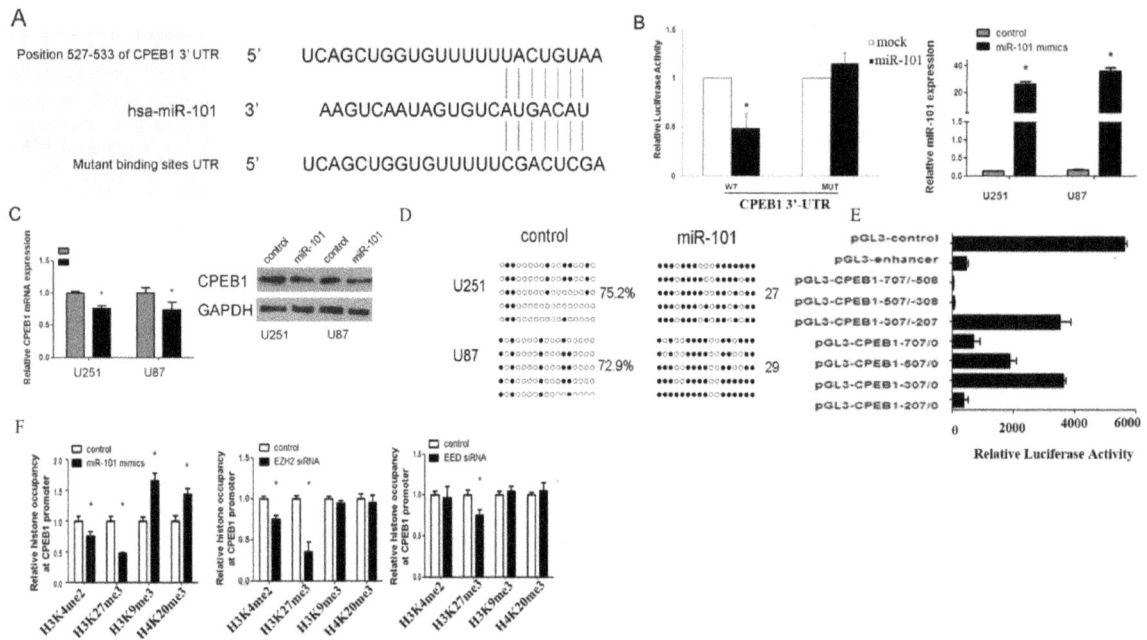

Figure 9: CPEB1 is a direct and epigenetical target of miR-101. (A) Predicted binding between miR-101 and the 7mer seed matches in CPEB1 3'UTRs. (B) miR-101 regulates CPEB1 3'UTR reporters. Luciferase reporter assays 48 h after transfection with indicated pMIR-Report plasmids and a renilla transfection control plasmid, co-transfected with miR-101, or relevant scramble controls. Data shown are the mean±s.d. of six replicates and were representative of two or three independent experiments. *$P<0.05$. (C) Expression of CPEB1 in glioma cell lines and 293T cells. (D) miR-101 reverses the methylation status by BSP. For each sample, at least five separate clones are sequenced and the results are shown here. Unmethylated CpG sites are shown as open circles whereas methylated CpG sites are indicated by closed circles. For each row of circles sequence results for an individual clone of the bisulfite-PCR product are given. The number of methylated CpGs divided by the total number of true CpGs analyzed was given as a percentage on the right of each bisulfite result. (E) Luciferase reporter assay defines the position of CPEB1 core promoter. 0 is the TSS. The core promoter ranged from -307 to -207. pGL3-control is the positive control, pGL3-enhancer is the negative control. Relative activity is compared to the pRL-TK plasmid. Relative luciferase ctivity higher than pGL3-enhancer is considered to embody core promoter region. (F) ChIP is performed to detect the enrichment of H3K4me2, H3K27me3, H3K9me3 and H4K20me3 at CPEB1 core promoter. U251 and U87 cells transfected with miR-101 mimics, EZH2 siRNA and EED siRNA are detected. *$P<0.05$.

(-307 to -207, -707 to 0, -507 to 0, and -307 to 0, 0 is the TSS) exhibited high activity, whereas the remaining three fragments (-707 to -508, -507 to -308, and -207 to 0) exhibited little activity (Figure 9E). Therefore, the data suggest that the core promoter ranged from -307 to -207, and a repressive element resided between positions -707 and -508. Next, following the miR-101 treatment of the U251 cells, we observed the enrichment of H3K27 methylation, a marker of DNA methylation at the CPEB1 active promoter locus. Using the chromatin immunoprecipitation (ChIP) assay, we observed that the H3K27 tri-methylation (H3K27me3) enrichment was decreased at the CPEB1 core promoter following the miR-101 treatment compared with the control group (Figure 9F). In addition, the DNA methylation-associated histone modifications, H3K9 tri-methylation (H3K3me3) and H4K20 tri-methylation (H4K20me3), were observed. The data demonstrated that the enrichment of H3K9me3 and H4K20me3 at the CPEB1 core promoter was upregulated by miR-101 compared with the control (Figure 9F). The H3K4 bi-methylation (H3K4me2) enrichment could be used as a marker to trace loci that have undergone DNA demethylation. The ChIP assay demonstrated that the H3K4me2 enrichment at the CPEB1 core promoter was reduced by miR-101 (Figure 9F). Next, we investigated whether miR-101 regulated the histone modification of the CPEB1 core promoter through inhibiting EZH2 and EED by examining the effect of EZH2 and EED on histone modification of the core promoter of CPEB1. As shown in (Figure 9F), the loss of expression of EZH2 decreased the enrichment of H3K4me2 and H3K27me3 at the CPEB1 core promoter; however, there was no effect on the H3K9me3 and H4K20me3 enrichment; only the EED knockdown reduced the H3K27me3 enrichment at the CPEB1 core promoter. The results indicated that miR-101 reversed the methylation status of CPEB1 by downregulating the enrichment of H3K4me2 and H3K27me3 and upregulating the enrichment of H3K9me3 and H4K20me3 at the core promoter of CPEB1.

4   Discussion

In this study, we combined the use of genome-wide CpG promoter microarrays and the novel and sensitive methyl-DNA immunoprecipitation (MeDIP) method to identify differentially methylated regions in glioma vs. normal brain white matter samples. The global profiling of a small number (n = 10) of samples yielded a large number of differentially methylated regions, a number of which were validated in a series of glioma samples using Sequenom's MassARRAY System. Therefore, the MeDIP-chip platform proved both efficient and effective.

In the glioma samples, 524 hypermethylation and 104 hypomethylation differential regions were identified. Of these regions, 216 hypermethylation and 60 hypomethylation regions mapped to gene promoters and may play an important role in regulating the transcription of these genes. The genes containing the hypermethylation and hypomethylation promoter regions are involved in a variety of important cellular processes, including the regulation of transcription, cell communication, neurological system processes, apoptosis, the negative regulation of biological processes, homeostatic processes, brain development, cell adhesion, ion transport and cytoskeletal protein binding. The data are vital for the further understanding of the complete molecular mechanism of glioma development. Many of these genes are novel discoveries that have not been associated previously with aberrant methylation in glioma or in other malignancies. Meanwhile, several of the promoter hypermethylated genes have been reported in various human cancers, which validate the assays used in this study.

Growing evidence indicates that gene promoter methylation manifests in a nonrandom fashion in cancers. Methylation patterns are specific to cell or tumor types and even to subtypes within the same tumor category (Costello *et al.*, 2000). In addition to determining the methylation patterns specific to glioma, we identified genomic hotspots, which harbor an overabundance of methylation in the gene promoter regions. In particular, we demonstrated that the methylated gene promoters on chromosomes 1, 2, 3, 17 and X tend to aggregate in a methylation hotspot. Others have reported that chromosome 19 is the hotspot for methylation in acute lymphoblastic leukemia (ALL) (Taylor *et al.*, 2007). It appears that certain regions of the genome are targeted for methylation, and these targets vary with the type of cancer. However, the mechanism responsible for the disease-specific targeting of methylated loci is unclear.

The eight genes (ANKDD1A, GAD1, HIST1H3E, PCDHA8, PCDHA13, PHOX2B, SST and SIX3) were confirmed and newly identified as promoter hypermethylation genes in glioma. Although a number of these genes have been shown to undergo methylation in other cancers, this is the first report of their methylation in glioma. The ANKDD1A (ankyrin repeat and death domain-containing protein 1A) protein contains 4 ankyrin repeats that mediate protein-protein interactions in diverse families of proteins and death domains associated with apoptosis. The function of ANKDD1A is unknown; however, another ankyrin repeat-containing gene, ANKRD15, is a candidate tumor suppressor for renal cell carcinoma (Lerer et al., 2005). In this study, the ANKDD1A promoter was more susceptible to methylation in low-grade glioma patients, suggesting that this gene may be involved in the early development of glioma. The glutamate decarboxylase 1 (GAD1) gene encodes glutamic acid decarboxylase, which is responsible for catalyzing the production of the inhibitory neurotransmitter gamma-aminobutyric acid from the excitatory neurotransmitter L-glutamic acid. An association between promoter methylation and the decreased expression of GAD1 has been demonstrated in schizophrenia (Huang & Akbarian, 2007). HIST1H3E, a member of the histone H3 family, interacts with the linker DNA between nucleosomes and functions in the compaction of chromatin into higher order structures. This protein is differentially expressed in the temporal lobe of patients with schizophrenia (Martins-de-Souza et al., 2009). PCDHA8 and PCDHA13 are members of the family of protocadherin alpha proteins. These neural cadherin-like cell adhesion proteins are integral plasma membrane proteins that likely play a critical role in the establishment and function of specific cell-cell connections in the brain. The protocadherin-gamma subfamily A11 (PCDH-gamma-A11) gene exhibits hypermethylation in astrocytomas compared to normal brain (Waha et al., 2005). The inactivation of this cell-cell contact molecule might be involved in the invasive growth of astrocytoma cells into normal brain parenchyma. PHOX2B (paired-like homeobox 2b), a member of the paired family of homeobox genes, encodes a DNA-associated protein localized in the nucleus. The PHOX2B protein functions as a transcription factor involved in the development of several major noradrenergic neuron populations and the determination of the neurotransmitter phenotype. The gene product is also linked to the enhancement of the second messenger-mediated activation of the dopamine beta-hydroxylase, c-fos promoters and several enhancers, including the cyclic amp-response element and the serum-response element. The aberrant methylation of the PHOX2B promoter region was observed in 12.9% of human neuroblastoma cell lines (de Pontual et al., 2007). SST (somatostatin) is expressed throughout the body and inhibits the release of numerous secondary hormones by binding to high-affinity G-protein-coupled somatostatin receptors. Somatostatin also affects the rates of neurotransmission in the central nervous system and the proliferation of both normal and tumorigenic cells. Recently, SST promoter methylation has been observed in various cancers including gastric cancer, cervical cancer and colon cancer (Zhang et al., 2010; Ongenaert et al., 2008; Mori et al., 2006). SIX3 (SIX homeobox 3) is a member of the sine oculis homeobox transcription factor family. SIX3 regulates the transcriptional activity of the orphan nuclear receptor NOR-1 (NR4A3), which is normally involved in the balance between cell proliferation and cell death and is implicated in oncogenesis as part of the EWS/NOR-1 fusion protein found in human extraskeletal myxoid chondrosarcoma (EMC) tumors (Laflamme et al., 2003). Taken together, the eight genes are novel promoter hypermethylated genes in glioma, and promoter methylation in these genes may be involved in the initiation and progression of glioma or may serve as a biomarker for prognosis and susceptibility to treatment.

DNA methylation in promoters has been implicated in the deregulation of gene expression, possibly through the formation of an altered chromatin structure that is resistant to transcription initiation. Our study demonstrated that the expression of the eight promoter hypermethylated genes was downregulated significantly in the glioma samples compared to the normal brain white matter samples. An inverse relationship between methylation and gene expression was also observed in the primary glioma samples. As expected, the treatment of the glioma cell lines with 5-aza-2'-deoxycytidine resulted in general gene reactivation in the methylated glioma cell lines. Moreover, it has become increasingly evident that DNA methylation and histone modification exhibit a complex interplay that contributes to gene regulation and to the establishment and maintenance of chromosomal domains. The results of our study indicate that gene promoter hypermethylation is always enriched in 3mK9H3 and depleted in H3 acetylation and 3mK4H3. In contrast, the level of 3mK9H3 decreased and the level of H3 acetylation and 3mK4H3 increased after treatment with 5-aza-2'-deoxycytidine. These data suggest that 3mK9H3 correlates directly and H3 acetylation and 3mK4H3 correlate inversely with promoter hypermethylation.

The deletion of the genomic interval encompassing miR-185 (22q11.2) is an extremely frequent event in diverse types of cancer (Takahashi *et al.*, 1993; Bian *et al.*, 2005). It has been reported that miR-185 induces cell cycle arrest in human non-small cell lung cancer (Takahashi *et al.*, 2009). In this study, we found that miR-185 was significantly down-regulated in glioma compared with normal brain tissue, and the reduced miR-185 expression was associated with the loss of 22q11.2 in glioma. These results suggest that the loss of miR-185 is a frequent event in glioma and raise the possibility that the miR-185 loss of function plays an important role in glioma.

Furthermore, we characterized the role of miR-185 in the regulation of DNA methylation in glioma. Our data demonstrated that miR-185 targets DNMT1, thereby resulting in global DNA hypomethylation, and the reexpression of the promoter hypermethylated genes coincided with the significant DNA demethylation of the promoter regions of these genes in glioma. In the primary glioma samples, the DNMT1 expression was the opposite of the miR-185 expression. Therefore, we speculated that the miR-185 downregulation led to the increased expression of DNMT1, which may contribute to aberrant DNA methylation and in turn to gliomagenesis.

Hypomethylation is a common mechanism of dysregulation in cancer. We performed BSP and MSP to identify the promoter methylation status of CPEB1. The analyses demonstrated the hypomethylation of the CPEB1 promoter in the glioma cell lines and tissues. We also demonstrated the overexpression of CPEB1 in the glioma tissues and cell lines, and the statistical analysis indicated that the overexpression of CPEB1 correlated with promoter hypomethylation. Therefore, we considered hypomethylation one of the mechanisms upregulating CPEB1. The Kaplan-Meier method verified that the glioma patients exhibiting the overexpression or hypomethylation of CPEB1 had a poor outcome. Therefore, CPEB1 overexpression and hypomethylation could be considered as potential markers of glioma prognosis.

We have demonstrated that CPEB1 is hypomethylated and overexpressed in glioma; however, the mechanism of its dysregulation is unclear. miRNAs play an important role in the process of glioma (Yue *et al.*, 2012; Tang *et al.*, 2011). Using bioinformatics, we predicted that miRNAs control CPEB1 and selected the tumor suppressor miR-101 to verify this hypothesis. The luciferase reporter assay, real-time PCR and Western blots indicated that CPEB1 was the direct target of miR-101; however, the mechanism of hypomethylation is unknown. Surprisingly, the histone methyltransferases EZH2 and EED are targets of miR-101(Chiang *et al.*, 2010; Leung-Kuen *et al.*, 2012). We hypothesized that the hypomethylation of CPEB1 was because of histone methylation modifications regulated by miR-101. First, we investigated whether the CPEB1 methylation status was regulated by miR-101, EZH2 and EED. To determine if miR-101 modulated histone modification at the CPEB1 promoter through EZH2 and EED, we identified that the core promoter of CPEB1 was at position -307 to -207. We tested the DNA methylation-related enrichment of the histones H3K4me2, H3K27me3, H3K9me3 and H4K20me3 after transfection with miR-101 mimics, EZH2 siRNA and EED siRNA. The ChIP analysis suggested that the enrichment of H3K4me2 and H3K27me3 was decreased and the enrichment of H3K9me3 and H4K20me3 was increased by the presence of miR-101, the knockdown of EZH2 reduced the enrichment of H3K4me2 and

H3K27me3, and only the knockdown of EED reduced the enrichment of H3K27me3. The analysis revealed that miR-101 regulated the enrichment of H3K4me2 and H3K27me3 by EZH2 and/or EED, and it modulated the enrichment of H3K9me3 and H4K20me3 by regulating other histone methyltranferases, such as the H3K9-specific SUV39H1/2 (Lehnertz *et al.*, 2003), G9a (Tachibana *et al.*, 2005) and H4K20-specific SUV4−20H (Gonzalo *et al.*, 2005).

In summary, this study provides comprehensive data for the identification of aberrant methylation in glioma using the MeDIP-chip and demonstrates that nine novel genes are epigenetically regulated by DNA methylation in glioma. Meanwhile, we also determined that miR-185 reduced global DNA methylation and restored promoter hypermethylation gene expression through the direct targeting of DNMT1. The miR-101 regulates the histone methylation modification of hypomethylated genes by targeting EZH2, EED and DNMT3A and affects their methylation level and expression in glioma. Taken together, miRNAs, as small noncoding RNAs, not only regulate the expression of hyper/hypo- methylation genes directly but also regulate methylation levels and gene expression through histone and DNA methylation modification.

Acknowledgements

This study was supported by grants from The 111 project (111-2-12), the National Science Foundation of China (81272297; 81171932), the Hunan Province Natural Sciences Foundations of China (11JJ1013), the research Fund for the Doctoral Program of Higher Education of China (20110162110037).

References

Amatya, V.J., Naumann, U., Weller, M., Ohgaki, H. (2005).TP53 promoter methylation in human gliomas. Acta Neuropathol, 110, 178-184.

Bartel, D.P. (2004). MicroRNAs: genomics, biogenesis, mechanism, and function. Cell, 116, 281-297.

Baylin, S.B., Esteller, M., Rountree, M.R., Bachman, K.E., Schuebel, K., Herman, J.G. (2001).Aberrant patterns of DNA methylation, chromatin formation and gene expression in cancer. Hum Mol Genet, 10, 687-692.

Benetti, R., Gonzalo, S., Jaco, I., Munoz, P., Gonzalez, S., Schoeftner, S., Murchison, E., Andl, T., Chen, T., Klatt, P., Li, E., Serrano, M., Millar, S., Hannon, G., Blasco, M.A.. (2008). A mammalian microRNA cluster controls DNA methylation and telomere recombination via Rbl2-dependent regulation of DNA methyltransferases. Nat Struct Mol Biol, 15,268-279.

Bian, L.G., Sun, Q.F., Tirakotai, W., Zhao, W.G., Shen, J.K., Luo, Q.Z., Bertalanffy, H.. (2005). Loss of heterozygosity on chromosome 22 in sporadic schwannoma and its relation to the proliferation of tumor cells. Chin Med J (Engl), 118, 1517-1524.

Burns, D.M., D'Ambrogio, A., Nottrott, S., Richter, J.D. (2011).CPEB and two poly(A) polymerases control miR-122 stability and p53 mRNA translation. Nature, 473, 105-108.

Chiang,C.W., Huang,Y., Leong, K.W., Chen, L.C., Chen, H.C., Chen, S.J., Chou, C.K.. (2010) .PKCalpha mediated induction of miR-101 in human hepatoma HepG2 cells. J Biomed Sci, 17, 35.

Costello, J.F., Fruhwald, M.C., Smiraglia, D.J., Rush,J., Robertson,G.P, Gao, X., Wright,F.A., Feramisco, J.D., Peltomäki, P., Lang, J.C., Schuller, D.E., Yu, L., Bloomfield, C.D., Caligiuri, M.A., Yates, A., Nishikawa, R., Su, Huang, H.,

Petrelli, N.J., Zhang, X., O'Dorisio, M.S., Held,W.A., Cavenee, W.K., Plass, C.(2000).Aberrant CpG-island methylation has non-random and tumour-type-specific patterns. Nature Genetics, 24, 132-138.

Datta, J., Kutay, H., Nasser, M.W., Nuovo, G.J., Wang, B., Majumder, S., Liu, C.G., Volinia, S., Croce, C.M., Schmittgen,T.D., Ghoshal, K., Jacob, S.T. (2008).Methylation mediated silencing of MicroRNA-1 gene and its role in hepatocellular carcinogenesis. Cancer Res. 68, 5049-5058.

De. Pontual, L., Trochet, D., Bourdeaut, F., Thomas, S., Etchevers, H., Chompret, A., Minard, V., Valteau, D., Brugieres, L., Munnich, A., Delattre, O., Lyonnet,S., Janoueix-Lerosey, I., Amiel, J. (2007). Methylation-associated PHOX2B gene silencing is a rare event in human neuroblastoma. Eur J Cancer, 43, 2366-2372.

Ehrich, M., Nelson, M.R., Stanssens, P., Zabeau, M., Liloglou, T., Xinarianos, G., Cantor, C.R., Field, J.K., van.den. Boom, D.. (2005). Quantitative high-throughput analysis of DNA methylation patterns by base-specific cleavage and mass spectrometry. Proc Natl Acad Sci USA, 102,15785-15790.

Ehrlich, M. (2002). DNA methylation in cancer: too much, but also too little. Oncogene, 21,5400-5413.

Fabbri, M., Garzon, R., Cimmino, A., Liu, Z., Zanesi, N., Callegari, E., Liu, S., Alder, H., Costinean, S., Fernandez-Cymering,C., Volinia, S., Guler, G., Morrison, C.D., Chan, K.K., Marcucci, G., Calin, G.A., Huebner, K., Croce, C.M.(2007). MicroRNA-29 family reverts aberrant methylation in lung cancer by targeting DNA methyltransferases 3A and 3B. Proc Natl Acad Sci USA ,104, 15805-15810.

Fanelli, M., Caprodossi, S., Ricci-Vitiani, L., Porcellini, A., Tomassoni-Ardori, F., Amatori, S., Andreoni, F., Magnani, M., De. Maria, R., Santoni, A., Minucci, S., Pelicci, P.G. (2008). Loss of pericentromeric DNA methylation pattern in human glioblastoma is associated with altered DNA methyltransferases expression and involves the stem cell compartment. Oncogene, 27, 358-365.

Foltz, G., Yoon, J.G., Lee, H., Ryken, T.C., Sibenaller, Z., Ehrich, M., Hood, L., Madan, A. (2009). DNA methyltransferase-mediated transcriptional silencing in malignant glioma: a combined whole-genome microarray and promoter array analysis. Oncogene, 28, 2667-2677.

Fukushima, T., Katayama, Y., Watanabe, T., Yoshino, A., Ogino, A., Ohta, T., Komine, C. (2005). Promoter hypermethylation of mismatch repair gene hMLH1 predicts the clinical response of malignant astrocytomas to nitrosourea. Clin Cancer Res, 11, 1539-1544.

Gieni, R.S., Hendzel, M.J.(2009) ,Polycomb group protein gene silencing, non-coding RNA, stem cells, and cancer. Biochem Cell Biol, 87, 711-746.

Gonzalo, S., Garcia-Cao, M., Fraga, M.F., Schotta, G., Peters, A.H., Cotter, S.E., Eguía, R., Dean, D.C., Esteller, M., Jenuwein, T., Blasco, M.A. (2005), Role of the RB1 family in stabilizing histone methylation at constitutive heterochromatin. Nat Cell Biol, 7, 420-428.

He, L., Hannon, G.J.(2004). MicroRNAs: small RNAs with a big role in gene regulation. Nat Rev Genet, 5,522-531.

Hegi, M.E., Diserens, A.C., Godard, S., Dietrich, P.Y., Regli, L., Ostermann, S., Otten, P., Van. Melle ,G., de, Tribolet, N., Stupp, R. (2004). Clinical trial substantiates the predictive value of O-6-methylguanine-DNA methyltransferase promoter methylation in glioblastoma patients treated with temozolomide. Clin Cancer Res, 10, 1871-1874.

Herman,J.G., Baylin,S.B.(2003).Gene silencing in cancer in association with promoter hypermethylation. N Engl J Med, 349, 2042-2054.

Hesson, L., Bieche, I., Krex, D., Criniere, E., Hoang-Xuan, K., Maher, E.R., Latif, F. (2004). Frequent epigenetic inactivation of RASSF1A and BLU genes located within the critical 3p21.3 region in gliomas. Oncogene, 23, 2408-2419.

Horiguchi, K., Tomizawa, Y., Tosaka, M., Ishiuchi, S., Kurihara, H., Mori, M., Saito,N. (2003). Epigenetic inactivation of RASSF1A candidate tumor suppressor gene at 3p21.3 in brain tumors. Oncogene, 22, 7862-7865.

Huang, H.S., Akbarian, S. (2007). GAD1 mRNA Expression and DNA Methylation in Prefrontal Cortex of Subjects with Schizophrenia. Plos One, 2, e809.

Huang, K.H., Huang, S.F., Chen, I.H., Liao,C.T., Wang, H.M., Hsieh, L.L. (2009). Methylation of RASSF1A, RASSF2A, and HIN-1 is associated with poor outcome after radiotherapy, but not surgery, in oral squamous cell carcinoma. Clin Cancer Res, 15, 4174-4180.

Huang, J., Lin, Y., Li, L.H. Qing, D., Teng, X.M., Zhang, Y.L., Hu, X., Hu,.Y, Yang, P., Han, Z.G. (2009). ARHI, As a Novel Suppressor of Cell Growth and Downregulated in Human Hepatocellular Carcinoma, Could Contribute to Hepatocarcinogenesis. Mol Carcinogenesis, 48, 130-140.

Hong, G.M., Bain, L.J. (2012). Sodium arsenite represses the expression of myogenin in C2C12 mouse myoblast cells through histone modifications and altered expression of Ezh2, Glp, and Igf-1. Toxicol Appl Pharmacol, 260, 250-259.

Jacinto, F.V., Ballestar, E., Esteller, M. (2008). Methyl-DNA immunoprecipitation (MeDIP): hunting down the DNA methylome. Biotechniques, 44: 35, 37, 39 passim.

Jeltsch, A. (2002). Beyond Watson and Crick: DNA methylation and molecular enzymology of DNA methyltransferases. Chembiochem, 3, 274-293.

Jenuwein, T., Allis, C.D.(2001) .Translating the histone code. Science, 293, 1074-1080.

Jones, P.A., Baylin, S.B. (2007). The epigenomics of cancer. Cell, 128, 683-692.

Kim, T.Y., Zhong, S., Fields, C.R., Kim, J.H., Robertson, K.D. (2006) .Epigenomic profiling reveals novel and frequent targets of aberrant DNA methylation-mediated silencing in malignant glioma. Cancer Res, 66, 7490-7501.

Komine,C.,Watanabe,T., Katayama ,Y., Yoshino, A., Yokoyama, T., Fukushima, T. (2003). Promoter hypermethylation of the DNA repair gene O6-methylguanine-DNA methyltransferase is an independent predictor of shortened progression free survival in patients with low-grade diffuse astrocytomas. Brain Pathol, 13, 176-184.

Kuang, S.Q., Tong, W.G., Yang, H., Lin, W., Lee, M.K., Fang, Z.H., Wei, Y., Jelinek, J., Issa, J.P., Garcia-Manero, G.. (2008). Genome-wide identification of aberrantly methylated promoter associated CpG islands in acute lymphocytic leukemia. Leukemia, 22, 1529-1538.

Laflamme, C., Filion, C., Bridge, J.A., Ladanyi, M., Goldring, M.B., Labelle, Y. (2003). The homeotic protein Six3 is a coactivator of the nuclear receptor NOR-1 and a corepressor of the fusion protein EWS/NOR-1 in human extraskeletal myxoid chondrosarcomas. Cancer Research, 63,449-454.

Laird, P.W. (2005) .Cancer epigenetics. Hum Mol Genet, 14 Spec No 1: R65-76.

Lehnertz, B., Ueda, Y., Derijck, A.A., Braunschweig, U., Perez-Burgos, L., Kubicek, S., Chen, T., Li, E., Jenuwein, T., Peters, A.H. (2003).Suv39h-mediated histone H3 lysine 9 methylation directs DNA methylation to major satellite repeats at pericentric heterochromatin. Curr Biol, 13, 1192-1200.

Lerer, I., Sagi, M., Meiner, V., Cohen, T., Zlotogora, J., Abeliovich, D. (2005). Deletion of the ANKRD15 gene at 9p24.3 causes parent-of-origin-dependent inheritance of familial cerebral palsy. Hum Mol Genet,14, 3911-3920.

Au, S.L., Wong, C.C., Lee, J.M., Fan, D.N., Tsang, F.H., Ng, I.O., Wong, C.M. (2012). Enhancer of zeste homolog 2 (EZH2) epigenetically silences multiple tumor suppressor miRNAs to promote liver cancer metastasis. Hepatology, 56, 622-631.

Lewis, B.P., Shih, I.H., Jones-Rhoades, M.W., Bartel, D.P., Burge, C.B. (2003). Prediction of mammalian microRNA targets. Cell, 115, 787-798.

Liu, Z., Liu, S., Xie, Z., Blum, W., Perrotti, D., Paschka, P., Klisovic, R., Byrd, J., Chan, K.K., Marcucci,G. (2007).Characterization of in vitro and in vivo hypomethylating effects of decitabine in acute myeloid leukemia by a rapid, specific and sensitive LC-MS/MS method. Nucleic Acids Res, 35, e31.

Louis, D.N., Ohgaki, H., Wiestler, O.D., Cavenee, W.K., Burger, P.C., Jouvet, A., Scheithauer, B.W., Kleihues, P. (2007) .The 2007 WHO classification of tumours of the central nervous system. Acta Neuropathol, 114, 97-109.

Lujambio, A., Calin, G.A., Villanueva, A., Ropero, S., Sanchez-Cespedes, M., Blanco, D., Montuenga, L.M., Rossi, S., Nicoloso, M.S., Faller, W.J., Gallagher, W.M., Eccles, S.A., Croce, C.M., Esteller, M. (2008). A microRNA DNA methylation signature for human cancer metastasis. Proc Natl Acad Sci USA ,105, 13556-13561.

Ma, Y.Y., Tao, H.Q. (2012) .Microribonucleic acids and gastric cancer. Cancer Sci, 103, 620-625.

Martins-de-Souza, D., Gattaz, W.F., Schmitt, A., Rewerts, C., Marangoni, S., Novello, J.C., Maccarrone, G., Turck, C.W., Dias-Neto, E. (2009). Alterations in oligodendrocyte proteins, calcium homeostasis and new potential markers in schizophrenia anterior temporal lobe are revealed by shotgun proteome analysis. J Neural Transm, 116, 275-289.

McCabe, M.T., Brandes, J.C., Vertino, P.M. (2009).Cancer DNA methylation: molecular mechanisms and clinical implications. Clin Cancer Res, 15, 3927-3937.

Morgan, M., Iaconcig, A., Muro, A.F. (2010). CPEB2, CPEB3 and CPEB4 are coordinately regulated by miRNAs recognizing conserved binding sites in paralog positions of their 3'-UTRs. Nucleic Acids Res, 38,7698-7710.

Mori ,Y,, Cai, K., Cheng, Y., Wang, S., Paun, B., Hamilton, J.P., Jin, Z., Sato, F., Berki, A.T., Kan, T., Ito, T., Mantzur, C., Abraham, J.M., Meltzer, S.J. (2006). A genome-wide search identifies epigenetic silencing of Somatostatin, Tachykinin-1, and 5 other genes in colon cancer. Gastroenterology, 131, 1659-1659.

Murata,T., Kondo,Y., Sugimoto, A, Kawashima, D., Saito, S., Isomura, H., Kanda, T., Tsurumi, T. (2012). Epigenetic histone modification of Epstein-Barr virus BZLF1 promoter during latency and reactivation in Raji cells. J Virol , 86 ,4752-4761.

Nakamura, M., Watanabe, T., Yonekawa, Y., Kleihues, P., Ohgaki, H. (2001). Promoter methylation of the DNA repair gene MGMT in astrocytomas is frequently associated with G:C --> A:T mutations of the TP53 tumor suppressor gene. Carcinogenesis, 22, 1715-1719.

Ohta, T., Watanabe, T., Katayama, Y., Yoshino, A., Yachi K., Ogino, A., Komine, C., Fukushima, T. (2006). Aberrant promoter hypermethylation profile of cell cycle regulatory genes in malignant astrocytomas. Oncol Rep, 16, 957-963.

Ongenaert,M., Wisman, GBA., Volders, H.H., Koning, A.J., van. Der. Zee, AGJ, Schuuring, E. (2008). Discovery of DNA methylation markers in cervical cancer using relaxation ranking. BMC Med Genomics, 1, 57.

Riemenschneider, M.J., Reifenberger, J., Reifenberger, G. (2008). Frequent biallelic inactivation and transcriptional silencing of the DIRAS3 gene at 1p31 in oligodendroglial tumors with 1p loss. Int J Cancer, 122, 2503-2510.

Saito, Y., Liang, G., Egger, G., Friedman, J.M., Chuang, J.C., Coetzee,G.A., Jones, P.A. (2006). Specific activation of microRNA-127 with downregulation of the proto-oncogene BCL6 by chromatin-modifying drugs in human cancer cells. Cancer Cell, 9, 435-443.

Saito, Y., Suzuki, H., Matsuura, M., Sato, A., Kasai, Y., Yamada, K., Saito, H., Hibi, T. (2012) . MicroRNAs in Hepatobiliary and Pancreatic Cancers. Front Genet, 2, 66.

Semaan, A., Qazi, A.M., Seward, S., Chamala, S., Bryant, C.S., Kumar, S., Morris, R., Steffes, C.P., Bouwman, D.L., Munkarah, A.R., Weaver, D.W., Gruber, S.A., Batchu, R.B. (2011).MicroRNA-101 inhibits growth of epithelial ovarian cancer by relieving chromatin-mediated transcriptional repression of p21(waf(1)/cip(1)). Pharm Res, 28, 3079-3090.

Sessa, L., Breiling, A., Lavorgna, G., Silvestri, L., Casari, G., Orlando, V. (2007). Noncoding RNA synthesis and loss of Polycomb group repression accompanies the colinear activation of the human HOXA cluster. RNA, 13, 223-239.

Shumaker, D.K., Dechat, T., Kohlmaier, A., Adam, S.A., Bozovsky, M.R., Eriksson, M., Goldman, A.E., Khuon, S., Collins, F..S, Jenuwein, T., Goldman, R.D. (2006) .Mutant nuclear lamin A leads to progressive alterations of epigenetic control in premature aging. Proc Natl Acad Sci USA, 103, 8703-8708.

Simon, J.A., Kingston, R.E. (2009). Mechanisms of polycomb gene silencing: knowns and unknowns. Nat Rev Mol Cell Biol, 10, 697-708.

Stone, A.R., Bobo, W., Brat, D.J., Devi, N.S., Van. Meir, E.G., Vertino, P.M. (2004). Aberrant methylation and down-regulation of TMS1/ASC in human glioblastoma. Am J Pathol, 165, 1151-1161.

Tachibana, M., Ueda, J., Fukuda, M., Takeda, N., Ohta, T., Iwanari, H., Sakihama, T., Kodama, T., Hamakubo, T., Shinkai, Y. (2005). Histone methyltransferases G9a and GLP form heteromeric complexes and are both crucial for methylation of euchromatin at H3-K9. Genes Dev, 19, 815-826.

Takahashi, K., Kudo, J., Ishibashi, H., Hirata, Y., Niho, Y. (1993). Frequent loss of heterozygosity on chromosome 22 in hepatocellular carcinoma. Hepatology, 17, 794-799.

Takahashi, Y., Forrest, ARR., Maeno, E., Hashimoto, T., Daub, C.O., Yasuda, J. (2009). MiR-107 and MiR-185 Can Induce Cell Cycle Arrest in Human Non Small Cell Lung Cancer Cell Lines. Plos One, 4, 2

Tang, H., Liu, X., Wang, Z., She, X., Zeng, X., Deng, M., Liao, Q., Guo, X., Wang, R., Li, X., Zeng, F., Wu, M., Li ,G. (2011). Interaction of hsa-miR-381 and glioma suppressor LRRC4 is involved in glioma growth. Brain Res, 1390, 21-32.

Taylor, K.H., Pena-Hernandez, K.E., Davis, J.W., Arthur, G.L., Duff, D.J., Shi, H., Rahmatpanah, F.B., Sjahputera, O., Caldwell, C.W. (2007). Large-scale CpG methylation analysis identifies novel candidate genes and reveals methylation hotspots in acute lymphoblastic leukemia. Cancer Res, 67, 2617-2625.

Toyota, M., Suzuki, H., Sasaki, Y., Maruyama, R., Imai, K., Shinomura, Y., Tokino, T. (2008). Epigenetic silencing of microRNA-34b/c and B-cell translocation gene 4 is associated with CpG island methylation in colorectal cancer. Cancer Res, 68, 4123-4132.

Varambally, S., Cao, Q., Mani, R.S., Shankar, S., Wang, X., Ateeq, B., Laxman, B., Cao, X., Jing, X., Ramnarayanan, K., Brenner, J.C., Yu, J., Kim, J.H., Han, B., Tan, P., Kumar-Sinha, C., Lonigro, R.J., Palanisamy, N., Maher, C.A., Chinnaiyan, A.M.(2008). Genomic loss of microRNA-101 leads to overexpression of histone methyltransferase EZH2 in cancer. Science, 322, 1695-1699.

Waha, A., Guntner, S., Huang, T.H., Yan, P.S., Arslan, B., Yamada, K., Saito, H., Hibi, T. (2005). Epigenetic silencing of the protocadherin family member PCDH-gamma-A11 in astrocytomas. Neoplasia, 7, 193-199.

Wiencke, J.K., Zheng, S., Jelluma, N., Tihan, T., Vandenberg, S., Tamgüney, T., Baumber, R., Parsons,R., Lamborn, K.R., Berger, M.S., Wrensch, M.R., Haas-Kogan, D.A., Stokoe, D. (2007).Methylation of the PTEN promoter defines low-grade gliomas and secondary glioblastoma. Neuro Oncol, 9, 271-279.

Wu, L., Zhou, H., Zhang, Q., Zhang, J., Ni, F., Liu, C., Qi, Y. (2010). DNA methylation mediated by a microRNA pathway. Mol Cell, 38, 465-475.

Wu, M., Huang, C., Gan, K., Huang, H., Chen, Q., Ouyang, J., Tang, Y., Li, X., Yang, Y., Zhou, H., Zhou, Y., Zeng, Z., Xiao, L., Li, D., Tang, K., Shen, S., Li .G. (2006) .LRRC4, a putative tumor suppressor gene, requires a functional leucine-rich repeat cassette domain to inhibit proliferation of glioma cells in vitro by modulating the extracellular signal-regulated kinase/protein kinase B/nuclear factor-kappaB pathway. Mol Biol Cell, 17, 3534-3542.

Wu, X., Rauch, T.A., Zhong, X., Bennett, W.P., Latif, F., Krex, D., Pfeifer, G.P. (2010) .CpG island hypermethylation in human astrocytomas. Cancer Res, 70, 2718-2727.

Yates, D.R., Rehman, I., Abbod, M.F., Meuth, M., Cross, S.S., Linkens, D.A., Hamdy, F.C., Catto, J.W. (2007). Promoter hypermethylation identifies progression risk in bladder cancer. Clin Cancer Res, 13, 2046-2053.

Yin, D., Xie, D., Hofmann, W.K., Zhang, W., Asotra, K., Wong, R., Black, K.L., Koeffler, H.P. (2003). DNA repair gene O6-methylguanine-DNA methyltransferase: promoter hypermethylation associated with decreased expression and G:C to A:T mutations of p53 in brain tumors. Mol Carcinog, 36, 23-31.

Yue, X., Wang, P., Xu, J., Zhu, Y., Sun, G., Pang, Q., Tao, R. (2012). MicroRNA-205 functions as a tumor suppressor in human glioblastoma cells by targeting VEGF-A. Oncol Rep, 27, 1200-1206.

Zhang, X., Yang, J.J., Kim, Y.S., Kim, K.Y., Ahn, W.S., Yang, S. (2010). An 8-gene signature, including methylated and down-regulated glutathione peroxidase 3, of gastric cancer. Int J Oncol, 36, 405-414.

Zhang, Z., Li, D., Wu, M., Xiang, B., Wang, L., Zhou, M., Chen, P., Li, X., Shen, S., Li, G. (2008). Promoter hypermethylation-mediated inactivation of LRRC4 in gliomas. BMC Mol Biol, 9, 99.

Effect of Water Molar Rate on the Properties and Delivery Profiles of Dopamine from Nanostructured Sol-gel Silica

Tessy López
Departamento de Atención a la Salud
UAM-Xochimilco, México
Laboratorio de Nanotecnología
Instituto Nacional de Neurología y Neurocirugía "MVS", México

Emma Ortiz
Laboratorio de Nanotecnología
Instituto Nacional de Neurología y Neurocirugía "MVS", México

Paola Ramírez
Departamento de Atención a la Salud
UAM-Xochimilco, México

Dulce Esquivel
Laboratorio de Nanotecnología
Instituto Nacional de Neurología y Neurocirugía "MVS", México

Jesús García
Departamento de Atención a la Salud
UAM-Xochimilco, México

Esperanza García
Laboratorio de Nanotecnología
Instituto Nacional de Neurología y Neurocirugía "MVS", México

1   Introduction

Parkinson's disease was first medically described as a neurological syndrome by James Parkinson in 1817, though "fragments of Parkinson" can be found in earlier descriptions (Parkinson, 1817). Parkinson's disease (PD) is a movement disorder characterized by shakiness that generally starts by hands, but it also affects jaw and feet; resistance or lack of muscular flexibility; loss of spontaneous and automatic movement which generates slowness; postural instability, which can be recognized by forwards or backwards inclination causing frequent falls; depression, constipation, lack of facial expression; total simultaneous immobility during a few minutes till an hour (Burch & Sheerin, 2005; Pfeiffer, 2007) (Figure 1b). PD is the second most common neurodegenerative disease occurring worldwide, with equal incidence in both sexes. About 5–10% of people develop PD and the condition appears before the age of 40 (young onset). The mean age of onset is around 65 years. Overall age-adjusted prevalence is 1% worldwide and 1.6% in Europe, rising from 0.6% at age 60–64 to 3.5% at age 85–89 (De Rijk *et al.*, 1997; Zhang & Roman, 1993).

PD is a severe and progressive neurodegenerative disease. It is the second most common neurodegenerative disease, after Alzheimer's disease. It is caused by the selective loss of dopaminergic neurons in the substantia nigra (SN) pars compacta (Chand, 2007) (Figure 1a). Although it has been subject to intensive research, the etiology of PD is still enigmatic and the treatment is basically symptomatic. Many factors are thought to operate in the mechanism of cell death of the nigrostriatal dopaminergic neurons in PD. In recent years, evidence for the role of apoptotic cell death in PD arises from morphological, as well as molecular, studies in cell cultures, animal models, as well as human studies on postmortem brains from PD patients. These studies indicate that apoptosis takes place in PD and that there is a proapoptotic environment in the nigrostriatal region of parkinsonian patients. It is important to conclusively determine the mode of cell death in PD because new "antiapoptotic" compounds may offer protection to neurons from cell death and slow the neurodegeneration rate and disease progression.

Most of the movement-related symptoms of PD are associated to the lack of dopamine due to the loss of dopamine producing cells, this substance acts as a messenger between two areas of the brain, the substantia nigra and the corpus stratum, to produce smooth and controlled movements. When the concentration of dopamine decreases, communication between the two areas becomes ineffective, and movement becomes impaired; the grater the loss of dopamine, the worse the movement related symptoms (Figure 1c).

Risk factors have been consistently identified; age is the main factor for the development of the disease, head trauma, illness and exposure to environmental toxins. Smoking and caffeine show strong inverse associations with the disease and family history show a positive association (Hernan *et al.*, 2002; Marder *et al.*, 1996). Other risk factors such as specific foods or nutrients have been identified in some studies, but not in others (Chen *et al.*, 2002; Hellenbrand *et al.*, 1996; Logroscino *et al.*, 1996; Zhang *et al.*, 2002).

The 'Gold-standard' treatment for PD is medication or drug therapy. Virtually all of the available drug therapies increase the level of dopamine in the brain. The treatment for PD with dopamine has several disadvantages. One of them is its low intrinsic stability because it easily oxidizes in the body. That makes it unable to cross the blood-brain barrier (BBB) (Andén *et al.*, 1964; Bisaglia *et al.*, 2007; Smythies & Galzigna, 1998). These circumstances have derived in the use of L-dopa (levodopa), the natural precursor of dopamine as the main drug for Parkinson´s treatment. L-dopa is able to cross the BBB and transforms into dopamine by enzymatic decarboxylation once in the brain as is shown in Figure 2.

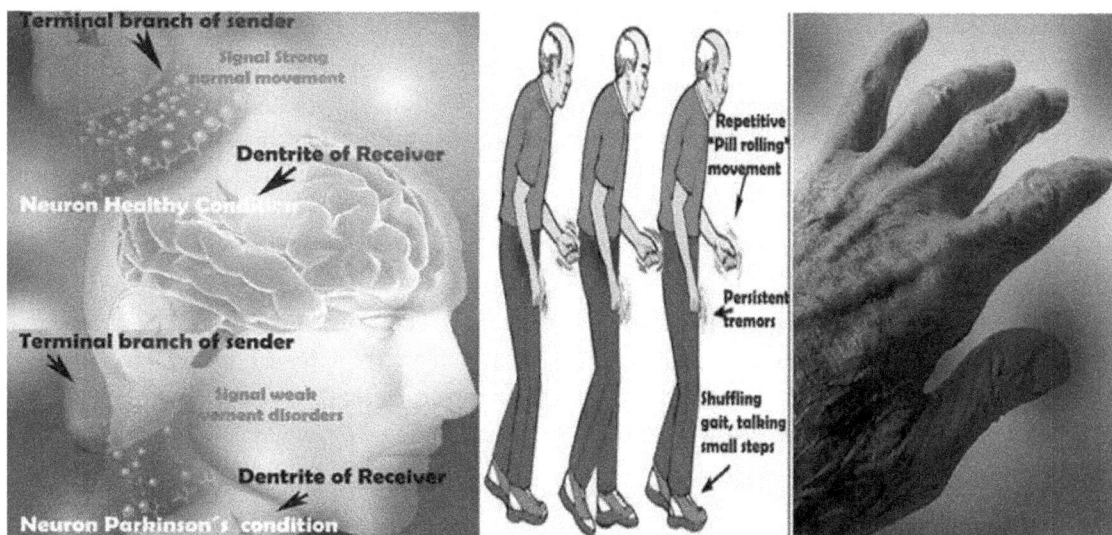

Figure 1: Parkinson's disease (PD) is developed due to the damage of dopaminergic neurons in the brain leading to a decrease in the production of the neurotransmitter dopamine, which controls movement. Involuntary movement is characteristic in PD.

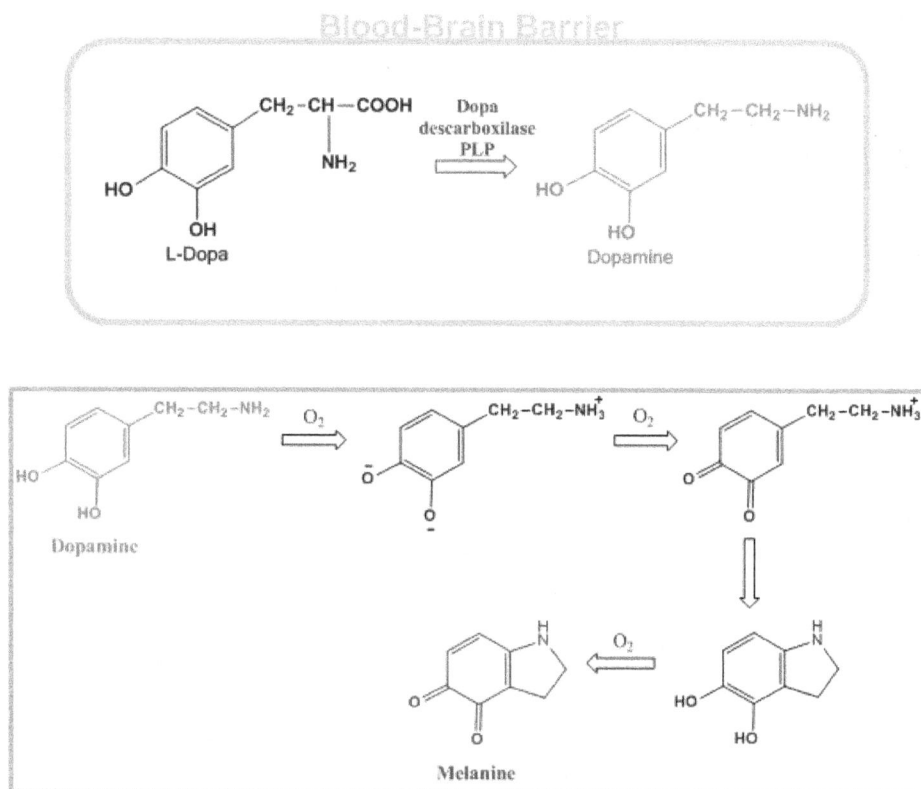

Figure 2: L-DOPA transformation by enzymatic catalysis to Dopamine and Dopamine's oxidation process.

Dopamine is one of three main neurotransmitters known as *catecholamines*, which help the body to respond to stress and prepare it for the fight-or-flight response. Loss of dopamine negatively affects the nerves and muscles that control movement and coordination, resulting in the major symptoms characteristic of Parkinson's disease. Dopamine also appears to be important for efficient information processing, and deficiencies may also be responsible for problems in memory and concentration that occur in many patients. Parkinson's disease is a multi-factor, complex disease. As is apparent from the 'upstream' factors (toxins, genes and energy metabolism), an integration of many mechanisms and cellular processes will be required to explain how PD can be developed and slowly drive a normally functioning healthy organism to 'unhealthy' conditions where α-synculein is accumulated into Lewy bodies. The complexity of Parkinson's disease development mechanisms requires an integrative approach to link together all the subcellular, cellular and cerebral systems. The Systems approach presented here thus consider the relevant subsystems and aims to show how their failures can lead to disease development. These systems are:

- Metabolic systems to handle energy requirements (glycolysis, mitochondria etc.) and stresses (oxidative stress response).

- Cellular systems to recycle damaged proteins.

- Electro-chemical systems associated with the motor circuit.

- Dopamine regulation systems.

- Relevant signalling systems (e.g. apoptosis).

The Systems of Parkinson's disease approach thus aims at building comprehensive models and methods to integrate scientific knowledge in order to better understand how a failure or a combination of failure can lead to disease development. Further details on the actual works on the specific systems are found in the relevant research subsections.

There is a suggestion that apoptotic autophagy may occur in the Substantia Nigra during Parkinson's disease. Moreover, since the dopaminergic neurons are the most affected by the apoptotic processes during PD development, links between cellular apoptosis in a tissue and the loss of dopamine 'functionality' in the surrounding area must be sought in order to get a better understanding of how the disease progress.

The way of administration is oral and implies further complications, it has been determined that a low quantity of the drug reaches the cerebrospinal fluid, and even less the substantia nigra pars compact ($\approx$ 4%) (Horstink, 1984; Freed *et al.*, 1983) (Figure 3), when L-dopa is administered orally, a large amount is lost before it reaches the brain because a big portion is renally excreted, another part goes through the liver to be metabolized into different toxic products and finally only a small part goes to the brain where it has to cross the BBB as L-dopa to be transformed into dopamine, as shown in Figure 3.

L-dopa has also side effects: dyskinesia (the inability to control muscles); low blood pressure, which is a common problem during the first weeks of treatment, particularly if the initial dose is too high, and in some cases, arrhythmia might occur. Although levodopa effectively treats the symptoms of Parkinson´s, the disease nevertheless progresses and gets worse over time. The disease damages neurons that manufacture dopamine or that convert levodopa into dopamine. As the disease progresses it gets more and more difficult to stimulate the brain production of dopamine (Hely *et al.*, 1994; Marsden *et al.*, 1981; García-Escrig & Bermejo-Pareja, 1999) (Figure 3).

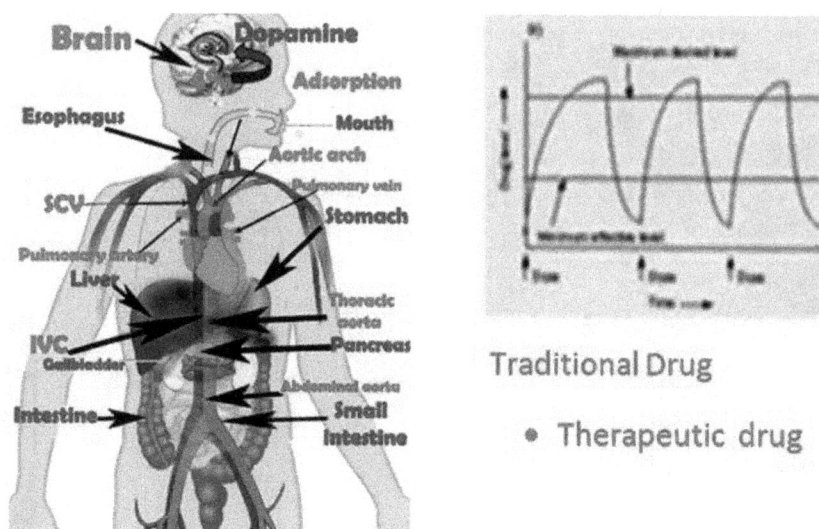

Figure 3: Traditional Parkinson's disease treatment. The figure on the left side shows that L-dopa only reaches the brain in approximately 4 % to become to dopamine.

Neurons from the striatum nucleus can be classified according to their morphology as spiny (GABA and substance p), which constitute the 95 % of the nucleus, and non-spiny (GABA and acetylcholine).

Cortical and subcortical afferents form synapses in type I and II neurons, at the same time type I neurons emit collateral signals responsible of lateral inhibition. The only afferent that produces pure excitatory potentials on the intrinsic striatal circuits is the median-par fascicular complex of the thalamus (cholinergic fibers). The rest cause both EPSP (excitatory postsynaptic potential) and IPSP (inhibitory postsynaptic potentials) sequentially, in accordance to the activation of inhibitory or recurring collateral neurons. Dopaminergic afferent in substance nigra excites silent neurons (which inhibit non spiny type ii neurons) and inhibit active spontaneous neurons (Benson *et al.*, 2001; Sesack & Grace, 2010).

One way to fight this problem is to use nanomedicine (1-100 nm), which has developed controlled drug-release systems for reducing drug dosage and to make the drug available at the target sites. We have proposed a drug-release device, which delivers dopamine directly in the brain, once implanted in the striatum, it releases dopamine in a controlled way ensuring a 100% delivery without causing side effects (López *et al.*, 2007, 2011), as shown in Figure 4.

The emphasis on the design of ideal drug delivery systems has evolved significantly over the past decades. Initial research efforts were focused on encapsulating therapeutic agents to protect them from degradation and to control drug release kinetics. Recently, the challenge has been to improve the efficiency of drug delivery, and therefore reduce side effects, such that drug carriers are preferentially releasing therapeutic agents at the desired site or damaged tissues.

The reservoirs prepared in our laboratory present a controlled release; the effect is a constant delivery of dopamine, because dopamine is stabilized into the silica network (Figure 4). The synthesis process allows the formation of hydroxyl-dopamine compounds which stabilizes the drug and protects neurons in the caudate nucleus. Brain is susceptible to free radicals attack so it produces oxidative products as other body organs. Our alternative to PD treatment is controlled administration of dopamine trough a

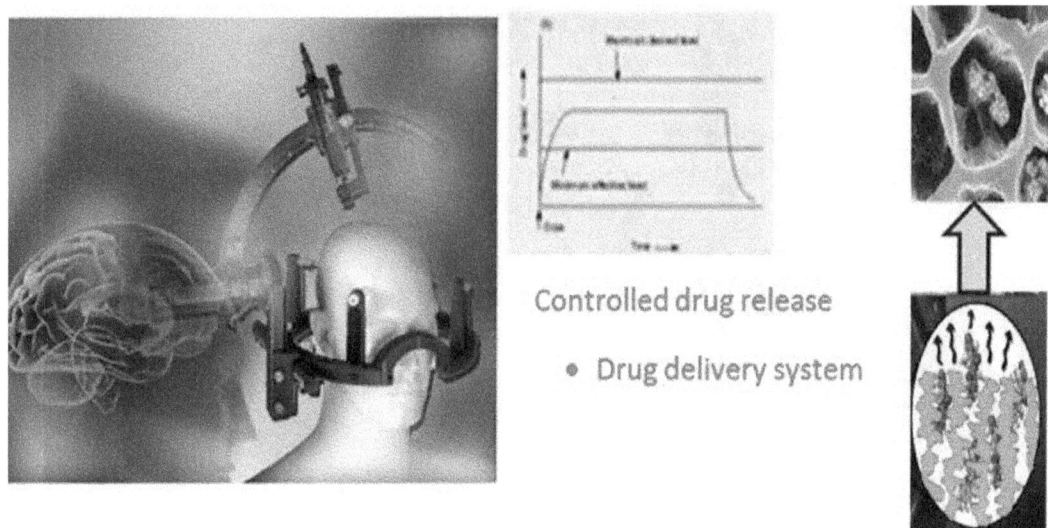

Figure 4: Nanomedicine as alternative treatment to PD, which makes it possible for 100 % of the dopamine administered to reach the damaged site by stereotactic surgery.

silica device (Figure 4). It was possible to deliver 100% of dopamine at the target site in the brain. Tests were performed on wistar rats by stereotactic surgery, "minimally invasive surgery", delivering dopamine during six months. It uses a three-dimensional coordinate system to localize small structures within body and also, to make actions such as ablation, biopsies, lesions, injections, stimulations, device's implantation, radiosurgery and others (Figure 4). The advantages of carrier systems are: (a) drug target, (b) no oxidation of dopamine, (c) *in vivo* drug stability, and others. Current drug-delivery systems are effective at releasing drugs in a controlled manner to produce a high local concentration; however, the scope is limited to targeting tissues rather than individual cells. Currently in the laboratory we are intending to reach dopamine control release over six months.

The development of new materials has enabled the use of porous solid supports for drug immobilization via encapsulation, due to the immobilization on a solid support the drug can maintaining their near-native activity and selectivity. These porous metal oxides have large surface areas, tailorable pore sizes, controlled particle size and shapes, and dual-functional surfaces (exterior and interior) (Yoshino *et al.*, 1990; Fidalgo & Ilharco, 2004; Innocenzi, 2003). These materials can be functionalized to increase or modify its access to specific cells, to deliver molecular payloads to their targets, and/or to report cellular activities and increase their biocompatibility (Figure 5).

Nanostructured silica obtained by the sol-gel process is chemically stable, morphology and porosity are easily controllable, is highly pure and it is possible to control its design from the beginning of the synthesis. It has been well demonstrated that xerogels, have the appropriate internal and external surface characteristics to interact with biomolecules, so they have been widely used.

We found that the drug release rate depends mainly on the pore diameter and drug interactions with the matrix surface (Hwang *et al.*, 2005; Tang *et al.*, 2006; Khedr *et al.*, 2012). On the other hand, biocompatibility depends on the chemical structure and physical properties. We suggest that SiO_2 materials have a great potential to stabilize dopamine and its later delivery in caudate nucleus using stereotactic surgery, which is a minimal invasion procedure, to administrate the 100% of the dose of pure dopamine

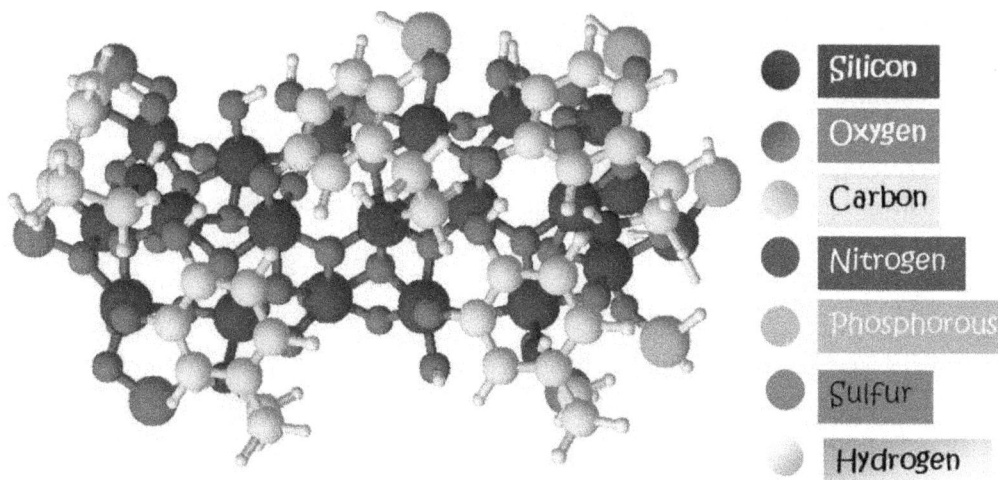

Figure 5: Silica nanoparticles functionalized with sulphate, phosphate and amine functional groups.

stabilized by nanosilanol groups and oxygen vacancies of the silica network synthesized by a special way using fine chemistry as Sol-Gel technique, which has been reported by our group.

2   Experimental

2.1   Sample Preparation

SiO_2 and the three different SiO_2-DA materials were prepared by the sol-gel method varying water/alkoxide molar ratio (r_{H2O}).   10, 20 and 40 water moles were used respectively while the alcohol/alkoxide molar ratio ($r_{EtOH/TEOS}$) and dopamine amount were maintained constant. The general procedure carried out to prepare one gram of each material is described below:

1. SiO_2. The adequate amount of water was added dropwise to a solution of 3.70 mL of tetraethoxysilane [TEOS] (Sigma-Aldrich, 98 %) dissolved in 19 mL of ethanol, maintaining constant stirring at room temperature and until gel formation. The gel was dried at 80 °C for three days.

2. SiO_2-DA-Xr_{H2O} (r=10, 20 and 40). 100 mg of dopamine (99%; Sigma-Aldrich) were dissolved in the adequate amount of water in accordance to the sample prepared. This solution was added dropwise to a solution of 3.70 mL of TEOS mixed with19 mL of ethanol. The final solution was continuously stirred at room temperature until the gel formation and finally the obtained gel was dried at 80°C. A N_2 atmosphere was used during the procedure to avoid dopamine oxidation, as we had reported before (López *et al.*, 2007, 2011).

2.2   Sample Characterization

Pore size, pore volume and surface area data, were obtained from the N_2 adsorption-desorption isotherms; analyses were performed with an ASAP 2010 Micromeritic apparatus. Pore size distribution and pore volume were calculated using the Barrett, Joyner, and Halenda (BJH) method from the desorption isotherm. Surface area was calculated using the Brunauer, Emmett, and Teller (BET) method. The Fourier Transformed-Infrarred (FTIR) spectra of translucent wafers consisting of a mix of KBr-sample (95 % weight) were obtained using an IR-Affinity Shimadzu Spectrophotometer. Transmission Electron Microscopy (TEM) was used to determine the morphology of the samples using an EM910 Carl Zeiss microscope with acceleration of 120KV. X-ray diffraction patterns were obtained using an EQUINOX-INEL diffractometer equipped with an X-ray tube and copper anodes operated at 30KV and 20 mA.

2.3   *In vitro* dopamine release test

A silica-dopamine device of approximately 2-3 mg was immersed in 50 ml of a solution of perchloric acid-sodium metabisulfite. At predetermined time, an aliquot of 3.0 µl was taken from the medium for its analysis. Dopamine concentration was quantified by High Performance Liquid Chromatography (HPLC) (Perkin Elmer). Peaks were integrated with a Perkin-Elmer Turbochrom Navigator 4.1 data station. Calibration curves were constructed by injection of several solutions with known concentrations of a dopamine standard into the 20 µl loop of the chromatograph. Dopamine concentrations were calculated by interpolation on the respective standard curve. Each experiment was realized by triplicate.

3   Results and Discussion

3.1   FTIR Spectra for SiO_2-Dopamine Samples

In a previous paper (López *et al.*, 2011) we reported the successful stabilization of dopamine within the silica network when silica-dopamine materials were studied by FT-IR and ^{13}CNMR techniques. Samples were prepared using 10, 20 and 40 moles of water, keeping alkoxide, dopamine and ethanol concentrations constant. At first we tried to stabilize dopamine into silica, however when testing with different concentrations of the support precursor, dopamine always get oxidized observing a yellow color on the final. Dopamine was added to the solvent under a nitrogen atmosphere using a stable relation of tetraethyl orthosilicate and 40 times less water concentrations, so we conclude that TEOS must be added dropwise to the primary solution under nitrogen atmosphere. Stabilization of dopamine molecule into silica matrix is the most important stage, that's why silica must be functionalized to prevent drug oxidation.

When this occurs a dopaminochrome is formed, dopamine-quinone, H_2O_2, OH^- and O_2; due to its high reactivity they could be the cause of apoptosis in dopaminergic neurons. In order to assure the integrity of the neurotransmitter a FTIR analysis was performed.

A wide band into the 2800–3700 cm^{-1} wavenumbers region is seen, this band is attributed to the stretching modes of residual Si–OH and some adsorbed water molecules. It can be observed in Figure 6 that when water amount used in the synthesis is greater, the silanol band is higher; the dotted line notes a displacement of the band corresponding to sample made with 10 water moles. On the other hand, physically adsorbed water in the silica network, shows a band at 1622 cm^{-1} due to H-O-H scissor bending vibrations (Yoshino *et al.*, 1990; Fidalgo & Ilharco, 2004; Innocenzi, 2003). The most important signals of dopamine were localized at 3350 cm^{-1}, 3205 cm^{-1}, and 3034 cm^{-1} corresponding to stretching vibrations of the O-H, C-N, and N-H functional groups present in its structure. The same peaks were identified in silica-dopamine materials suggesting that dopamine was successfully loaded in the silica sol–gel matrix and that the drug is stable. In Figure 6 we can see that the signal corresponding to the silanol groups ($\equiv$Si-OH) at approximately 3390 cm^{-1} shifts to higher energies, if water relation is greater, when the r_{H2O} increases gradually. It is due to the interaction produced between silica molecules and silanol groups present in the surface of tetrahedral and octahedral (Figure 14) silica as we previously reported (López *et al.*, 2007). We have identified all these signals observed on the samples as well as their wavenumbers of appearance and their assignment in greater detail as is reported in Table 1.

Wavenumber (cm⁻¹)			Assignment
Dopamine	SiO$_2$	SiO$_2$-DA	
	3000-2800$_{vw}$	3000-2800$_{vw}$	OH (SiO-H) asymmetric stretch
3348$_{(w)}$			OH asymmetric stretching
3150$_{(vs)}$			C-H asymmetricstretching (aromatics)
2957$_{(w)}$			C-H stretching (aromatics)
	1638	1638	O-H water molecule
1598$_{(vw)}$			C=C asymmetric stretching (aromatics)
1584			C-C asymmetric stretching (aromatic)
1504			C-C symmetric stretch (aromatic)
1472			C-C symmetric stretch (aromatic)
1322			C-O-H asymmetric bending
1260			C-OH symmetric bending
1206			C-C stretch
1192$_{(vs)}$			C-O symmetric stretch
1177(s)			C-C stretch
1115			C-C(NH$_2$) stretch
	1110$_{(VS, broad)}$	1110$_{(VS, broad)}$	Si-O-Si asymmetricstretching
1079			C-C-H symmetric bending
965			C-C(NH$_2$) symmetric bending
	957$_{(m)}$	957$_{(m)}$	Si-OH stretch
	798$_{(m)}$	798$_{(m)}$	O-H bending (SiOH)
600$_{(w)}$			C-C-C- symmetric bending
	560$_{(w)}$	560$_{(w)}$	
556			C-C-O symmetric bending
540			C-C-O asymmetric bending
476$_{(w)}$			C-C-OH symmetric bending
	462	462	Si-O oscillation

Table 1: Assignation of bands from the infrared spectra of SiO$_2$, Dopamine and SiO$_2$-DA. Where (w) is weak, (s) is stronger (vw) very weak and (vs) very strong.

These Si-OH groups interact with guest molecules through weak hydrogen bonds, which break easily via hydrolysis, releasing them and water. This feature allows us to incorporate specific molecules with different therapeutic effects. One example is dopamine (DA), which presumably is incorporated into silica xerogels by effect of its amino groups (Figure 6). The incorporation of dopamine has a clear effect over silica porosity which acts as the support, as well as in the pore size and the rate of release (Hwang *et al.*, 2005; Tang *et al.*, 2006). The objective in this work was to determine the effect of varying the molar ratio water/TEOS on the chemical-physical and release properties of silica-dopamine materials (SiO$_2$-DA). The aim was also to determine how the amount of water used during the TEOS hydrolysis affects the amount of Si-OH groups produced from the process, the effect on their porous structure and the re-lease kinetics of dopamine from a controlled-release device (Khedr *et al.*, 2012).

The bands at the minimal energy region (1000 a 400 cm^{-1}) are assigned to the flexion of -O-Si-O-, Si-OH and Si-O-Si silica network bonds.

The samples were functionalized with phosphates, nitrates and sulfates to obtain a biocompatible nanostructure with cell membrane. In this way the dopamine-silica is able to cross the BBB and then release the drug in the caudate nucleus cells.

The peaks at 949 cm^{-1}, 809 cm^{-1} correspond to phosphate and sulfate groups on the nanostructured support surface. As can be seen in Figure 6 L-dopa has different links compared to those present on do-pamine. We concluded that dopamine is well stabilized into the silica network without the presence of L-dopa.

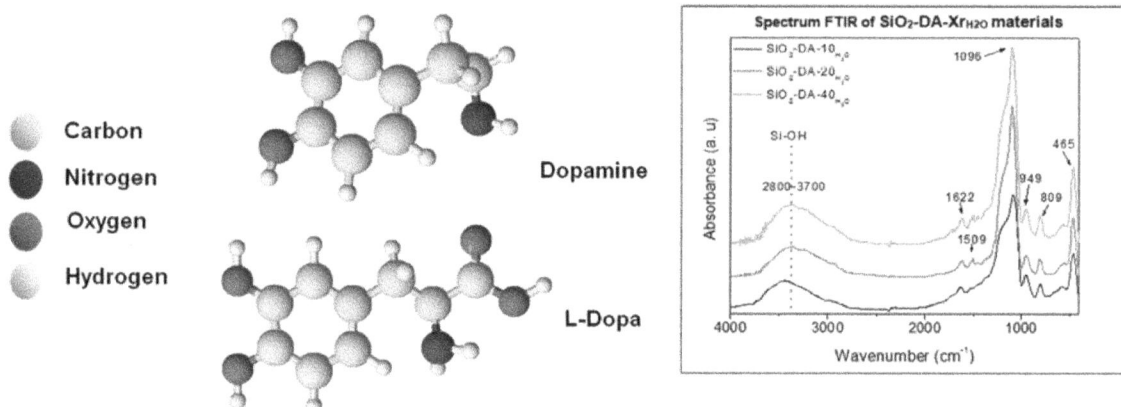

Figure 6: FTIR spectra of SiO$_2$-DA-Xr$_{H2O}$ materials, where X= 10, 20 and 40 respectively.

3.2   Textural Properties of the Materials

The N$_2$ adsorption-desorption isotherms of the SiO$_2$-DA materials are shown in Figure 7. According to the IUPAC classification all they correspond to the type IV isotherms, indicative that mesopores (pores sizes between 20 to 500 Å) were formed into each material (Brunauer *et al.*, 1940). However, it is possi-ble to observe several differences among them. From the nitrogen adsorption isotherms of the SiO$_2$-DA-10$_{H2O}$ and SiO$_2$-DA-40$_{H2O}$ samples is possible to identify only a sustained stage of nitrogen adsorption from the first relatives pressure to approximately 0.8 of relative pressure.This fact suggests that only mesopores in both samples were formed, it is possible to corroborate with the pore size distribution graphic shown in the insert of the Figure 7. Where, a narrow size pore distribution was obtained suggest homogeneous size pores in both sample were formed. In contrast, the isotherm of the SiO$_2$-DA-20$_{H2O}$ material shows nitrogen adsorptions at high relative pressures at approximately 0.9 indicative that both mesopores and macro-pores were formed. It is corroborated by the pore distribution graphic shown in the insert of the Figure 7, where a wide pore size distribution is observed. In all samples the adsorption and

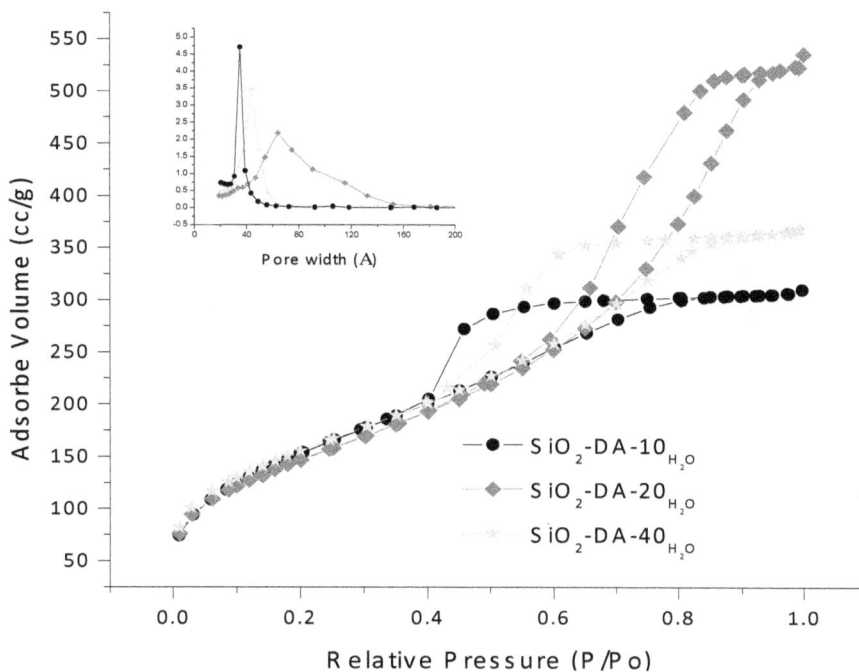

Figure 7: Nitrogen adsorption-desorption isotherms of the different SiO_2-DA-Xr_{H2O} sample, where Xr_{H2O}=10,\ 20 and 40 respectively. The insert shows the pore size distribution for each sample.

desorption isotherms formed a hysteresis loops due to capillary condensation in mesopores was carried out. This hysteresis is classified to according IUPAC as a H1 type, suggests there are open-ended cylinders pores in the silica network according to Barret, Joyner and Halenda (Barrett *et al.*, 1951).

The surface areas (S_{BET}) for all samples were determined from the N_2 adsorption isotherms in the region of relative pressures between 0.05 and 0.3 using the Brunauer–Emmett–Teller (BET) equation taking the N_2 cross sectional area of 16.2 $Å^2$ are given in Table 2 (Brunauer *et al.*, 1938; Sing *et al.*, 1985). The values of S_{BET} obtained were 569, 539 and 566 m²/g for each sample respectively to according in the water amount was increased. There is not a linear effect of the water quantity used during the silica-dopamine synthesis on the surface area values due to the surface area values did not change significantly. The average pore sizes calculated from the desorption branch using the BJH theory were 33, 59 and 39 Å in the order ascendant in that the water was used respectively. In the other hand, the pore volumes were 0.57, 0.85 and 0.55 cc/g in the same order that samples were prepared. These results were consisting with the pore sizes to high pore sizes high pore volume.

Samples	S_{BET} (m²/g)	D_p(Å)	V_p(cc/g)
SiO$_2$-DA-10$_{H2O}$	569	33	0.57
SiO$_2$-DA-20$_{H2O}$	539	59	0.85
SiO$_2$-DA-40$_{H2O}$	566	39	0.55

Table 2: Textural properties of SiO_2-dopamine materials, where S_{BET} is the specific surface area calculate from the BET equation, D_p is the average pore diameter, and V_p is the total pore volume calculated from the BJH equation.

3.3   X- ray Diffraction Patterns of SiO$_2$-DA Samples

Silica is an amorphous material that can only be transformed into a nanocrystalline material by treatment at high temperatures. The nanosilica material present in its structure both octahedral and tetrahedral (Figure 14) amorphous structure which yields a porous material adequate to host drugs as dopamine.Through X-ray diffraction studies, it was possible to identify the amorphous phase present in all samples (Figure 8). Diffraction patterns show a slowly shifted at peak maximum. A wide peak characteristic of amorphous silica is observed at 23 degrees (Figure 8). Signals derived from dopamine molecules were not observed due to two reasons: 1) dopamine molecules are highly dispersed into silica network and 2) The quantity of dopamine molecules is not sufficient to generate visible signals by x-ray. When the sample is analyzed by electronic diffraction a nanocrystallinity pattern can be observed (Figure 10). The X-ray diffraction results together with infrared suggest that dopamine molecules were occluded in the mesoporous nanostructure of silica without undergoing changes in their initial structure. It is possible to observe in Figure 7 the shift of the peaks indicated by a dotted line.

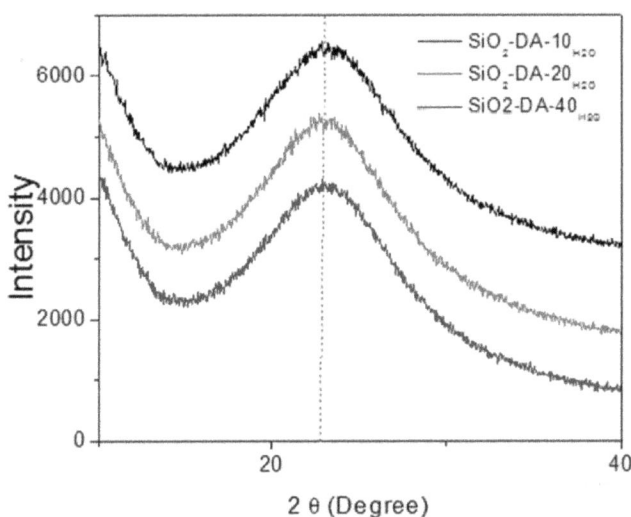

Figure 8: X-Ray Diffraction patterns of SiO$_2$-DA-Xr$_{H2O}$ materials (X= 10, 20 and 40), the wide peak indicates that an amorphous phase in silica was obtained.

3.4   Transmission and Scanning Electron Microscopy

Silica materials have a three-dimensional porous network when is obtained by the sol-gel process due to the dimmers and trimmers formed by the hydrolysis and condensation of tetraethoxysilane (TEOS) that rapidly condense into mostly cycle-tetrasiloxanes or cycle-hexasiloxanes. The three-dimensional network is built upon aggregation of the nanometric particles formed by condensation of those cycle siloxanes, yielding a porous wet gel that when dried, forms a powder with high surface area and high porosity. Figure 9 shows the scanning electron microscopy of SiO$_2$-DA where we can see that the nanoparticles formed have different sizes from 25 to 150 nm. It is possible to observe the nanoparticles aggregation when the gel formed was dried.

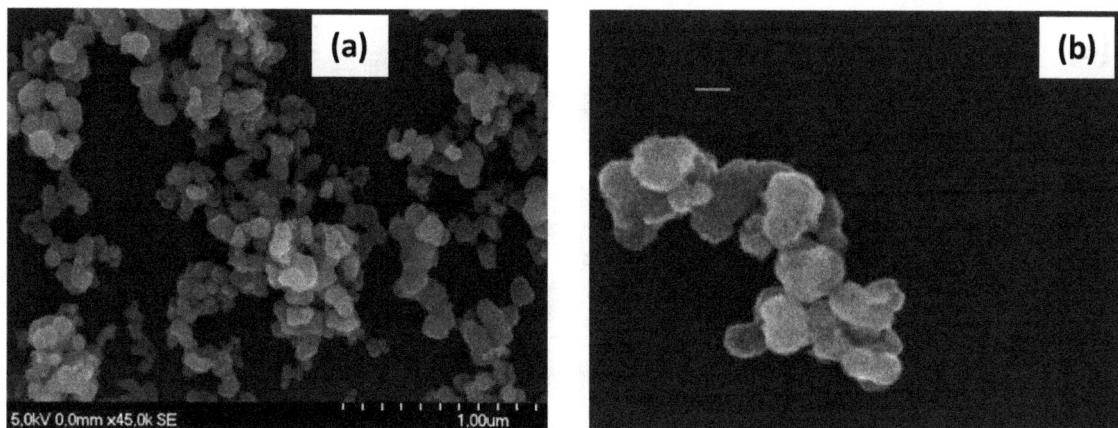

Figure 9: Scanning Electron Micrographs of silica-DA materials: (a) Nanoparticles formation and their aggregation, and (b) Individual nanoparticles with sizes by 100 nm.

From the micrographs taken with an electronic microscope we can note both the formation of the porous sol-gel silica network as well as the aggregation of the nanoparticles as is shown in Figures 12a, 12c and 12d. From these images is possible to determine that there is a heterogeneous size distribution between the aggregates, all fall into the nanometric scale. On the other hand, Figure 10b shows the diffraction pattern of the silica with DA, from which is possible to determine that there is a crystalline phase in this sample (Figure 10b). However, since silica is not crystalline when it is prepared at room temperature, we suggest that these diffractions are due to an atomic arrange in the silica network, instead of the formation of a crystalline phase. In this case dopamine molecules act as a structuring where the tetrasiloxane and hexasiloxane cycles were orderly formed around it during the synthesis process, in similar way as SBA-15 is prepared, but in this case dopamine was not eliminated by temperature action (Lopez *et al.*, 2011b).

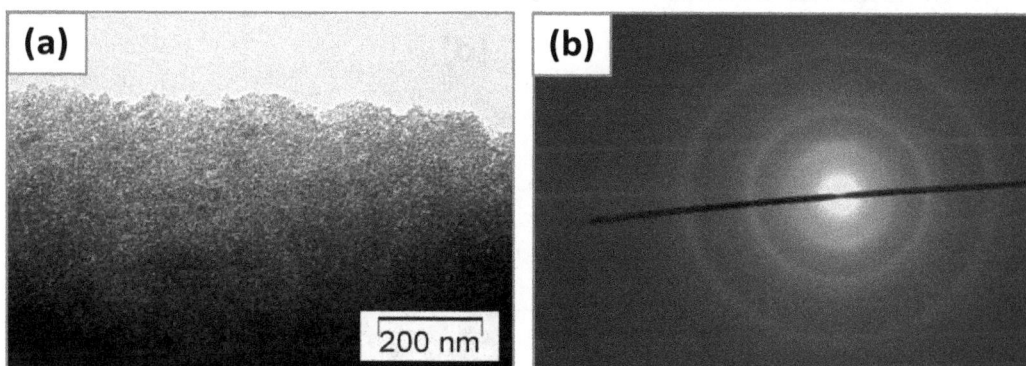

Figure 10: Transmission Electronic Micrograph of SiO_2-DA-10_{H2O} sample. (a) Taken at 80000 X, and (b) X-Ray Diffraction at 120 KV and 900 mm.

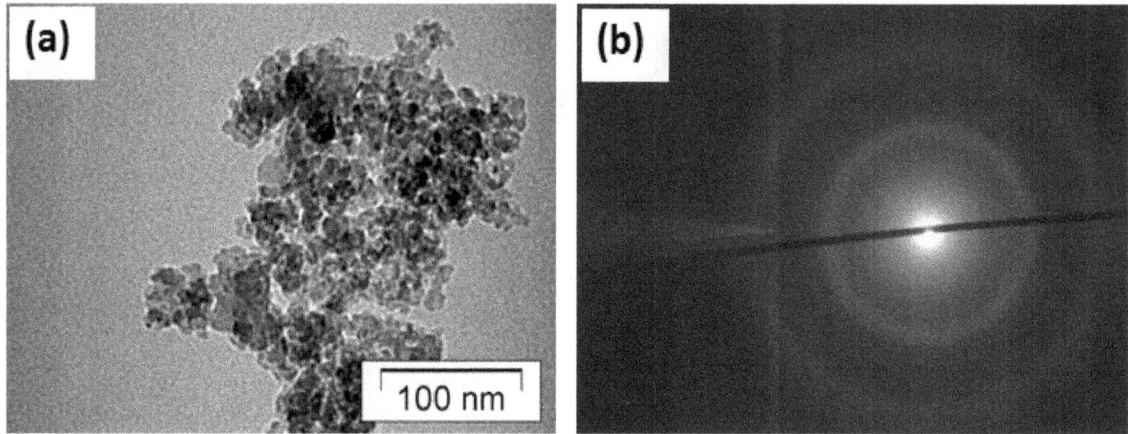

Figure 11: Transmission Electronic Micrographs of SiO_2-DA-20H_2O sample. (a) Taken at 80000 X, (b) X-Ray Diffraction at 120 KV and 900 mm.

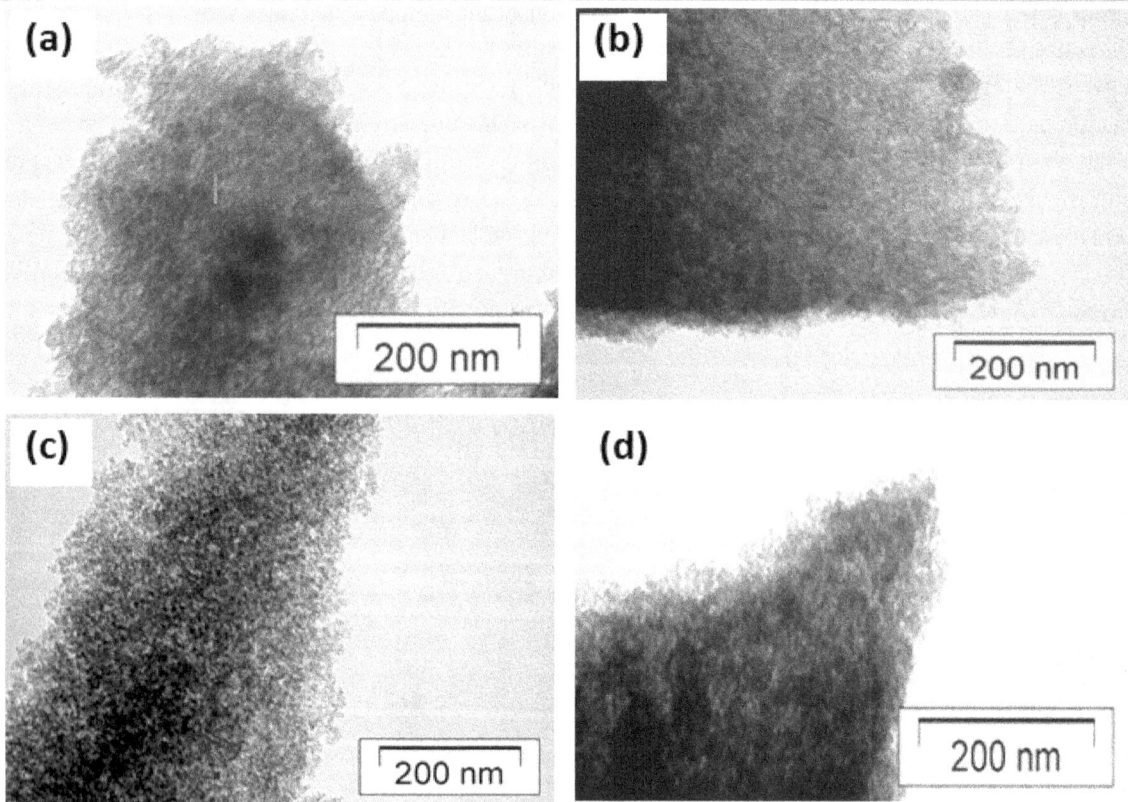

Figure 12: Transmission Electronic Micrographs of SiO_2-DA-40H_2O sample. (a)-(c) Were taken at 100000 X, and (d) Taken at 125000 X.

3.5   *In vitro* Release Test

In order to avoid the dopamine oxidation an acidic solution with pH=3 was used according with the suggests by Garcia *et al.* (Lugo-Huitrón *et al.*, 2011; Silva-Adaya *et al.*, 2011; Tobón-Velasco *et al.*, 2010). From Figure 13 is possible to observe that a sustained dopamine release in all samples occurs during the period in that the test was carried out. There was not a lineal effect of the r_{H2O} used on the release dopamine kinetic profiles. The dopamine molecules into the sample prepared with the smallest r_{H2O} were released slowly in the first hours, however, it sample released the largest amount of dopamine approximately a 95 % while the other two samples released approximately a 75 % of dopamine at the end of the test. We can explain dopamine release kinetic in terms of two factors: The pore size and the interactions between dopamine molecules and the superficial silanol groups ($\equiv$Si-OH) on silica.

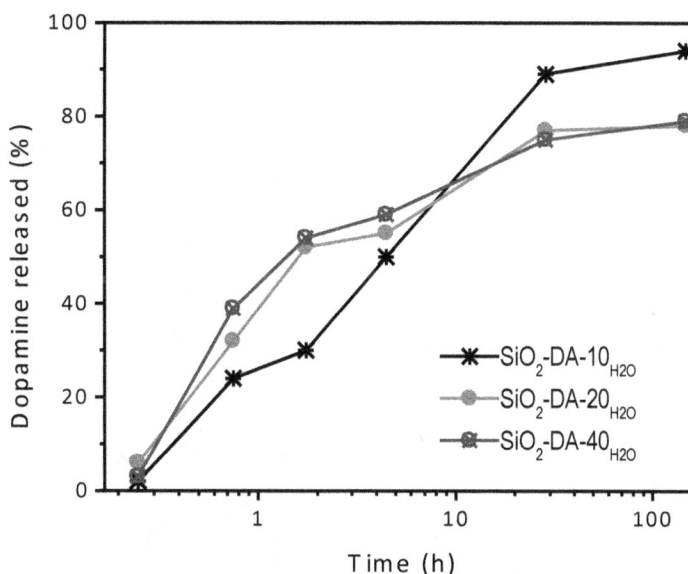

Figure 13: Dopamine release profiles from silica-dopamine materials prepared with different water concentrations.

It is well known that when silica is obtained by the sol-gel method its surface contains hydroxyl groups or silanol groups ($\equiv$Si-O-H) (López *et al.*, 2007, 2011a). This is one of the major advantages offered for this technique to prepared silica and used it as carrier of a variety of drugs due to its hydroxilated surface increases the chemical stability of the drug hosted in its network. In the literature has been reported that fully hydroxylated silica contains 4.6 OH/nm^2 and that this value can be considered as a physical constant for all existing types of silica (Mueller *et al.*, 2003). However is necessary to know others parameters that can be affecting the release of dopamine. Since silanol groups on silica can interact with hosted molecules, is important to control the surface nature of silica. In some works, the authors have mentioned that the degree of the metal oxide surface coverage with hydroxyl groups plays an important role in the strength of the drug-matrix interaction, therefore affecting the profile of the drug release (López *et al.*, 2001, 2010). In a previous work we have reported that dopamine forms weak hydrogen bonds with Si-OH groups of silica. From theoretical calculus was possible to determinate that these bonds can become preferably between N-H and O-H functional groups on dopamine and surface hydroxyl on silica (López *et al.*, 2011a).

On the other hand, the fundamental structural unit of pure silica is the tetrahedral SiO_4, in which a silicon atom is bonded to four oxygen atoms. However, octahedral unites can be formed (Luo *et al.*, 2004). In consequence the three-dimensional SiO_2 network consist of a random mixture of tetrahedral and octahedral unites. In the sol-gel process, during the early stages of hydrolysis and condensation of TEOS, those geometric unites are formed from the initially produced dimmers and trimmers which rapidly condense into siloxane (Si–O–Si) units (Yoshino *et al.*, 1990). The three-dimensional network is built upon by aggregation of the nanometric particles formed by condensation of those geometric unites as is shown in Figure 14. The formation of a high number of octahedral siloxanes allows the formation of larger primary particles due to the condensation is preferentially carried out. These big nanoparticles may form aggregates yielding a porous wet gel with larger pores with less surface OHs groups (Fidalgo & Ilharco, 2004). The final concentrations of terminal –OH depends the amount of water used during the hydrolysis and condensation of TEOS. If hydrolysis were not completed the xerogel could not contain a significant amount of silanol (Si–OH) groups on its surfaces.

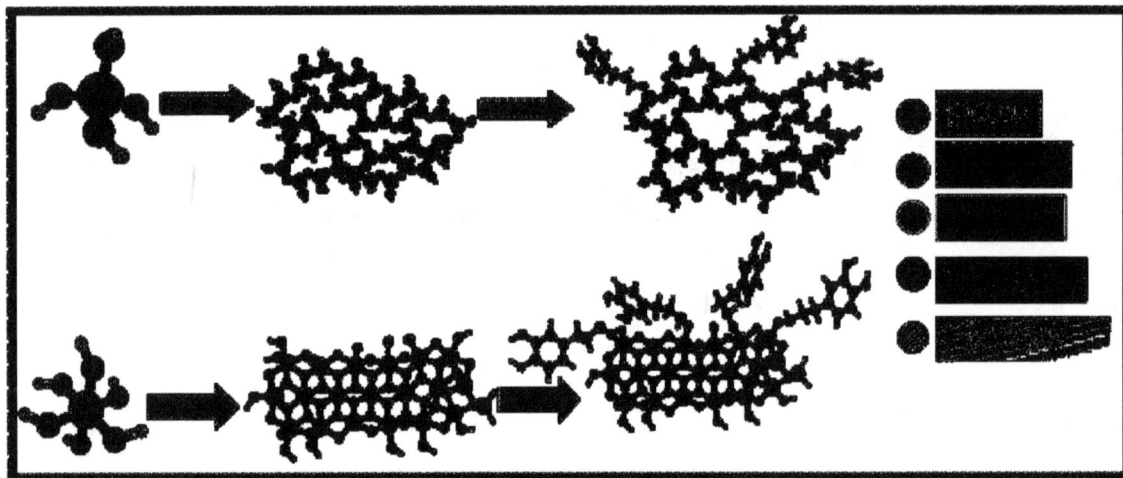

Figure 14: Schematic formation of tetrahedral and octahedral silica units, which make up the three-dimensional silica network. Schematic interactions between dopamine molecules and the silica's surface (silanol groups, ≡Si-OH) affect the dopamine release kinetic.

An increase on the r_{H2O} can lead to a high hydroxylation surface degree in consequence the interactions between the surface hydroxyl groups and dopamine should be increased. This increase in interactions should lead to a decrease in the rate of drug release (Figure 13). Under these ideas we can expect to the dopamine release should follow the increase order rate: $10r_{H2O} > 20r_{H2O} > 40r_{H2O}$. In the other hand, we can expect that with an increase in the pore size the dopamine release rate increase. Under this concept the dopamine release rate may be increased of the following way: $20r_{H2O} > 40r_{H2O} > 10r_{H2O}$. However, the dopamine released rate from the sample prepared with a $r_{H2O} = 10$ is slowly during the first hours due to it has the smallest pore sizes of all samples but it released a 94 % of dopamine at the end of the test. This behavior indicates the dopamine release kinetic is not governed by the interaction between dopamine and silica surface. The dopamine release kinetic is affected by the pore size in the sample. In the beginning the dopamine is released slowly because it occludes the pores but once them are free the dopamine is released fast. The sample with a $20r_{H2O}$ delivers dopamine faster in first hours because it has the highest pore size of all the samples, however at the end only a 75 % of dopamine was released. It is might due to the interaction drug-silica are increased causing a decrease in the amount of released dopamine. The samples prepared with a $40r_{H2O}$ delivers dopamine faster than the other two samples at the first hours of the test due to it has the intermediate value of pore size. After that the dopamine release is slowly because the dopamine-silica interactions are increased.

The values obtained for the dopamine release were adjusted to different models to establish the mechanism and the kinetics of the dopamine release. The criteria followed for the selection of the most appropriate kinetic model was based on the least squares adjustment approach of the *ln* of remaining drug as a function of time (Figure 15).

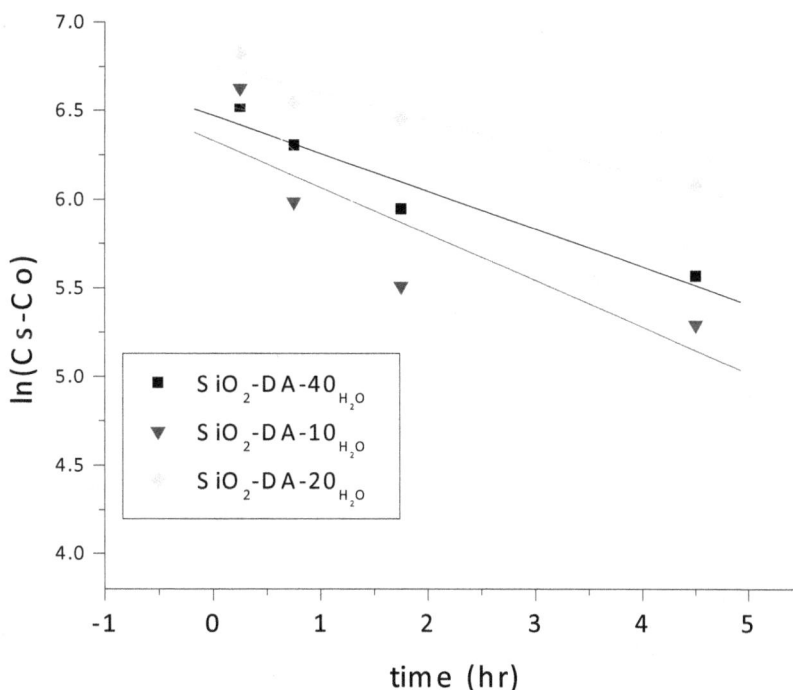

Figure 15: Noyes-Whitney equation fit to the dopamine release profiles of the different SiO_2-DA materials. This equation gives the rate of dissolution of a drug through a solid.

Higuchi´s model was selected and the results of the constant K from the modified Noyes-Whitney equation were obtained. This equation gives the rate of dissolution of a drug through a solid. It is assumed that there is a "stagnant layer" of liquid in immediate contact with the solid that is dissolving. The thickness of the stagnant layer is believed to be constant. There exists a concentration gradient within this layer or film and decreases as one move from the surface of the solid to the bulk. Table 4 includes the liberation constant K for the three samples; greater values of K, corresponding with variations in the slope, are indicative of a greater release rate.

4   Conclusions

SiO$_2$-DA materials were prepared by the variation of the r$_{H2O}$ and studied as drug release systems. Dopamine molecules were stabilized into the silica network when it was prepared by the sol-gel method varying the r$_{H2O}$ during the hydrolysis of TEOS. The materials had different textural properties each other; however, there was not a direct correlation between the increase on r$_{H2O}$ and the textural properties and dopamine release. Both the surface hydroxyl groups present on silica, and pore size, had an influence on the dopamine release kinetics. The formationof superficial ≡Si-OH groups and their interactions with dopamine molecules cause a slow dopamine release.

Acknowledgment

We would like to thank the ICyTDF for its financial support with the project number PCIDS08-12. We also thank Liliana Schifter for technical support.

References

Andén, N.E., Carlsson, A., Dahlstrom, A., Fuxe, K., Hillarp, N., Larsson, K. (1964). Demonstration and mapping out of nigro-neostriatal dopamine neurons. Life Sci.; 3:523-530.

Barrett, E.P., Joyner, L.G., Jalenda, P.P. (1951). TheDetermination of Pore Volume and Area Distributions in Porous Substances. I. Computations from Nitrogen Isotherms. J. Am. Chem. Soc. 73 373-380.

Benson, D.L., Colman, D.R., Huntley, G.W. (2001). Molecules, Maps and Synapse Specificity. Nature reviews. Neuroscience. 2: 899-909.

Bisaglia, M., Mammi, S., Bubacco, L. (2007). Kinetic and structural analysis of the early oxidation products of dopamine: analysis of the interactions with alpha-synuclein. J. of Biol. Chem.;282:15597-15605.

Brunauer, S., Deming, L.S., Deming, W.S., Teller, E. (1940). On a theory of the van der Waals adsorption of gases. J Am Chem Soc.; 62:1723-1732.

Brunauer, S., Emmett, P.H., Teller, E. (1938). Adsorption of Gases in Multimolecular Layers.J. Am. Chem. Soc.; 60:309-319.

Burch, D., Sheerin, F. (2005). Parkinson's disease. Lancet.; 365:622–627.

Chand, P., Litvan, I. (2007). Encyclopedia of Gerontology. Elsevier.

Chen, H., Zhang, S.M., Hernan, M.A., Willett, W.C., Ascherio, A. (2002). Diet and Parkinson's disease: a potential role of dairy products in men. Ann Neurol.; 52:793–801.

De Rijk, M.C., Tzourio, C., Breteler, M.M.B., Dartigues, J.F., Amaducci, L., Lopez-Pousa, S., Manubens-Bertran, J.M., Alperovitch, A., et al. (1997). Prevalence of parkinsonism and Parkinson's disease in Europe: the EUROPARKINSON collaborative study. J Neurol Neurosurg Psychiatry; 62:10–15.

Fidalgo, A., Ilharco, L.M. (2004). Correlation between physical properties and structure of silica xerogels . J. of Non-Cryst.Solids.; 347:128-137.

Freed, W.J., Karoum, F., Spoor, H.E., Morihisa, J.M., Olson, L., Wyatt, R.J. (1938). Catecholamine content of intercerebral adrenal grafts. Brain Research; 269:184-189.

García-Escrig, M., Bermejo-Pareja, F. (1999). Complicaciones motoras del tratamiento con levodopa en la enfermedad de Parkinson. Rev Neurol; 28:799–809.

Hellenbrand, W., Seidler, A., Boeing, H., Robra, B.P., Vieregge, P., Nischan, P., Joerg, J., Oertel, W.H., Schneider, E., Ulm, G. (1996). Diet and Parkinson's disease I: a possible role for the past intake of specific foods and food groups. Results from a self-administered food frequency questionnaire in a case-control study. Neurology; 47:636–43.

Hely, M.A., Morris, J.G., Reid, W.G., O'Sullivan, D.J., Williamson, P.M., Rail, D. (1994). The Sydney multicentre study of Parkinson's disease: A randomized, prospective 5 years study comparing low dose bromocriptine with low dose levodopa-carbidopa. J Neurol Neurosurg Psychiatr; 57:903–910.

Hernan, M.A., Takkouche, B., Caamano-Isorna, F., Gestal-Otero, J.J. (2002). A meta-analysis of coffee drinking, cigarette smoking, and the risk of Parkinson's disease. Ann Neurol; 52:276–84.

Horstink, M.W.I.M. (1984). Problems of levodopa treatment. Clin.Neurol, Neurosurg; 86:196-206.

Hwang, Y., Oh, C., Oh, S. (2005). Controlled release of retinol from silica particles prepared in O/W/O emulsion: The effect of surfactants and polymers. J. of Controlled Release;106 (3): 339-349.

Innocenzi, P. (2003). Infrared spectroscopy of sol–gel derived silica-based films: a spectra-microstructure overview. Journal of Non-Crystalline Solids; 316:309–319.

Khedr, E.M., Attar, G.S., Kandil, M.R., Kamel, N.F., Elfetoh, N.A., Ahmed, M.A. (2012). Assiut Governorate, Egypt: A community-Based Study. Neuroepidemiology; 38(3):154-163.

Logroscino, G., Marder, K., Cote, L., Tang, M–X, Shea, S., Mayeux, R. (1996). Dietary lipids and antioxidants in Parkinson's disease: a population-based case-control study. Ann Neurol; 39:89–94.

López, T., Bata-García, J.L., Esquivel, D., Ortiz-Islas, E., Gonzalez, R., Ascencio, J., Quintana, P., et al. (2011a). Treatment of Parkinson's disease: nanostructured sol–gel silica–dopamine reservoirs for controlled drug release in the central nervous system. International Journal of Nanomedicine; 6:19–31.

López, T., Espinoza, K.A., Kozina, A., Castillo, P., Silvestre-Albero, A., Rodriguez-Reinoso, F. et al. (2001). Langmuir; 27:4004.

López, T., Ortiz, E., Alexander-Katz, R., Odriozola, J.A., Quintana, P., Gonzalez, R.D., Lottici, P.P. et al. (2010). The Effect of Water on Particle Size, Porosity and the Rate of Drug Release From Implanted Titania Reservoirs. Journal of biomedical materials research part B: Applied Biomaterials; 93:401-406.

López, T., Ortiz, E., Meza, D., Basaldella, E., Bokhimi, X., Magaña, C., Sepulveda, C., Rodriguez, F., et al (2011b). Controlled release of phenytoin for epilepsy treatment from titania and silica based materials. Materials Chemistry and Physics. 2011; 126:922–929.

López, T., Quintana, P., Martínez, J.M., Esquivel, D. (2007). Stabilization of dopamine in nanosilica sol-gel matrix to be used as a controlled drug delivery system. Journal of Non-Crystalline Solids, 353, 8.

Lugo-Huitrón, R., Blanco-Ayala, T., Ugalde-Muñiz, P., Carrillo-Mora, P., Pedraza-Chaverrí, J., Silva-Adaya, D., et al. (2011). On the antioxidant properties of kynurenic acid: free radical scavenging activity and inhibition of oxidative stress. Neurotoxicol Teratology; 5:538-47.

Luo, L.N., Tschauner, O., Asimow, P.D., Ahrens, T.J. (2004). A new dense silica polymorph: A possible link between tetrahedrally and octahedrally coordinated silica. American Mineralogist; 89: 455–461.

Marder, K., Tang, M.X., Mejia, H., Alfaro, B., Cote, L., Louis, E., Groves, J., Mayeus, R. (1996). Risk of Parkinson's disease among first degree relatives: a community-based study. Neurology; 47:155–60.

Marsden, C.D., Parkes, J.D., Quinn, N. (1981). Fluctuations in disability in Parkinson's disease–clinical aspects. In: Marsden CD, Fahn S, editors. Movement Disorders. London: Butterworths.

Mueller, R., Kammler, H.K., Wegner, K., Pratsinis, S.E. (2003). Langmuir; 19:160.

Parkinson, J. (1817). An essay on the shaking palsy. Whittingham and Rowland for Sherwood, Needly

Pfeiffer, R.F. (2007). Non-motor parkinsonism. Parkinsonism Relat Disord; 13:S211–S220.

Sesack, S.R., Grace, A.A. (2010). Cortico-Basal Ganglia Reward Network: Microcircuitry. Neuropsychopharmacology;35(1): 27–47.

Silva-Adaya, D., Pérez-De La Cruz, V., Villeda-Hernández, J., Carrillo-Mora, P., González-Herrera, I.G., et al. (2011). Protective effect of L-kynurenine and probenecid on 6-hydroxydopamine-induced striatal toxicity in rats: implications of modulating kynurenate as a protective strategy Neurotoxicology and Teratology; 33:303-312.

Sing, K.S.W., Everett, D.H., Haul, R.A.W., Moscou, L., Pierotti, R.A., Rouquerol, J., Siemieniewska, T. (1985). Reporting physisorption data for gas/solid systems with Special Reference to the Determination of Surface Area and Porosity. Pure & Appl. Chem.; 57(4): 603-619.

Smythies, J., Galzigna, L. (1998). The Oxidative Metabolism of Catecholamines in the Brain: A Review. Biochimica Et Biophysica Acta.; 1380: 159-162.

Tang, Q., Xu, Y., Wu, D., Sun, Y. (2006). A study of carboxylic-modified mesoporous silica in controlled delivery for drug famotidine. J. of Solid State Chem; 179:1513-1520.

Tobón-Velasco, J.C., Silva-Adaya, D., Carmona-Aparicio, L., García, E., Galván-Arzate, S., Santamaría, A. (2010). The early effect of 6-hydroxydopamine on extracellular concentrations of neurotransmitters in the rat striatum: An in vivo microdialysis study. Neurotoxicology; 31:715-723.

Yoshino, H., Kamiya, K., Nasu, H. (1990). IR study on the structural evolution of sol-gel derived SiO$_2$ gels in the early stage of conversion to glasses. Journal of Non-Crystalline Solids; 126:68-78.

Zhang, S.M., Hernan, M.A., Chen, H., Spiegelman, D., Willett, W.C., Ascherio, A. (2002). Intakes of vitamins E and C, carotenoids, vitamin supplements, and PD risk. Neurology; 59:1161–9.

Zhang, Z., Roman, G. (1993). Worldwide occurrence of Parkinson's disease: an updated review. Neuroepidemiology; 12:195–208.

Industrial Food Process Water: Quality and Reuse Opportunities for Biorefinery Purposes

Kornsulee Ratanapariyanuch
Food and Bioproduct Sciences
University of Saskatchewan, Canada

Youn Young Shim
Plant Sciences
University of Saskatchewan, Canada

Robert T. Tyler
Food and Bioproduct Sciences
University of Saskatchewan, Canada

Martin J.T. Reaney
Plant Sciences
University of Saskatchewan, Canada

1   Introduction

Water is important for life (Leiknes, 2009). Population growth, improved living standards, climate change, increased industrialization, intensification of agriculture and urbanization have increased the demand for water. The United Nation predicted that by 2050 approximately 2-7 billion people would face chronic water shortages (Population Reference Bureau, 2012; Verstraete *et al.*, 2009). Water is a major resource for industrial processes and wastewater is an undesirable product of many industries. Industrial water consumption may create serious impacts on all water consumers as a wide variety of potentially toxic pollutants in the wastewater may not receive proper treatment before it is discarded (Gavrilescu *et al.*, 2008). Water consumers and natural water sources may be protected from the negative impacts of wastewater contamination by the logical use of water (Leiknes, 2009). In many jurisdictions, companies are compelled by regulations and cost constraints to decrease the quantity and environmental effects of their liquid waste. While treating liquid waste is a common approach, recycling or reuse of water with little treatment may be a strategy to preserve water and decrease the impact of water use (Kentish & Stevens, 2001).

2   Water and Industry

2.1   Current Uses of Water in Industry

Industries that produce metal, wood and paper products, chemicals, fuels, etc. rely on water resources. The properties of water, including its heat capacity and heat of vaporization (for cooling and heating), density and viscosity (for floating and sedimentation), chemical solvation and reactivity (for dissolving materials and in catalysis), and biocompatibility (for fermentation and nutrition), will be discussed.

2.1.1   Heat Transfer

Water is used as a medium for the transfer of heat energy in the form of steam or liquid water (Resource Dynamics Corporation, 2003). Steam is widely used to transfer energy from the source of its generation, i.e. a boiler, to the site of its use (Ellis *et al.*, 2012). Steam is used to drive machinery, for reactor heating and direct use, in low-temperature furnace heating ($\leq 800°C$), in the petroleum industry for distillation, desulfurization, alkylation and hydrogen production, and in major metal industries (Ellis *et al.*, 2012). In food processing, steam is utilized for cooking, sterilization, blanching, pasteurization and dehydration. Low-pressure steam has a number of applications in the pulp and paper industry. For many industrial chemical-manufacturing processes, liquid water is used as a coolant. Water is utilized to cool cooked meats (Wang & Sun, 2002) and fresh vegetables may be blanched using hot water (Wang & Sun, 2003).

2.1.2   Process Solutions

Water is used in process solutions for flotation, sedimentation, dispersion or dissolution. Singh *et al.* (1999) studied the recovery of fiber in a dry-grind corn ethanol process by flotation. Fiber flotation was optimized when the specific gravity of the solution was 1.090-1.098 (12-13 Bé). At this density, endosperm particles and coarse fiber were readily separated. Other valuable products, including corn fiber, corn oil and corn fiber gum could be extracted from the corn fiber fraction after separation (Singh *et al.*, 1999). Water is also utilized in the dissolution of material. Photographic products require a cross-linked gelatin matrix which can be prepared by dissolving swelled gelatin in water at 35°C (Keenan, 2003). Weiss (1997) noted that water could be used in the paint and coatings industries as a medium to disperse an alkyd resin, as the main volatile liquid component, as a viscosity reducer, and as a binder/dissolver in the formation of true solutions.

2.1.3   Catalytic Solutions

By definition, a catalyst is a compound or material that increases the rate of a reaction but is not consumed during the course of the reaction (Seager & Slabaugh, 2010). Catalysts are classified as being either homogeneous (catalyst dissolves in the reaction mixture) or heterogeneous (catalyst separates into its own phase) (Wijingaarden et al., 1998). Water is used to dissolve many homogeneous catalysts. According to Manabe et al. (2001), water is considered a good medium in lieu of organic solvents in organic reactions, as it is inexpensive, safe and environmentally friendly. In addition, water may provide reactivity that may not easily achieved in other media (Li & Chen, 2006). For these reasons, several studies of catalysis have been conducted in water and largely aqueous solutions. Lewis acid-surfactant-combined catalysts (LASCs), such as scandium tris(dodecyl sulfate) $Sc(DS)_3$, were developed as combined catalysts and surfactants for the synthesis of β-amino carbonyl compounds, which are versatile synthetic intermediates in the manufacture of pharmaceuticals and other products in water (Manabe et al., 2001). Amides produced by the hydration of nitriles may be utilized as intermediates and reagents in the production of plastics, detergents, lubricants, etc. Acrylamide may be produced by quantitative hydration of acrylonitrile in water using a ruthenium hydroxide catalyst ($Ru(OH)x/Al_2O_3$) (Li & Chen, 2006).

2.1.4   Fermentation

Fermentation of biomass with living organisms requires water. Preparation of maize for ethanol production often begins with wet milling, a technique that enables both the separation of grain constituents and the production of a starch-rich fermentation broth (Kohl, 2009). Wet milling yields a variety of primary products, including starch, corn gluten meal and feed, and corn germ from which corn oil and corn germ meal are extracted. In the initial steps of wet milling, the grain is cleaned and transferred to steep tanks, to which water is then added for the purpose of hydrating the grain. Additional fresh water is later added to the partially steeped grain. After use, a portion of the steep water is added to the incoming grain, and the rest, since it contains dissolved and suspended grain components, may be evaporated and sold as a nutrient source, either directly or after addition to other by-product streams. After steeping, the seed is ground to enable germ separation, germ washing and fibre removal, in that order. Each process step involves additional water use. Water is also required in processes that ready the fermentation broth for inoculation. These include mashing, cooking and liquefaction (Ingledew et al., 2009). Yeast are propagated separately by inoculation of active dry yeast into liquefied mash to increase the yeast cell mass, before pumping the yeast suspension into a fermentation tank (Bellissimi & Richards, 2009) containing the liquefied fermentation mash. Water is used extensively in the fermentation of maize.

2.1.5   Fertilizer Production

Water is employed in the production of fertilizer. Ammonia is a reagent used to produce urea, ammonium nitrate and ammonium sulfate fertilizers. Ammonia is manufactured by contacting nitrogen gas at high pressure and temperature with an iron catalyst. Ammonia synthesis is a reversible reaction that utilizes a condensation step to separate the product, ammonia, from unreacted nitrogen gas (Ahlgren et al., 2008).

The ammonium industry requires large volumes of steam for ammonia production and cooling water for ammonia condensation (Goodman, 1999). Nitric oxide is produced as a precursor of nitric acid by the exothermic reaction of ammonia and air over a noble metal catalyst, typically platinum rhodium. Water is utilized to absorb the nitric oxide gas produced by this reaction. Nitric acid solution and ammonia may then be reacted to produce ammonium nitrate solution in an exothermic reaction. The water in the solution may be evaporated to afford ammonium nitrate (Ahlgren et al., 2008). Phosphate fertilizer production also requires water. Phosphate rock is slurried with sulfuric acid in the presence of water (Pérez-López et al., 2007). Twenty moles of water are consumed for the production of six moles of phosphoric acid.

2.2   Water Consumption by Industry

It has been reported that 20% of global water is utilized by industry (Gavrilescu et al., 2008) and that industrial water consumption is increasing (Schroeder, 2012). World annual industrial water consumption was expected to increase from 156.9 km^3 in 1995 to 235.7 km^3 in 2025 (Rosegrant & Cai, 2002). For example, Canadian manufacturing industries had a total water intake of 3,806.2 million m^3 in 2009. Paper production consumed the most water (41.9%) followed by primary metal production (27.7%), chemical production (8.8%), food production (8.7%), and petroleum and coal processing (7.9%). These manufacturers and processors produced 3,450.6 million m^3 of wastewater, with paper industries accounting for the largest percentage (45.2%) followed by primary metal production at 26.4% and petroleum and coal industries at 7.9%; 75.1 and 11.0% of the wastewater was released to surface freshwater and tidewater, respectively (figures represent only high-level-treated wastewater) (Statistics Canada, 2012).

2.2.1   Ethanol Production

Yeast-based fermentation of grain to ethanol utilizes water in processes that include wet milling, mashing, cooking and liquefaction. According to the Renewable Fuels Association (2012), world ethanol production reached approximately 85.2 billion L by the end of 2012. Very high gravity fermentation with normal active dry yeast can be achieved in the laboratory, yielding an ethanol concentration of 23.8% (v/v) (Ingledew, 2009). It was estimated that 21 m^3 water was utilized to mill 1 ton of sugarcane with annex distillery (Macedo, 2005). Scholten (2009) reported that the average global total water footprint of ethanol production was 2,855, 1,355 and 1,004 L of water/L of ethanol produced when using sugar cane, sugar beet and maize, respectively. The production of one L of ethanol by dry and wet milling processes using maize as a raw material consumes 3.45 and 3.92 L of fresh water, respectively (Wu, 2008). Therefore, 464 billion L of water would be utilized to produce 116 billion L of ethanol by the wet mill process.

2.2.2   Vegetable Oil Refining

Vegetable oil production and refining consumes a considerable amount of water. Whereas vegetable oil is extracted from seed in a process that utilizes steam but little other process water, oil refining requires considerably more water. Refining crude oil is necessary in order to remove minor lipids such as free fatty acids, monoglycerides, phospholipids, lipid-soluble off-flavors, carotenoids and non-lipid materials from the triglycerides. Refining consists of degumming, neutralization, bleaching and deodorization processes. Degumming uses water and acid to remove phospholipids. Degumming involves contacting filtered oil with water (1-3%) at 60-80°C (McClements & Decker, 2008) to agglomerate hydratable phospholipids into a separable gum phase (Čmolík & Pokorný, 2000). The global production of vegetable oil increased to 154.3 million tons in 2012 (United States Department of Agriculture, 2012). Therefore, it would take 1.55-4.63 million tons of water for the degumming of vegetable oil. Similar amounts of water are used in alkali refining where an NaOH and water solution is mixed with the oil to remove free fatty acids. After acid and alkali refining, the oil is washed with water to prevent hydrolysis of triglycerides.

2.2.3   Barley Malting

The purpose of malting barley is to release the enzymes α- and β- amylase (Collicutt, 2009) during controlled germination. The enzymes convert seed carbohydrates to fermentable sugars (Petters *et al.*, 1988). In the malting process, barley is submerged in warm water and a supply of oxygen until the grain moisture content reaches 43-47% in a process called steeping. Typically, the water is drained periodically during steeping to increase the availability of oxygen. After steeping, the water is drained and the seed is germinated at 13.0-16.5°C for 5-6 days. After germination has maximized the hydrolysis of grain starch, the malt is dried at 50-70°C for up to 24 h in a process called kilning. Finally, the malt is heated briefly to reduce the moisture content to 3-4% (Petters *et al.*, 1988). The steeping process requires the use of 4.5-5.0 m^3 of water per ton of malt produced. This yields approximately 3.0-3.3 m^3 of wastewater per ton (EUREKA SWAN, 2012). Global barley malt production between 2011 and 2012 was 6.4 million tons (FAO, 2007); therefore, 28.8-32.0 billion L of water was needed for the malting process.

2.2.4   Starch Production

Corn, wheat, and potato are the primary starch products of the U.S. (Murray *et al.*, 1994).

2.2.4.1   Corn Starch Production

Corn is taken through a wet milling process to produce a starch slurry. The starch slurry is then passed through a hydrocyclone (hydroclone) separator to remove the lighter germ. Hulls, gluten, and starch components that remain suspended are sent to an additional series of grinding and screening processes. The hulls are then removed using screens. After hull removal, gluten and starch are separated by centrifugation following by washing and dewatering using by filtration or centrifugation (Murray *et al.*, 1994).

2.2.4.2   Wheat Starch Production

Commercial wheat starch production begins with dry milling of wheat to produce flour. Water is then applied to form a stiff dough from wheat flour. While the dough is rolled or kneaded over a screen, a water spray is applied to wash the starch and soluble from the dough, yielding gluten, which is then dried. Insoluble and soluble impurities are removed from the starch slurry by screening, centrifugation and washing. The purified starch suspension is then dried (Murray *et al.*, 1994).

2.2.4.3   Potato Starch Production

Stones and dirt are removed from potatoes by running water flumes. Potatoes are then taken through a washer for rigorous cleaning. The cleaned potatoes are ground or crushed to disintegrate the potato cells and free the starch grains. Fiber and potato skins are separated from the starch using a screen or rotary sieve. The starch slurry is then filtered and redispersed in water. The starch slurry passes through a settling step to remove insoluble impurities. Finally, starch is dewatered and dried (Murray *et al.*, 1994). It has been reported that potato starch production utilizes 0.3-0.5 m^3 of water/ton of potatoes (new washing system) to wash the potatoes and 0.4-0.5 m^3 of water/ton of processed potatoes is required for subsequent extraction and refining of starch (Bergthaller *et al.*, 1999). Jose (2010) stated that the starch market could reach 80 million tons in 2015. This increase in starch production will also increase water consumption.

2.2.5   Plant Protein Isolate Production

The combination of growth of the global population and increases in affluence has increased the demand for high quality food protein, especially meat, milk and eggs. Increases in production will be required to fulfill the increasing demand for protein. Therefore, plant protein resources, including vegetable and cereal sources, will be required to meet demand. It has been predicted that the supply of vegetable protein must be doubled while the supply of animal-based protein needs to quadruple to maintain human nutrition levels in the next decade (Xu & Diosady, 2003). Production of 1 kg of animal protein requires about 100 times more water than producing the same amount of plant protein (Pimentel & Pimentel, 2003). Therefore, it can be concluded that world plant protein production will be increased. According to Fauconneau (1983), world plant protein consumption was 44.8 g/day per person in 1977. The global population surpassed 7 billion in 2012, and now over 320,000 tons of plant protein is consumed daily. Water is used as a solvent for food component extraction and separation (Aguilera, 2003) and is particularly useful for separation of protein from other constituents (Sumner *et al.*, 1981). Protein solubility is an equilibrium process where protein-protein and protein-solvent interactions determine the amount of protein dissolved in water (Damodaran, 2008). There are several methods to produce plant protein isolates. Protein may be extracted in an alkaline solution followed by precipitation at the isoelectric point. The precipitated protein isolate is obtained by washing followed by spray drying. Neutralizing the precipitate prior to drying produces a more stable isolate, i.e. a sodium proteinate. Ultrafiltration and reverse osmosis are alternative methods for protein isolate production. Protein isolates have also been extracted in sodium chloride solution (salting in) and subsequently precipitated by dilution with additional water (Sumner at al., 1981). The optimum ratio of solid to liquid used for industrial protein production ranged from 1:10 to 1:20 (Berk, 1992). After protein extraction, water may also be utilized for protein isolation. According to Milanova *et al.* (2006), 15-fold (v/v) of chilled water was utilized to form a discrete protein (micelle) in the aqueous phase. The protein micelle was allowed to settle to form an amorphous, gelatinous, protein micelle mass. Based on the information above, it is clear that protein isolation processes consume large quantities of water.

2.2.6   Juice Production

In 2005, based on data from major juice and nectar consuming countries (U.S., Germany, Russia, China, United Kingdom, France, Japan, Canada, Spain and Mexico), approximately 21,725 million L of juices and nectars were consumed (Ashurst, 2007).

2.2.6.1   Citrus Juice Extraction

Citrus fruit is washed with water prior to juice extraction. There are two main types of citrus juice extractors used commonly by the citrus juice industry, the FMC extractor and the Brown extractor.

2.2.6.1.1   FMC Extractor

A hole is cut in the fruit and the juice and flesh are squeezed out (Höhn *et al.*, 2005). During juice extraction, peel oil is washed away with a water spray, yielding an oil-water emulsion. Water is then separated from the oil via a two-step centrifugation (Ashurst, 2007).

2.2.6.1.2   Brown Extractor

A stationary knife is used to cut the fruit in half (Ashurst, 2007) followed by reaming process to extract the juice and flesh from the fruit (Höhn *et al.*, 2005). Prior to juice extraction, peel oil is removed and recovered in a separate step by pricking the peel of whole fruit with needle-sharp spikes to release the oil. Water is utilized to wash the oil and recover it as an oil-water emulsion (Ashurst, 2007). After citrus juice extraction, the juice is forced through the screen by a screw action to remove the larger pulp particles. Washing and finishing the pulp separation are performed several times to produce a juice solution. The yield of juice can be increased be adding the juice solution to the juice (Ashurst, 2007). Based on the information above, wastewater is produced in juice production by washing fruit, cleaning machines and oil recovery.

2.2.6.2   Soft Fruit Processing

Fruits are washed and then go through a diversity of processes to release the juice depending on fruit structure, the clarity needed in the final product, enzymatic discoloration and destruction of pectin. Light crushing is utilized to break the fruit and release the juice in soft fruits. Milling and pressing cannot release juice from some types of fruit due to their cell structure. In such cases, breaking the cell structure and degrading pectin in the juice is accomplished by addition of a commercial pectolytic enzyme to improve extraction efficiency. The fruit pulp is then pressed to obtain the juice. In order to improve juice yield, water is added to the press cake, which is then repressed (Ashurst, 2007). After extraction, heating with steam or hot water in a heat exchanger pasteurizes the juice. Heated juice is then usually cooled with a heat exchanger using chilled water. In the case of hot container filling, the containers must be cooled immediately after pasteurization. A hot water spray may be utilized for preheating and pasteurizing, followed by cooling with a cool water spray (Ashurst, 2007). Both fruit juice and concentrated juice are available in the market. According to Ashurst (2007), steam is utilized to provide the heat to concentrate the juice. From the soft juice process, wastewater can arise from washing fruits, cleaning the machines, preheating, pasteurization and cooling after pasteurization.

2.3   Water from Natural Sources and Industrial Wastewater

Water from natural sources and industrial wastewater contains microorganisms, ionic solutes, organic materials, etc. Lactic acid bacteria, acetic acid bacteria, molds and/or anaerobic bacteria are present in liquid waste from the ethanol industry (Wheals *et al.*, 1999; Ratanapariyanuch *et al.*, 2011). In addition to microorganisms, liquid waste from fermentation contains organic compounds such as fatty acids (Frenkel, 2010). Aconitic and lactic acids were present in liquid waste from the sugar cane industry (Malmary *et al.*, 2000). Cheese production yields a whey co-product (liquid remaining after casein precipitation and removal) representing 85-90% of the milk volume and which contains a high organic matter content demonstrating chemical oxygen demand (COD) of 60,000-80,000 ppm (Athanasiadis *et al.*, 2002). Ratanapariyanuch and her co-workers (2011) discovered that wheat-based thin stillage contained several organic compounds, including isopropanol, lactic acid, 1,3-propanediol, acetic acid, succinic acid, glycerolphosphorylcholine (GPC), betaine phosphate, glycerol and 2-phenylethanol. In addition, thin stillage also contained protein and carbohydrate (dextrin, maltotriose and maltose monohydrate). According to Kentish and Stevens (2001), metals, including heavy metals, cations and anions, can be found in industrial wastewater. The heavy metals include zinc, cadmium, chromium and copper. Alkaline metals present in wastewater include sodium and potassium. They also mentioned that negatively-charged multivalent anions and monovalent salts were present in wastewater from the dairy, tanning, sugar and textile industries. The above information above shows that effluent from industry contains a number of contaminants and microorganisms. Therefore, the processing is required to remove these contaminants and microorganisms before wastewater is reused or discarded.

2.4   Wastewater Purification

Wastewater from industry has to be treated or purified prior to reuse or discard. Before treatment, biochemical oxygen demand (BOD) and COD should be measured. BOD is the quantity of oxygen (mg/L or ppm) that bacteria utilize from the water to oxidize organic matter (Hach *et al.*, 1997) whereas COD is "a measure of the oxygen equivalent of the organic matter content of a sample that is susceptible to oxidation by a strong chemical oxidant" (Boyles, 1997). In addition, total soluble solids should also be determined. Several processes, including sedimentation, flocculation, membrane techniques (microfiltration, ultrafiltration and reverse osmosis) and deionization may be used to remove bacteria, organic materials and ionic solutes. According to United States Environmental Protection Agency (2004), wastewater treatment involves several steps that can be divided into primary treatment and secondary/advanced treatment.

2.4.1   Primary Treatment

Debris and solids are removed by passing the wastewater through a screen. The remaining solids that are heavier than water can be removed from wastewater by sedimentation (United States Environmental Protection Agency, 2004).

2.4.1.1   Sedimentation

When particulate waste and the surrounding water have different densities, sedimentation occurs. Waste particulates sink when the specific gravity of particulates due to gravitational force without other disturbing influences is greater than 1. Particle surface dimensions and specific weight and flow velocity of the surrounding water are key to the settling velocity of suspended solids. The efficiency of sedimentation can be increased by decreasing flow velocity, increasing retention time in a sedimentation pond, shortening sedimentation distance and increasing the specific size and weight of particles (Sindilariu, 2007). However, Brostow and his co-workers (2009) stated that sedimentation by gravity alone would not succeed if the fine particles have diameters less than approximately 10 μm. Wastewater passes through a sedimentation tank with a low flow rate such that suspended solids sink to the bottom of the tank. Solids at the bottom are removed continuously or at intervals depending on the design of the system (González, 1996). The aqueous solution after primary treatment will be processed further during advanced treatment. Wastewater from the fishery industry contains fish scales, portions of fish muscle and offal (González, 1996). Primary treatment by sedimentation eliminates floatable and setting solids. The sedimentation process depends on the properties of the solids.

1. Discrete settling: If interactions between particles do not occur and wastewater is quite dilute.

2. Flocculent settling: If coalescence or flocculation of particles increases particle mass the settling rate increases.

3. Zone settling: If adherence of particles forms a separating interface with the liquid, zone settling occurs.

In some fishery processes, the amount of grease and oil may be too high. To separate oil and grease from wastewater, the emulsion must be broken. Therefore, heat may be applied using steam following the gravity separator. To remove oil and grease and suspended solids, a flotation technique using dissolved air flotation is applied.

2.4.2   Advanced Treatment

2.4.2.1   Flocculation

Particles have charged structures called Stern and Gouy-Chapman layers. The Stern layer is located at the particle surface and attracts a dispersed layer of oppositely-charged free ions (the Gouy-Chapman layer). The Stern layer has to be overcome in order for particles to make contact and aggregate. To overcome the potential energy at the Stern layer, enough kinetic energy must be provided to the particles. Subsequently, the dispersion stability to flocculate occurs. Furthermore, to eliminate the barrier a surface charge neutralization mechanism (double layer compression) and a bridge mechanism (adsorption of the flocculation onto the surface of particle) are involved (Tripathy & Ranjan De, 2006). Both inorganic and organic flocculants are used. Among the inorganic flocculants, salts of multivalent metals such as aluminum and iron are applied most often and at high concentrations. Synthetic flocculants are broadly divided into anionic, cationic and non-ionic categories. The quantity of organic flocculant used is usually much less than for inorganic flocculants. Several applications of flocculants in effluent treatment have been reported. They can be used to remove suspended solids, which cause turbidity in industry process water by gravity separation and flotation processes. Flocculants are used for water treatment in paper making processes. In order to provide opacity and whiteness to paper, clays, titanium dioxide, calcium carbonate, etc. are utilized as fillers. However, fine fiber loss may occur during drainage. Therefore, a reduction in the loss of valuable filler and fine fiber is achieved by adding flocculants, e.g. alum or cationic polymers (cationic starch, etc.) to neutralize the negative charge on paper fibers (Brostow et al., 2009).

2.4.2.2   Membrane Techniques

Two streams are generated when the inlet feed passes through a membrane, namely the permeate stream (which passes through the membrane) and the retentate stream (the fraction retained). The permeation rate (flux) and selectivity (retention or rejection) are the main performance parameters for a membrane process. The separation target, within the limitations of a specific application, is the primary consideration in membrane selection (Jirjis & Luque, 2010). Advanced membrane technologies untangle water management and water quality and are now offering practical, cost-effective and energy-saving solutions for large-, medium- or small-scale applications Leiknes (2009). Membrane processes are applicable to treatment of both municipal and industrial wastewater. Frenkel (2010) stated the advantages of using membranes for wastewater treatment from food processing compared to conventional technology:

1.   Complete removal of pathogenic organisms;

2.   Space savings due to a smaller footprint;

3.   Consistent effluent quality;

4.   Effluent of tertiary treatment quality with some types of recycling or reuse;

5.   Easy retrofit into an existing treatment system;

6.   Greater nitrification due to longer retention of nitrifying bacteria;

7.   Modular expansion capability;

8.   Lesser volumes of discharge waste due to long sludge age;

9.   Easy remote monitoring of operation; and

10.   Lower chlorine demand for post disinfection and UV intensity for inactivation due to high-efficiency of particulate removal.

Microfiltration, ultrafiltration, reverse osmosis and electrodialysis membranes have been developed for a variety of industrial applications (Baker, 2004). The primary focus in this section will be on the applications of microfiltration and ultrafiltration in wastewater treatment.

2.4.2.2.1   Microfiltration and Ultrafiltration

Microfiltration and ultrafiltration membranes have pore sizes of 0.05-1.0 μm and 0.01-0.005 μm, respectively (Jirjis & Luque, 2010). Therefore, colloidal particles and bacteria from 0.1 to 10 μm in size can be removed by a microfiltration membrane, whereas ultrafiltration can filter dissolved proteins and other macromolecules or viruses from solution (Baker, 2004; Jirjis & Luque, 2010).

The use of microfiltration and ultrafiltration membranes to treat wastewater has been reported by several researchers. An ultrafiltration-complexation process to remove metals from pulp and paper wastewater was employed by Vieira and his colleagues (2001). Water-soluble polymeric macroligands (polyethyleneimine and polyvinylalcohol) were used to remove trace metals (Fe, Mg, and Ca), and a polyvinylidene fluoride membrane to remove water-soluble polymeric ligands. The ultrafiltration system was operated at a pressure of 3 bars and 500 rpm agitation. The pH of the wastewater was adjusted with HNO_3 or NaOH. They concluded that the ultrafiltration-complexation process was able to remove metals and reduce COD. The ultrafiltration-complexation process showed better efficiency for metal removal than did ultrafiltration without the added ligands. Campos and co-workers (2002) studied oil field wastewater treatment using a combination of microfiltration and biological processes. They reported that wastewater from oil fields contained a number of organic pollutants, including xylenes (BTX), naphthalenes, phenol and total organic carbon (TOC), and a very high salt (NaCl) concentration. Therefore, hydroclones, microfiltration through ceramic membranes, ultrafiltration through polymer membranes, and coagulation and flocculation were explored as pretreatments to remove or recover the oil and suspended solids from oil field wastewater. The wastewater obtained from Campos Basin (Rio de Janeiro State, Brazil) had average COD, oil and grease (O&G), TOC and BOD contents of 1,622, 220, 386 and 695 mg/L, respectively. A microfiltration technique was utilized to remove insoluble, high-molecular-mass pollutants. A mixed cellulose ester membrane with a nominal pore size of 0.1 μm was chosen. The system was operated at pressure of 50 kPa with a feed tangential velocity of 0.43 m/s. After the membrane process, the wastewater was passed through an airlift reactor (biological removal) to remove the remaining organic pollutions. A ratio of COD: N: P of 200: 5: 1 was maintained by adding phosphorus to the influent. Air velocity was kept stable at 23 cm/s. They found that 25, 25, 92 and 35% of the COD, TOC, O&G and phenol, respectively, were removed by microfiltration. Passage of the permeate through the reactor at the lowest hydraulic retention time (12 h) yielded efficiencies of removal of COD, TOC, phenols and ammonium of 65, 80, 65 and 40%, respectively. The COD and TOD values of microfiltered and reacted wastewater were approximately 230 and 55 mg/L, respectively. Frenkel (2010) reported the use of ultrafiltration in an olive processing facility in North California where wastewater had high ferrous gluconate, acetic acid, salt, sodium benzoate, calcium chloride, soluble organic and organic particulate contents. This problem was addressed by installing an ultrafiltration system downstream of the pond system. As stated by Frenkel (2010), the United States Environmental Protection Agency set a limit for BOD_5 in effluent of 25 mg/L prior to discharge. As a result, a squid processing plant in Rhode Island was no longer able to discharge wastewater into a river system. To address the problem, an ultrafiltration membrane bioreactor was installed. Consequently, BOD_5, total suspended solid and total Kjeldahl nitrogen levels were reduced from 5,500 to 25 mg/L, 400 to 20 mg/L, and 400 to 10 mg/L, respectively. Kubota *et al.* (2008) stated that successful application of microfiltration and ultrafiltration required consideration of the degree to which membranes are resistant to clogging, possess the mechanical strength necessary to maintain performance over an extended period, and the chemical strength to resistant frequently cleaning with an oxidant, acid, alkali, etc.

2.4.2.2.2   Membrane Deionization

Deionization is the removal of positively- and negatively-charged ions from water (Euro Tech, 2012) and can be accomplished by several techniques. Only ion exchange resin electrodialysis (ion exchange membrane) and reverse osmosis will be discussed here.

Ion exchange resins are not soluble and bind ions electrostatically. Therefore, when a solution that contains the same charged species is passed over the resin, ion exchange occurs. Both cation and anion exchange resins are common and they may be used alone or in mixed beds. Resins may be regenerated and reused indefinitely. Industry utilizes ion exchange resins for wastewater treatment to reduce water hardness and to remove toxic metal (Alexandratos, 2009). Lin and Chen (1997) studied a combination of the Fenton process and ion exchange to purify textile wastewater effluent for reuse. In secondary wastewater treatment, color, turbidity and COD were removed/reduced via the Fenton process. Subsequently, COD and Fe ion concentrations, total hardness, conductivity, alkalinity, and levels of suspended and total dissolved solids were reduced by ion exchange. Wastewater was collected from a large textile dyeing and finishing mill. A screen was utilized to filter large suspended particulates. Wastewater was then passed through a Fenton reactor and into a sedimentation tank, which had a retention time 60 min. Chemical treatment using polyaluminum chloride and polymer then was carried out, followed by removal of coagulated flocculants. H-type Ambersep 132 and OH-type Ambersep 900 were utilized as strong acid cationic and strong base anionic exchange resins, respectively. It was found that after chemical coagulation percent color removal increased from 97.7 to 100% and that COD was reduced from 42.8 to 9.3 mg/L, conductivity from 5,450 to 1 µmho/cm, hardness from 45.8 to 8.9 mg/L, alkalinity from 72 to 4 mg/L, Fe from 0.11 to 0.03 mg/L, total dissolved solids from 3,490 to 30 mg/L, and suspended solids to 0 mg/L. The wastewater then met the required standard for reuse. Manahan (2005) reported that ion exchange is utilized in the metal plating industry to purify rinse water and spent plating bath solution. Cationic metal species such as Cu^{2+} are removed by cation exchangers, and anionic cyanide metal complexes species such as $Ni(CN)_4^{2-}$ and chromium (IV) species such as CrO_4^{2-} by anion exchange media. An electrodialysis system consists of a stacked series of anion- and cation-exchange membranes. Anion- and cation-exchange membranes are placed to form alternating individual cells between an anode and a cathode. Positively-charged ions in solution will move toward the cathode by permeating through the cation-exchange membrane, but are confined by the anion exchange membrane, and vice versa for negatively-charged ions. This results in an ion concentration increase in every other compartment; a depletion of ion concentration occurs concurrently in other compartments. Electromembrane processes are divided into three types, which are electromembrane separation processes, electromembrane synthesis, and electromembrane energy conversion processes (Strathmann, 2009). However, the focus here is the electromembrane separation process and the ionic constituents removed by this process (Strathmann, 2009). Nataraj and his colleagues (2007) studied treatment of paper industry effluent using a hybrid microfiltration/electrodialysis process. Microfiltration with a ceramic membrane was utilized as a pretreatment prior to electrodialysis (11 cell pairs consisting of 10 and 11 anion- and cation-exchange membranes, respectively). It was found that levels of total dissolved solids, conductivity and COD of 546 mg/L, 0.61 mS/c and less than 20 mg/L, respectively, were achieved at an applied potential 50 V.

Reverse osmosis membranes are utilized to remove monovalent salts and undissociated acids from water (Jirjis & Luque, 2010). Dissolved salts and water are separated by passing wastewater through a semi-permeable membrane with an applied pressure greater than the osmotic pressure generated by the dissolved salts in the wastewater (Lefebvre & Moletta, 2006). In addition, the solubility of salts in the feed water is much less than the solubility of water in the membrane. Therefore, the separation of salts and water occurs (Semiat & Hasson, 2009). Lefebvre and Moletta (2006) reported reverse osmosis was less selective when removing dissolved organics than other processes for demineralization. They also reported the disadvantages of reverse osmosis membrane to be high cost, limited operational history in industrial and domestic wastewater treatment, and a requirement for high quality effluent. Some industries produce saline effluent as wastewater. Examples are the food industry (e.g. pickling, vegetable and fish processing), the leather industry (e.g. the tanning process) and the petroleum industry (salinity up to three-fold that of sea water). Salts in wastewater can be removed by reverse osmosis (Lefebvre & Moletta, 2006). Baker (2012) provided the example of the high concentration of nickel and other plating chemicals in nickel-plating baths. After plating, parts are moved to countercurrent rinse tanks to obtain nickel-free parts. The water from the countercurrent tanks contained nickel at a concentration of 2,000-3,000 ppm. By passing the wastewater through a reverse osmosis unit, the concentration of nickel was reduced to 20-50 ppm, allowing the water to be reused in the plating tank. It should be noted that pretreatment of effluent to eliminate foulants should take place prior to passage through a reverse osmosis unit (Lefebvre & Moletta, 2006).

2.5   Trends in Water Use by Industry

Water use in industrial sectors creates problems in terms of sustainability, as industry is a major consumer of water. There are three principal factors to consider with respect to sustainable water management (Gavrilescu et al., 2008):

1.   Environmental considerations: water consumption and energy and chemical use should be reduced;

2.   Economic considerations: cleaner processes, increased water reuse and better energy efficiency can be achieved by employing new, lower-cost technologies; and

3.   Social considerations: environmental impacts and human health risks must be reduced.

Water conservation, minimizing water consumption, water recycling through wastewater treatment, and improvements in process integration and control all can reduce water consumption and the discharge of wastewater into the environment (Gavrilescu et al., 2008). Major trends in industry with respect to water use include both reduced water usage and greater recycling and reuse. It has been reported that the 70% of the water use in the paper industry in Europe is process water, and more than 95% of the wastewater produced goes to wastewater treatment (Gavrilescu et al., 2008). Although industry would ideally reuse or recycle more of its wastewater due to concern for the environment and social issues, the capital cost of wastewater treatment is high. Jiménez-González and Constable (2011) stated that although one or more hazards can be reduced by wastewater treatment, costs related to energy, transportation and chemical use are encountered. For instance, it has been reported that the cost to treat wastewater from a textile processing facility generating 250,000 m^3 of wastewater per year using ultrafiltration/reverse osmosis was 145,000 Euro annually, which included the cost of the membrane system (21%), and the cost of energy (34%), chemicals (17%) and membranes (28%, three-year lifetime) (Ciardelli *et al.*, 2000). Based on this information, it is clear that a major cost of wastewater treatment in the textile industry is the cost of energy, followed by the costs of membranes, system hardware and chemicals. Applying the biorefinery concept to water use might enable discharge of wastewater with little or no treatment, thus reducing costs.

2.6   Biorefining as a Tool to Utilize Aqueous Solutes

A biorefinery is a facility that integrates biomass conversion processes and equipment to produce fuels, power, and value-added chemicals from biomass. The biorefinery concept is analogous to today's crude oil refineries, which produce multiple fuels and products from petroleum. Biorefining refers to the conversion of biomass feedstock into a host of valuable chemicals and energy with minimal waste and emissions. In the broad sense, biorefineries process many kinds of biomass (organic residues, energy crops, aquatic biomass, etc.) into a wide variety of products (fuels, chemicals, power and heat, materials, food and feed, etc.) (Demirbas, 2010, Figure 1). Ohara (2000) stated that there are two types of biorefinery, namely the biomass-producing type and the waste-material-utilization type. The focus here will be on the latter.

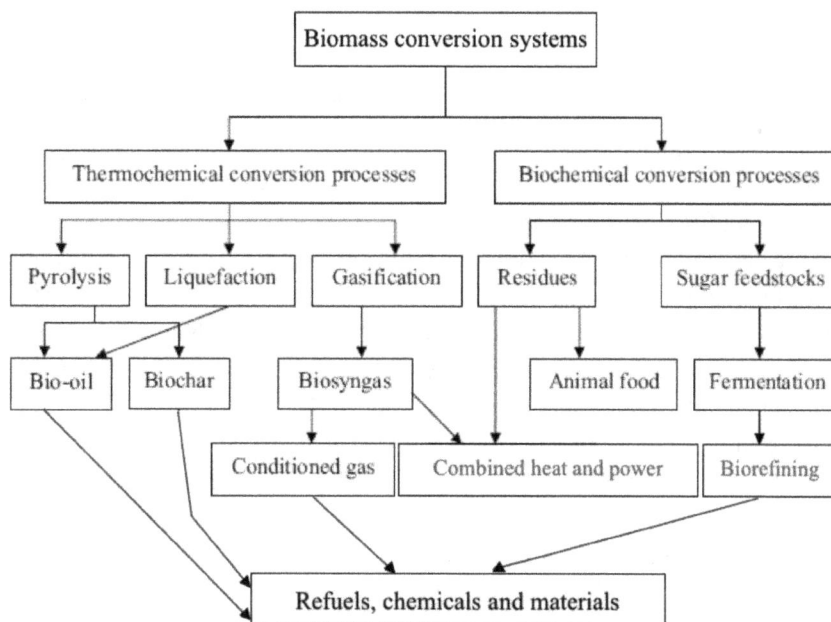

Figure 1: Schematic concept of biorefinery.

The design of a biorefinery is such that if wastewater can be employed in another process with little or no treatment, capital costs will be reduced. In addition, the volume of waste discharged into the environment and the amount of chemicals used for wastewater treatment will be decreased. Moreover, the industry might incorporate a new process line to produce or recover valuable compounds from the effluent. Both the industry and the environment would benefit. Borole (2011) studied the use of bioelectrochemical systems to improve energy efficiency and recovery and enable water recycling in biorefineries through the use of biochemical systems (microfuel cells and/or microbial electrolysis cells). Heat loss could be minimized, a higher value product could be generated, and the volume of water needed for ethanol production could be reduced drastically. In addition, energy could be produced in microfuel cells and/or microbial electrolysis cells using byproducts such as furans, phenolics and acetate from sugar- and lignin- degradation products. Ratanapariyanuch *et al.* (2011) determined that wheat-based thin stillage, a liquid by-product from the ethanol industry, contained metabolites from yeast, bacteria, and wheat, which included ethanol, isopropanol, lactic acid, 1,3-propanediol, acetic acid, succinic acid, betaine, GPC, glycerol and phenethyl alcohol (PEA). These compounds have value and application in other industrial processes:

1. Succinic acid in the manufacture of surfactants, detergent extenders and foaming agents (Zeikus *et al.*, 1999);

2. Acetic acid in the manufacture of vinyl acetate, acetic anhydride, esters, etc. (Global-Oneness, 2010);

3. GPC in the manufacture of moisturizers, emollients, elasticizers, restitutives, nutritive creams and other topical cosmetic and pharmaceutical compositions (Reaney *et al.*, 2011);

4. PEA in the manufacture of perfumes and cosmetics (Etschmann *et al.*, 2002); and

5. 1,3-propanediol in the manufacture of polyesters and polyurethanes (Biebl *et al.*, 1999), cosmetics, foods, transport fuels and medicines (Xiu & Zeng, 2008).

Reaney *et al.* (2011) studied the recovery of multiple compounds and the recycle of water from thin stillage. Thin stillage was condensed into thick syrup, which was then extracted with acetone to remove glycerol, a portion of the lactic acid and acetic acid, and a small portion of the betaine. The remaining solids were extracted with methanol to recover GPC and betaine. The remaining solids consisted of sugars and protein. In addition, PEA was recovered from thin stillage by extraction with canola oil and isopropyl alcohol (IPA), after distillation to remove trace levels of short-chain alcohols. Rather than using thin stillage to feed cattle, the fuel alcohol industry could earn additional income by recovering and selling these valuable compounds. Reaney and Ratanapariyanuch (2011) reported a process for the extraction of macromolecules from biomass using thin stillage. It was demonstrated that mucilage, beta-glucan and starch could be extracted by using thin stillage instead of water. Ratanapariyanuch *et al.* (2012) studied the use of thin stillage to extract protein from oriental mustard (*Brassica juncea* L. Czern.). The pH of the protein extraction system was adjusted using alkaline glycerol from the biodiesel industry. No differences were found in terms of extraction efficiency, SDS-PAGE profile, digestibility, lysine availability or amino acid composition when comparing protein extracted using thin stillage with protein extracted using saline water. The use of thin stillage would reduce energy and waste disposal costs for both fuel ethanol and biodiesel producers if strategically located. Clearly, biorefineries represent an alternative means to reuse/recycle liquid waste with little or no treatment, as mentioned previously. Methane production from wastewater represents another opportunity. Wagner *et al.* (2009) studied the use of microbial electrolysis cells to produce hydrogen and methane from full strength or diluted swine wastewater. Their process employed electrohydrogenesis in a single-chamber, microbial electrolysis cell with a graphite fiber brush anode. It was determined that 0.9-1.0 m^3/m^3/day of hydrogen gas could be produced from full strength or diluted swine wastewater. COD could be reduced by 69-75% in full strength wastewater over 184 h. Hydrogen represented $77\pm11\%$ of the gas produced with $28\pm6\%$ COD recovery and maximum production of methane of $13\pm4\%$.

3   Conclusions

Water is important for industry processes as it is consumed for many purposes including heat transfer, fermentation, etc. Consequently, a large amount of water has been employed in industries. However, environmental issues have been concerned especially sustainability. With this regard, industries have been trying to reduce water use and treat wastewater after processing. Therefore, wastewater can be recycled or discarded without creating any environmental problems. Primary and/or advanced techniques have been studied and used widely to treat wastewater from manufactures. Nonetheless, the cost of water treatment might be expensive/unaffordable for industries. Biorefinery approaches may be used to solve these problems as the system could utilize wastewater without treatment or with only slight treatment prior to use. Therefore, the factories can cut down the cost of wastewater treatments. In addition, it might allow the industries to create products that including valuable compounds or energy. Therefore, the full benefit of water use occurs when the water is used multiple times or is treated to recover previously unused products.

References

Ahlgren, S., Baky, A., Bernesson, S., Nordberg, Å., Norén, O., & Hansson, P-A. (2008). Ammonium nitrate fertiliser production based on biomass-environmental effects from a life cycle perspective. Bioresource Technology, 99(17), 8034–8041.

Alexandratos, S. D. (2009). Ion-exchange resins: a retrospective from industrial and engineering chemistry research. Industrial & Engineering Chemistry Research, 48(1), 388–398.

Ashurst, P. R. (2007). Fruit juices. In Seidel, A., Kirk-Othmer Encyclopedia of Chemistry Technology (5th ed.). Hoboken, NJ: John Wiley & Sons, Inc. (pp. 1–22).

Athanasiadis, I., Boskou, D., Kanellaki, M., Kiosseoglou, V., & Koutinas, A. A. (2002). Whey liquid waste of the dairy industry as raw material for potable alcohol production by kefir granules. Journal of Agricultural and Food Chemistry, 50(25), 7231–7234.

Baker, R. W. (2004). Overview of membrane science and technology. Membrane technology and applications (2nd ed.). Hoboken, NJ: John Wiley & Sons, Inc. (pp. 1–14).

Baker, R. W. (2012). Reverse osmosis. Membrane technology and applications (3rd ed.). Hoboken, NJ: John Wiley & Sons, Inc. (pp. 207–251).

Bellissimi, E. & Richards, C. (2009). Yeast propagation. In Ingledew, W. M., Kelsall, D. R., Austin, G. D., & Kluhspies, C. The alcohol textbook (5th ed.). Nottingham, UK: Nottingham University Press (pp. 1–6).

Berk, Z. (1992). Isolated soybean protein. In Technology of production of edible flours and protein products from soybeans. Food and agricultural industries services, Agricultural service division, Food and Agriculture Organization of the United Nations. Available from: http://www.fao.org/docrep/t0532e/t0532e07.htm.

Bergthaller, W., Witt, W., & Goldao, H-P. (1999). Potato starch technology. Starch-Stärke, 51(7), 235–242.

Biebl, H., Menzel, K., Zeng, A-P., & Deckwer, W-D. (1999). Microbial production of 1,3-propanediol. Applied Microbiological Biotechnology, 52(3), 289–297.

Borole, A. P. (2011). Improving energy efficiency and enabling water recycling in biorefineries using bioelectrochemical systems. Biofuels Bioproducts & Biorefining, 5(1), 28–36.

Boyles, W. (1997). The science of chemical oxygen demand. Technical information series-booklet No. 9. Loveland, Colorado: Hach Conpany.

Brostow, W., Hagg Lobland, H. E., Pal, P., & Sing, R. P. (2009). Polymeric flocculants for wastewater and industrial effluent treatment. Journal of Material Education, 31(3–4), 157–166.

Campos, J. C., Borges, R. M. H., Oliveira Filho, A. M., Nobrega, R., & Sant'Anna Jr., G. L. (2002). Oilfield wastewater treatment by combined microfiltration and biological process. Water Research, 36(1), 95–104.

Ciardelli, G., Corsi, L., & Marcucci, M. (2000). Membrane separation for wastewater reuse in the textile industry. Resources, Conservation and Recycling, 31(2), 189–197.

Čmolík, J. & Pokorný, J. (2000). Physical refining of edible oils. European Journal of Lipid Science and Technology, 102(7), 472–486.

Collicutt, H. (2009). The alcohol industry: How has it changed and matured? In Ingledew, W. M., Kelsall, D. R., Austin, G. D., & Kluhspies, C. The alcohol textbook (5th ed.). Nottingham, UK: Nottingham University Press (pp. 413–430).

Damodaran, S. (2008). Amino acids, peptides, and proteins. In Damodaran, S., Parkin, K. L., & Fennama, O. R. Food Chemistry (4th ed.). CRC Press Taylor & Fracis Group, BocaRaron, FL (pp. 155–216).

Demirbas, A. (2010). Biorefinery. In Biorefineries for biomass upgrading facilities. London, UK: Spring-Verlag London Ltd. (pp. 75–92).

Ellis, M., Dillich, S., & Margolis, N. (2012). Industrial water use and its energy implications. Available from: http://www1.eere.energy.gov/industry/steel/pdfs/water_use_rpt.pdf.

EUREKA SWAN. (2012). Recycle of malting process water. Retrieved from Executive of EUREKA SWAN project AR0916. Available from: http://www.ukmalt.com/sites/default/files/files/SWAN%20FINAL%20REPORT.pdf.

Euro Tech. (2012). DE Series deionization system. Available from: http://www.eurosanwatertreatment.com/product_detail_de_series_deionization_systems_.html.

Etschmann, M. M., Bluemke, W., Sell, D., & Schrader, J. (2002). Biotechnological production of 2-phenylethanol. Applied Microbiology Biotechnology, 59(1), 1–8.

FAO. (2007). Agribusiness handbook. Barley malt beer. Available from: ftp://ftp.fao.org/docrep/fao/012/i1003e/i1003e00.pdf.

Fauconneau, G. (1983). World protein supplies: the role of plant protein. Plant Foods for Human Nutrition, 32(3–4), 205–223.

Frenkel, V. S. (2010). Membrane technologies for food processing waste treatment. In Cui, Z. F. & Muralidhara, H. S. Membrane technology (1st ed.). Burlington, MA: Elsevier Ltd. (pp. 155–178).

Gavrilescu, M., Teodosiu, C., Gavrilescu, D., & Lupu, L. (2008). Strategies and practices for sustainable use of water in industrial papermaking processes. Engineering in Life Science, 8(2), 99–124.

Global-Oneness. (2010). Acetic acid-applications. Retrieved from: Global Oneness Co creating & happy world (April 26, 2010). Available from http://www.experiencefestival.com/acetic_acid_-_applications.

Goodman, W. H. (1999). Advanced water resource management in ammonia and fertilizer industries. Corrosion 99 conference. Paper No. 376. NACE international. Available from: http://www.onepetro.org/mslib/servlet/onepetropreview?id=NACE-99376.

González, J. F. (1996). Wastewater treatment in the fishery industry. Food and Agriculture Organization of the United Nations. Available from: http://www.fao.org/docrep/003/V9922E/V9922E01.htm.

Hach, C. C., Klein, Jr., R. T., & Gibbs, C. R. (1997). Introduction to biochemical oxygen demand. Technical information series-Booklet 7. Hach Technical Center for Applied Analytical Chemistry, Loveland, Colorado: Hach Company.

Höhn, A., Sun, D., & Francois, N. (2005). Enzymes in the fruit juice and wine industry. In Barrett, D. M., Somogyi, L., & Ramaswamy, H. Processing fruits: Science and Technology (2nd ed.). Boca Raton, FL: CRC press LLC. (pp. 197–112).

Ingledew, W. M. (2009). The alcohol industry: Yeast: physiology, nutrition and ethanol production. In Ingledew, W. M., Kelsall, D. R., Austin, G. D., & Kluhspies, C. The alcohol textbook (5th ed.). Nottingham, UK: Nottingham University Press (pp. 101–113).

Ingledew, W. M., Austin, G. D., Kersall, D. R., & Kluhspies, C. (2009). The alcohol industry: How has it changed and matured? In Ingledew, W. M., Kelsall, D. R., Austin, G. D., & Kluhspies, C. The alcohol textbook (5th ed.). Nottingham, UK: Nottingham University Press (pp. 1–6).

Jiménez-González, A. & Constable, D. J. C. (2011). Impacts of waste and waste treatment. Green chemistry and engineering: A practical design approach. Hoboken, NJ: John Wiley & Sons, Inc. (pp. 545–578).

Jirjis, B. F. & Luque, S. (2010). Practical aspects of membrane system design in food and bioprocessing applications. In Cui, Z. F., & Muralidhara, H. S. Membrane technology. Burlington, MA: Elsevier Ltd. (pp. 179–212).

Jose, S. (2010). Global starch consumption to reach 80 million metric tons by 2015, According to new report by Global Industry Analysis, Inc. Retrieved from: Vocus (May 27, 2010). Available from: http://www.prweb.com/releases/starch_market/dry_starch_market/prweb4047074.htm.

Keenan, T. R. (2003). Gelatin. In Seidel, A., Kirk-Othmer Encyclopedia of Chemistry Technology (4th ed.). Hoboken, NJ: John Wiley & Sons, Inc. (pp. 436–447).

Kentish, S. E. & Stevens, G. W. (2001). Innovations in separations technology for the recycling and re-use of liquid waste streams. Chemical Engineering Journal, 84(2), 149–159.

Kohl, S. (2009). Wet milling and mash preparation. In Ingledew, W. M., Kelsall, D. R., Austin, G. D., & Kluhspies, C. The alcohol textbook (5th ed.). Nottingham, UK: Nottingham University Press (pp. 177–192).

Kubota, N., Hashimoto, T., & Mori, Y. (2008). Microfiltration and ultrafiltration. In Li., N. N., A. G., Fane, W S., Winston Ho, & T., Matsuura. Advanced membrane technology and applications. Hoboken, NJ: John Wiley & Sons, Inc. (pp. 101–130).

Lefebvre, O. & Moletta, R. (2006). Treatment of organic pollution in industrial saline wastewater: a literature review. Water Research, 40(20), 3671–3682.

Leiknes, T. (2009). Wastewater treatment by membrane bioreactors. In Drioli, E., & Giorno, L. Membrane operations. Weinheim, Germany: Wiley-VCH Verlag GmbH & Co. KGaA (pp. 363–398).

Li, C-H. & Chen, L. (2006). Organic chemistry in water. Chemistry Society Reviews, 35(1), 68–82.

Lin, S. H. & Chen, M. L. (1997). Purification of textile wastewater effluents by a combined Fenton process and ion exchange. Desalination, 109(2), 121–130.

Macedo, I. C. (2005). Sugar cane's energy. Twelve studies on Brazilian sugar cane agribusiness and its sustainability. UNICA. Berlendis & Vertecchia. Saõ Paulo, Brazil.

Malmary, G., Albet, J., Putranto, A., Hanine, H., & Molinier, J. (2000). Recovery of aconitic and lactic acids from simulated aqueous effluents of the sugar-cane industry through liquid-liquid extraction. Journal of Chemical Technology and Biotechnology, 75(12), 1169–1173.

Manabe, K., Mori, Y., & Kobayashi, S. (2001). Three-component carbon-carbon bond-forming reactions catalysed by a Brønsted acid-surfactant-combined catalyst in water. Tetrahedron, 57(13), 2537–2544.

Manahan, S. F. (2005). *Industrial ecology for waste minimization, utilization, and treatment. In Environmental chemistry* (8th ed.) Boca Raton, FL: CRC Press LLC. (pp. 573–607).

McClements, D. J. & Decker, E. A. (2008). *Lipids. In Damodaran, S., Parkin, K. L., & Fennama, O. R. Food Chemistry* (4th ed.). BocaRaron, FL: CRC Press Taylor & Fracis Group (pp. 155–216).

Milanova, R., Murray, D., & Westdal, P. S. (2006). *Protein extraction from canola oil seed meal.* United States patent No. 6,992,173 B2.

Murray, B. C., Gross, D. H., & Fox, T. J. (1994). *Starch manufacturing: a profile.* Retrieved from U.S. Environmental Protection Agency. Available from: http://www.epa.gov/ttnecas1/regdata/IPs/Starch%20Manufacturing_IP.pdf.

Nataraj, S. K., Sridhar, S. Shaikha, I. N., Reddy, D. S., & Aminabhavi, T. M. (2007). *Membrane-based microfiltration/electrodialysis hybrid process for the treatment of paper industry wastewater. Separation and Purification Technology*, 57(1), 185–192.

Ohara, H. (2000). *Zero emission is realized by polylactate. In: United Nations. Preprints of zero emission symposium 2000.* United Nations, Tokyo (pp. 81–89).

Pérez-López, R., Álvarez-Valero, A. M., & Nieto, J. M. (2007). *Changes in mobility of toxic elements during the production of phosphoric acid in the fertilizer industry of Huelva (SW Spain) and environmental impact of phosphogypsum wastes. Journal of Hazardous Material*, 148(3), 745–750.

Petters, H. I., Flannigan, B., & Austin, B. (1988). *Quantitative and qualitative studies of the microflora of barley malt production. Journal of Applied Bacteriology*, 65(4), 279–297.

Pimentel, D. & Pimentel, M. (2003). *Sustainability of meat-based and plant-based diets and the environment. The American Journal of Clinical Nutrition*, 78 (suppl), 660S–663S.

Population Reference Bureau. (2012). *2012 world population data sheet.* Washington, DC. Available from: http://www.prb.org/pdf12/2012-population-data-sheet_eng.pdf.

Ratanapariyanuch, K., Shen, J., Jia, Y., Tyler, R. T., Shim, Y. Y., & Reaney, M. J. T. (2011). *Rapid NMR method for the quantification of organic compounds in thin stillage. Journal of Agricultural and Food Chemistry*, 59, 10454–10460.

Ratanapariyanuch, K., Shen, J., Jia, Y., Tyler, R. T., Shim, Y. Y., & Reaney, M. J. T. (2012). *Biorefinery process for protein extraction from oriental mustard (Brassica juncea L. Czern.) using ethanol stillage. ABS Express.* 2, 5.

Reaney, M. J. T. & Ratanapariyanuch, K. (2011). *Process for the extraction of macromolecules from a biomass using thin stillage.* United States Patent Application Publication No. US 2011/0237778 A1.

Reaney, M. J. T., Shen, J., Jia, Y., & Ratanapariyanuch, K. (2011). *Recovery of multiple compounds and recyclable water from thin stillage.* United States Patent Application Publication No. US 2011/0130586 A1.

Renewable fuels association. (2012). *Global ethanol production to reach 85.2 billion litres in 2012.* Available from: http://www.ethanolrfa.org/news/entry/global-ethanol-production-to-reach-85.2-billion-litres-in-2012.

Resource Dynamics Corporation. (2003). *Cooling, heating, and power for industry: a market assessment. Report.* Washington, DC: U.S. Department of Energy-Office of Energy Efficiency and Renewable Energy.

Rosegrant, M. W. & Cai, X. (2002). *Global demand and supply projections: Part 2. Results and Prospects to 2025. Water International*, 27(2), 170–182.

Statistics Canada. (2012). *Industrial water use: 2009. 16-401-X.* Ottawa, Canada, Statistics Canada: Environment Accounts and Statistics Division (pp. 11).

Schroeder, B. (2012). *Industrial water use.* Available from: http://academic.evergreen.edu/g/grossmaz/SCHROEBJ.

Scholten, W. (2009). *The water footprint of sugar and sugar-based ethanol.* Enschede, The Netherlands: University of Twente.

Seager, S. L. & Slabaugh, M. R. (2010). *Reaction rates and equilibrium. In Chemistry for today: general, organic & biochemistry,* Cengage Learning, CA: Books/Cole (pp. 239–263).

Semiat, R. & Hasson, D. (2009). Seawater and brackish-water desalination with membrane operations. In Drioli, E., & Giorno, L., Membrane operations. Weinheim, Germany: Wiley-VCH Verlag GmbH & Co. KGaA (pp. 221–244).

Sindilariu, P-D. (2007). Reduction in effluence nutrient loads from flow-through facility for trout production: a review. Aquaculture Research, 38(10), 1005–1036.

Singh, V., Moreau, R. A., Doner, L. W., Eckhoff, S. R., & Hicks, K. B. (1999). Recovery of fiber in the corn dry-grind ethanol process: a feedstock for valuable coproducts. Cereal Chemistry, 76(6), 868–872.

Strathmann, H. (2009). Foundamentals in electromembrane separation process. In Drioli, E. & Giorno, L. Membrane operations (pp. 83–119). Weinheim, Germany: Wiley-VCH Verlag GmbH & Co KGaA.

Sumner, A. K., Nielsen, M. A., & Youngs, C. G. (1981). Production and evaluation of pea protein isolate. Journal of Food Science, 46(2), 364–366.

Tripathy, T. & Ranjan De, B. (2006). Flocculation: a new way to treat the wastewater. Journal of Physical Sciences, 10, 93–127.

United States Department of Agriculture, Foreign Agricultural Service. (2012). Oil seeds: World market and trade. Available from: http://www.fas.usda.gov/psdonline/circulars/oilseeds.pdf.

United States Environmental Protection Agency. (2004). Primer for municipal wastewater treatment systems. Available from: http://water.epa.gov/aboutow/owm/upload/2005_08_19_primer.pdf.

Verstraete, W., Van de Caveye, P., & Diamantis, V. (2009). Maximum use of resources present in domestic "use water". Bioresource Technology, 100(23), 5537–5545.

Vieira, M., Tavares, C. R., Bergamasco, R., & Petrus, J. C. C. (2001). Application of ultrafiltration-complexation process for metal removal from pulp and paper industry wastewater. Journal of Membrane Science, 194, 273–276.

Wagner, R. C., Regan, J. M., Oh, S-E., Zuo, Y., & Logan, B. E. (2009). Hydrogen and methane production from swine wastewater using microbial electrolysis cells. Water Research, 43, 1480–1488.

Wang, L. & Sun, D-W. (2002). Evaluation of performance of slow air, air blast and water immersion cooling methods in the cooked meat industry by finite element method. Journal of Food Engineering, 51(4), 329–340.

Wang, L. & Sun, D-W. (2003). Recent developments in numerical modelling of heating and cooling processes in the food industry: a review. Trends in Food Science & Technology, 14(10), 408–423.

Weiss, K. D. (1997). Paint and coatings: a mature industry in transition. Progress in polymer science, 22(2), 203–245.

Wheals, A. E., Basso, L. C., Alves, D. M. G. & Amorim, H. V. (1999). Fuelethanolafter25years. Trends in Biotechnology, 17(12), 482–487.

Wijingaarden, R. J., Kringberg, A., & Westerterp, K. R. (1998). Introduction. In Industrial catalysis: optimizing catalyses and processes (pp. 1–8). Weinheim, Germany: Wiley-VCH Verlag GmbH & Co. KGaA.

Wu, M. (2008). Analysis of the efficiency of the U.S. ethanol industry 2007. Washington, DC: Renewable Fuels Association.

Xiu, Z. & Zeng, A. (2008). Present state and perspective of downstream processing of biologically produced 1,3-propanediol and 2,3-butanediol. Applied Microbiology and Biotechnology, 78(6), 917–926.

Xu, L. & Diosady, L. L. (2003). Protein from plant materials. In Tzia, G. & Liadakis, G. Extraction optimization in food engineering. New York, NY: Marcel Dekker, Inc.

Zeikus, J. G., Jain, M. K., & Elankovan, P. (1999). Biotechnology of succinic acid production and markets for derived industrial products. Applied Microbiology and Biotechnology, 51(5), 545–552.

Information Flow during Gene Activation by Signaling Molecules

José Díaz

Theoretical and Computational Biology Group, Facultad de Ciencias
Universidad Autónoma del Estado de Morelos, México

1   Introduction

Information Theory was firmly introduced in science by Claude Elwood Shannon in 1948. The original aim of this theory was to solve the problem of increasing the performance of communication systems against of interferences (noise) that diminish the quality of the transmitting information (Shannon, 1948). That is, *the theory deals only with the problem of transmitting with the maximal precision the symbols constituting a message.* This particular level of the whole subject of communication is often referred to as the syntactic level, the others being the semantic and the efficiency levels. In general the semantic problem would be to transmit with the maximum precision the intended meaning of the message, while maximizing the influence of a message on receptor's behavior is a problem about its efficiency (Weaver, 1949). Neither semantics nor message efficiency was considered in Shannon's original work, and they are not a part of present day Information Theory.

This fact is probably an important source for the disappointment amongst biologist that followed the initial great enthusiasm sparked by Information Theory along with Cybernetics (Johnson, 1970; Quatler, 1953) about its explanatory powers in fields like genetics, molecular and cellular biology, and evolution. However, in the last decade new intents of extending Information Theory to explain the transmission of information from the cell´s environment to its genetic network have been made (Díaz, 2011; González-Garcia and Díaz, 2011; Schulthess and Blüthgen, 2011; Cheong et al., 2011; Tkačik and Walczak, 2011).

Following this trend, this Chapter is oriented to show how the combination of system analysis and information theory can be a reliable strategy for the determination of the Shannon entropy, bitrate and capacity of signaling pathways and genetic networks.

2   Shannon Entropy in Genetic Networks

2.1   Entropy and Information

The flow diagram depicted in Figure 1 is the basic model of a communication system where the source S produces a message processed (coded) by the transmitter T in a suitable way to be sent through channel Ch, just the medium or physical support where the signal travels along and where it can be perturbed by noise N, before the receptor R receives and decodes the message to be delivered to its final destination, the user U of the information (González-García and Díaz, 2011). The basic problem in Information Theory is to send a message to U with the maximum fidelity possible, given the fact that noise can distort its content

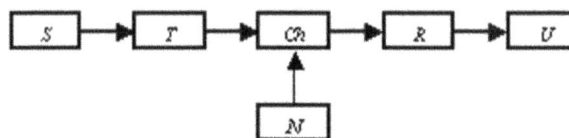

Figure 1: Diagram of a communication channel. Figure adapted from González-García and Díaz (2011).

Two issues are crucial to find a solution, the codification of the message at the source and its protection while traveling through a noisy channel. For example, the genetic code is known to be efficient in limiting the effect of mistranslation errors. A misread codon often codes for the same amino acid or one with similar biochemical properties, so the structure and function of the coded protein remain relatively unaltered (Watson et al., 2006). In signaling pathways the codification and protection of a message is achieved by the specific interaction between the protein components of the communication channel (Marks et al., 2009).

Classical Information theory deals with the problem of sending a message from a source that operates in a discrete time scale. Each symbol x_i of a message is sent one by one and picked out in an independent form from the set of n symbols that form an alphabet $A = \{x_1, x_2, ...,x_n\}$. Each symbol has a probability $p(x_i)$ of being emitted by the source, and the set:

$$\mathbf{P}_X = \left\{ p(x_1), p(x_2),...,p(x_n) \middle| \sum_{i=1}^{n} p(x_i) = 1 \right\}$$

is the discrete probability distribution for the symbols of the message emitted.

One of the purposes of the theory is to measure how information is lost by the effect of noise during its passage through the communication channel, it is clear that one needs a measure of the information content of each transmitted symbol. *A priori* it is reasonable to assume that rare events ($p(x_i)$ close to cero) give more information when they appear, rather than the common results of an experiment, for which $p(x_i)$ is close to one (Pierce, 1980; Ash, 1965; González-García and Díaz, 2011). A convenient elementary function that goes higher when $p(x_i)$ tends to zero and goes to zero when $p(x_i)$ approaches one is:

$$I(x_i) = -\log\left[p(x_i) \right] \tag{1}$$

where $I(x_i)$ is the amount of information that the symbol x_i has. In a general form, Equation (1) can be interpreted as the information content of an event when a random variable X takes a particular value x_i. The base of the logarithm establishes a unit of measure. When the base is 2 the information content is measured in bits. If the base is e the information content is measured in mers. This equation also measures uncertainty, since it depends on the probability of occurrence of events. Low probability events are highly uncertain and carry more information *per se* than very probable events.

According to its probabilities, each message x_i has particular information content. The average amount of information sent by the source S is just the weighted average of $I(x_i)$ given by:

$$H(X) = \sum_{i=1}^{n} p(x_i)I(x_i) = -\sum_{i=1}^{n} p(x_i)\log\left[p(x_i) \right] \tag{2}$$

in this Equation (2), since $p(x_i)$ may be zero, $p(x_i)\log[p(x_i)]$ could be indeterminate. So, when $p(x_i) = 0$ the value of zero is assigned to $p(x_i)\log[p(x_i)]$. Function H is also known as the entropy of the source S or Shannon entropy, $H(S)$, and is symbolized as such to honor the pioneering work of Ludwig Boltzmann who, in the 19th century, symbolized with an H a function similar to (2) in the context of statistical mechanics. Entropy H may be regarded as a measure of uncertainty. $H(X) = 0$ if and only if $p(x_i) = 1$ for some x_i, i.e., if an event occurs for sure, the entropy (uncertainty) vanishes, taking its minimum value. Furthermore, when all events are equally probable, the most uncertainty prevails as to which event will occur. That is $H(X)$ takes on its maximum value: $H(X) = \log(n)$, when $p(x_1) = p(x_2) =... = p(x_n) = 1/n$.

The entropy of the receiver R at the exit of the channel is the average amount of information received per symbol:

$$H(Y) = -\sum_{i=1}^{n} p(y_i) \log[p(y_i)] \tag{3}$$

where $p(y_i)$ is the probability of receiving the symbol y_i that belongs to the alphabet of reception $B = \{y_1, y_2, …, y_m\}$. Thus the receiver working is characterized by a discrete probability distribution:

$$\mathbf{P}_Y = \left\{ p(y_1), p(y_2), …, p(y_n) \left| \sum_{i=1}^{n} p(y_i) = 1 \right. \right\}$$

which means that R receives symbol y_j with probability $p(y_j)$.

2.2   The Communication Channel in the Cell

Cells perceive the state of its environment by a set of physicochemical mechanisms like the binding of growth factors and hormones to specific receptors in the cell surface, electrical flow through ionic channels, flow of small molecules and ions through gap junctions, among others (Speralakis et al., 2012). Each one of these mechanisms can generate a particular cell response by its own or in combination with other inputs.

Every input should be coded into a suitable code that is interpreted with precision by the cell. In the particular case of growth factors and hormones, the input signal is coded by cell-surface receptors that trigger an internal cascade of physico-chemical events that transmit the information to a series of molecular targets. These targets are proteins and genes that give rise to a specific response according to the information received from the source. As consequence, the cell communication channel is formed by signaling and genetic networks. Target proteins and genes of the cascade are the receivers and the novel synthesized proteins together with other modified molecules are the effectors. The diagram of flow of information for the cell communication channel is presented in Figure 2.

There are two main characteristics of the cellular communication channel: 1) the information flow is nonlinear and shows retroactivity between RNA and DNA, and between proteins and DNA. In the first case, retroactivity can be due, for example, to the action of viral reverse transcriptase that can reverse-transcribe viral RNA into the host DNA, modifying native genes and their expression. In the second case, proteins modify gene expression by positive and negative feedback loops (Watson et al., 2007; Lodish et al., 2012). 2) Genes act simultaneously as receivers and as effectors. Generally, signaling cascades act on transcription factors (TF) that activate or inhibit a series of immediate early genes (receivers). These TFs bind to the promoter site of their target genes by forming stable initiation complexes that allow or prevent the transcriptional activity of RNA polymerase. Once these early genes are activated, they can generate a cascade of genetic and cytoplasmic events that controls the amount and timing of production of the new synthesized proteins. These proteins distribute in the cytoplasm producing a specific response according to the message encoded at the cell surface (Marks et al., 2009). Genes, regulatory proteins, molecular transcriptional and translational machineries, and input signaling pathways assemble an open genetic network.

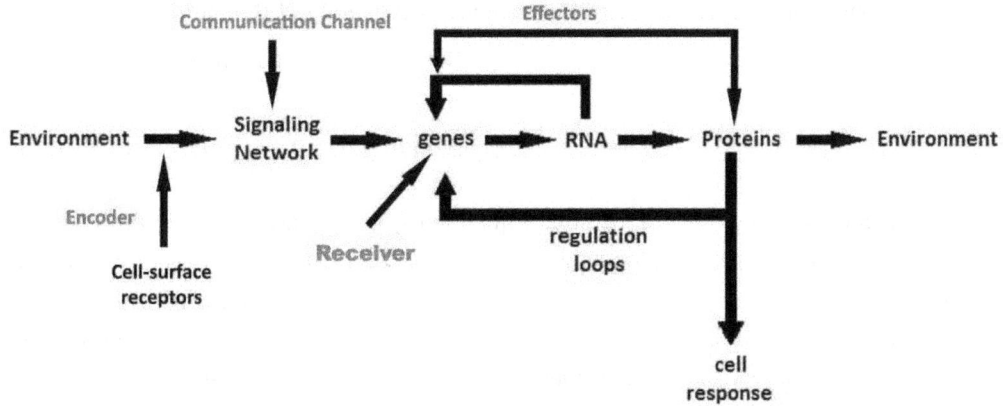

Figure 2: Diagram of the cell communication channel. The information flow in this channel has retroactivity between RNA and genes, and between proteins and genes.

An additional characteristic of cellular communication channels is that the message is not sent in form of symbols to the receiver, but through a cascade of chemical reactions. This fact avoids the direct application of classical Information Theory to measure the Shannon entropy of genetic networks. Equation (3) cannot be directly applied due to the fact that is impossible to assign a probability value to each symbol of a message. Furthermore, in living systems the transmission of information from the emitter to the receiver and effector genes occurs in different time scales, and in the particular case of the cellular communication channels activated by growth factors and hormones, the time lag between the emission of the message and the appearance of the first novel transcripts in the system can be of the order of minutes to hours (Spiller et al., 2010; Marks et al., 2011). In contrast, in classical communication systems the transmission of a message occurs instantly. However, classical Information Theory can be adapted to analyze the particular form in which information flows in cells.

Assuming that for every particular signal from the environment exists a genetic configuration of the genetic network in response to this signal at time t, it is possible to denote this particular genetic configuration by the set:

$$\mathbf{G} = \left\{ g_k^i\left(t\right) \middle| i = 1, 2, ..., m; k = 1, 2, ..., n \right\},$$

where $g_k^i\left(t\right)$ denotes the gene k in state i at time t, and n is the number of genes that are responsive to a particular signal. In most of the cases, the state i of the gene k can be either expressed ($i = on$) or not expressed ($i = off$). However, sometimes a gene can be over expressed and in such case k could have more than two states of activation, but this case is not considered in this work. In this form, $\mathbf{G}$ represents a state of the regulatory genetic network under a specific environmental condition. Depending on the strength, duration and form of the input signal, the genetic response will have dynamical features that reflect these input cues (Díaz and Álvarez-Buyllá, 2006).

However, instead of considering the absolute state of expression of a gene, an alternative approach to measure the Shannon's entropy of a genetic network is to define the set:

$$\mathbf{P} = \left\{ p_k^i\left(t\right) \middle| i = off, on; k = 1, 2, ..., n \right\},$$

where $p_k^i(t)$ is a continuous function of time that represents the probability that the gene k is in state i of expression at time t. In this form, the Shannon entropy of this set can be established as:

$$H(\mathbf{P}) = -\sum_{k=1}^{n}\sum_{i} p_k^i(t) \log\left[p_k^i(t)\right] \quad i = off, on \tag{4}$$

Although $p_k^i(t)$ is a continuous function of time, Equation (4) is evaluated over the probabilities of each gene activation state and over the number of genes responsive to the input signal, which are discrete quantities. Equation (4) represents the entropy of a genetic network and links cell biology with Information Theory and takes into consideration the dependence on time of the transmission of a message in the cellular communication channel. This Equation assumes that for each signal exits a specific genetic configuration with a probability configuration set $\mathbf{P}$ for which a Shannon entropy value can be assigned.

In a similar form, we can define an information value I for this set as:

$$I = H_{max} - H(\mathbf{P}) = H_{max} - \left(-\sum_{k=1}^{n}\sum_{i} p_k^i(t) \log\left[p_k^i(t)\right]\right) \quad i = off, on \tag{5}$$

where H_{max} is the maximum entropy value for the set $\mathbf{P}$. Equation (5) means that the amount of information generated by a signal input is the difference between the maximum uncertainty that the genetic network can have about the content of a message, and the actual value of uncertainty at time t.

Equations (4) and (5) allow the calculus of H and I once $\mathbf{P}$ is known. However, the experimental determination of the probabilistic distribution of a particular genetic configuration corresponding to an input signal could be a difficult task. An alternative method is the mathematical modeling of genetic networks, as it will be explained in the following section.

2.3   Determination of Probabilistic Distribution for a Genetic Network

The modeling of genetic networks is generally done in either of two complementary approaches: 1) discrete models based on the logical rules of the Boolean algebra (Albert, 2004) and 2) continuous models by using differential stochastic equations (Díaz and Álvarez-Buylla, 2006; Samad et al., 2005).

2.3.1   Boolean Genetic Networks

The Boolean models are based on the steady state interaction of the genes of a genetic network and were introduced in biology by Kauffman (1969). This approach is used to model $\mathbf{G}$ dynamics considering that the genes act like switches that can be either *on* or *off*. In this theory, the number "1" represents the *on* state of a gene and the number "0" represents its *off* state. The interaction between genes is modeled with logical Boolean rules. For example, if the initial state of $\mathbf{G}$ at time $t = 0$ is given by the states distribution:

$$\mathbf{G_0} = \left\{g_1^1(0), g_2^0(0), g_3^0(0), ..., g_m^1(0)\right\},$$

after a short number of steps of logical interactions the genetic network could reach either a stable steady state or a limit cycle (Greil, 2009). If after a short number τ of transitions between intermediate states the system of the example reaches a steady final state of the form:

$$\mathbf{G}^{\infty} = \left\{ g_1^0(\tau), g_2^1(\tau), g_3^1(\tau), ..., g_m^0(\tau) \right\},$$

this state represents a punctual attractor of the system. The change $\mathbf{G}_0 \rightarrow \mathbf{G}^{\infty}$ of the genetic configuration of the system represents the response of the system to an input, which is not explicitly modeled, that drives the system into a state that is implicitly related to a new physiological or developmental condition of the cell. In this theory, the basin of attraction of a given attractor $\mathbf{G}^{*}$ is the set of genetic configurations that lead to $\mathbf{G}^{*}$ after some transitions, including $\mathbf{G}^{*}$ itself.

This kind of discrete modeling has been successful, for example, in describing the dynamics of the genetic network that controls flowering in *Arabidopsis thaliana* (Álvarez-Buylla et al., 2010). Other applications have been intended in plant physiology (Li et al., 2006) and animal development (Huang and Kauffman, 2009).

2.3.1 Probabilistic Genetic Networks

The probabilistic approach takes into account the probability of expression (activation) of each gene. In the case of one gene we have:

$$p_1^{on}(t) + p_1^{off}(t) = 1 \Rightarrow p_1^{off}(t) = 1 - p_1^{on}(t). \tag{6}$$

In order to calculate $p_1^{on}(t)$ is necessary to estimate the number of molecules of a particular TF that is activated in response to a given input. Thus the probability of occupation of the promoter site of the gene is proportional to the number of activated TF molecules (N_{TF}). Denoting the velocity of transition from the gene *off* state to the *on* state by κ_1 and the transition for the gene *on* state to the *off* state by κ_2 the differential stochastic equation for the probability of state *on* of the gene can be written as:

$$\frac{dp_1^{on}(t)}{dt} = \kappa_1 N_{TF} p_1^{on}(t) - \kappa_2 p_1^{off}(t) \quad \text{as } \Delta t \rightarrow \infty,$$
$$p_1^{off}(t) = 1 - p_1^{on}(t). \tag{7}$$

By numerically solving Equation (7), subject to the initial condition $p_1^{on}(0) = p_o$, is possible to obtain the probabilistic distribution of activation of the gene:

$$\mathbf{P} = \left\{ p_1^{on}(t), p_1^{off}(t) \right\}.$$

Once $\mathbf{P}$ is obtained, the Shannon entropy and the amount of information corresponding to the activation of this gene is, from Equations (4), (5) and (6):

$$H = -p_1^{on}(t)\log p_1^{on}(t) - \left(1 - p_1^{on}(t)\right)\log\left(1 - p_1^{on}(t)\right),$$
$$I = H_{max} - \left[-p_1^{on}(t)\log p_1^{on}(t) - \left(1 - p_1^{on}(t)\right)\log\left(1 - p_1^{on}(t)\right) \right]. \tag{8}$$

In this case $H_{max} = \log 2$, because there are two mutually exclusive gene states. Figure 3 shows the graphics corresponding to Equation (8).

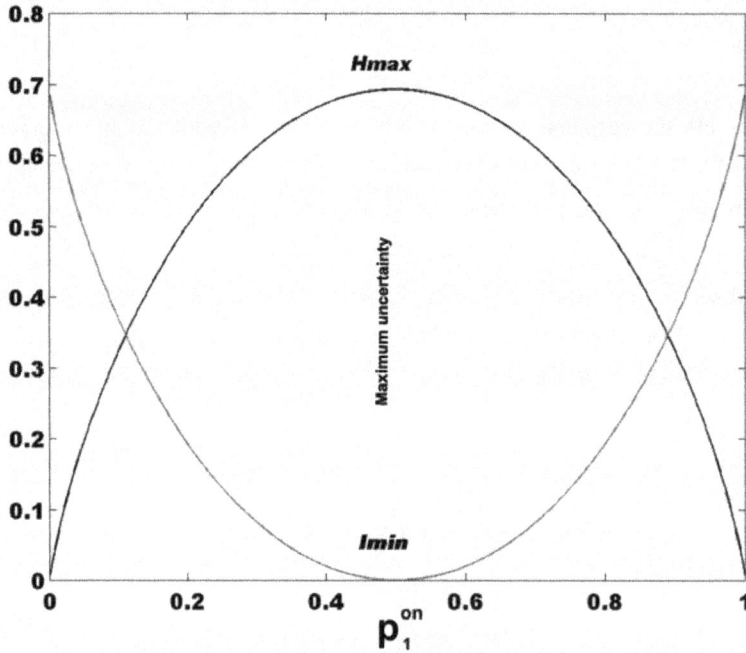

Figure 3: Relationship between H and I for one gene. The maximum value of uncertainty (minimum value of information) is obtained when the probability of expression of the gene is 0.5.

From Figure 3, it is clear that the maximum uncertainty is not obtained when $p_1^{on}(t) = 0$, but when $p_1^{on}(t) = 0.5$. This probably means that the system has not enough information to decide the correct response to a given input, i.e., the instructions from the emitter are ambiguous.

In the case of a two genes system, gene A produces protein A which is a transcription factor for gene B. If there is not retroactivity between gene A and gene B, we obtain the coupled system of differential stochastic equations, where gene A is denoted as gene 1 and gene B is denoted as gene 2:

$$\frac{dp_1^{on}(t)}{dt} = \kappa_1 N_{TF} p_1^{off}(t) - \kappa_2 p_1^{on}(t)$$

$$p_1^{off}(t) = 1 - p_1^{on}(t)$$

$$\frac{dmRNA}{dt} = V_{trans}^{max} p_1^{on}(t) - \kappa_3 mRNA$$

$$\frac{dproteinA}{dt} = \kappa_4 mRNA - \kappa_5 proteinA \tag{9}$$

$$N_{TFA} = f.(proteinA) V_{Nuc} N_{Avogadro}$$

$$\frac{dp_2^{on}(t)}{dt} = \kappa_6 N_{TFA} p_2^{off}(t) - \kappa_7 p_2^{on}(t)$$

$$p_2^{off}(t) = 1 - p_2^{on}(t)$$

subject to: $p_1^{on}(0) = p_{10}$ and $p_2^{on}(0) = 0$. In these equations, N_{TF} represents the number of TFs that bind to the promoter site of gene A, and N_{TFA} represents the number of TFs that are produced by gene A and bind to gene B promoter site.

In this set of equations, V_{trans}^{max} represents the maximum rate of transcription of gene A; $mRNA$ is the concentration of mRNA transcribed from gene A, and $proteinA$ is the cytoplasmic concentration of the protein A synthesized from the mRNA produced.

N_{TFA} can be calculated from the concentration of protein A considering the adjust factor f, which is used to scale cytoplasmic concentration of protein A with respect to the nuclear volume V_{nuc}, which is generally smaller that the cytoplasmic volume. Thus $f = V_{cyt} / V_{nuc}$ when protein A is transported into the nucleus. Finally, $N_{Avogadro}$ is the Avogadro's number (6.023×10^{23} molecules/mol).

From the numerical solution of the set of Equations (9), is possible to obtain the probabilistic distribution of the two genes system:

$$\mathbf{P} = \left\{ p_1^{on}(t), p_1^{off}(t), p_2^{on}(t), p_2^{off}(t) \right\}.$$

Once $\mathbf{P}$ is obtained, the Shannon entropy and the amount of information corresponding to the activation of this genetic system is, from Equations (4), (5) and (9):

$$H = -\sum_{k=1}^{2} \sum_{i} p_k^i(t) \log p_k^i(t)$$

$$I = H_{max} - \left[-\sum_{k=1}^{2} \sum_{i} p_k^i(t) \log p_k^i(t) \right] \qquad i = off, on$$

(10)

in this case H_{max} can be evaluated by considering that:

$$p_1^{on}(t) = 1 \text{ then } p_2^{on} = p\left(B^{on} \Big/ A^{on} \right) p_1^{on} + p\left(B^{on} \Big/ A^{off} \right) p_1^{off},$$

where $p_2^{on}(t)$ is a conditional probability that represents the probability of activation of gene B (even B^{on}) given the fact that the gene A is either in state *on* or in state *off* (events A^{on} and A^{off}). When $p_1^{on}(t) \approx 1 \Rightarrow p_1^{off} \approx 0$ and $p_2^{on}(t) \sim 1$, giving rise to the configuration:

$$\mathbf{P}_1 = \left\{ p_1^{on}(t) \approx 1, p_1^{off}(t) \approx 0, p_2^{on}(t) \sim 1, p_2^{off}(t) \sim 0 \right\} = \left\{ 1, 0, 1, 0 \right\}.$$

On the contrary, when $p_1^{on}(t) \approx 0$ we obtain the configuration:

$$\mathbf{P}_2 = \left\{ p_1^{on}(t) \approx 0, p_1^{off}(t) \approx 1, p_2^{on}(t) \sim 0, p_2^{off}(t) \sim 1 \right\} = \left\{ 0, 1, 0, 1 \right\}.$$

Thus, there are two mutually exclusive configurations of the genetic system and then: $H_{max} = \log 2$. Figure 4 shows an example.

A different scenario arises when a negative feedback loop between gene A and gene B exists. In this case gene A activates gene B, and gene B inhibits gene A. If it is assumed that protein B competes with TF for the promoter site of gene A, then the set of Equations (9) must be modified in the following form as shown in Equation (11).

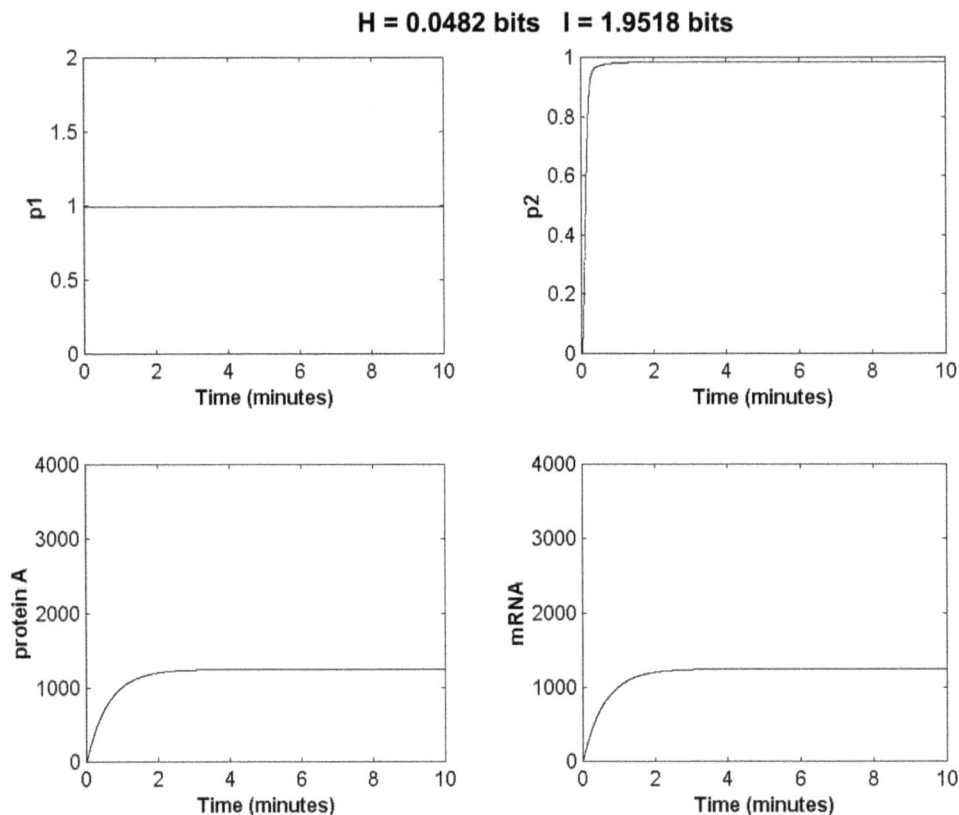

Figure 4: Numerical solution of the set of Equations (9), showing the probability of activation of genes A and B in a cascade of gene activation. In these graphics p_1 represents the probability of activation of gene A, p_2 the probability of activation of gene B. The graphics at bottom of the figure show the number of molecules of protein A and mRNA. In all graphics time is measured in minutes. The values of H and I of the steady probabilistic distribution are calculated using Equations (10). The values of the parameters of the set of Equations (9) are: $\kappa_1 = 0.02$ s^{-1}; $\kappa_2 = 0.05$ s^{-1}; $V_{trans}^{max} = 35$ molecules/s; $\kappa_3 = 0.028$ s^{-1}; $\kappa_4 = 2$ s^{-1}; $\kappa_5 = 2$ s^{-1}; $\kappa_6 = 0.001$ s^{-1}; $\kappa_7 = 0.02$ s^{-1}; $N_{TF} = 500$ molecules. In this case, $N_{TFA} = protein\ A$.

$$\frac{dp_1^{on}(t)}{dt} = \kappa_1 \frac{N_{TF}}{N_{TF} + \kappa_I\left(1+\frac{N_{TFB}}{\kappa}\right)} p_1^{off}(t) - \kappa_2 p_1^{on}(t)$$

$$p_1^{off}(t) = 1 - p_1^{on}(t)$$

$$\frac{dmRNA_A}{dt} = V_{transA}^{max} p_1^{on}(t) - \kappa_3 mRNA_A$$

$$\frac{dproteinA}{dt} = \kappa_4 mRNA_A - \kappa_5 proteinA$$

$$N_{TFA} = f.\left(proteinA\right)V_{Nuc}N_{Avogadro}$$

$$\frac{dp_2^{on}(t)}{dt} = \kappa_6 N_{TFA} p_2^{on}(t) - \kappa_7 p_2^{on}(t)$$

$$p_2^{off}(t) = 1 - p_2^{on}(t)$$

$$\frac{dmRNA_B}{dt} = V_{transB}^{max} p_2^{on}(t) - \kappa_8 mRNA_B$$

$$\frac{dproteinB}{dt} = \kappa_9 mRNA_B - \kappa_{10} proteinB$$

$$N_{TFB} = f.\left(proteinB\right)V_{Nuc}N_{Avogadro}$$

(11)

From the numerical solution of the set of Equations (11), it is possible to obtain the probabilistic distribution of the two genes system:

$$\mathbf{P} = \left\{ p_1^{on}(t), p_1^{off}(t), p_2^{on}(t), p_2^{off}(t) \right\}.$$

Once **P** is obtained, the Shannon entropy and the amount of information corresponding to the activation of this system of genes can be calculated with Equation (10). However, in this case H_{max} must be numerically estimated for each probabilistic distribution. Numerical solution of the system of equations (11) is shown in Figure 5. This procedure can be extended to more complex genetic networks by adding new terms to the set of Equations (11), which can include mathematical expressions for a variety of negative and positive feedback processes like auto-activation and competitive inhibition.

2.4   Noise in the Communication Channel

All communication channels are subject to noise, i.e., random fluctuations in the transmission media that can distort the content of a message transmitted to the receiver. If ξ is the noise level in the communication channel then the fidelity of transmission of the message is $1-\xi$. For example, if the transmitter sends a binary message composed by the symbols 1 0 through a noisy channel, the receiver will get the first correct symbol 1 with probability $1-\xi$. However, noise can alter this message and the receiver could get the incorrect symbol 0 with a probability ξ. In a similar form, the second symbol of the message will be correctly received with probability $1-\xi$ and incorrectly received with probability ξ. Thus, the probability of receiving the correct message is $(1-\xi)^2$, assuming that each symbol is sent in an independent form. For example, if $\xi = 0.1$, then the probability of receiving the correct message is $(1-\xi)^2 = 0.81$. In this form, the goal of every communication channel is to increase fidelity by diminishing the noise source that decreases the probability of receiving the correct message.

H = 0.6355 bits   I = 1.3645 bits

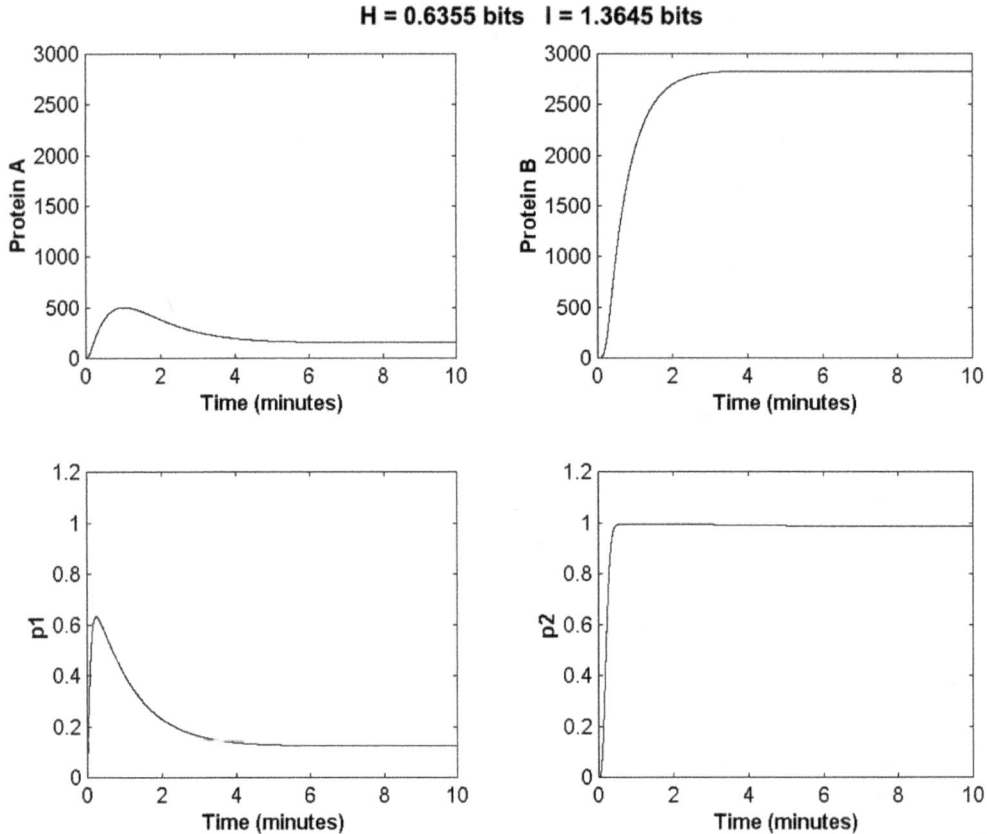

Figure 5: Numerical solution of the set of Equations (11), showing the probability of activation of genes A and B in a negative feedback loop. In these graphics p_1 represents the probability of activation of gene A, p_2 the probability of activation of gene B. The graphics at bottom of the figure show the number of molecules of protein A and mRNA. In all graphics time is measured in minutes. The values of H and I of the steady probabilistic distribution are calculated using the couple of Equations (10). The values of the parameters of the set of Equations (10) are: $\kappa_1 = 0.12$ s^{-1}; $\kappa_I = 0.01$; $\kappa = 0.015$; $\kappa_2 = 0.015$ s^{-1}; $V_{transA}^{max} = 35$ molecules/s; $\kappa_3 = 0.028$ s^{-1}; $\kappa_4 = 2$ s^{-1}; $\kappa_5 = 2$ s^{-1}; $\kappa_6 = 0.001$ s^{-1}; $\kappa_7 = 0.002$ s^{-1}; $V_{transB}^{max} = 40$; $\kappa_8 = 0.008$ s^{-1}; $\kappa_9 = 2$ s^{-1}; $\kappa_{10} = 1$ s^{-1}; $NTF = 500$ molecules; $H_{max} = 2$. In this case, $N_{TFA} = protein\ A$ and $N_{TFB} = protein\ B$.

As far as this point, it has been possible to calculate the uncertainty of a message at the receiver, i.e., it is possible to determine the probability distribution of the state of activation of the genes of a genetic network under a given signal and its entropy. However, this entropy at the output of the communication channel depends both on the input to the channel and the errors (noise) made during transmission. On the contrary, entropy at the source $H(X)$ depends only on the input to the communication channel and measures the uncertainty in the generation of the message that will be transmitted.

If there is any fidelity in the transmission of information through the channel, one expects to find a relationship between the processes going on at the source (X) and at the receiver (Y), since the output of the channel depends on its input. Such dependence can be described by the joint distribution P_{XY} which is the set of all the $n \cdot m$ probabilities $p(x_i, y_j) = \Pr\{X = x_i, Y = y_j\}$. In this case, the joint entropy of the source and the receiver is:

$$H(XY) = -\sum_{i=1}^{n}\sum_{j=1}^{m} p(x_i, y_j) \log\left[p(x_i, y_j) \right] \tag{12}$$

and $H(XY)$ is the amount of uncertainty about the state of S and R taken together.

If the events at the S and R (Figure 1) were independent, the joint probability distribution is just the product of P_X and P_Y and the joint entropy decomposes into the sum of each separated entropy: $H(XY)$ = $H(X) + H(Y)$. On the other hand if there is certain fidelity in the transmission, there will be some correlation between X and Y and so there will be a degree of knowledge about the state of one variable given the state of the other. That is, some uncertainty is dissipated when a correlation exists. Therefore the joint entropy will be less than $H(X) + H(Y)$ in such situation. The amount of information gained by correlation between X and Y is:

$$\mathbf{I}(X:Y) = H(X) + H(Y) - H(XY) \tag{13}$$

that can also be interpreted as the amount of information that the receiver has about the state of the source (and vice versa). Thus, mutual information $\mathbf{I}(X:Y)$ measures the deviation from independence emerging out of mutual knowledge, the amount by which the entropy of X or Y is reduced by knowing the other, Y or X. Equation (13) can be modified by introducing the concept of conditional entropy $H(X/Y)$, which is the average amount of uncertainty per source symbol when the received symbol is known, and is given by:

$$H(X/Y) = H(XY) - H(Y) \tag{14}$$

$H(X/Y)$ represents the equivocation or error size, a measure of the average ambiguity in the received signal, since it is the uncertainty at R about the symbol x_i sent to S given that symbol y_j has been received. Substituting Equation (14) into Equation (13) we obtain:

$$\mathbf{I}(X:Y) = H(X) - H\left(\frac{X}{Y}\right) \tag{15}$$

which is the average amount of information transmitted through a noisy channel, a measure of the information preserved after crossing it.

The capacity C of a noisy channel is defined as the maximal amount of information I that can be obtained over all possible information sources S and represents the maximum value of $I(X:Y)$. C depends only on the channel (Arbib, 1964). Codification and protection of the message are two key problems to be solved in order to maximize the fidelity of transmission. Shannon's theorem defines precisely the conditions in which this is possible and it says that if the average amount of entropy per symbol at the source $H(X)$ overflows channel capacity C, there is an error level, equal to $H(X) - C$, that cannot be further reduced by an adequate code selection, although there are codes that close to such level as needed. Otherwise, if $H(X) - C < 0$ there are codes that make it possible to reduce the effects of noise down to zero.

Shannon's theorem only establishes conditions for the existence of adequate codes that tend to minimize equivocation down to a certain level, but does not find them nor gives a procedure to build them. A technical drawback of the theorem is that it relies on long symbol sequences for its demonstration. Thus, its conclusions are applicable only after the reception of such messages, implying long delays.

In other words, error free transmission is accomplished at the expense of long time delays. Therefore, in practice a tradeoff is established between reliability and transmission time (Jones, 1979).

2.4   Noise in the Cellular Communication Channel

In cells noise is due to random fluctuations in the population of signaling molecules due to the stochastic process of birth and death of molecules like proteins and mRNA's (Paulson 2004). There are two sources of noise in living cells: intrinsic and extrinsic noise.

Intrinsic noise (η_{in}^2) is due to the inherent stochasticity of biochemical processes like transcription, protein synthesis and cascades of signaling molecules, among others. Extrinsic noise (η_{ext}^2) is due to fluctuations in the amount or state of other cellular components that can influence gene expression or signaling pathways (Swain et al., 2002). In this form, it is possible to sum up both noise sources in order to estimate the total noise (η_{tot}^2) present in a cellular communication channel as (Swain et al., 2002; Elowitz et al., 2002):

$$\eta_{tot}^2 = \eta_{in}^2 + \eta_{ext}^2. \tag{16}$$

Noise of a population of molecules can be estimated as:

$$\eta^2 = \frac{\sigma^2}{\mu}, \tag{17}$$

where σ^2 is the variance in the amount of molecules and μ is the average number of molecules. Equation (17) is also known as the Fano factor. For example, fluctuations (noise) in the number of molecules of mRNA in a cell can be calculated as:

$$\eta^2 = \frac{\sigma^2}{\mu} = \frac{\left\langle mRNA^2 \right\rangle - \left\langle mRNA \right\rangle^2}{\left\langle mRNA \right\rangle}. \tag{18}$$

There is a variety of forms of estimate noise in biological systems, depending on the particular system under analysis (Bruggeman et al., 2009; Paulson, 2004; Elowitz et al., 2002).

In cellular systems the problem of codification of a message is quite different from electrical or mechanical devices. The message from the environment is generally written in the form of a concentration of a hormone or growth factor, and is coded in terms of the number of specific receptors activated per unit of area of membrane. Furthermore, the message has temporal and spatial components that have to be taken into account by the encoder in order to transmit the correct message to the receiver.

Most of the membrane receptors have high affinity by their ligand, and saturate at low concentration of it (from picomolar (pM) to nanomolar (nM)), giving a full respond to low levels of the input signal. Thus, if we consider that each receptor can be in the state j of activation at time t, then the probability that a receptor is in state j of activation at time t can be estimated as $p^{(j)}(t) = N_j(t) / N(t)$, where $N_j(t)$ is the number of receptors in state j of activation and $N(t)$ is the total number of receptors on the cell surface. Generally, there are two mutually exclusive states of activation due to the high affinity of receptors for their ligand, and thus $j = 1, 2$. However, if a receptor could be in either one of m states of activation, j runs from 1 to m. This leads to the probability distribution:

$$\mathbf{Px} = \left\{ p^{(1)}\left(t\right), p^{(2)}\left(t\right), ..., p^{(m)}\left(t\right) \right\}.$$

Assuming a two state receptor, the entropy at the source can be calculated as:

$$H(\mathbf{Px}) = -\sum_{j=1}^{2} p^{(j)}\left(t\right) \log p^{(j)}(t), \tag{19}$$

which is analog to a binary communication system. From the Equations (4), (12), (13) and (19) we can write:

$$I\left(X:Y\right) = -\sum_{j=1}^{2} p^{j}\left(t\right) \log p^{j}(t) - \sum_{k=1}^{n}\sum_{i} p_{k}^{i}\left(t\right) \log\left(p_{k}^{i}\left(t\right)\right) - H\left(XY\right) \quad i = off, on, \tag{20}$$

and the capacity of the cell communication channel can be calculated as:

$$C = \max_{\mathbf{Px}} I\left(X:Y\right). \tag{21}$$

The calculation of the capacity of a channel is a difficult problem in general, since $H(XY)$ should be established for each particular system. However, it has been possible to calculate C experimentally in mouse fibroblast cells. Cheong et al., (2011), using immunochemistry, assayed different concentrations of nuclear NF-κB in thousands of fibroblast cells after 30 min of exposition to TNF and found that the NF-κB response value (capacity) yield ~ 1.92 bits of information, which is equivalent to resolving only 2 levels of TNF, i.e., the system has a bottleneck for the flow of information caused by noise.

Once a message has been encoded, it should be transmitted with fidelity to the nucleus where it triggers a specific genetic response. In cells, the communication channel is composed by a series of signaling pathways that links the information from the receptors to the early response genes (Section 2.2). These pathways form an intricate signaling network due to the "*crosstalk*" between them. For example, in animal cells the MAPK signaling pathway interacts with the IP3-Ca^{2+}, Wnt and PI3-kinase signaling pathways, among others. In vegetal cells, the ethylene signaling pathway interacts with the auxin and jasmonate signaling pathways.

However, the important fact, from the Information Theory point of view, is the flow of information that generates the probabilistic set **P** of gene states of activation. This set represents the most probable phenotype in response to environmental signals. For example, FGF is a potent mitogen that can activate and regulate cell division by signals of relative short duration. However, under the action of sustained FGF signals cells undergo differentiation. Thus, depending on the concentration and timing of the FGF input signal, a particular set **P** of gene states of activation is set up.

Most of the signaling pathways are structurally and functionally protected against noise, assuring the fidelity of the information that they are carrying into the nucleus. In this case, "*structure*" not only means the molecular structure of the signaling proteins, which produces their high degree of specificity, but also the topological structure of the signaling pathway. The fidelity of transmission of information is a property of the structure of the communication channel, thus the structure of the signaling pathway determines its fidelity in the transmission of information. For example, noise practically does not affect cascades of proteins with sigmoid kinetics, i.e., ultra sensitivity to the input (Díaz and Álvarez-Buylla, 2006; Marks et al., 2009; Kholodenko, 2000). On the contrary, noise has a stronger effect on cascades with linear and hyperbolic dynamics, which are more sensitive to signals of small intensity. (Marks et al., 2009).

The structure of the signaling pathway includes molecular switches, which are proteins with sigmoid dynamics of activation, and logical gates AND, OR, NOT and NOR assembled by proteins interacting in a specific form. Molecular switches are natural filters of noise, while positive and negative feedback loops assure the high-fidelity spatio-temporal integration of the information flowing through the logical gates (Marks et al., 2009).

In most cases, the information from the surface receptors is coded in two forms: amplitude modulated (AM) signals and frequency modulated (FM) signals. For example, the ethylene signaling pathway codes its information in amplitude modulated signals (Díaz and Álvarez-Buylla, 2006), while the FGF receptor in Xenopus presumptive mesoderm cells can split the input signal into an AM signal that is transmitted through the canonical Ras-Raf MAPK cascade, and a FM signal that is transmitted by the IP3-Ca^{2+} signaling system (Díaz et al., 2002; Díaz and Martínez-Mekler, 2005). However, both signals can be integrated at the Ras and Raf levels (Cullen and Lockyer, 2002; Corbit et al., 2003) affecting gene expression (Li et al., 2011).

Experiments by Dolmetsch et al. (1997, 1998), show that AM and FM signals affect gene expression, and that some transcription factors like NFAT can operate as either an AM or an FM integrator of the input signal. For example, in self-tolerant B cells, low amplitude steady calcium signals activate the NFAT transcription factor and the ERK pathway, whereas high amplitude steady calcium signals activate NF-κB transcription factor and JNK. Thus, this differential effect of the amplitude of the calcium signal conveys a differential gene expression. Genes that respond to the amplitude of the calcium signal are called *AM genes*.

In similar form, in T lymphocytes (Jurkat cells), the transcription factors NFAT and Oct/OAP are inactivated by calcium signals with a period > 400 s, whereas NF-κB remains active even at periods of ~ 1800 s. Dolmetsch et al. (1998), shown, by using transfected cells with luciferase reporter constructs driven by the IL-2 and IL-8 promoters, that the IL-2 gene exhibits the same response pattern that NFAT and Oct/OAP. In contrast, the IL-8 gene follows NF-κB frequency dependence. Thus, this differential effect of the frequency of the calcium signal also conveys a differential gene expression. Genes that respond to the frequency of the calcium signal are called *FM genes*.

Recent experimental results show that frequency encoding is not only related to the IP3-Ca^{2+} signaling pathway, but also the MAPK can exhibit oscillations. ERK oscillates between the nucleus and the cytoplasm in human mammary epithelial cells under the action of the Epidermal Growth Factor (EGF). The periodicity of these oscillations is of the order of ~ 900 s (Weber et al., 2010). These oscillations are proposed to be produced by a negative feedback loop between dually phosphorylated ERK and the MAPK cascade input. Mouse epidermal JB6 cells also show ERK oscillations in response to stimulation with FGF, and these oscillations are robust at a high cell population density. On the contrary, EGF induced oscillations in mammary cells are damped under low cell population density (Weber et al., 2010). Shin et al. (2009), also report ERK oscillations in COS-1 cells. These oscillations have a period that depends on the doses of EGF or FGF.

AM encoding is robust against noise in the case of molecular switches (Díaz and Álvarez-Buyllá, 2006; Mark et al., 2009). In contrast, FM encoding is more susceptible to noise when the signal-noise ratio (SNR) is under a threshold value named the noise-threshold level. However, above this noise-threshold value the signal-noise ratio can be improved, even more than in the case of the AM encoding, and the FM signal becomes more robust to noise. In most of the biological FM encoding systems, SNR is unknown and has not been determined yet.

3   Information Flow in the Ethylene Signaling Pathway

3.1   Information Flow in the Ethylene Signaling Pathway

Ethylene is a gaseous plant-specific growth regulator that mediates developmental responses. In the particular case of the ethylene signaling system of *Arabidopsis thaliana*, its structure is formed by two mutually exclusive modules. A molecular switch determines the "*on*" and "*off*" states of these modules.

The ethylene receptors ETR1,2 are located at the endoplasmic reticulum (ER) of plant cells, and in absence of ethylene are in their active state ("*on*"). In this state, the MAPK kinase CTR1 is active and positively influences the expression of the *POLARIS* (*PLS*) gene that promotes the auxin dependent growth response of the root cell (Liu et al., 2010). When ethylene binds to these receptors they are turned off and inactivates CTR1, activating the downstream protein EIN2, which induces the transcription of the gene *ERF1* (Díaz and Álvarez-Buylla, 2006; Díaz, 2011). The transcription factor ERF1 promotes the transcription of genes with a GCC box in their promoter sequence (Figure 6a) like *PDF1,2* (Brown et al., 2003) and *HLS1* (Rahman et al., 2002).

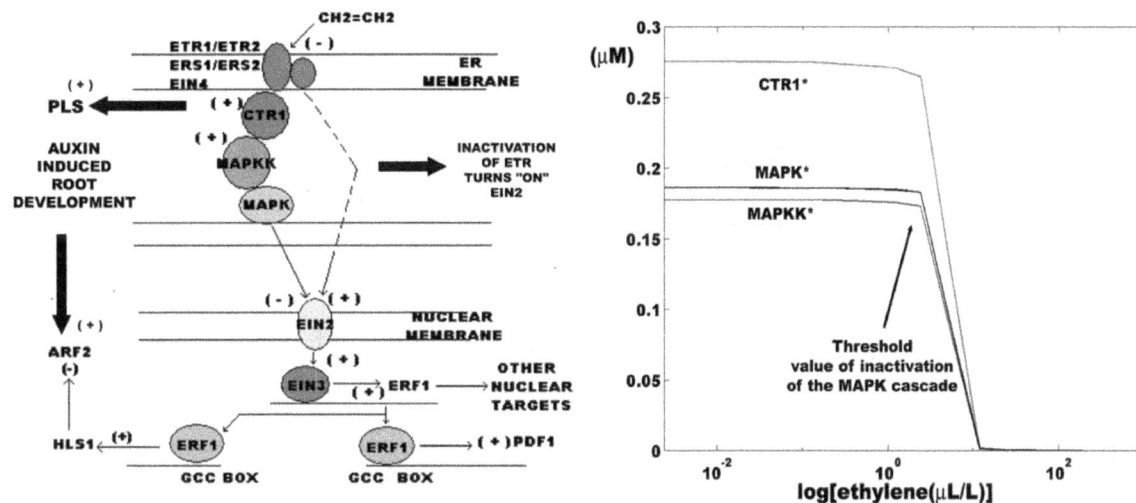

Figure 6: a) The ethylene signaling pathway. PLS links the CTR1 MAPK cascade with the auxin signaling system. Inactivation of ETR 1,2 turns "*on*" EIN2 giving rise to the ethylene-dependent control of root development. b) Doses-dependent inactivation of the CTR1 MAPK by ethylene. The threshold value of activation is about ~ 1 μL/L, above this value the amount of activated CTR1 (denoted by CTR1*) sharply falls to cero. In panel (b) the horizontal axis represents the logarithm base 10 of the ethylene concentration (μL/L).

From the work of Díaz and Álvarez-Buylla (2006) it has been possible to establish a plausible mathematical model of the activation of the ethylene signaling pathway (Figure 6a), which is shown in Table 1. This model has been extended to model the crosstalk between auxin and ethylene (Liu et al., 2010). In this model ordinary differential equations and two-state Markov chains are used to model the activation dynamics of ***ERF1*** in response to ethylene signaling. The numerical solution of this model shows that in absence of ethylene the ethylene receptors (ETR) are in their active state and the MAPK cascade (CTR1, MAPKK and MAPK) reaches a steady state of activation after a brief transient. This sta-

1. Equations describing inactivation of the ethylene receptor: $$\frac{\det r^{(-)}}{dt} = \kappa_1(ET - etr^{(-)})\left(etr_T - etr^{(-)}\right) - \kappa_2 etr^{(-)}$$ $$etr_T = etr^{(+)} + etr^{(-)}$$	**2. Equations describing the CTR1 module:** $$\frac{dctr1^*}{dt} = \kappa_3\left(etr_T - etr^{(-)}\right)\left(ctr1_T - ctr1^*\right) - \kappa_4 ctr1^*$$ $$\frac{dmapkk^*}{dt} = \kappa_5 ctr1^*\left(mapkk_T - mapkk^*\right) - \kappa_6 mapkk^*$$ $$\frac{dmapk^*}{dt} = \kappa_7 mapkk^*\left(mapk_T - mapk^*\right) - \kappa_8 mapk^*$$
3. Equations describing the EIN2 module: $$\frac{dein2^{(-)}}{dt} = \kappa_9 mapkc^*\left(ein2_T - ein2^{(-)}\right) -$$ $$\kappa_{10} ein2^{(-)} \frac{etr^{(-)}}{etr^{(-)} + \beta}$$ $$ein2_T = ein2^{(+)} + ein2^{(-)}$$ $$\frac{dein2^{(+)}}{dt} = -\frac{dein2^{(-)}}{dt}$$ $$\frac{dein3^*}{dt} = \kappa_{11} ein2^{(+)}\left(ein3_T - ein3^*\right) - \kappa_{12} ein3^*$$ $$\frac{dmRNA}{dt} = \frac{p^{on}(t) V_{trans} mRNA}{mRNA + \kappa_{15}} - \kappa_{16} mRNA$$ $$\left.\frac{derf1}{dt}\right|_{ER} = \kappa_{17} mRNA - D_{erf1} erf1$$ $$\left.\frac{derf1}{dt}\right|_{nucleus} = D_{erf1} erf1n - \kappa_{18} erf1n$$	**4. Equations describing the activation of _ERF1,HLS1_ and _ARF2_ genes:** $$\frac{dp_{ERF1}^{off}}{dt} = -\kappa_{13} N_{ein3} p_{ERF1}^{off} + \kappa_{14} p_{ERF1}^{on}$$ $$\frac{dp_{ERF1}^{on}}{dt} = \kappa_{13} N_{ein3} p_{ERF1}^{off} - \kappa_{14} p_{ERF1}^{on}$$ $$N_{ein3} = 602.3 V_{nucleus} EIN3^*$$ $$\frac{dp_{HLS1}^{on}(t)}{dt} = \kappa_{19} N_{ERF1n} p_{HLS1}^{off}(t) - \kappa_{20} p_{HLS1}^{on}(t)$$ $$p_{HLS1}^{off} = 1 - p_{HLS1}^{on}$$ $$p_{ARF2}^{on}(t) = \begin{cases} 0, & \text{if } 0.75 < p_2^{on}(t) \le 1 \\ 0.5, & \text{if } 0.5 < p_2^{on}(t) \le 0.75 \\ 1, & \text{if } 0 \le p_2^{on}(t) \le 0.5 \end{cases}$$ $$p_{ARF2}^{off}(t) = 1 - p_{ARF2}^{on}(t)$$
5. Adjustment of the MAPK concentration from ER to nucleus: $$n_{MAPK} = 5 \times 10^{-21} mapk^*$$ $$mapkc^* = 1.908 \times 10^{18} n_{MAPK}$$ **Adjustment of ERF1 concentration from ER to nucleus:** $$n_{erf1} = 5 \times 10^{-21} erf1$$ $$erf1n = 1.908 \times 10^{18} n_{erf1}$$	**6. Initial conditions:** $ctr1^*(0) = 0.3\,\mu M;$ $erf1(0) = 0;$ $etr^{(-)}(0) = 0;$ $erf1n(0) = 0;$ $p_{ERF1}^{on}(0) = 0;\ p_{HLS1}^{on}(0) = 0;\ p_{ARF2}^{on}(0) = 0;$ $p_{ERF1}^{off}(0) = 1;\ p_{HLS1}^{off}(0) = 0;\ p_{ARF2}^{off}(0) = 0;$ $mapkk^*(0) = 0.5\,\mu M;\qquad mapk^*(0) = 0.5\,\mu M;$ $ein2^{(-)}(0) = 0.005\,\mu M;\ ein3^*(0) = 0;$

7. Parameter values:	8. Variables:

7. **Parameter values:**

$k_1 = 5\mu M^{-1} s^{-1}$; $k_2 = 0.0003 s^{-1}$; $\kappa_3 = 3\mu M^{-1} s^{-1}$;

$\kappa_4 = 0.085 s^{-1}$; $\kappa_5 = 9.196\mu M^{-1} s^{-1}$; $\kappa_6 = 4.598 s^{-1}$;

$\kappa_7 = 0.318\mu M^{-1} s^{-1}$;

$\kappa_8 = 0.0954 s^{-1}$; $\kappa_9 = 2\mu M^{-1} s^{-1}$; $\kappa_{10} = 0.005 s^{-1}$;

$\kappa_{11} = 5\mu M^{-1} s^{-1}$;

$\kappa_{12} = 0.005 s^{-1}$; $\kappa_{13} = 0.003 s^{-1}$; $\kappa_{14} = 0.09 s^{-1}$;

$\kappa_{15} = 0.0001\mu M$;

$\kappa_{16} = 0.0009 s^{-1}$; $\kappa_{17} = 0.1972 s^{-1}$; $\kappa_{18} = 0.198 s^{-1}$;

$\kappa_{19} = 0.003 s^{-1}$; $\kappa_{20} = 0.65 s^{-1}$ $\beta = 6\mu M$;

$V_{trans} = 0.000003 \mu M s^{-1}$; $D_{erfl} = 0.99 s^{-1}$; $etr_T = 0.3\mu M$;

$ctrl_T = 0.3\mu M$; $mapkk_T = 0.5\mu M$; $mapk_T = 0.5 \mu M$;

$ein2_T = 0.005\mu M$; $ein3_T = 0.005\mu M$; $V_{nucleus} = 524\mu m^3$.

8. **Variables:**

etr = concentration of ethylene receptor at the cell membrane; ET = total concentration of ethylene outside the cell (**control variable**); $ctrl*$ = concentration of activated constitutive triple response1 protein; $mapkk^*$ = concentration of activated mitogen-activated protein kinase kinase; $mapk^*$ = concentration of activated mitogen-activated protein kinase; $ein2$ = concentration of ethylene-insensitive protein 2; $ein3*$ = concentration of activated ethylene-insensitive protein 2; $mRNA$ = concentration of messenger RNA in nucleus; $erfl$ = concentration of ERF1 transcription factor; N_{ein3} = number of activated EIN3 molecules in the nucleus; N_{erfl} = number of activated ERF1 molecules in the nucleus; $V_{nucleus}$ = nuclear volume; n_{MAPK} = number of moles of activated MAPK; $mapkc^*$ = concentration of MAPK in the nucleus; n_{erfl} = number of moles of activated ERF1 molecules; $erfln$ = concentration of activated ERF1 transcription factor in the nucleus.   The symbol (+) means the activated form of the corresponding receptor and EIN2 molecule, while the symbol (-) represents their inactivated form. The subscript T stands for the total concentration of the corresponding molecule. The superscript * means the active state of the molecule.

Table 1: Equations and parameters of the ethylene signaling pathway model. The probability of the activated state of genes *ERF1*, *HLS1* and *ARF2* are denoted by $p^{on}_{ERF1}(t)$, $p^{on}_{HLS1}(t)$, $p^{on}_{ARF2}(t)$. The superscript "*off*" denotes the inactivated state of each gene. The symbol (+) means the activated form of the corresponding receptor and EIN2 molecule, while the symbol (-) represents their inactivated form. The subscript T stands for the total concentration of the corresponding molecule. The superscript * means the active state of the molecule.

ble state of the MAPK cascade represents the ground state in which the system remains steadily in absence of ethylene (Figure 6b).

In the presence of ethylene, the model predicts a threshold value of ethylene concentration of ~ 1 μL/L, above of which the MAKP cascade is completely inactivated and the activity of the cascade in the ER sharply falls with ethylene concentration. As consequence, ethylene produces its effects even when the MAPK cascade has not been completely inactivated and *PLS* is still expressed. In this state, both the auxin signaling system and the ethylene signaling system exerts their action on the root development.

In figure 7a, it is shown how the probability of activation of **ERF1**, denoted by p^{on}_{ERF1}, changes as the concentration of ethylene increases. From this figure is clear that *the probability of activation of* **ERF1** *slowly increases according to a sigmoid curve when the concentration of ethylene is increased*.

The dose-response curve of Figure 7a can be adjusted to a Hill function as follows:

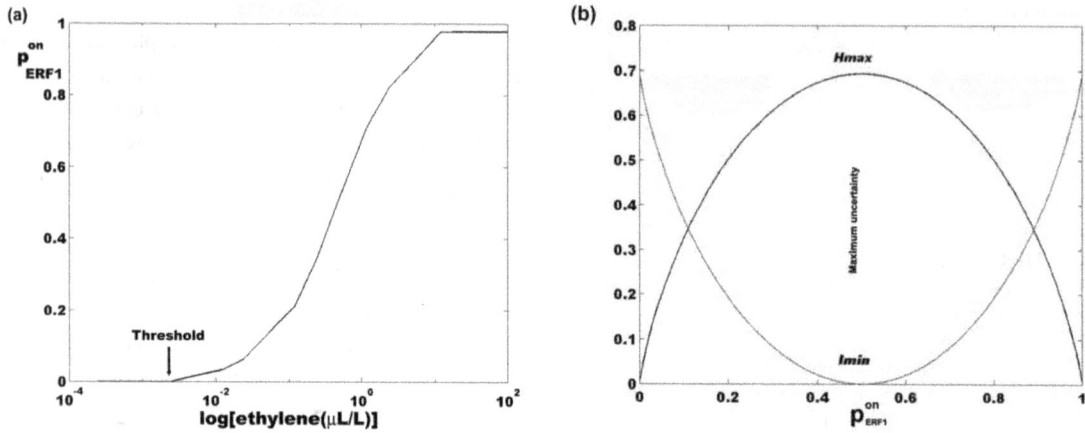

Figure 7: a) Doses-response graph for the probability of activation of *ERF1*. According to the model, the threshold ethylene concentration at which *ERF1* is activated is ~ 1 μL/L. The curve of activation of *ERF1* is a smooth sigmoid that saturates at ~ 10 μL/L. b) Graphic of *H* (black line) and *I* (red line) vs p_{ERF1}^{on}. H has its maximum value when $p_{ERF1}^{on} = 0.5$, as expected from Figure 3. The extremes of the curves correspond to the full action of the hormones auxin and ethylene. In panel (a) the horizontal axis represents the logarithm base 10 of the ethylene concentration (μL/L). In panel (b), the vertical axis represents the values of *H* and *I*, which were calculated by using the logarithm base *e* in the set of equations (23).

$$p_{ERF1}^{on} = \frac{0.9924\,ET^{0.97}}{ET^{0.97} + 0.46} \quad \text{with a } R^2 = 0.9942 \tag{22}$$

for which the Hill coefficient is 0.97 ± 0.029. This range contains the value of 0.99 reported by Chen and Bleeker (1995) for the experimentally documented dose-response curve of the wild-type *Arabidopsis* root The Hill coefficient ~ 1 indicates that it would not be adequate to model the activation kinetics of **ERF1** with a Boolean function because there is a wide interval of ethylene concentrations values, from 0.01 to 10 μL/L, for which the probability of the state *on* of the gene takes values that are less than 1 but not close enough to zero to postulate an all or none response (Figure 7a). This equation directly links the environmental information (concentration of ethylene *ET*) with the respective genetic response, i.e., the probability of expression of the master gene *ERF1*.

In this form, for each concentration of ethylene there is a value of p_{ERF1}^{on} and the amount of uncertainty *H* and *I* associated to each value of probability of expression of *ERF1* at time *t* is given by the set of Equations (10):

$$\begin{aligned} H &= -p_{ERF1}^{on} \log p_{ERF1}^{on} - \left(1 - p_{ERF1}^{on}\right) \log\left(1 - p_{ERF1}^{on}\right) \\ I &= \log(2) + p_{ERF1}^{on} \log p_{ERF1}^{on} + \left(1 - p_{ERF1}^{on}\right) \log\left(1 - p_{ERF1}^{on}\right) \end{aligned} \tag{23}$$

the corresponding graphics of *H* and *I* are presented in Figure 7b.

From Figure 7b, is clear that there is a switch that turns on either the auxin signaling system or the ethylene signaling pathway depending on the concentration of ethylene. When *ERF1* is expressed with $p_{ERF1}^{on} = 0$, the uncertainty in the message from the ethylene receptor is also zero and the root cell phenotype completely corresponds to an auxin induced one. As p_{ERF1}^{on} increases, H increases because the message from the ethylene receptors is composed by a fraction of activated receptors that sustain the activation of the MAPK module, which positively promotes *PLS* expression, and a smaller fraction of inactivated receptors that maintain the activity of the ethylene module. This point implies that the message is not clear enough to drive the root cell into an ethylene-induced phenotype. At $p_{ERF1}^{on} = 0.5$ (ethylene concentration of ~ 0.9 μL/L) the fraction of inactivated receptors equals the fraction of activated receptors and the root cell has the maximum uncertainty about its fate. At this point a bifurcation occurs and the system must decide which phenotype predominates according to the environmental conditions. However, when $p_{ERF1}^{on} > 0.5$ (ethylene concentrations > 0.9 μL/L) the fraction of inactivated receptors that sustains the activation of the ethylene module is larger than the fraction of the activated ones, thus the uncertainty in the root cell fate decreases as the ethylene module drives the cell into a full ethylene dependent-phenotype. Furthermore, ethylene has a circadian rhythm of production, with a peak at midday (Yakir et al., 2007; Taiz and Zeiger, 2010) and the existence of this limit cycle in ethylene emission implies a continuous switching between the auxin-dependent and the ethylene-dependent control of hypocotyl elongation. These results suggest that plants can also use simultaneously both signaling pathways to regulate the differentiation and elongation of the root system.

Once *ERF1* is activated, a cascade of activation of downstream genes initiates (Figure 6a). In the model (Table 1; Díaz and Álvarez-Buylla, 2006), the genes *HLS1* and *ARF2* (responsive to auxin) are considered. In this form, it is possible to define the probabilistic distribution for the activation of these genes under the action of ethylene as: $\mathbf{P_E} = \left\{ p_1^{on}(t), p_1^{off}(t), p_2^{on}(t), p_2^{off}(t), p_3^{on}(t), p_3^{off}(t) \right\}$, where *ERF1* is denoted as gene 1, *HLS1* as gene 2 and *ARF2* as gene 3. $\mathbf{P_E}$ presents two mutually exclusive configurations $\mathbf{P_{E1}} = \left\{1,0,1,0,0,1\right\}$ and $\mathbf{P_{E2}} = \left\{0,1,0,1,1,0\right\}$, which corresponds to the full ethylene response $\mathbf{P_{E1}}$ and the full auxin response $\mathbf{P_{E2}}$. From Equation (10), uncertainty H and information I can be calculated as:

$$H = -\sum_{k=1}^{3}\sum_i p_k^i(t)\log p_k^i(t)$$

$$I = H_{max} - \left[-\sum_{k=1}^{3}\sum_i p_k^i(t)\log p_k^i(t) \right] \quad i = off, on \tag{24}$$

The activation of genes *ERF1* and *HLS1* is modeled using the set of stochastic-differential equations shown in section 4 of Table 1, while the activation of ARF2 is modeled in a discrete form (Díaz-Álvarez-Buylla, 2006) given by the expression:

$$p_3^{on}(t) = p_{ARF2}^{on}(t) = \begin{cases} 0, & \text{if } 0.75 < p_2^{on}(t) \leq 1 \\ 0.5, & \text{if } 0.5 < p_2^{on}(t) \leq 0.75 \\ 1, & \text{if } 0 \leq p_2^{on}(t) \leq 0.5 \end{cases} \tag{25}$$

The numerical solution of the model at different ethylene concentrations (*ET*), allows the characterization of the form in which H varies as a function of *ET* and the estimation of $H_{max} \sim 1.8$ mers (Figure 8). As *ET* increases, the curve $H(t) = H(p^{on}_{ERF1}(t), p^{on}_{ARF2}(t))$ moves to a limit curve obtained when $ET = 0.5$ μM. Above this value not further changes in the position or in the form of the curve are produced by an increase in ET concentration. The plateau observed in the set of curves is due to the fact that p^{on}_{ARF2} is modeled as a continuous piecewise function. Figure 8 also shows the value of H for each configuration of $\mathbf{P_E}$ at a given ET concentration, i.e., the form in which the genetic network responds to each input and the uncertainty that the receiver has received the correct message.

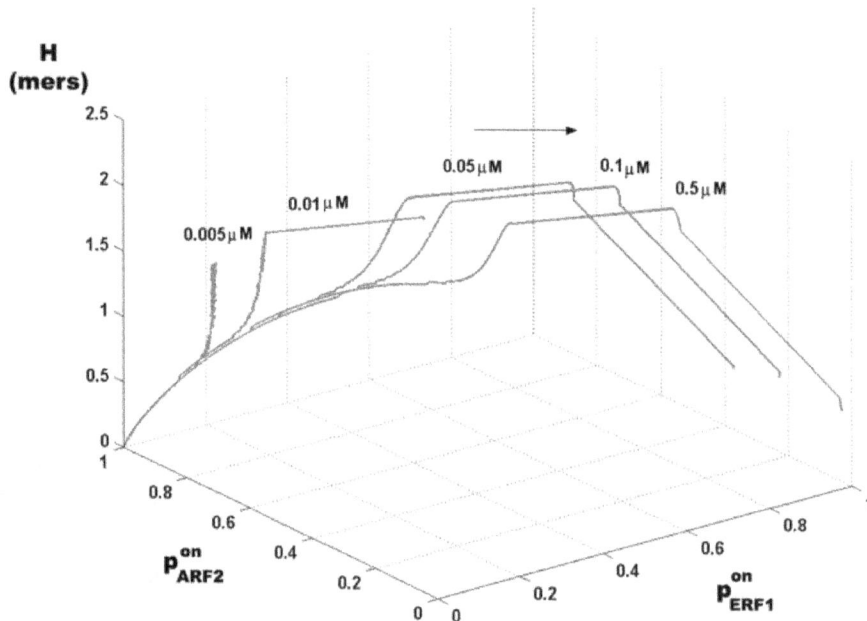

Figure 8: Value of $H(t)$ for each configuration of the genetic network of the ethylene responsive system. The vertical axis represents the values of H, which were calculated by using the logarithm base e in the set of equations (25), as a function of $p^{on}_{ERF1}(t)$ and $p^{on}_{ARF2}(t)$. The arrow indicates the direction of increase of the ethylene concentration (μM). H reaches its maximum value of the series (H_{max}) at an ethylene concentration of ~ 0.1 μM.

These results show that is possible to measure the amount of information that the ethylene signaling pathway manages during the transmission of a message from the environment to the nucleus of the cell. Although the procedure in this section is applied only to measure the value of H at the receiver, this value gives a deeper insight of how the cell perceives the ethylene signal by correlating the concentration of ethylene in the medium with the probability distribution of activation of the genes target of this hormone. At low ethylene concentrations, the system mainly perceives the auxin signal ($p^{on}_{ARF2} \sim 1$) (Figure 8), and as ET is increased some perception of the ethylene signal arises. Although this signal is not sufficiently strong to overcome the auxin signal, it increases the value of H, and the probabilistic distribution $\mathbf{P_E}$ shows low values of probability of activation of the genes $ERF1$ and $HLS1$ and high probability of activation of the gene $ARF2$. On the contrary, elevated concentrations of ethylene increase the perception of the signal ($p_{ERF1}^{on} \rightarrow 1$) in such form that the signal is intense enough to overcome the auxin signal and decrease the value of H to its minimum (Figure 8). In this point, a question arises: is this behavior robust enough to overcome the effects of noise or is sensible to temporal fluctuations in ethylene concentration?

3.2   Noise in the Ethylene Signaling System

In the particular case of the ethylene signaling system, its topological structure formed by two mutually exclusive modules produces a switch like behavior that controls the expression of the ethylene response of the root cell (Figure 6). This dynamical behavior provides robustness to noise, as it was mentioned in section 2.4. Thus, the ethylene signaling pathway has filtering properties that cleans any random fluctuation of the signal transmitted into the nucleus (Díaz and Álvarez-Buylla, 2006; Díaz, 2011; González-García and Díaz, 2011).

In response to a periodic input signal to the model of Table 1, the ethylene signaling pathway cuts off extremely low and very high frequencies, allowing a window of frequency response in which the nucleus reads the incoming message as an oscillatory input. Outside of this window the nucleus reads the input message as an approximately non-varying one. This window of frequency response includes the circadian rhythm of ethylene production in not stressed, wild type Arabidopsis seedlings (Thain et al., 2004; Yakir et al., 2007). In this form, the genetic network of Arabidopsis cells may respond to the circadian frequency of variation of the input. The information carried by the frequency of the ethylene signal may regulate the activation of *ERF1* and downstream genes, giving rise to an oscillatory response with the same frequency of the input signal but with different amplitude and form (Figure 9) (Díaz and Álvarez-Buylla, 2006; Díaz, 2011). These genetic periodic responses could underlie visible periodic changes in the plant physiology or morphological adjustments to the varying environment.

Slow fluctuating chaotic signals induce a chaotic response of the ethylene genetic system. However, the signal only affects the probability of expression of *ERF1*. The probability of the state *on* of the remained genes does not substantially fluctuate and the system evolves to a chaotic attractor generated by p_{ERF1}^{on} in a probability subspace of $\mathbf{P_E}$ (Figure 10a). Additionally, the model of Table 1 predicts that the ethylene response system filters fast fluctuating chaotic signals, responding to them as if they were constant inputs. Furthermore, the translational machinery downstream *ERF1* filters all kind of chaotic signals.

In the case of slow random fluctuations in the ethylene input signal, the trajectory of the system in the probability space is a smooth curve that leads the system to a probability subspace of $\mathbf{P_E}$ in which the state of the system changes randomly as consequence of the random changes in p_{ERF1}^{on} (Figure 10b). Thus, the fluctuating environmental conditions are reflected only in the activation of the gene *ERF1* and apparently do not affect the expression of the genes downstream *ERF1*.

These results suggest that functions H and I are not constant when cells are immersed in a fluctuating environment (Figure 10c), pointing out to the fact that plant cells live submerged in a sea of uncertainty about their fate, i.e., plant cells are adaptive information-processing units by necessity (González-García and Díaz, 2011).

The response of cells to random slow ethylene signals suggest that low level noise has a little effect on the translational machinery downstream *ERF1* due to its filtering properties (González-García and Díaz, 2011) while fast random ethylene signals are completely ignored., i.e., high level noise is completely filtered. Thus, the ethylene signaling pathway is a high fidelity system of transmission and processing of information that can distinguish between noise and smooth periodical signals (Figures 9 and 10).

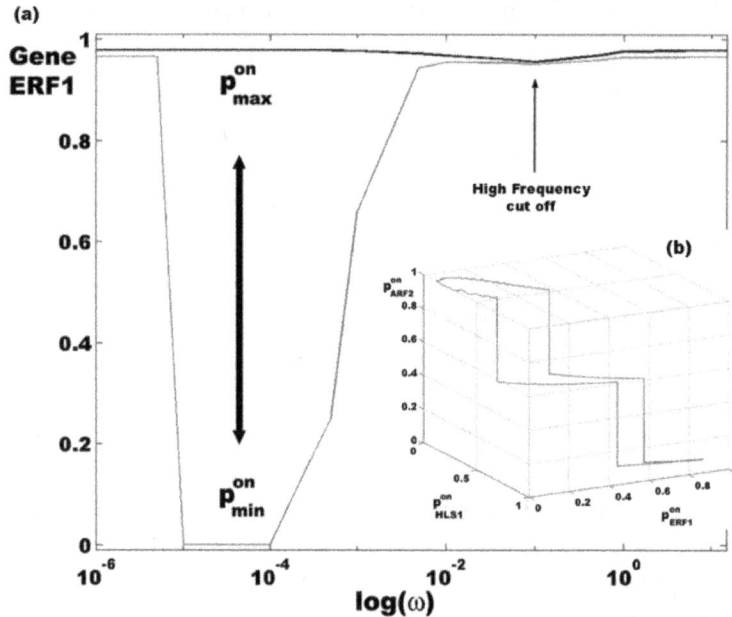

Figure 9: Effect of an oscillatory input on the probability of activation of the genes *ERF1*, *HLS1* and *ARF2*. (a) An oscillatory input of ethylene given by the function $ET(t) = 0.5 + 0.5\sin(\omega t)(\mu M)$ produces periodic variations in the probability of expression of the gene *ERF1*, the bandwidth of frequency response is the interval 0.00001 s^{-1} $< \omega < 0.001$ s^{-1}. The minimum value of $p_{ERF1}^{on} \sim 0$, indicating that *ERF1* is inactivated during a short interval of time during the circadian cycle ($\omega = 0.0000727$ s^{-1}); (b) The periodic ethylene input produces a periodic variation in the genetic configuration of the cell with the same frequency of the input ($\omega = 0.00005$s^{-1} in the example). Figure adapted from Díaz and Álvarez-Buylla, 2006.

By using systems analysis tools, in this section it has been possible to link the temporal pattern of a stimulus - in this case eliciting an ethylene response - with the probability of expression of a set of genes that can mediate a particular cellular response to the original stimulus, and to determine the form in which the functions *H* and *I* change in function of the temporal variations of the input signal (Díaz and Álvarez-Buylla, 2006; Díaz and Álvarez-Buylla, 2009).

3.3   Estimating the bitrate

Systems analysis tools can also be used to estimate the bitrate (bps), which is a measure of the rate of information processing in the communication channel. In the case of a cell, it is of interest the estimation of the rate of information processing during the synthesis and utilization of proteins.

By using the model of the ethylene signaling pathway is possible to make a theoretical estimation of the number of bits that are transferred into the nucleus or the cytoplasm for each novel protein synthesized under the command of the phytohormone ethylene. In order to make the estimation is necessary to use a smooth oscillatory signal. The frequency of this signal must lie in the bandwidth of response of the system (See section 3.2 and Figure 9).

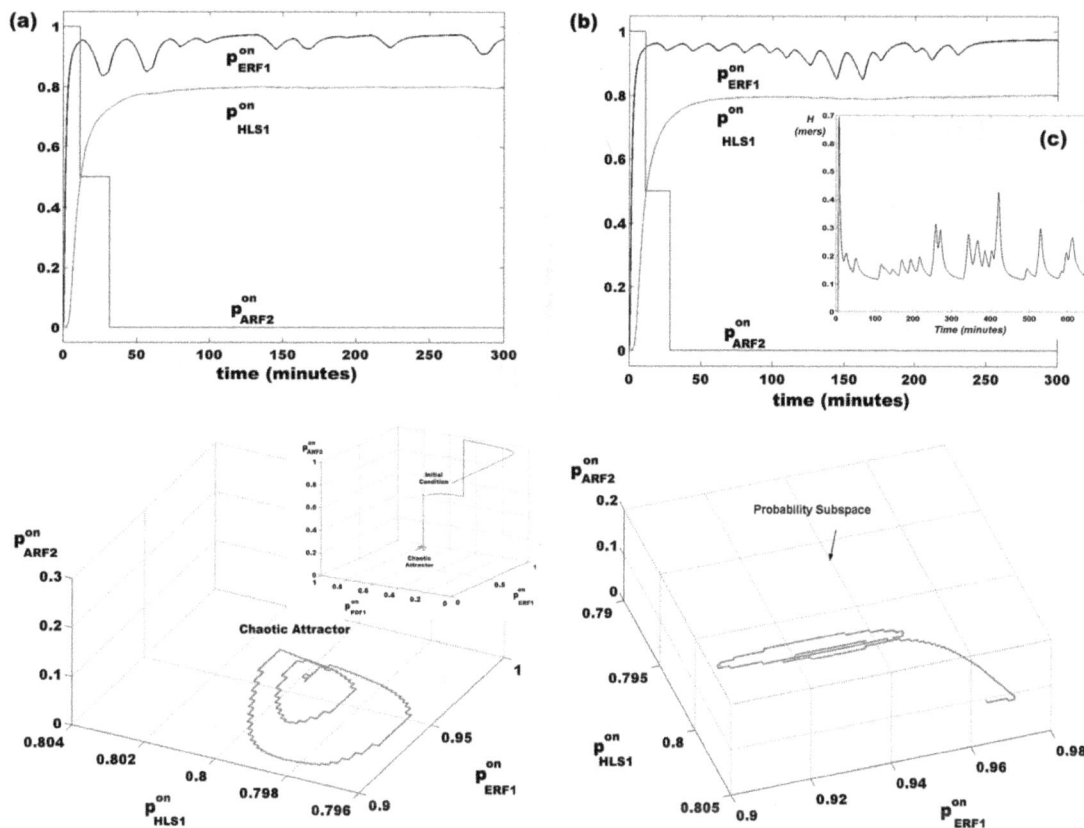

Figure 10: Effect of non oscillatory ethylene inputs on the probability of activation of the genes *ERF1*, *HLS1* and *ARF2*. (a) Chaotic logistic input, represented by the function $ET(j+1) = rET(j)(1-ET(j))$ (μM), where $r = 3.99$, $j = 0, 1, 2, 3,...$, and j changing each 360 s. The trajectory is a smooth curve that drives the system to an attracting basin generated by the chaotic fluctuations in p_{ERF1}^{on}. (b) Slow fluctuations of ethylene produce only random variations in p_{ERF1}^{on}, which exhibits large fluctuations around its steady value. Genes *HLS1* and *ARF2* are unaffected by the ethylene fluctuations. (c) As a consequence, H also exhibits large fluctuations around a steady value. Random changes in ethylene concentration, between 0 and 1 μM, are produced every 360 s.

From Figure 11, it is also clear that when the oscillating input signal has an angular frequency $\sim$0.0005 s^{-1}, the time between the minimum and the maximum values of the cycle can be used to estimate the time needed for the protein synthesis machinery to recover from a decrease in its activity. The amplitude of the peak is $\sim$1.3 nM and the recovery time is approximately 150 min, so that in 9000 s an expected total of $\sim$423 ERF1 molecules are produced assuming that the nuclear volume is on the order of 540 μm^3 (Díaz and Álvarez-Buylla, 2006). This implies that the rate of protein synthesis is $\sim$0.047 molecules/s; in other words, each ERF1 molecule is synthesized and returned to the nucleus in $\sim$21.3 s.

During this recovery time, the amount of information increases by $\sim$0.5 mers, which means that each new molecule of ERF1 protein carries 0.0018 *mers* [0.0026 bits $\approx$ 2.6 millibits (mb)] of information

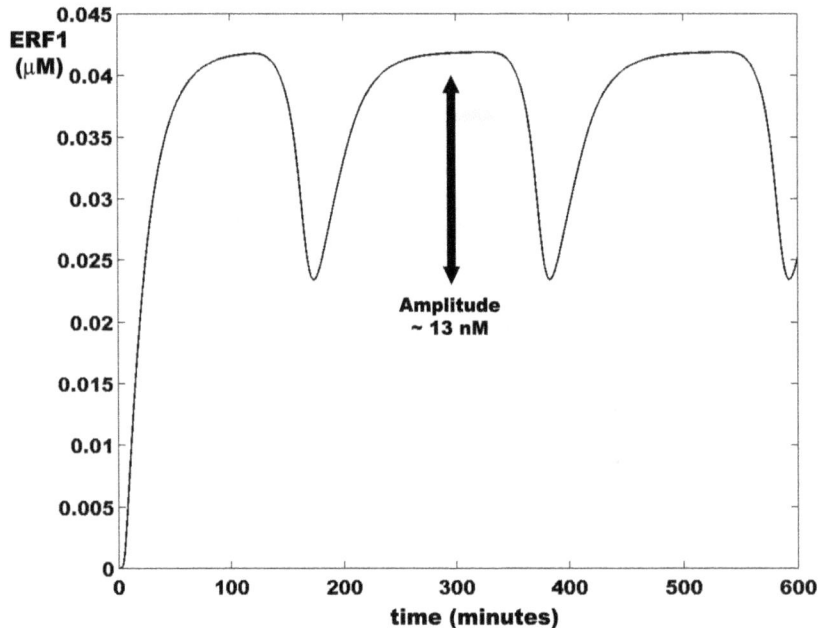

Figure 11: Production of protein ERF1 under the command of an oscillatory input of ethylene given by $ET(t) = 0.5 + 0.5\sin(\omega t)$ (μM), with $\omega = 0.0005$ s^{-1}. The amplitude of the steady signal is ~ 13 nM.

into the nucleus at a rate of 8.45 x 10^{-5} mers/s (1.22 x 10^{-4} bits/s $\approx$ 0.1 mb/s) in the presence of periodic ethylene stimulation with $\omega = 0.0005$ s^{-1}. In addition, once it becomes possible to measure these rates within single cells, the predictions of the model presented here may be tested experimentally and used to improve the model.

Although the circadian cycle is not sinusoidal, the procedure used above can be extended to estimate the bitrate during the daily production of ethylene. In Díaz (2011) the amount of information driven into the nucleus for each novel molecule of ERF1 synthesized during 1 h of the circadian cycle ($\omega = 0.0000727$ s^{-1}) was estimated to be of the order of 0.07 milibits (mb) at an average rate of 0.12 mb/s.

In this form, is possible to estimate, at least from a theoretical point of view, the bitrate of the ethylene communication channel. This procedure can be extended to other signaling systems, and can eventually be experimentally tested.

4   Conclusions

Cells are immersed in a noisy environment in which the necessary information for surviving must have high reception fidelity in order to produce the required specific genetic response. The specificity of the response depends on the capacity of the signaling pathway to distinguish between different signal intensities under noisy conditions.

The ethylene signaling system has a topological structure that minimizes the effects of noise, and its sequence of biochemical processes has filtering properties that define a bandwidth in which the system is highly responsive to the frequency of periodical signals and can discriminate between different concentrations and temporal variations of the input.

However, low rate background noise could eventually induce stochastic resonance in the system when coincides with a sinusoidal input, increasing the level of expression of *ERF1* but decreasing the capacity of the system. In the ethylene system, low rate noise added to a sinusoidal signal produces the elimination of the periodic variations in p_{ERF1}^{on} and drives it to a steady constant value of ~ 1, i.e., stochastic resonance changes a cycle into a steady point in the probabilistic space associated to $\mathbf{P_E}$ (data not shown). On the other hand, the circadian cycle is a stable limit cycle and fluctuations around it are damped, i.e., the response to the ethylene circadian is robust to noisy perturbations.

In this Chapter, it has been shown that modeling gene expression with a stochastic approach allows the use of Information Theory to understand how cells use their signal transductions pathways to transmit information with fidelity, and to estimate the values of *H* and *I* during the data processing by the communication channel.

Hormonal input is probably coded in the form of the fraction of active (represented by 1) and inactive (represented by 0) ethylene receptors at a given time *t*. From the probabilistic distribution of activation of the receptor it is possible to estimate *H* at the source (Equation (19)). This code is written out in the form of a point in the space of probabilities defined by the set $\mathbf{P} = \left\{ p_k^i(t) \middle| i = off, on; k = 1, 2, ..., n \right\}$, where *k* represents the number of genes responsive to ethylene, *i* the state of expression of each gene and $p_k^i(t)$ represents the probability that the gene *k* is in the state *i* at time *t*. Given this probabilistic distribution it is possible to calculate the entropy *H* at the receiver (Equation (4)). However, it seems that is necessary to estimate experimentally the capacity of the ethylene communication channel due to the difficult of calculating *H(XY)* from theoretical procedures (Cheon et al., 2011).

In this Chapter, it is also shown that the combination of Information Theory with the frequency response analysis of dynamical systems allows the determination of the cell's genetic response to input signals with varying frequencies, amplitude and form, in order to determine if the cell can distinguish between different regimes of information flow from the environment. This approach allows the estimation of the bitrate of some steps of the data processing by the ethylene signaling system.

The type of stochastic modeling presented in this work is also an alternative to other models that apply Information Theory to cells. Chen & Li (2010) propose that the interplay between entropy and robustness of gene networks is a core mechanism of systems biology. They propose that entropy in gene networks is due to the fluctuations in the network parameters and to environmental noise, while robustness is a structural property of the network that tries to attenuate the environmental noise. In their work, Chen and Li present a measure of the randomness of a genetic network and the also obtain an expression for the entropy of the network. Formally, the model presented in this Chapter, given by Equations (9) and (11), is quite different from the Chen & Li model, which is based on Ito's stochastic differential equations. The expression for entropy in Chen & Li model is of a very general type, and when is applied as such to a particular model it implies to solve the corresponding Ito's stochastic differential equations. In the model presented in this work, the equivalent entropy expression is Equation (4), which could be easier to evaluate, at least numerically, and represents an approach to circumvent the technical difficulties found in the Ito's model. It has been shown for particular models that, under certain conditions, the predictions of both approaches can closely agree between them and with experimental results (Ekanayakea et al., 2010). However, it is not known if such situation will hold in general.

The above conclusion suggests that one of the problems which difficult the finding of the general principles that govern the flow and storage of information in the living cells is, paradoxically, the uncertainty of a unique an appropriate measure of information (Gatenby and Frieden, 2007). Furthermore, in living cells information denotes a dynamical variable, and the information content of a message deeply depends on the particular dynamical structure of the system. Thus, information flow depends on: 1) the form in which instructions are encoded at the source, 2) the capacity of the receiver to interpret and use this instruction to perform a specific function and 3) the energy cost of the processes that convey to the correct use of the information (Gatenby and Frieden, 2007).

During the information flow process in living cells, hormonal or growth factor inputs could produce drastic rearranges of the genetic and proteic networks within the cell, i.e., changes in the dynamical structure of the system, as suggested by Luscombe et al. (2004). Throughout the rearrange some hubs of the network will remain stables, while other nodes and their respective links will be added or removed from the net. For example, a node and its connections will be lost when the protein is not expressed, or if its concentration falls below some threshold (Luscombe et al., 2004). Similarly, a gene can be removed from the active gene regulatory network when it is silenced in response to the input signal. As consequence, cell communication channels can exhibit memory of the past processes that driven it into the actual state. Hysteresis and limit cycles are examples of dynamical processes with memory that cells can exhibit in response to hormonal and growth factor inputs.

In order to find an appropriate measure of information for living cells, it is necessary to adopt a quantitative expression that could take into account time as a variable and could be experimentally tested. Traditional information measures relay on the Kullback-Leibler (K-L) information, which measures the distance between two curves: an unknown $p(y_i)$ curve, which is the subject probability low for the events y_i, $i = 1, 2, 3,..., N$ and a curve $r(y_i)$ which represents a known input probability law. The mathematical expression of K-L information is:

$$K_{KL}(p/r) = -\sum_i p(y_i) \log_b \frac{p(y_i)}{r(y_i)}$$

(26)

In the especial case in which $r(y_i) = 1$, Equation (26) becomes:

$$K_{KL}(p/r) = H(y) = -\sum_i p(y_i) \log_b p(y_i)$$

(27)

which is the Shannon entropy. For the K-L information the Fisher information can also be obtained from a different value of the reference function $r(y_i)$. Thus, different metrics are available for their application to biological systems (Gatenby and Frieden, 2007). However, this metrics must be modified in order to take into consideration the variable t. In equations (26) and (27) the probability distribution for the set of values of y_i is generally constant over time. However, the probability value for the state of expression of each gene of a regulatory network could depend on time. For example, the transition through different values of the set $\mathbf{P_E} = \{ p_{ERF1}^{on}, p_{ERF1}^{off}, p_{HLS1}^{on}, p_{HLS1}^{off}, p_{ARF2}^{on}, p_{ARF2}^{off} \}$ along a circadian cycle implies different values of Shannon entropy at different times according to Equation (4) (see also Figure 10c). Furthermore, the lag between stimulation and the start of expression of the target genes within a cell can generate delays in the transmission of information, which are not taken into account by classical metrics. In consequence, the metrics proposed by Chen & Li (2010), together with the metrics proposed in this Chapter

(Equation 4), can be options for the measure of information in living systems. These measures can be applied even to cell communication channels with memory and time delays.

Finally, the technique for the modeling of genetic networks with stochastic continuous equations allows the estimation of H and I in the cases of a cascade of gene activation, and the presence of positive and negative feedback mechanisms (Section 2.3.1). This theoretical procedure is still in development but it could be the necessary link for the full application of Information Theory to biological systems and for the experimental verification of the corresponding theoretical predictions.

Acknowledgments

I thank Dr. Barry Commoner for useful discussions concerning this work. I also thank Erika Juarez Luna for technical and logistical assistance. Financial support for this work was from CONACYT (Consejo Nacional de Ciencia y Tecnología) grant 105678.

References

Albert, R. (2004). *Boolean Modeling of Genetic Regulatory Networks. Lect. Notes Phys., 650, 459–481.*

Álvarez-Buylla, E.R., Benítez, M., Corvera-Poiré, A., Chaos, A., de Folter, S., Gamboa, A., Garay-Arroyo, A., García-Ponce, B., Jaimes-Miranda, F., Pérez-Ruiz, R.V., Piñeyro-Nelson, A., & Sánchez-Corrales, Y.E. (2010). *Flower Development. The Arabidopsis Book, 8, 1-57.*

Arbib M. (1964). *Brains, machines and mathematics. Ney York: MacGraw-Hill.*

Brown, R., Kazan, K., McGrath, K., Maclean, D., & Manners, J. (2003). *A Role for the GCC-Box in Jasmonate-Mediated Activation of the PDF1.2 Gene of Arabidopsis.* Plant Physiology, 132, 1020–1032.

Bruggeman, F.J., Blüthgen, N., & Westerhoff, H.V. (2009). *Noise Management by Molecular Networks. PLoS Comput Biol , 5(9): e1000506.*

Chen, Q., & Bleecker, A. (1995). *Analysis of ethylene signal-transduction kinetics associated with seedling-growth response and chitinase induction in wild-type and mutant Arabidopsis. Plant Physiol., 108, 597-607.*

Chen, B., & Li, C. (2010). *On the Interplay between Entropy and Robustness of Gene Regulatory Networks. Entropy 12:1071-1101.*

Cheong, R., Rhee, A., Wang, C.J., Nemenman, I., & Levchenko, A. (2011). *Information Transduction Capacity of Noisy Biochemical Signaling Networks. Science, 334, 354-358.*

Corbit, K.C., Trakul, N., Eves, E.M., Diaz, B., Marshall, M., & Rosner, M.R. (2003). *Activation of Raf-1 Signaling by Protein Kinase C through a Mechanism Involving Raf Kinase Inhibitory Protein.* The Journal of Biological Chemistry, 278, 13061–13068.

Cullen, P. J., & Lockyer, P. J. (2002). *Integration of calcium and Ras signalling. Molecular Cell Biology, 3, 339-348.*

Diaz, J., Baier G., Martinez-Mekler, G., & Pastor, N. (2002). *Interaction of the IP3-Ca2+ and the FGF-MAPK Signaling Pathways in the Xenopus laevis Embryo: A qualitative Approach to the Mesodermal Induction Problem. Biophys. Chem., 97, 55-72.*

Díaz, J., & Martínez-Mekler, G. (2005). *Interaction of the IP3-Ca2+ and MAPK Signaling Systems in the Xenopus blastomere: a possible frequency encoding mechanism of control of the Xbra gene expression. Bulletin of Mathematical Biology, 67, 433-465.*

Diaz, J., & Álvarez-Buylla Elena R. (2006). *A model of the ethylene signaling pathway and its gene response in Arabidopsis thaliana: pathway cross-talk and noise-filtering properties. Chaos, 16, 023112.*

Díaz, J., & Álvarez-Buylla, E.R. (2009). *Information flow during gene activation by signaling molecules: ethylene transduction in Arabidopsis cells as a study system. BMC Systems Biol, 3, 48.*

Díaz, J. (2011). *Information flow in plant signaling pathways. Plant Signaling & Behavior, 6, 1-5.*

Dolmetsch, R.E., Lewis, R.S., Goodnow, C.C., & Healy, J.I. (1997). *Differential activation of transcription factors induced by Ca^{2+} response amplitude and duration. Nature, 386, 855-858.*

Dolmetsch, R. E., Xu, K., & Lewis, R. S. (1998). *Calcium oscillations increase the efficiency and specificity of gene expression. Nature, 392, 933-936.*

Ekanayakea, A.J., Linda, J., & Allena, S. (2010). *Comparison of Markov Chain and Stochastic Differential Equation Population Models Under Higher-Order Moment Closure Approximations. Stochastic Analysis and Applications, 28, 907 – 927.*

Elowitz, M.B., Levine, A.J., Eric D. Siggia, E.D., & Swain, P.S. (2002). *Stochastic Gene Expression in a Single Cell. Science, 297, 1183-1186.*

Gatenby, A.R., & Frieden, B.R. (2007). *Information theory in living systems, Methods, Applications, and Challenges. Bulletin of Mathematical Biology, 69, 635-657.*

González-García, J.S., & Díaz, J. (2011). *Information Theory and the Ethylene Genetic Network (Review). Plant Signaling and Behavior, 6, 1483-1498.*

Greil, F. (2009). *Dynamics of Boolean Networks. Darmstadt: PhD-Thesis.*

Huang, S., & Kauffman, S. A. (2009). *Complex Gene Regulatory Networks - from Structure to Biological Observables: Cell Fate Determination. Encyclopedia of Compexity and Systems Science. R. A. Meyers, Editor. Encyclopedia of Complexity and Systems Science, New York, Springer.*

Johnson, H.A. (1970). *Information Theory in Biology after 18 Years. Science, 168, 1545 –50.*

Jones, D.S. (1979). *Elementary information theory. Oxford applied mathematics and computing science series. Oxford: Oxford University Press.*

Kauffman, S. A. (1969). *Metabolic stability and epigenesis in randomly constructed genetic nets. Journal of Theoretical Biology, 22, 437-467.*

Kholodenko, B.N. (2000). *Negative feedback and ultrasensitivity can bring about oscillations in the mitogen activated protein kinase cascades. Eur. J. Biochem, 267, 1583-1588.*

Li, S., Assmann, S.M., & Réka, A. (2006). *Predicting Essential Components of Signal Transduction Networks: A Dynamic Model of Guard Cell Abscisic Acid Signaling. PlosBiol , 4, e312.*

Liu, J., Mehdi, S., Topping, J., Tarkowski, P., & Lindsey K. (2010). *Modelling and experimental analysis of hormonal crosstalk in Arabidopsis. Mol Syst Biol, 6, 373.*

Lodish, H., Berk, A., Kaiser, C.A., Krieger, M., Bretscher, A., Ploegh, H., Amon, A., & Scott, M.P. *Molecular Cell Biology, Seventh Edition. New York: W. H. Freeman.*

Luscombe, N.M., Babu, M.M., Yu, H., Snyder, M., Teichman, S.A., & Gerstein, M. (2004). *Genomic analysis of regulatory dynamics reveals large topological changes. Nature, 431, 308-312.*

Marks, F., Klingmüller, U., & Müller-Decker, K. (2008). *Cellular Signal Processing: An Introduction to the Molecular Mechanisms of Signal Transduction. New York: Garland Science.*

Paulsson, J. (2004). *Summing up the noise in gene networks. Nature, 427, 415-418.*

Quastler, H. (1953). *Information Theory in Biology. Urbana: University of Illinois Press.*

Rahman, A., Hosokawa, S., Oono, Y., Amakawa, T., Goto, N., & Tsurumi, S. (2002). *Auxin and ethylene response interactions during Arabidopsis root hair development dissected by auxin influx modulators. Plant Physiol, 130, 1908– 1917.*

Samad, H.E., Khammash, M., Petzold, L., & Gillespie, D. (2005). Stochastic modelling of gene regulatory networks. Int. J. Robust Nonlinear Control, 15, 691–711.

Schulthess, P., & Blüthgen, N. (2011). From reaction networks to information flow—using modular response analysis to track information in signaling networks. Methods Enzymol, 500, 397-409.

Shannon, C.E. (1948). A mathematical theory of communication. Bell Systems Technical Journal, 27, 379-423.

Shin, S., Rath, O., Choo, S., Fee, F., McFerran, B., Kolch, W., & Cho, K. (2009). Positive- and negative-feedback regulations coordinate the dynamic behavior of the Ras-Raf-MEK-ERK signal transduction pathway. Journal of Cell Science, 122, 425-435.

Sperelakis, N. (2012). Cell Physiology Source Book, Fourth Edition: Essentials of Membrane Biophysics. New York: Academic Press.

Spiller, D.G., Wood, C.D., Rand, D.A., & White, M.R.H. (2010). Measurement of single-cell dynamics. Nature, 465, 736-745.

Swain, P.S., Elowitz, M.B., & Siggia, E.D. (2002). Intrinsic and extrinsic contributions to stochasticity in gene expression. Proc Natl Acad Sci U S A, 99, 12795-800.

Taiz, L., & Zeiger, E. (2010). Plant Physiology. Sunderland: Sinauer Associates, Inc.

Thain, S.C., Vandenbussche, F., Laarhoven, L.J.J., Dowson-Day, M.J., Wang, Z., Tobin, E.M., Harren, F.J.M., Millar, A.J., & Van Der Straeten, D. (2004). Circadian rhythms of ethylene emission in Arabidopsis. Plant Physiol, 136, 3751-3761.

Tkačik, G., & Walczak, A.M. (2011). Information transmission in genetic regulatory networks: a review. arXiv:1101.4240v1 [physics.bio-ph].

Watson, J.D., Baker, T.A., Bell, S.P., Gann, A.A.F., Levine, M., & Losick, R.M. (2007). Molecular Biology of the Gene, Sixth Edition. New York: Cold Spring Harbor Laboratory Press.

Weaver, W. (1949). Recent contributions to the mathematical theory of communication. In Shannon C.E., Weaver, W., Mathematical theory of communication. Urbana: University of Illinois Press.

Weber, T.J., Shankaran, H., Wiley, H.S., Opresko, L.K., Chrisler, W.B., & Quesenberry, R.D. (2010). Basic fibroblast growth factor regulates persistent ERK oscillations in premalignant but not malignant JB6 cells. J Invest Dermatol, 130, 1444-1456.

Yakir, E., Hilman, D., Harir, Y., & Green, R.M. (2007). Regulation of output from the plant circadian clock. FEBS J, 274, 335-45.

Yi, M., Zhao, Q., Tang, J., & Wang, C. (2011). A theoretical modeling for frequency modulation of Ca2+ signal on activation of MAPK cascade. Biophysical Chemistry, 157, 33–42.

www.ingramcontent.com/pod-product-compliance
Lightning Source LLC
Chambersburg PA
CBHW080929220326
41598CB00034B/5727